ANNALS OF THE NEW YORK ACADEMY OF SCIENCES

Volume 873

EDITORIAL STAFF

Executive Editor
BILL BOLAND

Managing Editor
JUSTINE CULLINAN

Associate Editor
STEFAN MALMOLI

The New York Academy of Sciences
2 East 63rd Street
New York, New York 10021

NEW YORK ACADEMY OF SCIENCES
(Founded in 1817)

BOARD OF GOVERNORS, October 1998–September 1999

ELEANOR BAUM, *Chairman of the Board*
BILL GREEN, *Vice Chairman of the Board*
RODNEY W. NICHOLS, *President and CEO* [ex officio]

Honorary Life Governors
WILLIAM T. GOLDEN   JOSHUA LEDERBERG

JOHN T. MORGAN, *Treasurer*

Governors

D. ALLAN BROMLEY	LAWRENCE B. BUTTENWIESER	PRAVEEN CHAUDHARI
JOHN H. GIBBONS	RONALD L. GRAHAM	HENRY M. GREENBERG
ROBERT G. LAHITA	MARTIN L. LEIBOWITZ	JACQUELINE LEO
WILLIAM J. McDONOUGH	KATHLEEN P. MULLINIX	SANDRA PANEM
CHARLES RAMOND	SARA LEE SCHUPF	JAMES H. SIMONS
	TORSTEN WIESEL	

RICHARD A. RIFKIND, *Past Chairman of the Board*
HELENE L. KAPLAN, *Counsel* [ex officio]   CRAIG PURINTON, *Secretary* [ex officio]

ELECTRICAL BIOIMPEDANCE METHODS:
APPLICATIONS TO MEDICINE AND BIOTECHNOLOGY

ANNALS OF THE NEW YORK ACADEMY OF SCIENCES

Volume 873

ELECTRICAL BIOIMPEDANCE METHODS:
APPLICATIONS TO MEDICINE AND BIOTECHNOLOGY

Edited by Pere J. Riu, Javier Rosell, Ramon Bragós, and Óscar Casas

The New York Academy of Sciences
New York, New York
1999

Copyright © 1999 by the New York Academy of Sciences. All rights reserved. Under the provisions of the United States Copyright Act of 1976, individual readers of the Annals are permitted to make fair use of the material in them for teaching and research. Permission is granted to quote from the Annals provided that the customary acknowledgment is made of the source. Material in the Annals may be republished only by permission of the Academy. Address inquiries to the Executive Editor at the New York Academy of Sciences.

Copying fees: *For each copy of an article made beyond the free copying permitted under Section 107 or 108 of the 1976 Copyright Act, a fee should be paid through the Copyright Clearance Center, Inc., 222 Rosewood Drive, Danvers, MA 01923. The fee for copying an article is $3.00 for nonacademic use; for use in the classroom it is $0.07 per page.*

∞ *The paper used in this publication meets the minimum requirements of American National Standard for Information Sciences—Permanence of Paper for Printed Library Materials, ANSI Z39.48-1984.*

Library of Congress Cataloging-in-Publication Data

Electrical bioimpedance methods: applications to medicine and biotechnology/edited by Pere J. Riu ... [et al.].
    p. cm. — (Annals of the New York Academy of Sciences: v. 873).
   Includes bibliographical references and index.
   ISBN 1-57331-190-1 (cloth: alk. paper). — ISBN 1-57331-191-X (paper: alk. paper).
    1. Impedance, Bioelectric—Congresses. 2. Impedance, Bioelectric–Diagnostic use—Congresses. I. Riu, Pere J. II. Series.
Q11.N5 vol. 873
[QP341]
500 s—dc21
[612'.01442]

99-22308
CIP

TT/BM
Printed in the United States of America
ISBN 1-57331-190-1 (cloth)
ISBN 1-57331-191-X (paper)
ISSN 0077-8923

ANNALS OF THE NEW YORK ACADEMY OF SCIENCES

Volume 873
April 20, 1999

ELECTRICAL BIOIMPEDANCE METHODS: APPLICATIONS TO MEDICINE AND BIOTECHNOLOGY[a]

Editors and Conference Organizers
PERE J. RIU, JAVIER ROSELL, RAMON BRAGÓS, AND ÓSCAR CASAS

CONTENTS

Preface. *By* PERE J. RIU	xi
The Practical Success of Impedance Techniques from an Historical Perspective. *By* HERMAN P. SCHWAN	1

Part I. Organ State and Tumors

Monitoring Temperature-Induced Changes in Tissue during Hyperthermia by Impedance Methods. *By* EBERHARD GERSING	13
Application of Linear Circuit Models to Impedance Spectra in Irradiated Muscle. *By* K. SUNSHINE OSTERMAN, KEITH D. PAULSEN, and P. JACK HOOPES	21
A Review of Parameters for the Bioelectrical Characterization of Breast Tissue. *By* JACQUES JOSSINET and MICHEL SCHMITT	30
Ex Vivo Discrimination between Normal and Pathological Tissues in Human Breast Surgical Biopsies Using Bioimpedance Spectroscopy. *By* N. CHAUVEAU, L. HAMZAOUI, P. ROCHAIX, B. RIGAUD, J. J. VOIGT, and J. P. MORUCCI	42
In Vivo and *In Situ* Ischemic Tissue Characterization Using Electrical Impedance Spectroscopy. *By* O. CASAS, R. BRAGÓS, P. J. RIU, J. ROSELL, M. TRESÀNCHEZ, M. WARREN, A. RODRIGUEZ-SINOVAS, A. CARREÑO, and J. CINCA	51

[a]This volume is the result of the Tenth International Conference on Electrical Bio-Impedance, which was sponsored by the International Committee for Promotion of Research in Bio-Impedance and held on April 5–9, 1998, in Barcelona, Spain.

Dielectric Properties of Skeletal Muscle during Ischemia in the Frequency Range from 50 Hz to 200 MHz. *By* M. SCHÄFER, H-J. KIRLUM, C. SCHLEGEL, and M. M. GEBHARD.. 59

Quantitative Analysis of Impedance Spectra of Organs during Ischemia. *By* MIHAELA GHEORGHIU, EBERHARD GERSING, and EUGEN GHEORGHIU....... 65

Part II. Body Composition

Requirements for Clinical Use of Bioelectrical Impedance Analysis (BIA). *By* HENRY C. LUKASKI... 72

Study of the Relation between Fluid Distribution Change in Tissue and Impedance Change during Hemodialysis by Frequency Characteristics of the Flowing Blood. *By* K. SAKAMOTO, R. SUNAGA, K. NAKAMURA, Y. SATO, M. FUJII, H. KANAI, T. TSUCHIDA, A. UENO, N. KANAI, and K. HASEGAWA.......... 77

Bioimpedance: Is It a Predictor of True Water Volume? *By* B. J. THOMAS, B. H. CORNISH, L. C. WARD, and A. JACOBS....................... 89

Fat-Free Mass Qualitative Assessment with Bioelectric Impedance Analysis (BIA). *By* T. TALLURI, R. J. LIETDKE, A. EVANGELISTI, J. TALLURI, and G. MAGGIA... 94

Estimation of Extracellular Volume by a Two-Frequency Measurement. *By* H. G. GOOVAERTS, TH. J. C. FAES, G. W. DE VALK–DE ROO, M. TEN BOLSCHER, J. C. NETELENBOSCH, W. J. F. VAN DER VIJGH, and R. M. HEETHAAR....... 99

The RXc Graph in Evaluating and Monitoring Fluid Balance in Patients with Liver Cirrhosis. *By* FRANCESCO WILLIAM GUGLIELMI, TECLA MASTRONUZZI, LORENA PIETRINI, ALBA PANARESE, CARMINE PANELLA, and ANTONIO FRANCAVILLA... 105

Part III. Cardiovascular System

Measurement of Leg Arterial Compliance of Normal Subjects and Diabetics Using Impedance Plethysmography. *By* DEOK WON KIM and SOO CHAN KIM...... 112

A Meta-analysis of Published Studies Concerning the Validity of Thoracic Impedance Cardiography. *By* E. RAAIJMAKERS, TH. J. C. FAES, R. J. P. M. SCHOLTEN, H. G. GOOVAERTS, and R. M. HEETHAAR........... 121

Towards a Theoretical Understanding of Stroke Volume Estimation with Impedance Cardiography. *By* TH. J. C. FAES, E. RAAIJMAKERS, J. H. MEIJER, H. G. GOOVAERTS, and R. M. HEETHAAR............................ 128

Lead Field Theoretical Approach in Bioimpedance Measurements: Towards More Controlled Measurement Sensitivity. *By* PASI K. KAUPPINEN, JARI A. HYTTINEN, TIIT KÖÖBI, and JAAKKO MALMIVUO................ 135

Impedance Stroke Volume Compared with Dye and Electromagnetic Flowmeter Values during Drug-Induced Inotropic and Vascular Changes in Dogs. *By* ROBERT P. PATTERSON, DAVID A. WITSOE, and ARTHUR FROM 143

A Comparison of Bioimpedance and Echocardiography in Measuring Systolic Heart Function in Cardiac Patients. *By* H. J. JURN KERKKAMP and ROB M. HEETHAAR... 149

Thoracic Bioimpedance as a Basis for Pacing Control. *By* MART MIN, TOOMAS PARVE, and ANDRES KINK 155

Evaluation of Systolic Performance by Automated Impedance Cardiography. *By* ARMIN W. SCHERHAG, JANA STASTNY, STEFAN PFLEGER, WOLFRAM VOELKER, and DIETER L. HEENE............................ 167

Impact of Cardiovascular Reactions Using the Impedance Cardiography Method in Borderline Hypertension. *By* T. NAWARYCZ, L. OSTROWSKA-NAWARYCZ, and J. KACZMAREK... 174

Stroke Volume Variability—Cardiovascular Response to Orthostatic Maneuver in Patients with Coronary Artery Diseases. *By* JANUSZ SIEBERT, JERZY WTOREK, and JAN ROGOWSKI.. 182

Assessment of Left Ventricular Systolic Function and Diastolic Time Intervals by the Bioimpedance Polyrheocardiographic System. *By* MICHAIL ZUBAREV, ANDREY DUMLER, VLADIMIR SHUTOV, and NICOLAY POPOV 191

Part IV.   Skin Impedance

In Vivo ac Impedance Spectroscopy of Human Skin: Theory and Problems in Monitoring of Passive Percutaneous Drug Delivery. *By* A. H. LACKERMEIER, E. T. MCADAMS, G. P. MOSS, and A. D. WOOLFSON..................... 197

On Assessment of Skin Reactivity Using Electrical Impedance. *By* MIRUNA NYRÉN, LENA HAGSTRÖMER, and LENNART EMTESTAM........................ 214

Electrical Bioimpedance Related to Structural Differences and Reactions in Skin and Oral Mucosa. *By* INGRID NICANDER and STIG OLLMAR........... 221

Stress Action on Biological Tissue and Tissue Models Detected by the P_y Value. *By* FRITZ PLIQUETT and UWE PLIQUETT............................... 227

Part V.   Cells and Cultures

From Concept to Market in Industrial Impedance Applications. *By* CHRISTOPHER DAVEY, ROBERT TODD, and JOHN BARRETT 239

Orientation and Deformation of Erythrocytes in Flowing Blood. *By* MAMIKO FUJII, KENGO NAKAJIMA, KATSUYUKI SAKAMOTO, and HIROSHI KANAI.......... 245

On the Limits of Ellipsoidal Models when Analyzing Dielectric Behavior of Living Cells: Emphasis on Red Blood Cells. *By* EUGEN GHEORGHIU.............. 262

Electrical Impedance Tomography Study of Biological Processes in a Single Cell. *By* TERRY C. CHILCOTT and HANS G. L. COSTER 269

New Light-Scattering and Field-Trapping Methods Access the Internal Electric Structure of Submicron Particles, like Influenza Viruses. *By* JAN GIMSA... 287

Biomass Monitoring Using Impedance Spectroscopy. *By* R. BRAGÓS, X. GÁMEZ, J. CAIRÓ, P. J. RIU, and F. GÒDIA 299

Part VI. Instrumentation

Improvement of a Front End for Bioimpedance Spectroscopy. *By* DAVID YÉLAMOS, ÓSCAR CASAS, RAMON BRAGÓS, and JAVIER ROSELL..................... 306

Virtual Biopsies in Barrett's Esophagus Using an Impedance Probe. *By* C. A. GONZÁLEZ-CORREA, B. H. BROWN, R. H. SMALLWOOD, N. KALIA, C. J. STODDARD, T. J. STEPHENSON, S. J. HAGGIE, D. N. SLATER, and K. D. BARDHAN 313

Inductively Coupled Wideband Transceiver for Bioimpedance Spectroscopy (IBIS). *By* HERMANN SCHARFETTER, WOLFGANG NINAUS, BERNHARD PUSWALD, GALIDIA I. PETROVA, DIMITER KOVACHEV, and HELMUT HUTTEN.......... 322

Magnetic Induction Tomography: A Measurement System for Biological Tissues. *By* H. GRIFFITHS, W. R. STEWART, and W. GOUGH 335

Progress in Realization of Magnetic Induction Tomography. *By* ALEXANDER V. KORJENEVSKY and VLADIMIR A. CHEREPENIN............. 346

Magnetic Impedance Tomography. *By* J. C. TOZER, R. H. IRELAND, D. C. BARBER, and A. T. BAKER... 353

Part VII. Electrical Bioimpedance Methods and Applications

Evaluation of Impedance Technique for Detecting Breast Carcinoma Using a 2-D Numerical Model of the Torso. *By* MICHAL M. RADAI, SHIMON ABBOUD, and MOSHE ROSENFELD 360

A Comparison of the Siconolfi and Cole-Cole Procedures for Multifrequency Impedance Data Analysis. *By* LEIGH WARD, NIGEL FULLER, BRUCE CORNISH, MARINOS ELIA, and BRIAN THOMAS 370

Practical Limits of the Kramers-Kronig Relationships Applied to Experimental Bioimpedance Data. *By* PERE J. RIU and CRISTINA LAPAZ 374

Experimental Assessment of Phase Magnitude Imaging in Multifrequency EIT by Simulation and Saline Tank Studies. *By* ANTHONY FITZGERALD, DAVID HOLDER, and HUW GRIFFITHS. 381

Some Design Concepts for Electrical Impedance Measurement. *By* H. G. GOOVAERTS, TH. J. C. FAES, E. RAAIJMAKERS, and R. M. HEETHAAR 388

Impedance Modulation by Pulsed Ultrasound. *By* JACQUES JOSSINET, BERNARD LAVANDIER, and DOMINIQUE CATHIGNOL. 396

Focused Impedance Measurement (FIM)—A New Technique with Improved Zone Localization. *By* K. S. RABBANI, M. SARKER, M. H. R. AKOND, and T. AKTER. 408

Impedance Parameter Characterizing Apple Bruise. *By* ESZTER VOZÁRY, PÉTER LÁSZLÓ, and GÁBOR ZSIVÁNOVITS 421

Part VIII.   EIT Reconstruction

State Estimation in Time-Varying Electrical Impedance Tomography. *By* JARI P. KAIPIO, PASI A. KARJALAINEN, ERKKI SOMERSALO, and MARKO VAUHKONEN 430

A Parametric Method to Resolve the Ill-Posed Nature of the EIT Reconstruction Problem: A Simulation Study. *By* J. C. DE MUNCK, TH. J. C. FAES, A. J. HERMANS, and R. M. HEETHAAR. 440

EIT Reconstruction of Static Images by a Genetic Algorithm Approach. *By* R. OLMI, M. BINI, S. MANETTA, and S. PRIORI. 454

Uniqueness, Shape, and Dimension in EIT. *By* WILLIAM R. B. LIONHEART 466

Static Three-Dimensional Electrical Impedance Tomography. *By* PÄIVI J. VAUHKONEN, MARKO VAUHKONEN, TUOMO SAVOLAINEN, and JARI P. KAIPIO. 472

Development of a Reconstruction Algorithm for Imaging Impedance Changes in the Human Head. *By* A. GIBSON, R. H. BAYFORD, and D. S. HOLDER 482

Part IX.   EIT Applications

Monitoring Regional Lung Ventilation by Functional Electrical Impedance Tomography during Assisted Ventilation. *By* INÉZ FRERICHS, GÜNTER HAHN, HOLGER SCHIFFMANN, CORD BERGER, and GERHARD HELLIGE 493

Gastric Emptying in Patients with Type I Diabetes Mellitus. *By* NACHUM VAISMAN, NOAMI WEINTROB, ALEXANDER BLUMENTAL, ZEEV YOSEFSBERG, and PNINA VARDI. 506

Assessment and Calibration of a Low-Frequency System for Electrical Impedance Tomography (EIT), Optimized for Use in Imaging Brain Function in Ambulant Human Subjects. *By* D. S. HOLDER, C. A. GONZÁLEZ-CORREA, T. TIDSWELL, A. GIBSON, G. CUSICK, and R. H. BAYFORD 512

Impedance Mammograph 3D Phantom Studies. *By* JERZY WTOREK, JAROSLAW STELTER, and ANTONI NOWAKOWSKI. 520

Can We Optimize Electrode Placement for Impedance Pneumography? *By* N. KHAMBETE, P. METHERALL, B. BROWN, R. SMALLWOOD, and R. HOSE. 534

Index of Contributors 543

Financial assistance was received from:

- COMISSIONAT PER A UNIVERSITATS I RECERCA—GENERALITAT DE CATALUNYA
- DIRECCIÓN GENERAL DE ENSEÑANZA SUPERIOR—MINISTERIO DE EDUCACIÓN Y CULTURA
- UNIVERSITAT POLITÈCNICA DE CATALUNYA

> The New York Academy of Sciences believes it has a responsibility to provide an open forum for discussion of scientific questions. The positions taken by the participants in the reported conferences are their own and not necessarily those of the Academy. The Academy has no intent to influence legislation by providing such forums.

Preface

Bioimpedance techniques were born with the century. They are easy to apply and low in cost. In addition, impedance is a characteristic property of any material, including biological materials. With that premise, one might be expecting that bioimpedance techniques are currently used in all sorts of clinical and laboratory applications. However, these techniques have failed to find their place in the routine clinical and industrial world, with few, remarkable, exceptions.

In his paper, Herman P. Schwan analyzes the potential problems from an historical point of view, emphasizing technical aspects. It is worth reading. I would like to address a different, also historical, problem: the wheel. The problem is not the wheel itself, though. The problem is that we are reinventing it. Except for the lifelong works of some outstanding people—Geddes, Baker, Schwan, Cole, and few others—there is nothing like a "body of knowledge" related to bioimpedance. When my students ask me about reference materials to learn about these techniques, I feel ashamed. There is almost nothing. Of course, there are numerous excellent papers, but you cannot give a hundred papers to a freshman Ph.D. student and expect he or she will learn the basics from there.

Fortunately, things are changing. The International Conferences on Electrical Bio-Impedance (ICEBI) started in 1969 and a permanent Committee was created some years later. However, materials from these conferences, which represent the state of the art in the field, have had little diffusion. Development of new techniques, such as impedance imaging, has been a driving force for the last years, especially in Europe, where EU funding allowed for meetings, courses, and publication of the results. Also, the efforts of a few individuals (namely, groups from INSERM U305 in Toulouse and the Universidad Nacional de Tucumán) contributed to the compilation and diffusion of the knowledge in the field by publishing a volume in *Critical Reviews in Biomedical Engineering* devoted to bioimpedance techniques. In the last months, I also noticed a sharp increase in the number of papers in several journals dealing with applications of bioimpedance techniques to medical or biotechnological areas. All these are signs of a change in the (small) bioimpedance scientific community.

I would like to express my gratitude to the Executive Editor, Bill Boland, of the *Annals of the New York Academy of Sciences* for allowing us to publish a selection of the papers presented at the Tenth ICEBI as a volume of the *Annals*. I also wish to thank Stefan Malmoli for his excellent editorial duties in relation to this volume. This surely will make available to many researchers the latest developments in the area and will contribute to the establishment of a body of knowledge in bioimpedance, which will prevent future researchers and us from reinventing the wheel.

Pere J. Riu

The Practical Success of Impedance Techniques from an Historical Perspective

HERMAN P. SCHWAN[a]

Department of Bioengineering, University of Pennsylvania, Philadelphia, Pennsylvania 19104

ABSTRACT: Future problems are based on achievements of the past. They may be unresolved problems of a more basic nature or future practical applications made possible by recent technical innovations. The introductory part of this paper deals with recent history and its many significant advances. This is followed by a survey of the bioimpedance field. Past advances include contributions of the bioimpedance field to electrophysiology, biophysics, and biochemistry. More practical contributions include the data necessary for the development of diathermy techniques and modern dosimetry in the field of electromagnetic biohazards. A large array of practical applications relate to monitoring physiological events such as impedance plethysmography, impedance encephalography, impedance tomography, and body water, lung, and heart function parameters. Unresolved problems of a basic nature include topics that relate to mechanisms responsible for observed dielectric dispersions and membrane biophysics. Practical applications that can now be realized include several new electronic laboratory diagnostic techniques. Tissue spectroscopy of small biopsy samples and tissue culture samples should permit rapid extraction of valuable cellular data. This can be done for both normal and abnormal states, thus providing new diagnostic techniques. Possible sophistication of the Coulter counter principle should permit rapid investigations of many individual cell parameters, including cellular shape, using multielectrode techniques (microimpedance tomography). The theory of field-evoked force effects is well established now and can be used to develop electronic cell manipulation and new electronic cell sorting technologies. Additional significant practical applications to the biomedical field are now possible.

INTRODUCTION

There has been some concern about the future of the biological impedance field. It was therefore a good idea when Pere Riu suggested that I speak about the practical successes of the field during the past. I shall gladly do so. I also intend to include a summary of the significant advances in the more basic oriented fields of electrophysiology and biophysics. Finally, I discuss the promise that the future holds.

Permit me to briefly indicate the motivation for my interest in the bioimpedance field. While in Frankfurt at the Institute for Physical Foundations of Medicine, I learned about the bioimpedance field as it existed at the time. I studied the seminal works of Fricke, Cole, and Curtis with care. I joined the University of Pennsylvania in 1950 and, perhaps naively, formulated the ambitious program indicated in TABLE 1. It included the determination of the electrical and acoustic properties of tissues and cell suspensions over an extended frequency range, clarification of underlying mechanisms, and applications to medicine and biology. The study of the interactions of electromagnetic fields with biomatter became a particularly fascinating subject matter to us. This program kept us busy for

---

[a]Address for correspondence: 99 Kynlyn Road, Radnor, Pennsylvania 19087.

TABLE 1. Research Activities[a]

Study of the physical properties of biomatter with dielectric and acoustic spectroscopy includes
- Measurement of physical properties
  electrical (Hz to GHz)
  acoustic (kHz to MHz)
- Clarification of mechanisms
  (responsible for properties)
- Mechanism of field interactions with biological substances
  (biomolecules, membranes, cells)
- Applications to medicine and biology
  plethysmography
  electrocardiography
  electrodes
  ultrasonic diathermy and imaging (echocardiography)
  nonionizing radiation hazards and standards of safety

[a]Some coworkers include E. Carstensen, K. Foster, E. Franck, D. Geselowitz, H. Pauly, L. Sher, F. Sauer (Max Planck Institute), and S. Takashima.

most of my life as a scientist. I benefited greatly from many outstanding colleagues who joined my laboratory, including Ed Carstensen, Dave Geselowitz, Helmut Pauly, Gerhard Schwarz, Shiro Takashima, Jack Reid, Ken Foster, and others.

PAST ACHIEVEMENTS

Earlier activities since the turn of the century and of particular significance to the development of the bioimpedance field are summarized in TABLES 2–4. They present our attempt to summarize the scope of the bioimpedance field.

Hoeber was the first to compare the high- and low-frequency conductivity of erythrocytes.[1] He established from their difference in three significant papers (1910–13) the existence of biological membranes and was able to provide a first estimate for the conductivity of the erythrocyte interior. Hoeber left Germany when Hitler came to power. I met him at the University of Pennsylvania shortly after my arrival in the United States. He invited me to give a seminar about my extension of his work. This event led to my appointment to Penn's faculty.

Fricke, Cole, and Curtis laid the basis for our understanding of the β-dispersion.[2] They did this by applying the relevant Maxwell equations to cell suspensions surrounded by membranes. I had the good fortune to meet them shortly after coming to the United States. Fricke and Cole became friends and coauthors in due time and I profited from frequent discussions.

Cole and Curtis extended the bioimpedance work to the nonlinear level. They observed that the membrane conductance of the squid axon changes strongly with excitation. This started a new branch of biology: membrane biophysics. Hodgkin and Huxley studied in greater detail the nonlinear response first noted by Cole and Curtis. They established the

TABLE 2. Some Past Basic Achievements

Hoeber (1911):
    First demonstration of membrane and ery-interior led to discovery of β-dispersion.

Fricke, Cole & Curtis (1930s):
    Explanation of β-dispersion, caused by membranes (Maxwell Wagner effect).

Cole & Curtis (1938):
    First nonlinear membrane study. Strong conductivity change with excitation.

Hodgkin & Huxley (1952):
    Equations and model for membrane. Nobel prize. Beginning of membrane biophysics.

Schwan *et al.* (1947–57):
    Discovery of α-dispersion: muscle tissue (1950), colloids (1957).
    First tissue data at 100–1000 MHz, γ-dispersion (1947).
    Introduction to the α-β-γ notation for the dielectric response of tissues and cell suspensions from 1 Hz to 100 GHz.

Schwan *et al.* (Carstensen, Pauly, Takashima, Foster, ...), Hanai & Grant:
    Dielectric spectroscopy: cells, vesicles, organelles, membranes, bacteria, proteins, DNA, ...
    Principles of α-β-γ dispersions.

---

existence of Na- and K-channels. Their equivalent circuit and system of nonlinear differential equations became world famous. Their work was recognized by a Nobel prize.

I discovered the α-dispersion.[3] I was the first to extend measurements to 1 GHz, thus noting the existence of the γ-dispersion. I introduced the α-β-γ notation that states the dielectric response of tissues and cell suspensions from 1 Hz to 100 GHz. Many additional valuable contributions were made by the laboratories of Carstensen, Grant, Hanai, and myself (see references 4–7). Extensive reviews of the field are listed in references 2–8.

TABLE 3 summarizes significant techniques. Bioimpedance investigations of tissues and cell suspensions began before the turn of the century after the invention of the Wheatstone bridge. Extensive work on tissues and cell suspensions was carried out. We introduced high-resolution techniques at low frequencies and discovered the α-effect.[9] Single cell work gained popularity after the introduction of the microelectrode technique. Further significant advances in the nonlinear region required the development of the voltage clamp technique by Cole.[2] The detailed study of ion channels in the membrane benefited from the patch clamp technique introduced by Sackmann and Neher. They also received a Nobel prize.

Electrode polarization must be considered in bioimpedance work and was discussed at the linear and nonlinear level by McAdams and myself.[10] In 1963, I introduced four-electrode AC systems in order to avoid electrode problems.[9]

Applications that developed after World War I are summarized in TABLE 4. Let me first mention two applications of impedance data that are not widely appreciated. Ultrahigh frequency (UHF) therapy was introduced in the 1930s. It had become apparent that higher frequencies provided better penetration into body tissues. Better therapeutic effects could be achieved than with conventional therapy introduced by d'Arsonval. However, understand-

TABLE 3. Dielectric Spectroscopy Techniques

(A) Bulk + Suspension Techniques:
Wheatstone bridge
High-resolution LF techniques (Schwan, Wada)
Microwave technology
Network analyzers
Time domain spectroscopy (TDS)
(B) Single Cell Techniques:
Microelectrode, internal-external electrodes
Voltage clamp (Marmont & Cole)
Patch voltage clamp (Neher & Sackmann)
Electrorotation (Arnold & Zimmermann)
Levitation (dielectrophoretic effect) (Jones)
(C) Electrodes:
Polarization impedance (Geddes, Schwan, McAdams, ...)
Polarization impedance nonlinearity
Mechanisms (fractal, electrochem)
Four-electrode technique

ing of the achieved clinical success required relevant dielectric data for a variety of body tissues. Such data were collected by Rajewsky et al.[11] They enabled Schaefer to determine the subcutaneous fat to muscle heat development ratio as a function of frequency and to suggest optimal frequency choice.[11] Debates about thermal and speculated nonthermal benefits took place. Molecular resonance effects and cellular point heating effects were suggested. All this demanded collection of more molecular and cellular dielectric data.

After World War II, interest shifted from beneficial to feared detrimental effects. Microwave technology was rapidly advancing well above 100 MHz. Many dielectric measurements for body tissues were collected at the Mayo Clinic and by my laboratory, covering the range from 0.1 to 10 GHz.[3] These data formed the basis of modern dosimetry in the microwave-frequency range. They permitted determination of absorption coefficients, reflections at tissue interfaces, and first relative absorption cross sections for biological spheres and models of humans.[12,13] This work led to the development of safety standards for nonionizing radiation exposure.

A large number of clinical diagnostic techniques were introduced. They are numerous and, hence, will be only briefly mentioned.

(1) Investigations of single cells: The Coulter counter became an essential tool of the modern biology laboratory, permitting counting and sizing of cell populations. The electronic hematocrit that I developed with colleagues permits instant determination of hematocrit values. It met only with modest success since blood conductivity depends not only on cell concentration, but also on ion concentrations in the medium. An electronic hematocrit utilizing the permittivity of blood would not be affected by ion concentrations in the medium.

TABLE 4. Applications

Therapy (advances due to better impedance data):
UHF-therapy (Rajewsky & Schaefer)
Microwave therapy (Mayo Clinic & Schwan)
Laboratory:
Coulter counter (Coulter)
Electronic hematocrit (Schwan *et al.*)
Diagnostic:[a]
Electrocardiography (Eindhoven, Franck, ...)
Impedance imaging
Electrodiagnosis + myography (electrodiagnosis, chronaxy, skin resistance, electroretinography)
Detection of physiological events by impedance (impedance plethysmography; rheoencephalography; body fluid shift; respiration; blood flow: cardiac output, ventricular emptying, stroke volume, pulsative flow by plethysmograph, thoracic impedance cardiograph, ...)

[a]Many of these diagnostic techniques suffer from difficulties of quantification.

(2) Diagnostic techniques: Electrocardiography became a great success of well-established diagnostic value. So did encephalography. Other techniques met with limited success. These include electrodiagnosis and myography, chronaxy, skin resistance, electroretinography, and additional diagnostic techniques of modest utility.

(3) Monitoring of physiological events by impedance became a subject matter of great interest. Items monitored include body fluid shifts, respiration, blood flow, cardiac output, ventricular emptying, stroke volume, pulsative flow, and thoracic impedance. Impedance plethysmography was introduced by Nyboer to monitor changes in blood volume. Rheoencephalography measured pulsatile changes in brain impedance. In both cases, success was limited. This was probably due to the fact that attempts of rigorous quantification did not succeed.

The problem with most of these techniques is the complexity of the human body and its distribution of tissues of varying conductivity and permittivity, anisotropic properties at that. Even with sophisticated numerical techniques, it is almost impossible to do justice to this situation. The impedance signals received depend critically on this complex arrangement and simple models will not suffice.

Bioimpedance tomography is a new emerging visualization technique presently under intense study. It is discussed in several papers of this volume. I include it in my list of future goals since this field continues to be actively advanced.

FUTURE GOALS

Topics that deserve attention may be divided into two classes: important problems remaining from the past and entirely new possibilities, in part due to recent technological advances. In each category, we may subdivide between basic and applied aspects.

Problems from the Past

The mechanisms responsible for the α-dispersion of tissues need further elaboration. Recognized contributions include counterion relaxation, membrane structures connected to the cell membrane (e.g., the tubular system), membrane properties as predictable from the Hodgkin-Huxley equations, and gap junctions demonstrated recently by Gersing and discussed by him at this meeting. Little is known about the relative contribution of these mechanisms to various tissues. Much can be learned from a perusal of the extensive literature available about the electrical properties of cell suspensions observed at low frequencies.

Another puzzle is posed by the fact that α-dispersions determined by electrorotation and dielectric spectroscopy differ significantly.[14] Apparently, both techniques "see" different properties. This could be due to the fact that counterions move differently in the presence of either a rotating or a stationary alternating field. If so, exploitation of this difference should shed light on the details of the ion cloud's movement and resulting dielectric properties.

Other well-known and important unresolved problems are posed by membrane channel operation and muscle contraction. Both probably involve nonlinear and time-dependent macromolecular responses to local high field strength values. (See TABLE 5.)

New Possibilities

Diagnostic and laboratory tools are indicated in TABLES 6 and 7. We discuss first some emerging technologies that merit particular attention: harmonic analysis, impedance tomography, tissue water determinations, and Hall effect imaging. We conclude with a survey of some new laboratory techniques that are now emerging or possible.

Harmonic Analysis

The harmonic analysis technique used by Moussadi *et al.* for the electrode interface and by Kell for cell suspensions opens new fields of inquiry.[9] The technique exposes the sample of interest to a field strong enough to evoke a weak nonlinear response and evalu-

TABLE 5. Basic Problems from the Past[a]

(1) Sorting out the mechanisms causing α-dispersions [counterions, membrane relaxations (HH), tubular systems, gap junction]

(2) Counterion relaxation theory for cells

(3) Electrorotation versus dielectric spectroscopy: different techniques show different properties—Why?

(4) Membrane channel operation

(5) Muscle contraction

(6) Macromolecules and strong fields

[a]In cases 3–6, contributions of field-induced forces to the conformation of macromolecules require consideration.

TABLE 6. Some Future Applications

Nonlinear studies
    The harmonic technique as applied in the weakly nonlinear range (Kell, Moussadi-Schwan)
    (When does onset of nonlinearity indicate irreversible change?)

Impedance tomography
    Ultimate potential of imaging
    Anisotropy
    Frequency dependence

Hall effect imaging
    Need for defining proper frequency choice

Body water content

Laboratory techniques (see TABLE 7)

---

ates the harmonics. Harmonics can be readily measured at field strength values where the nonlinear contribution is still weak. This nonlinear approach could be used to study the onset of nonlinear properties of proteins. This problem has defied conventional approaches since they require fields too high to prevent thermal damage. Furthermore, many tissues

TABLE 7. Laboratory Techniques

Multielectrode advanced Coulter counter for cell shape, protein, and water content
    (size distributions of all these parameters)

Sedimentation, coagulation, ...
    (feasibility established)

Electronic hematocrit
    (based on permittivity)

Cellular (microscopic) imaging
    (microimpedance tomography)

Tissue structural analysis + diagnostics
    (by taking small tissue samples and analyzing their α-β-γ spectrum on-line for cell parameters)

Cell + macromolecular manipulation by electromagnetic fields

Cell + macromolecular sorting
    (AC electrophoresis using inhomogeneous alternating fields)

Taking advantage of polarization impedance
    (based on electrode impedance sensitivity)

Giaever's technique to study cell adhesion

Biosensor microelectrodes

---

and the electrode polarization impedance are frequently exposed to fields above 1 V/cm, the approximate limit of linearity. Thus, their nonlinear behavior should be of interest.

Impedance Imaging

A large amount of fairly sophisticated effort has been made to explore the potential of "macroscopic" impedance imaging. This includes hardware, reconstruction algorithms, and potential medical applications. I briefly comment on one aspect that appears to have been somewhat neglected. The potential of "microscopic" imaging will be described later.

Many tissues are highly anisotropic. The degree of anisotropy depends on frequency. For example, the low-frequency conductivity ratio for muscle is about five. Electricity will preferably flow along paths of high conductivity current. Therefore, current density and potential distributions are anticipated to differ markedly from those calculated without taking anisotropy into account. Anisotropy deserves attention in bioimpedance imaging and in nonionizing radiation dosimetry.

Tissue Water Estimates

Effort has been spent to extract information from an impedance determination at two frequency values, chosen below and above the anticipated β-dispersion range. The low-frequency value is believed to indicate only extracellular content and the high-frequency value total electrolyte content. However, the proper choice of the limits is beset with problems. Only a careful analysis of the total dielectric admittance spectrum will yield good results since β-dispersion conductivity contributions from organelles, protein-bound water, and macromolecular dipoles can be significant at high frequencies. At the low-frequency end, there exist contributions from the surface conductance of cells and other mechanisms contributing to the α-dispersion.

Hall Effect Imaging (HEI)

This new technique has been proposed recently. It is based on the Hall effect, which occurs when different charge carriers diverge, thereby creating a voltage. The movement may be induced by an ultrasonic field and the voltage depends on the tissue conductivity. The images are claimed to be better than those obtained by ultrasound. Further work needs to be done to evaluate the merits of the HEI technique. The method's strength is its sensitivity to tissue conductivity variations.

Future Laboratory Techniques

A number of new techniques are of potential great usefulness and are presented in TABLE 7.

The Electrode Masking Effect

Many years ago, we noted the masking effect of erythrocytes on the polarization impedance.[9,10] We also noted that the volume fraction dependence curve of the electrode polarization parameters was strikingly different depending on the state of platinum deposits. We never continued this sort of work and still don't understand it. Similar work with other cells and colloidal particles should be carried out. Giaever *et al.* conducted excellent studies of a variety of cell types.[15] They took advantage of the masking effect while studying their adhesion to the electrode surface. This work shows great promise and may give insight into the circumstances that dictate the adhesion of normal and abnormal cells and its relevance to the spread of cancer. Another example of this sort of work is provided by Hesketh, Hardeman, and coworkers.[16-18] They developed microelectrodes whose impedance changes with small amounts of glucose and buffer ionic strength. Other electrodes sense the specific binding of some enterotoxins. Their electrode preparations may well serve as sensitive microbiosensors for many different specific purposes. More work is needed to understand the interaction of the electrode surface and biological materials.

Sedimentation Rate

The sedimentation of erythrocytes can be monitored electronically. I first demonstrated this in 1948.[19] The technique was later advanced to a state where sedimentation rate could be obtained within a few seconds. I also know of some more recent developments and improvements, including evaluating the permittivity. I became aware of this work last summer (1997) when Bertil Jacobson from the Karolinska Institute in Stockholm brought it to my attention.

The Coulter Counter

The Coulter counter provides a typical example of electronic cell counting. Its principle is simple. It is based on the fact that biological cells conduct low-frequency alternating currents poorly, at least as compared with typical biological fluids. It is used to rapidly count cells and to measure their individual sizes. Almost every biological laboratory now has one since it became a valuable tool in cellular studies. The Coulter counter has become a sophisticated device with time. However, its full potential has not yet been realized. For example, consider the use of two electrode pairs, one placed across and the other at both ends of the orifice through which the cells pass. This permits a shape determination, assuming that the cells can be approximated by ellipsoids of revolution and are aligned by streaming forces. This technique was already successfully employed by Velick and Gorin in the 1940s.[20] High frequencies could be added so that the cell interior is sensed, providing a protein estimate.

Cell Imaging

Cell imaging using multielectrode arrangements should be now possible. Advances in the manufacture of microelectrodes permit them to be placed in small cavities containing single cells. This technique has been already applied by Arnold and Zimmermann.[21] They used small four-electrode chambers to generate rotating AC fields and deduced electrical cell properties from the observed rotational response. Electronic imaging techniques at the microscopic level now appear entirely feasible with the tools that have become available recently. The cells can be kept centered using cleverly designed field configurations and "cages". Jones *et al.* in Rochester, New York,[22] and Fuhr, Gimsa, and colleagues in Germany have done excellent work, demonstrating the ability to contain single cells by appropriate field configurations, manipulating them for various purposes, and further advancing spectroscopy via rotating and inhomogeneous fields.[23–25]

It is possible to measure cell impedances from different directions by use of some electrode pairs as source and others as receiving elements. This information could be obtained at different frequencies using on-line impedance analyzer or time domain spectroscopy (TDS) equipment. Thus, pictures showing the cell at different frequencies and from different directions could be obtained. This microimpedance tomography has much in common with macroimpedance tomography and should greatly benefit from what has been accomplished already in the latter case. Another approach can combine the well-established electrorotation technique with dielectric spectroscopy by combining a rotating field used to spin the cell with a sensing stationary electrode pair. This would permit the study of different cellular properties as seen from different directions.

The use of multiple electrodes, network analyzers, or time domain spectroscopy can help to provide rapid evaluation of cellular parameters. The quantities that can be obtained include extracellular and cytoplasmic conductivity, membrane capacitance and conductance, protein content, cell size, and shape. Distribution functions of these parameters representing the variance of these properties when large cell populations are evaluated sequentially could also be obtained. A first step in this direction is the Coulter counter.

Tissue Structural Analysis

The above proposed techniques could be applied also to cultured cells, establishing data that show how cellular dielectric properties and shape quantities depend on cell type and abnormality. The emergence of new rapid diagnostic technologies in the pathology laboratory appears possible.

The use of microelectrode bioimpedance investigations should be of value in determining the dielectric properties of small tissue samples for searching for different cell types, both normal and abnormal. Once established, such knowledge can be applied to electronic microbiopsies in order to rapidly perform a variety of diagnostic tasks.

Cellular Manipulation by Electromagnetic Fields

It has been known for some time that electromagnetic fields impart forces on cells. This can lead to such effects as destruction, fusion, shape changes, rotation, or cytoplasmic streaming. Until recently, these effects were of interest only as a curiosity, and little research was done to understand them fully. Our work on the threshold field strength needed to cause cellular "pearl chain" formation was probably the first quantitative study of these effects.[26] In more recent times, cell fusion and poration have become of prime importance in one of the most important fields to affect future health programs, namely, the biotechnology concerned with transfer and manipulation of genetic information. The electrical cell fusion technique, using alternating current fields, has developed as a promising tool to combine cells and their genetic contents. Further refinements of this technique, and the electromagnetic manipulation of cells for all sorts of purposes, are promising new biophysical research tools.

The theoretical basis of the forces that cells experience when exposed to electrical fields is well established.[27,28] Cells move in inhomogeneous AC fields. This effect can be used in precisely the same manner as DC fields are used in electrophoresis. It should yield different and complementary information. Furthermore, these field-evoked forces can be used to develop new cell sorting techniques since it is anticipated that different cells will experience different forces and, hence, move differently.

More examples could be listed to illustrate therapeutic and diagnostic advances, as well as emerging biophysical technologies based on bioimpedance data. Technologies related to health care such as pacemakers, artificial organs/limbs, and prosthetic devices will always be of particular interest to the public. However, the contributions of electrical engineering to biology, such as the electron microscope, evolving cell fusion techniques, and application of electric field theory to the understanding of cellular functions and electric responses, are just as important. It appears to me that the future of the bioimpedance field could be very bright indeed. Still, it will take determined effort combined with excellent biophysical insight and equally outstanding engineering to succeed. It will also take patience and conviction before the potential of the bioimpedance field is more widely appreciated.

REFERENCES

Space limitations will not permit a detailed list of references. Instead, we list pertinent review articles and books. We also list some seminal papers and a few recent biosensor articles, which are perhaps not widely known to the bioimpedance community. A few comments are added, perhaps helpful to the reader.

1. HOEBER, R. 1910. Eine Methode die elektrische Leitfaehigkeit im Innern von Zellen zu messen. Arch. Ges. Physiol. **133**: 237–259; 1912. Ein zweites Verfahren die Leitfaehigkeit im Innern von Zellen zu messen. Arch. Ges. Physiol. **148**: 189–221; 1913. Messungen der inneren Leitfaehigkeit von Zellen III. Arch. Ges. Physiol. **150**: 15–45. These articles were the first to determine internal cell conductivities. They furthermore established the existence of the β-dispersion and membranes by demonstrating the difference between low- and high-frequency conductivity values.
2. COLE, K. S. 1968. Membranes, Ions, and Impulses. University of California Press. Berkeley/Los Angeles. This is an often-quoted detailed reference to the cellular work done by Fricke, Cole, Curtis, and Schwan and the important extension to the nonlinear level leading to the Hodgkin-Huxley equations.
3. SCHWAN, H. P. 1957. Electrical properties of tissue and cell suspensions. In Advances in Biological and Medical Physics. Vol. 5, p. 147–209. Academic Press. New York. This often-quoted review summarizes dispersion principles, mechanisms, and dielectric data for biological matter.
4. GRANT, E. H., R. J. SHEPPARD & G. P. SOUTH. 1978. Dielectric Behavior of Biological Molecules in Solution. Oxford University Press (Clarendon). London/New York. This and the following reference concentrate on macromolecular dielectric phenomena.
5. TAKASHIMA, S. 1989. Electrical Properties of Biopolymers and Membranes. Adam Hilger. Bristol/Philadelphia.
6. FOSTER, K. R. & H. P. SCHWAN. 1995. Dielectric properties of tissues—a review. In Handbook of Biological Effects of Electro-Magnetic Radiation, p. 25–102. CRC Press. Boca Raton, Florida. This reference concentrates on cellular aspects.

7. SCHWAN, H. P. & S. TAKASHIMA. 1992. Electrical conduction and dielectric behavior in biological systems. *In* Encyclopedia of Applied Physics. Vol. 5, p. 177–200. VCH Pub. Weinheim.
8. PETHIG, R. & D. B. KELL. 1987. The passive electrical properties of biological systems: their significance in physiology, biophysics, and biotechnology. Phys. Med. Biol. **22:** 933–977.
9. SCHWAN, H. P. 1963. Determination of biological impedances. *In* Physical Techniques in Biological Research. Vol. 6, p. 323–406. Academic Press. New York.
10. SCHWAN, H. P. 1992. Linear and nonlinear electrode polarization and biological materials. Ann. Biomed. Eng. **20:** 269–288.
11. RAJEWSKY, B. 1938. Ergebnisse der Biophysikalischen Forschung. Vol. 1. Thieme. Leipzig. Perhaps the first detailed text dealing with frequency-dependent properties of tissues and a review of the state of the art at the time.
12. SCHWAN, H. P. 1958. Biophysics of diathermy. *In* Therapeutic Heat. Second edition, chapter 3, p. 63–125. Licht Pub. New Haven, Connecticut.
13. SCHWAN, H. P. 1986. Research on biological effects of nonionizing radiations: contributions to biological properties, field interactions, and dosimetry. D'Arsonval Medal Lect., Bioelectromagnetic Soc., Bioelectromagnetics **7:** 113–128.
14. ARNOLD, W. M., H. P. SCHWAN & U. ZIMMERMANN. 1987. Surface conductance and other properties of latex particles measured by electrorotation. J. Phys. Chem. **91:** 5093–5098.
15. GIAEVER, I. & C. R. KEESE. 1986. Use of electric fields to monitor the dynamical aspect of cell behavior in tissue culture. IEEE Trans. Biomed. Eng. **33**(No. 3): 242–247.
16. KASAPHASIOGLU, B., P. J. HESKETH, W. C. HANLY, G. J. MACLAY & E. N. ESFAHANI. 1993. A novel ultra-thin film glucose sensor. Sens. Actuators **14:** 749–751.
17. HARDEMAN, S., T. H. NELSON, D. BEIRNE, M. DE SILVA, P. J. HESKETH, G. J. MACLAY & S. M. GENDEL. 1995. Sensitivity of novel ultrathin platinum film immunosensors to buffer ionic strength. Sen. Actuators **B24–25:** 98–102.
18. DE SILVA, M., Y. U. ZHANG, P. J. HESKETH, G. J. MACLAY, S. GENDEL & J. R. STETTER. 1995. A novel biosensor for staphylococcal enterotoxin. Biosen. Bioelectronics **10:** 675–682.
19. SCHWAN, H. 1948. Sedimentation determinations by electrical resistance measurement. Kolloid-Z. **III:** 53.
20. VELICK, S. & M. GORIN. 1940. The electrical conductance of suspensions of ellipsoids and its relation to the study of avian erythrocytes. J. Gen. Physiol. **23:** 753–771.
21. ARNOLD, W. M. & U. ZIMMERMANN. 1982. Rotation of an isolated cell in a rotating electric field. Naturwissenschaften **69:** 297.
22. KALER, K. V. I. S. & T. B. JONES. 1990. Dielectrophoretic spectra of single cells determined by feedback-controlled levitation. Biophys. J. **57:** 173–182.
23. FUHR, G., T. H. SCHNELLE, R. HAGEDORN & S. G. SHIRLEY. 1995. Dielectrophoretic field cages: technique for cell, virus, and molecule handling. Cell. Eng. **1:** 47–57.
24. FUHR, G., W. P. ARNOLD, R. HAGEDORN, T. MUELLER, W. BENECKE, B. WAGNER & U. ZIMMERMANN. 1992. Levitation, holding, and rotation of cells within traps made by high-frequency fields. Biochim. Biophys. Acta **1108:** 215–223.
25. GIMSA, J., B. PRUEGER, P. ERPMANN & E. DONATH. 1995. Electrorotation of particles measured by dynamic light scattering—a new dielectric spectroscopy technique. Colloids Surf. **A98:** 243–249.
26. SCHWAN, H. P. & L. D. SHER. 1969. Electrostatic field induced forces and their biological implications. *In* Dielectrophoretic and Electrophoretic Deposition, p. 107–126. The Electrochemical Society. New York.
27. CHIABRERA, A., C. NICOLINI & H. P. SCHWAN, Eds. 1984. Interactions between Electromagnetic Fields and Cells, p. 1–18. Plenum. New York. The theory of field-induced force effects is presented by F. Sauer in two articles and experimental data are presented in an article by Schwan.
28. FOSTER, K. R., F. A. SAUER & H. P. SCHWAN. 1992. Electrorotation and levitation of cells and colloidal particles. Biophys. J. **63:** 180–190.

Monitoring Temperature-Induced Changes in Tissue during Hyperthermia by Impedance Methods[a]

EBERHARD GERSING

Department of Anesthesiological Research, University Hospital Göttingen, D-37075 Göttingen, Germany

ABSTRACT: The electrical conduction in living tissue depends on temperature in two ways: (1) the temperature coefficients of conductivity of the intra- and extracellular electrolytes and (2) temperature-induced fluid volume shifts in the tissue. Measurements in rat skeletal muscle and tumors (DS sarcoma) during hyperthermic treatment reveal that the contribution of fluid volume shifts to changes in conductance is of the same order of magnitude as the change in fluid conductivity. In skeletal muscles, blood volume changes are caused by the temperature-dependent regulation of the vessel diameter (vasodilatation). In tumors, fluid content changes irregularly. These effects render temperature measurements by impedance methods, for example, electrical impedance tomography (EIT), questionable. However, monitoring fluid volume changes in tissue and the state of cell membranes is an interesting application of impedance (or admittance) spectroscopy and tomography as well.

INTRODUCTION

The electrical admittance in organ tissue in the frequency range up to about 10 MHz depends on the fluid volume distribution of the intra- and extracellular compartments, the ion concentration and mobility in each of both spaces, and the properties of the membranes separating the compartments. Therefore, changes in the conductivity of the fluids, the volumes and dimensions of their compartments, or the conductance and capacitance of the membranes are reflected in the impedance or admittance spectra of the tissue under investigation. Hence, it seemed promising to introduce measurements of the electrical properties of tissue into the research on tumors, particularly alterations in tumor tissue caused by hyperthermic treatment. (Experiments on excised tumors during hyperthermia have been described by McRae.[1]) On the one hand, information on fluid volume shifts in the tissue and the state of the membranes could be expected; on the other, the question as to whether it is possible to obtain temperature coefficients of the conductivity of various living tissues reliably, in order to provide tissue temperature measurements based on the impedance method, could be answered. Already in the early days of electrical impedance tomography (EIT), Griffith[2] proposed the application of EIT in order to determine the temperature distribution inside a body. Especially during microwave treatment, it is necessary to monitor the temperature distribution because of the possible occurrence of hot spots. Currently, a noninvasive and sufficiently accurate temperature measuring method is still not available.

---

[a]This research was supported by the Dr.med.h.c. Erwin Braun Foundation, Basel, Switzerland (Grant No. 5.7).

In the following, admittance data obtained from tumors and skeletal muscles of rats during hyperthermic treatment are evaluated and compared in order to determine the contributions of changing extracellular and total fluid content and of the temperature coefficients (TC) of tissue fluid conductivity.

METHODS

Admittance measurements are carried out on rat skeletal muscles of the upper thigh and on experimental tumors (DS sarcoma) grown on the hind feet. The experimental set-up is described in reference 3. The warmth was produced by infrared radiation from two 150-W halogen lamps equipped with water filters[4] to suppress wavelengths above 1400 nm.

Heating was controlled automatically by a switching regulator and an insulated thermocouple inserted into the tumor (or skeletal muscle). Besides the temperature of the tissue under investigation, the temperatures of the untreated tumor and the body core were recorded, as well as the arterial blood pressure. Because tissue fluid content depends on blood pressure, where possible, only admittance data gained during a stable state of circulation of the animal were used for further evaluation. After warming up at a rate of 0.3, . . ., 0.5 °C per minute, the temperature was held constant at 42.5 °C over a period of 60 minutes and, thereafter, heating was switched off.

The admittance was measured in the frequency range of 100 Hz to 3 MHz using a Solartron 1260 Impedance Analyzer with a special active probe connected with an electrode set that consisted of two titanium needles, diameter 0.3 mm, 4 mm apart, with fractal surfaces (sputtered with iridium) in order to reduce the polarization impedance.[5] In some cases, a set of four needle electrodes (made from stainless steel, with smooth surfaces) arranged in a row was applied in order to extend the frequency range down to 3 Hz. Alternately, the admittance spectra of the treated and an untreated tissue were measured by means of a multiplexer in order to establish a reference in view of the state of the animal.

The conductance values measured during the hyperthermic treatment are normalized by division by the corresponding data at the beginning of the warming-up period. The changes in conductance are expressed as percentages. In this way, the data of different tissues or experiments can be readily compared.

RESULTS

Skeletal Muscle

In FIGURE 1a, the time course of the temperature measured inside the muscle during hyperthermic treatment is given. FIGURE 1b presents the corresponding courses of the measured relative changes in conductance G(LF) at 100 Hz (open circles) and G(HF) at 3 MHz (open triangles). The two curves do not coincide: during warming up from 37 to 42.5 °C, the conductance G(LF) of the extracellular compartment increases by 20%, and the total conductance G(HF) by 13%. Since intra- and extracellular fluids should exhibit TCs of the conductivity of about 2%/ °C, an increase in conductance of about 11% only is expected.

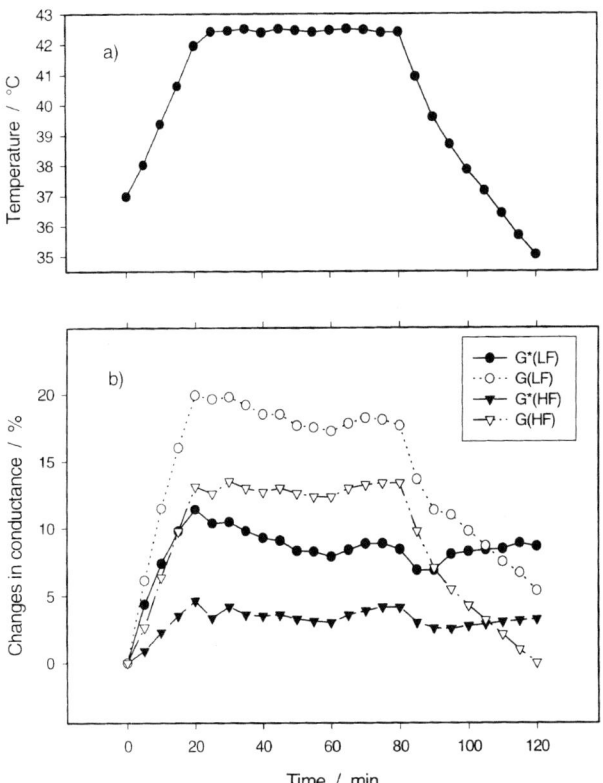

FIGURE 1. Skeletal muscle during hyperthermic treatment: (a) time course of temperature, (b) corresponding changes in conductance; for details, see text.

Assuming that the changes in conductance measured during the hyperthermic treatment are caused not only by the TCs of the intra- and extracellular fluids, but also by a changing extracellular and total fluid content, a way must be found to separate the contributions of both causes because no easily applicable real-time measurement method for the determination of the extra- and intracellular fluid content is available. Therefore, starting from the normal condition (temperature) with the conductances $G_o(LF)$ and $G_o(HF)$, at each point in time (or temperature) a change in conductance was calculated for each momentary temperature, based on an assumed TC value in the possible range of 1.5–2.5%/°C. This value of change in conductance caused by the TC of fluid conductivity was subtracted from the measured values G(LF) and G(HF) of the conductivity. The results were then changes in conductances $G^*(LF)$ and $G^*(HF)$ mainly reflecting fluid volume alterations—with a more or less vanishing contribution of the temperature-dependent conductivity changes of the fluids. This procedure was applied to the conductances G(LF) at 100 Hz and G(HF) at 3 MHz, corresponding to the extracellular compartment and the total tissue volume under test. The temperature coefficients TC_{LF} of the extracellular fluid and TC_{HF} of the total fluid volume were successively varied in the range mentioned above and the most appropriate value was chosen for calculating the changes in conductance $G^*(LF)$ and $G^*(HF)$, which represent the intracellular and total fluid volume changes during the time course:

residual changes in extracellular conductance: $G^*(LF) = G(LF) - (\Delta T \cdot TC_{LF})$

residual changes in total conductance: $G^*(HF) = G(HF) - (\Delta T \cdot TC_{HF})$.

For the skeletal muscle, TC_{LF} and TC_{HF} were ascertained to be 1.7%/°C. The curves plotted in FIGURE 1b (leaving out the contribution of the TC of the conductivity of the fluids) show that, with rising temperature, $G^*(LF)$ (solid circles), the residual conductance in the extracellular compartment, increases by about 10%, and $G^*(HF)$ (solid triangles) of the total volume increases by about 4%. These changes correspond to an increasing extracellular fluid volume due to temperature-induced vasodilatation. It is noteworthy that the regulatory effect begins immediately with the rise in temperature. Even after the return to normal temperature, the fluid volume remains augmented for some time.

During the experiment, the average blood pressure decreased slowly from about 120 to 90 mmHg, exhibiting some dips, for example, after 20, 60, and 80 minutes. Obviously, these events also influenced the conductance values G and G^* of the muscle tissue. In addition, the slowly decreasing pressure (especially between 20 and 60 minutes) can be observed in the course of $G(LF)$ and $G^*(LF)$.

Tumor Tissue

Tumor tissue (both cases presented are DS sarcoma) exhibits a completely different behavior. In contrast to the case of muscles, the curves (FIGURE 2b) presenting the measured changes in extracellular $G(LF)$ (open circles) and total conductance $G(HF)$ (open triangles) coincide during the warming-up period and, partially, during the cooling-down period. The temperature coefficients TC_{LF} and TC_{HF} of conductivity have been determined as 1.7%/°C. Initially, there is no change in the residual conductances $G^*(LF)$ (solid circles) of the extracellular pathways and $G^*(HF)$ (solid triangles) of the total tissue—not affected by the temperature-dependent contribution of the fluid conductivities. The increase in the measured conductances $G(LF)$ and $G(HF)$ is due to the temperature coefficients of the extra- and intracellular fluids only. This behavior indicates missing regulation of blood circulation in tumor vessels. However, during the hyperthermic period, 10 minutes after having reached the final temperature of 42.5 °C, a large increase in conductance occurred followed by a great decrease. In the case presented, $G^*(LF)$ (solid circles) rises by nearly 20% and $G^*(HF)$ (solid triangles) by about 7%. This indicates an increase in fluid in the tissue volume under investigation.

The behavior of another tumor of the same kind is presented in FIGURE 3. During warming up and cooling down, the measured conductances $G(LF)$ and $G(HF)$ changed identically. As explained before, there is no temperature-dependent blood flow regulation. However, after a steep increase in the residual conductance $G^*(LF)$ up to 26% and $G^*(HF)$ up to 5%, the values dropped again—still during the period of elevated temperature. This effect can be explained as an increase and subsequent decrease in fluid inside the tumor tissue, at least in the limited region covered by the admittance measurement.

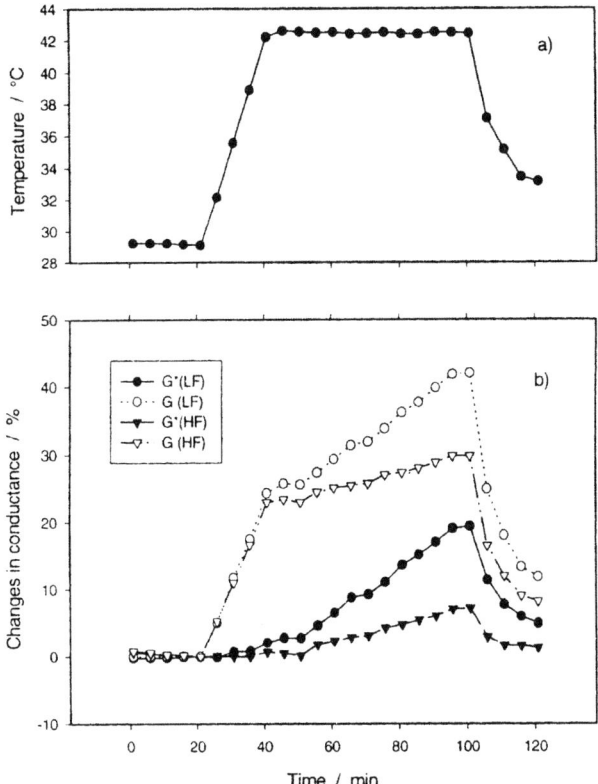

FIGURE 2. DS sarcoma (1) during hyperthermic treatment: (a) time course of temperature, (b) corresponding changes in conductance.

Membrane Disintegration

In order to follow damaging effects of temperatures exceeding 42.5 °C to healthy muscle tissue, the data of another experiment were used during which the temperature controller failed and a maximum temperature of 44.0 °C was reached. Once the failure was detected, the heating was turned off immediately. FIGURE 4a shows the time course of the temperature in the skeletal muscle under test. FIGURE 4b shows the corresponding courses of the extracellular space index (ECSI) and the phase angle of admittance at 72 kHz. The ECSI is defined as the quotient of the conductances at a low frequency (3 Hz) and a high frequency (3 MHz). It describes in a rough approximation the behavior of the extracellular space volume and is almost unaffected by temperature. Its value is 1.0 in the case of a pure electrolyte without cells if no α- or β-dispersion exists. The phase angle (e.g., at 72 kHz) itself, changing only slightly with temperature, is also a suitable indicator of the state of the cell membranes. Beyond 43 °C, the phase angle begins to decrease and the ECSI

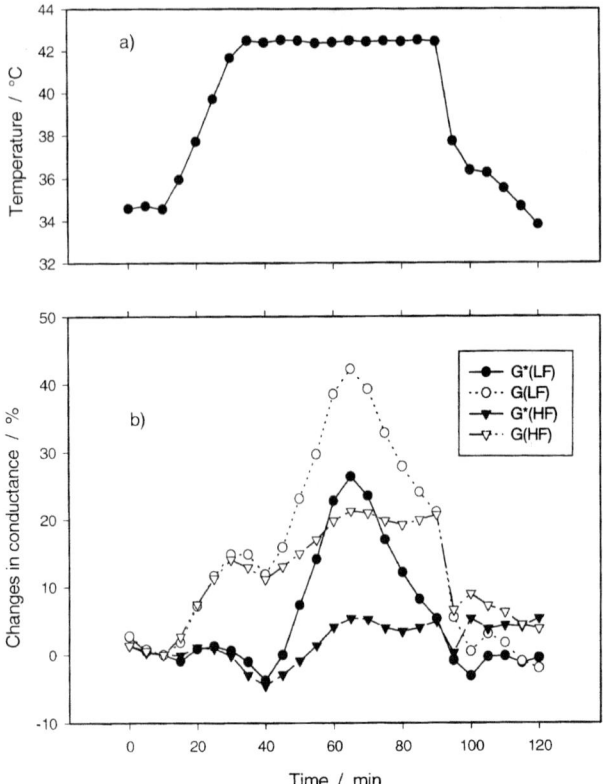

FIGURE 3. DS sarcoma (2) during hyperthermic treatment: (a) time course of temperature, (b) corresponding changes in conductance.

increases, revealing the growing extracellular volume—that is, the onset of the disintegration of cell membranes. Finally, the phase angle decreased to half the original value, but not to zero, and did not rise again. Correspondingly, the ECSI rose to a value near 65% and did not return to the original value. Both results indicate that numerous membranes are destroyed, although not all cells covered by the measuring process.

DISCUSSION

The changes observed in tissue conductance during hyperthermic treatment are caused by the temperature coefficient of conductivity of the material and by fluid volume shifts in the tissue—in other words, a material property and a process.

The curves $G^*(LF)$ and $G^*(HF)$ plotted in FIGURES 1b, 2b, and 3b reflect in a first approximation the changes in fluid content in the extracellular compartment and in the total tissue volume under test, irrespective of the change in conductivity with temperature.

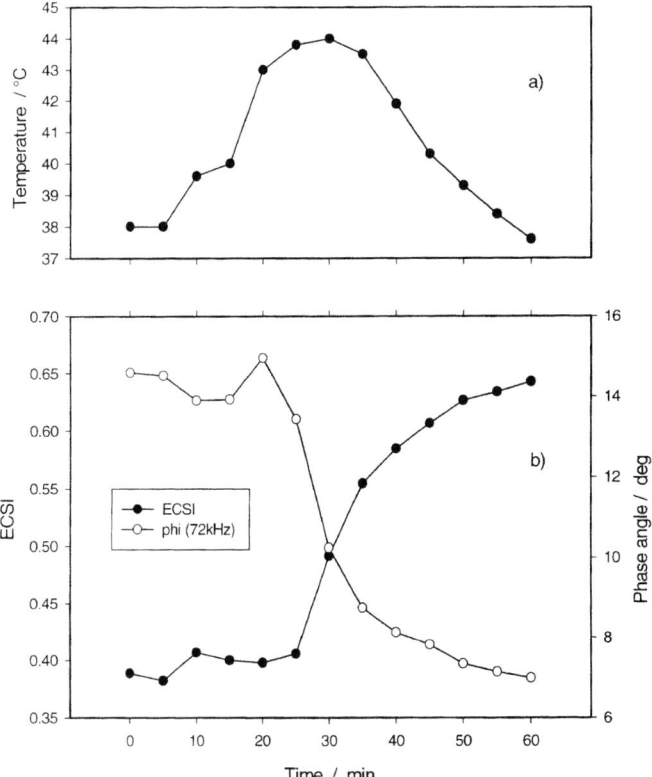

FIGURE 4. Skeletal muscle subjected to elevated temperatures: (a) time course of temperature, (b) extracellular space index (ECSI) and phase angle of admittance at 72 kHz.

In the case of the skeletal muscle in FIGURE 1b, the changing intravasal volume caused by regulation of the diameter of the vessels dependent on temperature is clearly demonstrated.

In contrast, as reported by Brockhoff,[6] excised canine myocardium (after perfusion with cardioplegic solution HTK) beyond the limit of viability, but with cell membranes still intact, does not exhibit such regulation phenomena. He determined (in the temperature range of 8 to 35 °C) the following temperature coefficients:

TC of resistivity at 200 Hz: –2.2%/°C

TC of resistivity at 2 MHz: –1.9%/°C

TC of phase angle at 5 kHz: –0.5%/°C

TC of the characteristic frequency of impedance: +2.0%/°C.

Only three cases are presented here as examples—a skeletal muscle and two DS sarcoma.

As in other experiments with tumors of the same type (DS sarcoma), as well as with Yoshida tumors, a similar typical behavior could be found, despite the individual differences in the behavior during treatment: earlier or later in the hyperthermic period, the conductance of the extracellular pathways always increases considerably, as presented by $G^*(LF)$. $G^*(HF)$ follows to a reduced extent (but not always correlated). This demonstrates the common finding that, during the hyperthermic treatment, the fluid content especially in the extracellular compartment (including the intravasal volume) is augmented. However, as in the examples of FIGURES 3b and 4b, the accumulated fluid can disappear again—at least it is shifted outside the small tissue region covered by the admittance measurement.

The relation between $G^*(HF)$ and $G^*(LF)$ is not yet completely physiologically understood. Hereby, it must be considered that membrane conductance itself is neither zero nor constant under changing external conditions. An increasing membrane conductance causes an increase in the conductance measured at low frequencies like an increasing extracellular space volume. Unfortunately, with macroscopic impedance measurements, we do not have any immediate access to the membranes in order to ascertain their conductance.

With respect to the determination of changes in the temperature distribution inside a body using EIT, what is the maximum error allowed? Above 43 °C, healthy tissue will be damaged, but the tumor should be treated with the highest possible temperature, for example, 42.5 °C. Consequently, the error must not exceed ±0.5 °C. Starting from a normal temperature of about 36.5 °C, a span of 6 °C remains. Thus, for a TC of 2%/°C, a deviation of the TC of only ±0.2%/°C leads to an error larger than ±0.5 °C. However, in the case of skeletal muscle, a deviation of about 2%/°C occurs because of fluid volume shifts and, in tumors, a still larger deviation may be found.

Therefore, a sufficiently accurate determination of tissue temperature using impedance or admittance measurements seems to be impossible. However, even if the temperature determination by impedance or admittance spectroscopy and also EIT is questionable, the method allows us to follow fluid volume shifts and developing edema, as well as the onset of membrane disintegration.

REFERENCES

1. ESRICK, M. A. & D. A. MCRAE. 1992. Temperature coefficients versus hyperthermia-induced changes in the electrical conductivity of tissues. Hyperthermic Oncol. **1:** 209.
2. GRIFFITH, H., I. ANTAL & A. AHMED. 1985. Non-invasive thermometry using applied potential tomography. Strahlentherapie **161:** 534.
3. GERSING, E., W. KRÜGER, M. OSYPKA & P. VAUPEL. 1995. Problems involved in temperature measurements using EIT. Physiol. Meas. **16:** A153–A160.
4. VAUPEL, P., D. K. KELLEHER & W. KRÜGER. 1992. Water-filtered infrared-A-radiation: a novel technique to heat superficial tumors. Strahlenther. Onkol. **168:** 633–639.
5. GERSING, E., M. SCHÄFER & M. OSYPKA. 1995. The appearance of positive phase angles in impedance measurements on extended biological objects. Innov. Technol. Biol. Med. **16**(Spec. issue 2): 71–76.
6. BROCKHOFF, C. 1988. Messung der elektrischen Impedanz des Herzmuskels zur Abschätzung der Ischämiebelastung des Myokards bei induziertem Herzstillstand. Thesis, Medical Faculty, University of Göttingen, Germany, pp. 85–86 and 131.

Application of Linear Circuit Models to Impedance Spectra in Irradiated Muscle[a]

K. SUNSHINE OSTERMAN,[b] KEITH D. PAULSEN,[b] AND P. JACK HOOPES[c]

[b]Thayer School of Engineering, Dartmouth College, Hanover, New Hampshire 03755-8000

[c]Department of Surgery, Dartmouth-Hitchcock Medical Center, Hanover, New Hampshire 03766

ABSTRACT: We have applied a number of modeling schemes to previously reported *in vivo* electrical impedance measurements on irradiated and normal muscle in the hind legs of rats. Specifically, seven-parameter parallel pathways and embedded membrane circuit models have been fit to group averages of impedance spectra measured at different doses and time points. Correlations between histologically scored tissue sections and model parameters have also been determined. The results show that both models produce good fits to the experimental observations, especially in the case of the irradiated tissues. The correlations between histology scores and circuit parameters were, however, higher with the embedded model. Trends in the spectra and the model parameters were found to agree with the expected changes in tissue pathophysiology associated with the progression of tissue injury from radiation exposure. Quantitative correlations with specific histological criteria were less conclusive, suggesting that more information may be needed to refine the model architecture if model parameters are to be explicitly related to the types and extent of tissue damage induced by radiation treatments.

INTRODUCTION

Normal tissue is always present within the radiation field during cancer treatment and it is the response of this normal, healthy tissue that limits the dose that can be administered. Present techniques for monitoring patient response to treatment, for example, biopsy or other imaging modalities, are costly, often invasive, and subject to significant measurement error. If the architectural integrity of the treatment site could be accurately assessed, the success rates of radiation therapy would likely increase.

Different tissue types have different electrical impedance signatures that are known to change with pathology, but it is often difficult to determine which components of these signatures are important and how their changes relate back to even the most basic physiological parameters.[1,2] In order to deploy electrical impedance spectroscopy (EIS) as a noninvasive tool for radiation response tracking, one would hope to develop a model that is able to fit the data well and that demonstrates a parametric variation that can be related to changes associated with the progression of tissue injury.

When a material has only a single relaxation frequency, its impedance can be accurately modeled by an Re (extracellular resistance) in parallel with a series Ri (intracellular resistance) and Cm (membrane capacitance). The curves generated from this simple three-element circuit model, however, must be semicircular and centered on the real axis.

[a]This work was supported in part by NIH Grant No. R01 CA64588, awarded by the National Cancer Institute.

Changes in the bulk capacitance of the muscle (as well as changes in the resistive components) will cause the center frequency to shift, but cannot alter the shape of this curve. The impedance data associated with muscle, as shown below, and biological tissue more generally, form a depressed semicircular arc when plotted in the impedance plane.

Parameterization of EIS data using the empirical Cole-Cole model is common. Gabriel *et al.* recently used the Cole-Cole model approach to successfully compile and describe the dielectric behavior of biological tissues over a broad frequency range.[3] The existence of a specific and continuous distribution of relaxation times, assumed with this model, is often attributed to nonuniformity of the cell size and shape or to the presence of some nonlinear process. There are, however, numerous relaxation functions, which will produce similar results in the impedance domain, and a total dielectric response can also be produced using a compartmental model.[4] Dissado *et al.* propose a self-similar hierarchical model for the cell with interconnected and leaky internal membrane structures to accurately describe dielectric data.[5] Hence, there are any number of ways to produce model-based matches to experimental impedance data that can be considered and may prove useful in determining tissue functional status.

It is likely that both the intracellular complexity and range of cell shapes and sizes within our measurement field, which contains varying degrees of irradiated tissue, will impact impedance readings. To gain better appreciation for the magnitude and importance of these different influences, we applied two relatively simple models to impedance data recorded on normal and irradiated muscle tissue. These results are compared to histological findings in these same animals to explore whether systematic model changes can be related to histological measures of tissue injury.

METHODS

Impedance readings were obtained on a total of 15 rats. The gastrocnemius and biceps femoris muscles in one leg of each animal were exposed to a single radiation dose of 70, 90, or 150 Gy, which was directed to the muscle with a 2-cm-diameter cone. The cone was positioned to block radiation to the femur. The skin was spared by retracting it out of the radiation field; an incision was made in the skin along the back of the leg and distal to the measurement site. After irradiation, the incision was surgically closed. All protocol procedures, except irradiation, were performed on the opposite leg to provide a control.

Readings were performed at 50 frequency points between 1 kHz and 1 MHz using a PC interfaced Hewlett-Packard 4284A precision LCR meter. Two disk electrodes, mounted on the parallel arms of a caliper, were positioned on either side of the thigh. The muscle was compressed slightly in this procedure and an AC current of 0.15 mA was applied to the skin or muscle surface. Readings through the skin were made at all monthly time points, while measurements directly on the muscle surface were confined to time points immediately prior to irradiation and at sacrifice.

Recessed, 8-mm-diameter, platinized stainless steel and solid matrix Ag-AgCl electrodes (In Vivo Metric, Healdsburg, California) were employed. The cavities of these electrodes were filled with electrode gel and residual polarization impedances were measured by shorting the electrode pairs across the gel. This polarization correction procedure allowed us to combine the data from both electrode types.

Using a parallel plate dielectric model, the relative real and imaginary components of impedance (a function of electrode separation) were converted to appropriate units of ohm-m. Fringing effects, which differ with separation, were not corrected for, but were assumed to be fairly constant between readings. Complex plots were generated and fit with STEPIT (J. P. Chandler, Quantum Chemistry Program Exchange, Indiana University); the sum of squared error between the model-generated impedance and the data was minimized. The two models to be considered are shown in FIGURE 1. For this initial phase of the study, the number of circuit elements has been chosen to be small in order to retain a certain level of model simplicity while providing the flexibility needed to achieve reasonably good fits to the experimental data. Each model contains seven fitting parameters.

The rats, one per dose group, were sacrificed at monthly end points and histology performed. Six histopathologic criteria—edema, congestion, necrosis, fibroplasia, inflammation, and hemorrhage—were established. Three distinct regions of the tissue—the subcutis, the muscle, and the interstitium—were identified. Each region was scored separately. An injury score ranging between 0 (normal) and 4 (severe, diffuse damage) was assessed for each criterion within a region. If the change within a category (e.g., edema) was minimal and focal, a numerical score of 1 was given. If damage was minimal but multifocal, or severe but focal, it received a score of 2. Likewise, a score of 3 was awarded for damage that was deemed minimal but diffuse, or severe but multifocal. Evaluations were made, in blinded fashion, by a trained research pathologist (P. J. Hoopes). The overlap built into the scoring scheme minimizes the need for a subjective assessment. While it is clear, for example, that minimal damage that is multifocal is more significant than minimal damage that is focal, the impact of multifocal minimal damage may be greater or lesser than severe focal damage. The scoring described above forces the latter two cases to receive the same injury rating, while effectively separating and ranking the former two conditions.

Impedance spectra from all animals at a specific time postirradiation and irradiation dose level were pooled and correlation coefficients between histological scores and fitting parameters were calculated.

Correlation coefficients were calculated using the following equation:

$$\rho_{XY} = \sum_i [(X_i - \mu_X)(Y_i - \mu_Y)] / \left[\sqrt{\sum_i (X_i - \mu_X)^2 \sum_i (Y_i - \mu_Y)^2} \right],$$

where μ_X and μ_Y are the means calculated from measurements on the normal nonirradiated legs. The variable X, in this case, would be the summation of histological scores in the

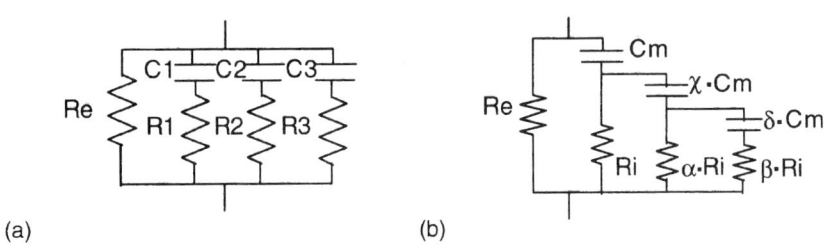

FIGURE 1. Tissue-equivalent circuit models: (a) multiple parallel pathways; (b) single cell pathway with embedded membrane structure.

muscle and interstitium for a given criterion (e.g., fibroplasia) and there would be 18 observations of this variable. Nine of the observations are from nonirradiated tissue and 9 are from irradiated tissue at the different radiation doses and times. The second variable, Y, is a circuit parameter generated by fitting the spectral data from the corresponding dose and time. Again, there are 18 observations of this variable since there are 18 spectral curves that were fit with each circuit model.

RESULTS AND DISCUSSION

The complex impedance spectra from measurements on rats sacrificed at two months postirradiation are shown in FIGURE 2. At 1 kHz, the resistivity for the control legs has a real component, Re[Z], of about 2.4 ohm-m, with an imaginary component, Im[Z], around 0.1 ohm-m. As the frequency increases, the real component decreases and the imaginary component increases until it reaches a peak at about 40 kHz. Above this frequency, Im[Z] begins to decrease while the value of Re[Z] continues to fall. Thus, the curve should be interpreted from right to left as the frequency increases. At the lower end of the spectrum used here, the current is confined to the extracellular space, explaining the higher resistance. The capacitance of intact cell membranes prevents the passage of current through the cell interior. However, as the frequency increases, more current is able to flow through the cell interior and the overall resistance drops. Charge buildup at the lipid interfaces accounts for most of the reactance seen in this frequency range, 1 kHz–1 MHz.

At all three doses, the real and reactive components of impedance in the irradiated leg have decreased and there is a clear separation of impedance spectra between the exposed and control legs. The error bars are +/–1 standard deviation, based on 32 measurements, and there is no overlap between irradiated and nonirradiated tissue impedance in the low frequency end of the spectrum. For clarity, error bars are only shown for the 90 Gy exposure. At 150 Gy, there are differences in impedance values at the highest frequencies, which may be significant as well. The frequency at which the imaginary component reached its maximum value was 48 kHz for the 70 Gy dose case averages, 70 kHz for the 90 Gy case, and 96 kHz for the 150 Gy exposures; the corresponding frequency for all of the control legs was 36 kHz. There has been some indication in the literature that the value of this peak frequency may be more stable than the absolute real or imaginary components of the impedance signature.[6]

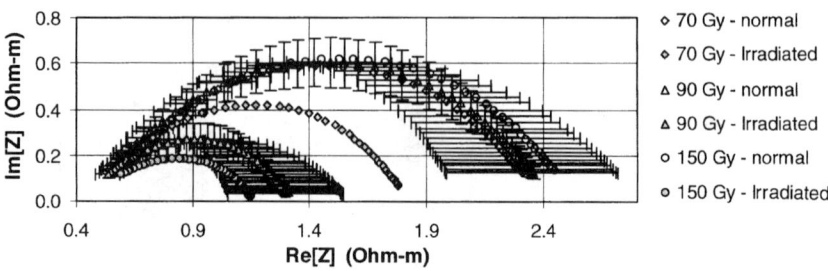

FIGURE 2. Average impedance spectra from data collected at 2 months postirradiation. Thirty-two measurement sets averaged; error bars are +/–1 SD.

TABLE 1. Histopathological Scoring of Irradiated Muscle Tissue at Two Months Postirradiation

Doses (Gy)	Edema	Congestion	Necrosis	Fibroplasia	Inflammation	Hemorrhage	Total Score
70	2.5	1.0	4.0	1.0	5.0	1.0	14.5
90	3.0	1.0	3.5	5.0	4.0	2.0	18.5
150	6.0	6.0	5.5	5.5	6.0	4.0	33.0
control	1.5	0.5	0	1.0	0.5	0.5	4.0

Tissue sections from these animals received the histological evaluations shown in TABLE 1. The scores from the control legs were averaged and the resulting values are presented in the last row of the table. The numerical values shown are the combined scores for injury within the muscle and interstitium. The general progression of injury predicted by EIS is reflected in the histological rankings.

The scores in the tissue exposed at the 70 Gy level are not very different from those in the tissue exposed to 90 Gy. There is, however, a much larger extent of fibroplasia, more widespread necrosis, and less inflammation observed with the higher dose at two months postirradiation. The tissue section taken from the 70 Gy exposed leg showed more diffuse necrosis, while the 90 Gy exposed tissue evidenced more focal but severe necrosis; thus, a similar score was applied in each case. The large extent of fibroplasia in the 90 Gy case also indicated that some early, and possibly more diffuse, areas of necrosis had already begun to be replaced by this two month end point. The dynamic nature of the radiation response is also evident in the inflammation scores: the initially high value at 70 Gy, a lower score at 90 Gy, and a high score again at the 150 Gy level. It is important to note that the types of physiological change observed with these high radiation doses, although they occur on a much shorter timescale, are not unlike late radiation effects seen with smaller, fractionated dose schedules typically applied clinically.

In an attempt to identify contributions to the shape of the spectral curves from each of the six criteria, the spectra (a subset is shown in FIGURE 2) were parameterized using the two circuit models illustrated in FIGURE 1. The same data subset is shown with the fits from the parallel model superimposed (FIGURE 3). The best-fit curves generated using the embedded element model are visually indistinguishable from the parallel model plots and

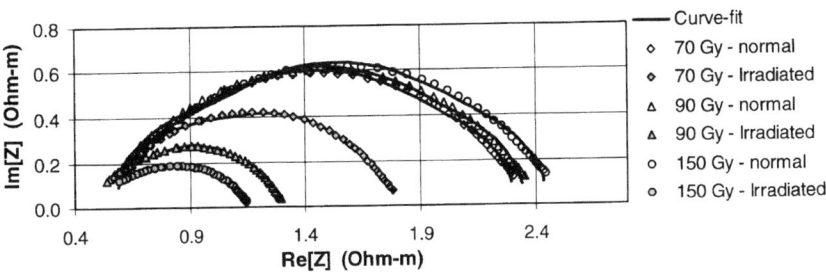

FIGURE 3. Average impedance spectra data for animals measured at 2 months postirradiation with superimposed circuit model curve fits on all six sets of data.

TABLE 2. Multiple Parallel Pathways (Optimized Parameters)

Tissue	Re	R1	C1	R2	C2	R3	C3
70 Gy–control	1.53	13.2	$2.06e{-}6$	2.35	$1.18e{-}6$	1.04	$5.05e{-}7$
90 Gy–control	1.59	12.5	$1.68e{-}6$	2.46	$1.01e{-}6$	1.03	$4.91e{-}7$
150 Gy–control	1.64	16.0	$1.58e{-}6$	2.79	$0.99e{-}6$	1.09	$4.92e{-}7$
70 Gy	1.20	22.4	$1.19e{-}6$	3.47	$0.82e{-}6$	1.09	$4.87e{-}7$
90 Gy	1.04	12.8	$1.04e{-}6$	2.05	$0.79e{-}6$	1.54	$2.00e{-}7$
150 Gy	0.911	14.9	$0.62e{-}6$	2.76	$0.43e{-}6$	2.07	$1.00e{-}7$

are not shown. It is interesting to note that we were consistently able to achieve fits that were closer to the damaged tissue than to the normal tissue regardless of which model was used. A reduction of the least squares error by a factor on the order of 10 was observed with curve fits to the 150 Gy case.

The presence of edema should cause a reduction in the extracellular resistance. Muscular and vascular damage should be expressed as changes primarily in capacitance values, as cell membranes break down. Fibroplasia, from previous experiments in our lab, appears to be more conductive than normal muscle tissue. The presence of interstitial fibroplasia may be providing a short around the muscle tissue, reducing the intracellular structural effects of muscle, which are more electrically complex despite the need to add an additional dispersive element to the model. This could account for our ability to achieve closer fits to the spectra of irradiated tissue.

The optimized circuit parameters are reported in TABLES 2 and 3 for the parallel and embedded models, respectively. We see a gradual decrease in extracellular resistance, Re, with increasing radiation dose in both models, as would be expected with fiber shrinkage and edema (see TABLE 1). There is a corresponding reduction in all capacitance values attributable to cell membrane breakdown in the vasculature and musculature. The values intended to correlate with intracellular resistances in the multiple pathway model (TABLE 2) are also interesting. There is an increase in the value of R3 at 90 and 150 Gy, while increases in R1 and R2 only occur at 70 Gy. Similarly, the most significant change in Ri is observed at 70 Gy in the embedded membrane model (TABLE 3), although the largest changes in Re and Cm occur at 150 Gy. The capacitances of the internal membranes are smaller than those associ-

TABLE 3. Embedded Membranes, Single Cell Pathway (Optimized Parameters)

Tissue	Re	Ri	Cm	α	β	χ	δ
70 Gy–control	1.53	4.19	$3.71e{-}6$	0.366	0.612	0.428	0.109
90 Gy–control	1.60	4.23	$3.30e{-}6$	0.352	0.677	0.424	0.117
150 Gy–control	1.63	4.27	$2.96e{-}6$	0.375	0.691	0.473	0.114
70 Gy	1.12	3.09	$1.99e{-}6$	0.529	0.697	0.863	0.088
90 Gy	1.03	3.52	$1.99e{-}6$	0.511	0.634	0.752	0.071
150 Gy	0.908	3.56	$1.01e{-}6$	0.746	0.482	1.040	0.058

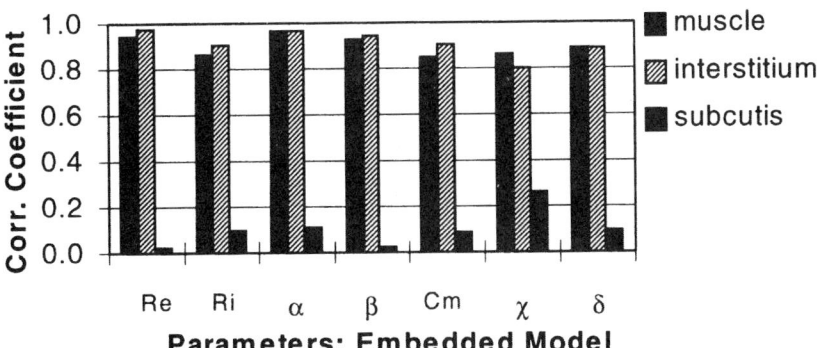

FIGURE 4. Correlation coefficients calculated between total histologic scores in each of the three tissue regions (summed across all injury types) and best-fit curve parameters from the embedded membrane circuit model (based on 18 observations).

ated with the outer cell membrane. This is expected since the surface area of internal structures such as nuclei or mitochondria will be smaller and capacitance will decrease proportionally. There does appear to be a proportional increase in the intracellular resistances for the exposed group above the controls when the embedded model was applied. Whether this is indicative of a real effect in the irradiated tissue warrants further study.

The correlation between the subcutaneous region and circuit parameters is universally low, reaching a maximum value of 0.32 (FIGURES 4 and 5). The small correlation between subcutaneous injury and parameterized EIS curves was encouraging. Since the objective was to measure radiation-induced changes in the bulk tissue, it was important to know that the EIS readings were not substantially impacted by changes in the skin, or the thin region immediately underlying it.

Except for R2's minimal correlation with histology scores in the muscle and interstitium, correlation coefficients for both of these deeper regions and all other circuit parameters are above 0.55 (FIGURES 6 and 7). The average correlation coefficient for these regions

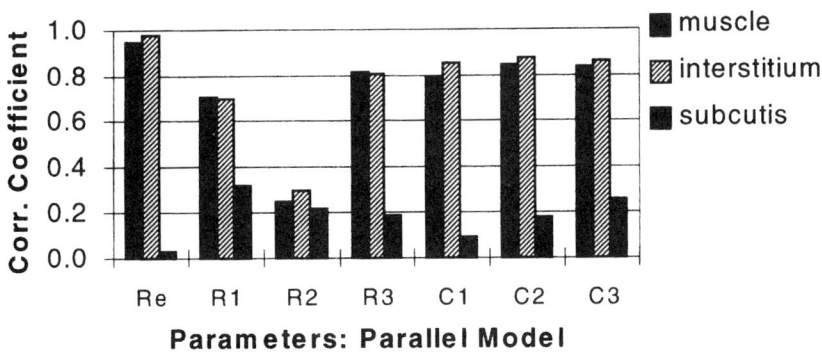

FIGURE 5. Same as FIGURE 4 for the parallel pathways circuit model.

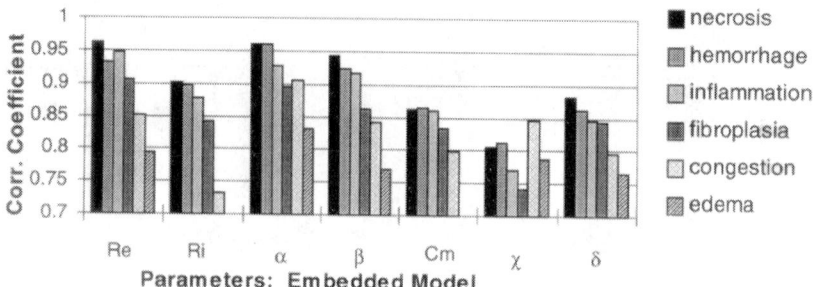

FIGURE 6. Correlation factors between histological rankings in six injury categories (summation of injury scores in muscle and interstitium) and best-fit parameter values for the embedded membrane circuit model (based on 18 observations).

is 0.78. When examining the relationship between the presence and severity of a specific injury and circuit parameter variation, the histologic scores in the muscle and interstitium were combined to give one value indicative of overall injury within the measured site.

Correlation coefficients between histological scores within specific categories (e.g., necrosis) and circuit parameter values are, in general, higher when using the embedded model. With the embedded membrane model, necrosis rankings correlate with six of the seven parameter values at a level above 0.8. There is a suggestion of preferential correlation between fibroplasia with the C3 and R1 parameters of the parallel model, which is encouraging, but not conclusive. Neither of these simple models demonstrates a clear ability to differentiate between types of physiological change. Both are, however, able to reflect the magnitude of radiation-induced tissue alterations.

CONCLUSIONS

The correlation between EIS readings and histological evaluations is encouraging. We are still some distance from being able to extract definitive parameters that theoretically, or even empirically, correlate with a specific physiological change observed in muscle's

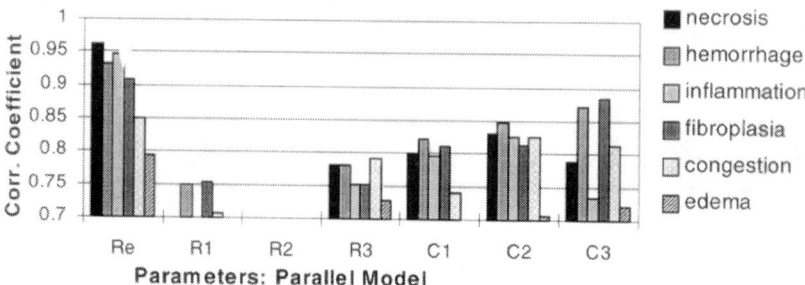

FIGURE 7. Same as FIGURE 6 for the parallel pathways circuit model.

response to radiation. Both models examined independently allow us to fit the data with a high degree of accuracy and provide some clues as to the underlying pathology. By combining the two into a single, more complicated model, it is likely that we may be able to isolate the effects that a specific physiological change (e.g., fibrosis versus necrosis) has on the spectral plots. It would also be desirable to increase the number of histologically scored animals and make measurements at more closely spaced time intervals. The data at this point are sparse; thus, while certain general trends are clear, more specific conclusions can only be drawn after more data have been collected.

In modeling, the next logical step may be to determine the actual distribution of cell sizes and shapes from frozen sections and insert this information into a model instead of relying on curve fitting or the Cole-Cole distribution function. The impact of specific cell size ranges could be examined more precisely in this manner. This may be the process through which we can integrate and evaluate the relative importance of parallel pathways and embedded structures on the impedance spectra of tissues.

REFERENCES

1. SCHWAN, H. P. 1985. Analysis of dielectric data: experience gained with biological materials. IEEE Trans. Electr. Insul. **EI-20.6:** 913–922.
2. HEROUX, P. & M. BOURDAGES. 1994. Monitoring living tissues by electrical impedance spectroscopy. Ann. Biomed. Eng. **22:** 328–337.
3. GABRIEL, S., R. W. LAU & C. GABRIEL. 1996. The dielectric properties of biological tissues: III. Parametric models for the dielectric spectrum of tissues. Phys. Med. Biol. **41:** 2271–2293.
4. FOSTER, K. R. & H. P. SCHWAN. 1986. Dielectric properties of tissues. *In* CRC Handbook of Biological Effects of Electromagnetic Fields, p. 27–96. CRC Press. Boca Raton, Florida.
5. DISSADO, L. A., J. ALISON, R. HILL, D. MCRAE & M. ESRICK. 1995. Dynamic scaling in the dielectric response of excised EMT-6 tumours undergoing hyperthermia. Phys. Med. Biol. **40:** 1067–1084.
6. BLAD, B. 1996. Clinical applications of characteristic frequency measurements: preliminary *in vivo* study. Med. Biol. Eng. Comput. **34:** 362–365.

A Review of Parameters for the Bioelectrical Characterization of Breast Tissue

JACQUES JOSSINET AND MICHEL SCHMITT

Institut National de la Santé et de la Recherche Médicale,
INSERM U281, 69424 Lyon Cedex 03, France

ABSTRACT: In the data set collected by the authors in freshly excised breast tissue, the admittance loci generally differed from circular arcs, rendering the calculation of the usual set of parameters impossible. Alternative parameters were used for the analysis of these data. The present study consists of the definition and evaluation of a set of such parameters aimed at the characterization and differentiation of breast tissues. These parameters were defined so that their calculation does not require the fit of circular arcs to the experimental points and is independent of any equivalent circuit model. The results of the statistical analysis showed significant differences between most of the tissue groups, especially between cancerous tissue and all the other groups, which confirmed that impedance spectroscopy can be considered as potentially suitable for breast cancer detection.

INTRODUCTION

The conduction of electric current through a tissue can be affected by changes in the tissue's structure and composition due to, for example, cell proliferation and tumor growth. The electric and dielectric properties of normal and pathological breast tissue have been investigated over a wide frequency range under various experimental conditions. Significant differences between normal and tumorous tissue in the raw measured data, in the elements of the Cole model of multifrequency loci, and in the calculated elements of equivalent circuit models have been reported in the literature. Fricke first reported the increase in the capacitive properties in tissue for tumors of the breast.[1] In the range of 20 kHz–100 MHz, Surowiec found "significant differences in dielectric properties between samples taken from different locations" while comparing the relative permittivities of infiltrating breast carcinoma and the surrounding tissues.[2] Morimoto, based on *in vivo* impedance measurements at frequencies up to 200 kHz, found that the elements of the Fricke equivalent circuit model for breast tumors differed significantly from those for benign tumors.[3] Heinitz found "highly significant differences between carcinoma and mastopathy forms" in the values in the resistances of the Fricke equivalent circuit model of impedance data collected in breast tissue samples.[4] From dielectric measurements at 3.2 GHz using the resonant cavity technique, Campbell commented on the "similarity of the dielectric properties of benign and malignant breast tumors",[5] which confirmed the lack of specificity of the dielectric mechanisms occurring at such frequencies. In the range of 100 Hz–10 MHz, Stelter observed in Bode plots that "the difference between characteristic frequencies of normal and cancerous tissues is significant".[6] In the same frequency range and using four aligned acupuncture needles, Chauveau[7] observed in *ex vivo* samples that "the behavior of mammary gland is very specific, with a quite constant real part versus frequency and an increasing imaginary part at high frequency". This finding is in agreement with the form of the multifrequency loci recorded by the authors in glandular tissue and fibroadenoma where, "in certain cases, the loci formed quasi-linear arcs, with a very small curvature".[8]

The above findings justified the development of multifrequency systems for breast examination.[9] However, no reliable method for the unequivocal identification of the bioelectrical spectrum for an unknown tissue has yet been proposed. The present study was based on a set of impedivity data collected by the authors.[8] Most of the recorded loci strongly differed from the "classical" semicircular arcs, which rendered impossible the calculation of the usual set of bioelectrical parameters, namely, the low-frequency and high-frequency limit resistances (or conductances), the fractional power α, and the apex frequency f_A (or characteristic frequency, f_C). This may be attributed to several factors including the presence of different tissues within the examined sample, the complex tissue structure involved (e.g., the lobular structure of breast glandular and connective tissues, tumorous tissue interpenetrating normal tissue), and the presence of several dielectric relaxation mechanisms within the measurement frequency range.

Special techniques, such as deconvolution,[10] have been used to separate the relaxation phenomena underlying such complex loci. The CNLS (Complex Nonlinear Least Squares) data-fitting method developed by Macdonald[11] enables the calculation of the elements of equivalent circuit models comprising more components than the simple two-resistor, one-capacitor model. All these calculations require a sufficient number of measurement points and a sufficiently wide frequency range to cover the different relaxation domains. Hence, this latter approach presents several drawbacks including the difficulty in ensuring low measurement errors over the wide frequency range involved and the existence of several equivalent circuits, all of which have identical impedances, thus making their choice and physiological interpretation ambiguous. This point has been emphasized by Aligne[12] while discussing the use of equivalent circuit models: "The main difficulty is in finding a realistic electrical model to biological processes." For the above reasons, "alternative parameters" were considered for the analysis of the present set of data and are proposed for the characterization and differentiation of breast tissues or other body tissues. Such parameters were defined so that their calculation does not require the fit of circular arcs to the experimental points and is independent of any equivalent circuit model. The present study consists of the definition, the analysis, and the evaluation of a set of such parameters.

THE CONDUCTION OF ELECTRICITY IN TISSUE

Although the calculation of the proposed parameters does not require circular loci, their interpretation is qualitatively based on the properties of circular arcs. Circular loci result from the electric and dielectric properties of biological media. The admittance of a tissue sample is the sum of its conductance and its susceptance. The "specific admittance" or "admittivity" is independent of the sample size and can be expressed as in equation 1:[13,14]

$$\sigma^* = \sigma + j\omega\varepsilon_0\varepsilon' \tag{1}$$

where
    σ^* tissue admittivity
    σ tissue conductivity
    ε' tissue permittivity

ε_0 dielectric constant of free space
ω angular frequency (rd/s).

The properties of the tissue can also be written in terms of its complex permittivity ε^*:

$$\varepsilon^* = \varepsilon' - j\sigma/\omega\varepsilon_0 \quad \text{with} \quad \sigma^* = j\omega\varepsilon_0\varepsilon^*. \tag{2}$$

According to Cole's empirical relationship for dielectrics and liquids,[15] the permittivity of biological media can be represented by equation 3:

$$\varepsilon' = \varepsilon_\infty + \frac{\varepsilon_S - \varepsilon_\infty}{1 + (j\omega\tau)^\alpha} \tag{3}$$

where ε_S and ε_∞ are the low-frequency and high-frequency limit permittivities, respectively, and τ is the average time constant of the medium. Finally, the expressions of the admittivity and dielectric permittivity of a medium are[13,14]

$$\varepsilon^* = \varepsilon_\infty + \frac{\varepsilon_S - \varepsilon_\infty}{1 + (j\omega\tau)^\alpha} - j\frac{\sigma_0}{\omega\varepsilon_0} \tag{4a}$$

$$\sigma^* = \sigma_\infty + \frac{\sigma_0 - \sigma_\infty}{1 + (j\omega\tau)^\alpha} + j\omega\varepsilon_0\varepsilon_\infty \tag{4b}$$

with

$$\varepsilon_0(\varepsilon_S - \varepsilon_\infty) = (\sigma_\infty - \sigma_0)\tau. \tag{4c}$$

At low frequency, the dielectric term in equation 4b can be neglected. In a limited frequency range (corresponding to a given relaxation), a tissue's frequency response is then described by equation 5, the locus of which on the complex plane is a depressed arc of a circle:

$$\sigma^* \approx \sigma_\infty + \frac{\sigma_0 - \sigma_\infty}{1 + (j\omega\tau)^\alpha}. \tag{5}$$

By inversion ($\rho = 1/\sigma$), admittivity loci form impedivity loci. The latter are also circular arcs, the centers of which are shifted from the horizontal axis, and obey equation 6a:

$$\rho = \rho_\infty + \frac{\rho_0 - \rho_\infty}{1 + \left(j\frac{f}{f_A}\right)^\alpha} \tag{6a}$$

where

$$\rho_0 = 1/\sigma_0, \quad \rho_\infty = 1/\sigma_\infty, \quad f_A = f_C\left(\frac{\sigma_0}{\sigma_\infty}\right)^{\frac{1}{\alpha}}, \quad \text{and} \quad f_C = 1/2\pi\tau. \tag{6b}$$

Finally, the fit of circular arcs to the measurement points reduces the multifrequency data to a set of four so-called bioelectrical parameters. Three of them result from the geometry of the circular arc, namely, the low-frequency intercept (σ_0 or ρ_0), the high-frequency intercept (σ_∞ or ρ_∞), and α, characterizing the shift of the center from the horizontal axis. The fourth parameter, the apex frequency, equal to the characteristic frequency of the tissue, f_C, in admittivity (or admittance) arcs, is related to the distribution of the frequency points on the arc (FIGURE 1).

The parameters of circular arcs can be used for the calculation of the components of equivalent circuit models comprising resistances and capacitive elements. A range of equivalent circuits have been proposed since the beginning of multifrequency impedance measurements and their interpretation has progressively been refined.[16] The model of Fricke, a resistance (representing the resistance of the interstitial space) in parallel with the series combination of a resistance (representing the intracellular medium) and a capacitive element, has been widely used to describe the response of body tissues. Today, a "constant phase element" also termed "pseudocapacitance" is often used as the capacitive element.[17]

ALTERNATIVE PARAMETERS

The Impedivity of Excised Breast Tissue

Experimental Data

The collection of the data set used in the present study has been described in previous publications.[18,19] Impedance measurements were carried out in freshly excised tissue samples at 12 frequencies halving successively from 1 MHz to 0.488 kHz. The same probe, which consisted of four aligned needle electrodes, was used in all the experiments.[18] As the electrode geometry factor was known, impedivity data could be calculated from

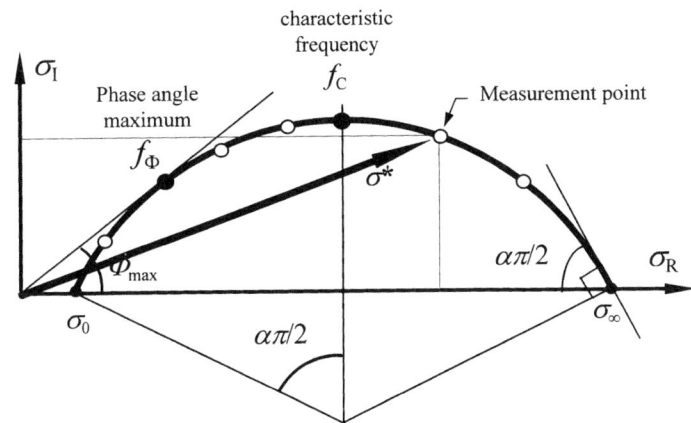

FIGURE 1. Geometrical properties of conductivity arcs. The frequency f_Φ at which the phase angle passes through a maximum (Φ_{max}) is lower than the characteristic frequency f_C (at which the imaginary part passes through a maximum). The magnitudes of the slopes of the tangents at σ_0 and σ_∞ are equal and can be used to determine the fractional power α.

impedance measurements. The minimum size of the samples was 1 cm^3, corresponding to the volume sensed by the electrodes.

The data set consisted of 120 spectra spread between three groups of normal tissues and three groups of pathological tissues. Normal tissue groups were glandular tissue MG (mammary gland), connective tissue CT, and adipose tissue AT. The pathological tissues were classified into groups MA (mastopathy: general term covering various benign breast diseases), FA (fibroadenoma: benign tumors of the breast), and CA (carcinoma: malignant tumors).

The consistency and the variability of the collected data were analyzed[19] prior to statistical analysis. The statistical analysis consisted of multiple intergroup comparisons carried out at every measurement frequency using the magnitude, phase angle, real part, and imaginary part of the measured impedivity and calculated admittivity. The most salient result of this study was the detection of a significant difference between the phase angle of group CA and those of all the other groups at the frequencies of 125 kHz, 250 kHz, 500 kHz, and 1 MHz.

Multifrequency Loci of Breast Tissue

In the present study, the measured impedivity spectra were transformed into admittivity spectra, as this representation is directly related to the conductivity and permittivity of a tissue. The loci to which it was impossible to fit circular arcs were termed "distorted loci". The loci in which no maximum in the imaginary component was observed were termed "incomplete loci". The loci covering two relaxation domains were termed "composite loci". Such loci were characterized by a frequency termed "notch frequency" at which the imaginary component passed through a minimum.

Some examples of admittance loci of excised breast tissues are given in FIGURE 2. Fatty tissues (connective tissue and adipose tissue, groups CT and AT) have low conductivity values that enable, in these particular cases, these groups to be distinguished from the others. This observation leads to the introduction of the concept of an "absolute parameter",

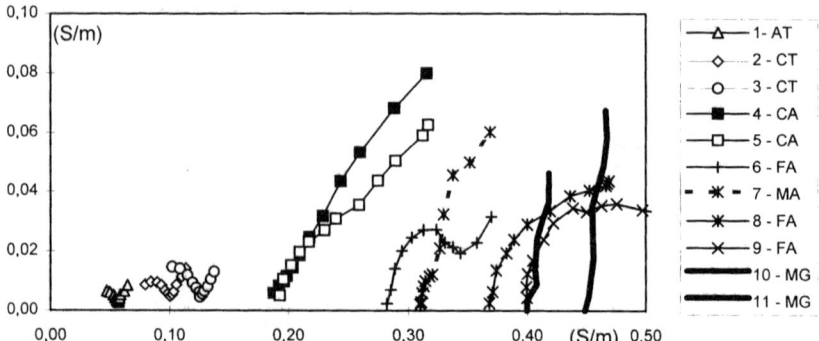

FIGURE 2. Typical admittivity arcs of the six groups of excised breast tissues. Loci 1, 2, 3, and 6 are "composite" loci. Loci 4, 5, 7, 8, 10, and 11 are "distorted" and "incomplete" loci. Locus 9 is distorted, not incomplete, and not composite. Loci 2, 6, and 9 exhibit a characteristic frequency.

that is, a parameter that represents a physical quantity. "Relative parameters" can also be used. Such parameters are dimensionless and independent of any proportionality coefficient such as electrode factor or device calibration factor. Although only admittance loci were used in the present study, the "alternative parameters" described in the following sections can be calculated using either admittivity (or admittance) or impedivity (or impedance) arcs. This does not affect the definition and interpretation of these parameters.

A Set of Proposed Alternative Parameters

A range of parameters can be defined based on the features of circular or distorted loci in relation to the tissues to be discriminated. However, the number of independent parameters depends on the complexity of the locus. For instance, circular arcs are characterized by four parameters. In loci with two relaxation domains, up to seven parameters are potentially calculable. In the present study, eight parameters were considered. This set is not exhaustive and has been selected as it appeared potentially suitable for breast tissue discrimination.

Parameter σ_0: Low-Frequency Limit Admittivity

This parameter, denoted σ_0, is an "absolute" parameter. Its use can be justified for several reasons, such as the successful discrimination of fatty tissues as in the reduced data set of FIGURE 1. In the present set of data, it was possible to extrapolate the low-frequency limit admittivity from all forms of loci using a second-order polynomial fitted to the five low-frequency points of each spectrum. In group MG, however, the frequency points at 15.625 kHz and above were used due to the presence of an artifact previously discussed[8] in the phase angle measured at low frequency in this group of tissue. It is presumed that this did not change appreciably the calculated values of σ_0 due to the generally small curvature of the admittivity arcs in this group.

Parameter α: Fractional Power

This relative parameter is calculable from both admittance and admittivity arcs. Classically, the interpretation of the fractional power is related to the dispersion of time constants within a tissue[14] and to the presumed presence of several different relaxation mechanisms.[20] It was calculated (at the same time as the above parameter, σ_0) as the slope of the extrapolation polynomial at the intersection point with the horizontal axis. This parameter is denoted α_{low} as it corresponds to the low-frequency end of the spectrum.

Parameter Q_{LH}: Ratio σ_0/σ_∞

As the low-frequency current flows only through the interstitial space, whereas the volume passed through by high-frequency current is predominantly intracellular medium, the ratio σ_0/σ_∞ (or ρ_∞/ρ_0) has been frequently used for tissue characterization. However, as the limit values are generally not available (as was the case in the present study for σ_∞), they are generally replaced with values measured at finite frequencies, generally around 10 kHz and 1 MHz. In the present study, the ratio $Q_{LH} = |\sigma_{LF}|/|\sigma_{HF}|$ was calculated using frequencies of 15.625 kHz and 1 MHz (the highest measurement frequency used).

Parameter D_A: Distance to the Low-Frequency Intercept

The positions on an admittance circular arc of the frequency points acquired at fixed frequencies depend on the value of the characteristic frequency. The length L_A of the circular arc limited by the low-frequency intercept and the point measured at a given frequency increases as this frequency tends towards the characteristic frequency f_C of the arc. Conversely, for a fixed measurement frequency, the higher the f_C, the shorter the arc length. Although it also depends on the other characteristics of the arc, this parameter is thus an index related to the characteristic frequency of the admittivity locus. For regular arcs, the length L_A and the chord D_A between the frequency point and the point σ_0 vary in similar proportions. In the present study, D_A was preferred to L_A as this parameter is not affected by the increase of arc length in composite loci. This parameter can be weighted by the dimension of the arc (ideally by the increment $\sigma_0 - \sigma_\infty$, or simply by σ_0 if σ_∞ is not available).

Parameter Φ_{500}: Magnitude of the Phase Angle at 500 kHz

The phase angle is a relative parameter that has the additional advantage of being calculable from either impedance or admittance data. This parameter characterizes the high-frequency part of a spectrum. Furthermore, significant differences in phase angle were found between group CA and all the other groups at the measurement frequencies of 125 kHz, 250 kHz, 500 kHz, and 1 MHz.[8] Hence, this parameter appeared suitable for the discrimination of cancerous tissue. As the use of all four frequency points gave redundant information for tissue discrimination, only one frequency among these four was selected for the definition of this parameter. The mean value of phase angle in group CA increased with frequency, but the standard deviation also increased, limiting the benefit of a large difference from the other tissue groups. The ratio of standard deviation to the mean value of phase angle in group CA had a minimum at 500 kHz (TABLE 1), which determined the choice of this frequency.

TABLE 1. Mean, Standard Deviation (STD), and Ratio STD/Mean of the Phase Angle, Φ_{CA}, for Group CA at the Four Highest Measurement Frequencies

Φ_{CA}	125 kHz	250 kHz	500 kHz	1 MHz
mean	7.975	10.055	12.170	14.747
STD	2.701	2.803	3.128	3.932
STD/mean	0.339	0.279	0.257	0.267

Parameter S_{HF}: High-Frequency Slope in Phase Angle

This parameter, denoted S_{HF}, was used to give an estimate of the high-frequency response of tissues with incomplete loci where f_C was unknown and the calculation of σ_∞ impossible. S_{HF} was defined as the slope of the phase angle against frequency in the high-frequency region of a spectrum. The empirical justification of this parameter is as follows: the more capacitive the response of the tissue, the larger the phase angle (cf. parameter Φ_{500}) and the more marked the increase in phase angle with frequency.

This parameter leads to two different situations if either a circular impedivity or admittivity arc is used. In an impedivity locus, the frequency f_Φ at which the phase angle passes through a maximum (contact point of the tangent to the circle passing by the origin of coordinates) is larger than the apex frequency. In this case, below the apex frequency, the phase angle increases monotonically, and one can write, if f_M denotes a measurement frequency, $f_M < f_A < f_\Phi$. In an admittivity locus, the characteristic frequency f_C is larger than f_A (equation 6b). Simple geometric considerations show that $f_A < f_\Phi < f_C$. In this case, the presence of a maximum in phase angle within the measurement frequency range is possible, even if the measurement points are below the characteristic frequency f_C with $f_\Phi < f_M < f_C$ (incomplete admittivity loci). In this case, the impedivity arc is not an incomplete locus and exhibits an apex frequency. This feature of S_{HF} is not an obstacle to the use of this parameter for discrimination purposes. In the present study, S_{HF} was calculated as the slope of the linear regression of the three uppermost frequency points (250 kHz, 500 kHz, and 1 MHz).

Parameter K_Φ: Integrated Phase Angle Ratio

The capacitive response of the tissue can also be estimated by comparing the "low-frequency" and "high-frequency" regions of a given spectrum. It can be expected that these regions would be "similar" in a resistive medium and would differ in the presence of a capacitive response. Blad[21] has proposed a relative parameter "based on the plot of the imaginary part of impedance against log-frequency". This parameter is the ratio between the areas below the curve in two adjacent frequency domains, 10 kHz–100 kHz and 100 kHz–1 MHz. The calculation proposed requires that "the impedance (Z) of a tissue follows the Cole model".

In the present study, a modified expression for this parameter was used. According to the features of the alternative parameters, the calculation of K_Φ does not require any particular hypothesis upon the frequency response of the tissue and is independent of any equivalent circuit model. Another difference is that the phase angle was used instead of the reactance. The two adjacent frequency domains were 15.625 kHz–125 kHz (frequency points 6 to 9) and 125 kHz–1 MHz (frequency points 9 to 12), with equally spaced log-frequency points. The surface area below the curve was estimated according to equation 7 using the trapezoidal rule, based on the discrete measurement frequencies. Φ_k denotes the phase angle at measurement frequency k:

$$K_\Phi = \frac{\dfrac{\Phi_6 + \Phi_9}{2} + \Phi_7 + \Phi_8}{\dfrac{\Phi_9 + \Phi_{12}}{2} + \Phi_{10} + \Phi_{11}}. \quad (7)$$

RESULTS AND DISCUSSION

The mean values and standard deviations of the eight parameters in the six groups of tissue considered in the present study are given in TABLE 2.

The dispersion of these parameters around their central values is, in general, relatively large, making the values of several groups overlap. This prevents the unequivocal recognition of a spectrum using a single parameter even if statistically significant differences between groups can be found. It can thus be anticipated that the differentiation of tissue would require the use of several parameters. However, if no significant difference is found between two groups with a given parameter, the latter can obviously not be used to determine to which group a particular spectrum belongs. The presence of significant differences between groups is thus necessary, but not sufficient, for the classification of spectra.

Significant differences between groups were looked for using two-by-two comparisons employing Student's t test. Although ANOVA or multiple comparison procedures such as Kruskal-Wallis are more sensitive than two-by-two comparisons when more than two groups are to be compared, the t test was used in the present study as the purpose was the detection of manifest differences usable for tissue discrimination.

The results of the comparisons between groups for each parameter are given in TABLE 3. The presence of a significant difference (at risk 1%) is denoted "#" and the absence of it is denoted "=". The principal results of this analysis are the following: With σ_0, the two groups of fatty tissues (CT, AT) differ significantly from all other groups. With α_{low} and Q_{LH}, the glandular tissue (MG) differs from all the other groups. With Q_{LH}, Φ_{500}, and S_{HF}, cancerous tissue (group CA) differs from all other groups. With D_A, adipose tissue (group AT) differs from all the other groups. With parameter D_A/σ_0, group CA differs from all nonfatty tissue (FA, MA, MG); while with D_A, a significant difference is only observed with fatty tissues (CT, AT). With S_{HF}, group CA differs from all groups, except for adipose tissue AT. Parameter K_Φ only yields a difference between groups MG and FA. None of the parameters considered in the present study yielded a significant difference between groups FA and MA. The significant differences between groups are summarized in TABLE 4.

TABLE 2. Mean and Standard Deviation Values of the Parameters for the Six Groups of Breast Tissues

	CA	FA	MA	MG	CT	AT
σ_0 (S/m)	0.28 ± 0.11	0.44 ± 0.13	0.39 ± 0.16	0.50 ± 0.22	0.09 ± 0.04	0.04 ± 0.01
α_{low} (–)	0.41 ± 0.14	0.50 ± 0.16	0.46 ± 0.22	0.70 ± 0.16	0.49 ± 0.09	0.54 ± 0.12
Q_{LH} (–)	0.71 ± 0.14	0.87 ± 0.05	0.87 ± 0.10	0.95 ± 0.04	0.90 ± 0.04	0.914 ± 0.05
D_A (S/m)	0.21 ± 0.17	0.12 ± 0.04	0.14 ± 0.08	0.12 ± 0.17	0.05 ± 0.03	0.02 ± 0.01
D_A/σ_0 (–)	0.80 ± 0.64	0.28 ± 0.07	0.37 ± 0.25	0.15 ± 0.07	1.35 ± 2.90	0.45 ± 0.23
Q_Φ	2.09 ± 0.40	1.50 ± 0.61	2.03 ± 0.70	3.03 ± 1.83	1.86 ± 0.57	1.84 ± 0.71
S_{HF} (deg/oct)	12.17 ± 3.13	5.46 ± 3.03	7.05 ± 2.99	5.99 ± 2.13	4.02 ± 1.54	4.22 ± 2.18
K_Φ	2.09 ± 0.40	1.50 ± 0.61	2.03 ± 0.70	3.03 ± 1.83	1.86 ± 0.57	1.84 ± 0.71

TABLE 3. Significant Differences between Groups for the Eight Considered Parameters[a]

(a)

σ_0	CA	FA	MA	MG	CT	AT
CA	–	#	=	#	#	#
FA	#	–	=	=	#	#
MA	=	=	–	=	#	#
MG	#	=	=	–	#	#
CT	#	#	#	#	–	#
AT	#	#	#	#	#	–

(b)

α_{low}	CA	FA	MA	MG	CT	AT
CA	–	=	=	#	=	#
FA	=	–	=	#	=	=
MA	=	=	–	#	=	=
MG	#	#	#	–	#	#
CT	=	=	=	#	–	=
AT	#	=	=	#	=	–

(c)

Q_{LH}	CA	FA	MA	MG	CT	AT
CA	–	#	#	#	#	#
FA	#	–	=	#	=	=
MA	#	=	–	#	=	=
MG	#	#	#	–	#	#
CT	#	=	=	#	–	=
AT	#	=	=	#	=	–

(d)

D_A	CA	FA	MA	MG	CT	AT
CA	–	=	=	=	#	#
FA	=	–	=	=	#	#
MA	=	=	–	=	#	#
MG	=	=	=	–	=	#
CT	#	#	#	=	–	#
AT	#	#	#	#	#	–

(e)

D_A/σ_0	CA	FA	MA	MG	CT	AT
CA	–	#	#	#	=	=
FA	#	–	=	#	=	#
MA	#	=	–	#	=	=
MG	#	#	#	–	=	#
CT	=	=	=	=	–	=
AT	=	#	=	#	=	–

(f)

Φ_{500}	CA	FA	MA	MG	CT	AT
CA	–	#	#	#	#	#
FA	#	–	=	=	=	=
MA	#	=	–	=	#	#
MG	#	=	=	–	#	#
CT	#	=	#	#	–	=
AT	#	=	#	#	=	–

(g)

S_{HF}	CA	FA	MA	MG	CT	AT
CA	–	#	#	#	#	=
FA	#	–	=	=	=	=
MA	#	=	–	=	=	=
MG	#	=	=	–	=	=
CT	#	=	=	=	–	=
AT	=	=	=	=	=	–

(h)

K_Φ	CA	FA	MA	MG	CT	AT
CA	–	#	=	=	=	=
FA	#	–	=	#	=	=
MA	=	=	–	=	=	=
MG	=	#	=	–	=	#
CT	=	=	=	=	–	=
AT	=	=	=	#	=	–

[a]Student's t test, risk 1%. See text for details, including the meaning of the symbols.

TABLE 4. Parameters Yielding Significant Differences between Tissue Groups[a]

	FA	MA	MG	CT	AT
CA	$\sigma_0\ Q_{LH}\ D_A/\sigma_0\ \Phi_{500}\ S_{HF}\ K_\Phi$	$Q_{LH}\ D_A/\sigma_0\ \Phi_{500}\ S_{HF}$	$\sigma_0\ \alpha_{low}\ Q_{LH}\ D_A/\sigma_0\ \Phi_{500}\ S_{HF}$	$\sigma_0\ Q_{LH}\ D_A\ \Phi_{500}\ S_{HF}$	$\sigma_0\ \alpha_{low}\ Q_{LH}\ D_A\ \Phi_{500}$
FA	*	---	$\alpha_{low}\ Q_{LH}\ D_A/\sigma_0\ K_\Phi$	$\sigma_0\ D_A$	$\sigma_0\ D_A\ D_A/\sigma_0$
MA		*	$\alpha_{low}\ Q_{LH}\ D_A/\sigma_0$	$\sigma_0\ D_A\ \Phi_{500}$	$\sigma_0\ D_A\ \Phi_{500}$
MG			*	$\sigma_0\ \alpha_{low}\ Q_{LH}\ \Phi_{500}$	$\sigma_0\ \alpha_{low}\ Q_{LH}\ D_A/\sigma_0\ \Phi_{500}\ K_\Phi$
CT				*	$\sigma_0\ D_A$

[a] The table is symmetrical with respect to the diagonal. For clarity, data are given only for the upper half of the table.

These results show that the considered groups of breast tissue differ significantly from each other with two parameters or more, except for the absence of any significant difference between groups FA and MA (with the present set of data and the used statistical test). A Kruskal-Wallis multiple comparison procedure carried out using the same set of data confirmed all the significant differences found with the t test and also detected additional significant differences, especially between groups FA and MA with σ_0. However, although this difference was significant for the used test, it can be expected that it would not enable the classification of individual spectra (cf. TABLE 2).

As several parameters yield significant differences between groups, there is presumably a certain redundancy between these parameters. This redundancy can originate either from the definition of the parameters (for instance, parameters controlled by the same features of the arcs) or by the redundancy in the control of these parameters by the biophysical properties of the tissue. The optimization of procedures for the differentiation of tissue would therefore involve the reduction of redundancy and the selection of the most efficient parameters according to each tissue group to be recognized.

CONCLUSIONS

The proposed alternative parameters enabled the detection of significant differences between certain groups of breast tissue, principally between cancerous tissue and the other groups. It can thus be expected that these parameters are potentially usable for tissue differentiation. However, none of them was found sufficient alone for the discrimination of any one individual group of tissue. It is therefore expected that several parameters will be needed for the classification of spectra. The further developments planned include the reduction of redundancy, the assessment of the most efficient set of parameters for the recognition of each tissue group, and the development of data processing techniques aimed at the discrimination between normal and pathological breast tissue. The significant differences found between cancerous tissue and all the other groups with most of the studied parameters confirmed that impedance spectroscopy can be considered as potentially suitable for breast cancer detection.

REFERENCES

1. FRICKE, H. & S. MORSE. 1926. The electric capacity of tumors of the breast. J. Cancer Res. **10:** 340–376.
2. SUROWIEC, A. J., S. S. STUCHLY, J. R. BARR & A. SWARUP. 1988. Dielectric properties of breast carcinoma and the surrounding tissues. IEEE Trans. **BME-35:** 257–263.
3. MORIMOTO, T., Y. KINOUCHI, T. IRITANI, S. KIMURA, Y. KONISHI, N. MITSUYAMA, K. KOMAKI & Y. MONDEN. 1990. Measurement of the electrical bio-impedance of breast tumors. Eur. Surg. Res. **22:** 86–92.
4. HEINITZ, J. & O. MINET. 1995. Dielectric properties of female breast tumors. *In* Proc. Ninth Int. Conf. on Electrical Bio-Impedance, Heidelberg, p. 356–359.
5. CAMPBELL, A. M. & D. V. LAND. 1992. Dielectric properties of female breast tissue measured *in vitro* at 3.2 GHz. Phys. Med. Biol. **37:** 193–210.
6. STELTER, J., J. WTOREK, A. NOWAKOWSKI, A. KOPACZ & T. JASTRZEMBSKI. 1998. Complex permittivity of breast tumor tissue. *In* Proc. Tenth Int. Conf. on Electrical Bio-Impedance, Barcelona, p. 59–62.
7. CHAUVEAU, N., L. HAMZAOUI, P. ROCHAIX, B. RIGAUD, J. J. VOIGT & J. P. MORUCCI. 1999. Ex vivo discrimination between normal and pathological tissues in human breast surgical biopsies using bioimpedance spectroscopy. This volume.
8. JOSSINET, J. 1998. The impedivity of freshly excised human breast tissue. Physiol. Meas. **19:** 61–75.
9. JOSSINET, J., C. TRILLAUD, F. RISACHER & E. T. MCADAMS. 1993. A high frequency electrical impedance tomograph using distributed parallel input channels. Med. Prog. Technol. **19:** 167–172.
10. MCRAE, D. A. & M. A. ESRICK. 1996. Deconvolved electrical impedance spectra track distinct cell morphology changes. IEEE Trans. **BME-43:** 607–618.
11. MACDONALD, J. R. 1992. Impedance spectroscopy. Ann. Biomed. Eng. **20:** 289–305.
12. ALIGNE, C., N. CHAUVEAU, B. RIGAUD & J. P. MORUCCI. 1995. Normal and tumoral tissue modelling from *in vivo* spectrometric measurements of electrical bioimpedance. ITBM Thematic Issue **16:** 689–693.
13. SCHWAN, H. P. & S. TAKASHIMA. 1993. Electrical conduction and dielectric behavior in biological systems. Encycl. Appl. Phys. **5:** 177–200.
14. FOSTER, K. R. & H. P. SCHWAN. 1989. Dielectric properties of tissues and biological materials: a critical review. Crit. Rev. Biomed. Eng. **17:** 25–104.
15. COLE, K. S & R. H. COLE. 1941. Dispersion and absorption in dielectrics. I. Alternating current characteristics. J. Chem. Phys. **9:** 341–351.
16. MCADAMS, E. T. & J. JOSSINET. 1995. Epidermal/tissue impedance: an historical overview. Physiol. Meas. **16:** A1–A14.
17. MCADAMS, E. T. & J. JOSSINET. 1996. Problems in equivalent circuit modelling of the electrical properties of biological tissues. Bioelectrochem. Bioenerg. **40:** 147–152.
18. JOSSINET, J., A. LOBEL, C. MICHOUDET & M. SCHMITT. 1985. Quantitative technique for bio-electrical spectroscopy. J. Biomed. Eng. **7:** 289–294.
19. JOSSINET, J. 1996. Variability of impedivity in normal and pathological breast tissue. Med. Biol. Eng. Comput. **34:** 346–350.
20. SCHWAN, H. P. 1985. Analysis of dielectric data: experience gained with biological material. IEEE Trans. **EI-20:** 913–922.
21. BLAD, B., P. WENDEL, M. JÖNSSON & K. LINDSTRÖM. 1998. An electrical impedance index to distinguish between normal and cancerous tissue. *In* Proc. Tenth Int. Conf. on Electrical Bio-Impedance, Barcelona, p. 51–54.

Ex Vivo Discrimination between Normal and Pathological Tissues in Human Breast Surgical Biopsies Using Bioimpedance Spectroscopy

N. CHAUVEAU,[a] L. HAMZAOUI,[b] P. ROCHAIX,[c] B. RIGAUD,[a] J. J. VOIGT,[c] AND J. P. MORUCCI[a]

[a]*INSERM U455, CHU Purpan, 31059 Toulouse, France*

[b]*Laboratoire Conception et Systèmes, Université Mohammed V, Rabat, Morocco*

[c]*Laboratoire d'Anatomie et Cytologie Pathologique, Institut Claudius Regaud, Toulouse, France*

ABSTRACT: *Ex vivo* bioimpedance data measured on normal and cancerous female breast tissues are reported. They clearly show that the electrical properties of normal tissues, surrounding tissues, and carcinoma are different. These differences lie in the conductivity, in the characteristic frequency (frequency of the maximum of the imaginary part of the bioimpedance), and also in the shape of the Bode plots. Modeling using an R-S-Z_{cpe} model is reported as well as indexes extracted from the real and imaginary parts of the bioimpedance. Even if a classification of the different types of tissues remains a difficult task and leads to much less precise diagnosis than microscopic examination, the electrical behavior of mammary tissue could be used to develop a noninvasive technique for early breast cancer detection.

INTRODUCTION

Variation of the electrical properties between normal and pathological breast tissues has already been reported. Surowiec et al.[1] measured dielectric changes at high frequencies up to 100 MHz, using the input reflection coefficient of the sample. They found higher conductivity in tumor tissue (2 to 3 mS/cm) than in normal breast tissue (lower than 1 mS/cm). The variation of conductivity versus frequency was also higher for the tumor. Using a two-electrode system placed in a needle electrode and applying an impulse, Heinitz and Minet[2] provided a classification of measurements carried out in normal and pathological breast tissues. This system exhibited a high capacitance coupling because of the small surface contact. From the electrical response, the parameters of the Cole model,[3] that is, the intracellular resistance, the extracellular resistance, and the membrane capacitance of the measured tissue equivalent circuit, were extracted. It is possible to define five kinds of tissues: carcinoma, fibroadenoma, mastopathy I, mastopathy II, and normal tissue. Jossinet[4] also proposed a very similar classification of the impedance plots versus their shape for data obtained with conventional spectroscopy on *ex vivo* measurement with a four-needle probe. The only difference was that three groups for normal tissue were defined instead of one: mammary gland, connective tissue, and adipose subcutaneous fatty tissue. Blad and Baldetorp[5] proposed to use the characteristic frequency (Fc) to distinguish between normal and cancerous tissues measured in mice tissues. They found higher Fc (more than 100 kHz) in cancerous tissues compared with 20 kHz in normal tissue, which corresponds to what we have observed in previous studies.[6] In all these papers, the authors try to extract information from the real and imaginary plots of the measured impedance in order to establish a "diagnosis" index. This data reduction can be achieved by modeling, shape recognition, indexes of measurements at different frequencies, ..., with each approach being adapted to the specific measurement conditions.

In this presentation, we report some examples of *ex vivo* measurements of normal and pathological breast tissues achieved in the first 30 minutes following the excision for histological analysis after surgery.

METHODS

A four-electrode probe was used, including acupuncture needles coupled to a Solartron SI 1260 gain phase analyzer with a special active front end as described in reference 7. Needle electrodes were preferred to the measurement cell technique, owing to the problem posed by the adaptation in size and volume of the biological sample. In this study, the frequency range was 10 kHz to 10 MHz.

In order to evaluate our electrode system, three conductive solutions were prepared by dilution of a well-known solution of 112 mS/cm at 25 °C. The measurement of the solutions with an HI8733 conductivity meter (Hanna Instruments) gave 112 mS/cm, 11.5 mS/cm, 0.97 mS/cm, and 0.13 mS/cm. The four electrodes were inserted to the same depth (13 mm) in the different solutions. The dimensions of the reservoir containing the conductive solutions were larger than those of the electrodes. A calibration coefficient K was optimized for the solution of conductivity of 0.97 mS/cm. Then, we applied it to the other solutions, which made it possible to estimate the other conductivity values. If the measured resistance R is defined as

$$R = \rho \frac{L}{S} = \frac{1}{\sigma} \times \frac{L}{S},$$

then the geometric factor K taking into account the geometry of the volume sensed by the measurement can be written as

$$K = R \times \sigma = \frac{L}{S}.$$

FIGURE 1 shows results after calibration in the range of 0.13 to 112 mS/cm. The 112 mS/cm point presents a 40% error at low frequency, probably owing to the high value compared to the reference point at 0.97 mS/cm used to calculate K. For the physiological range (1 to 10 mS/cm), the error on the real part of the impedance versus conductivity was less than 1% at low frequency, also with 3% variation over the frequency range for 0.97 mS/cm and 14% for 11.5 mS/cm. Different volumes of conductive solutions were used in order to check the effect of the size of the sample to be measured. It was found that this volume has to be larger than the one delimited by the electrodes in order to obtain good reproducibility. The estimated volume used for the measurements is in fact delimited by the length of the needles (13 mm), the distance between the middle electrodes (each 2.54 mm in diameter), and a width of about 8 mm on each side perpendicular to the electrode plane.

RESULTS

Breast tissue is composed of both epithelial and connective structures (FIGURE 2). The former are arranged in lobules and ducts. The latter are a compound of adipocytes, fibro-

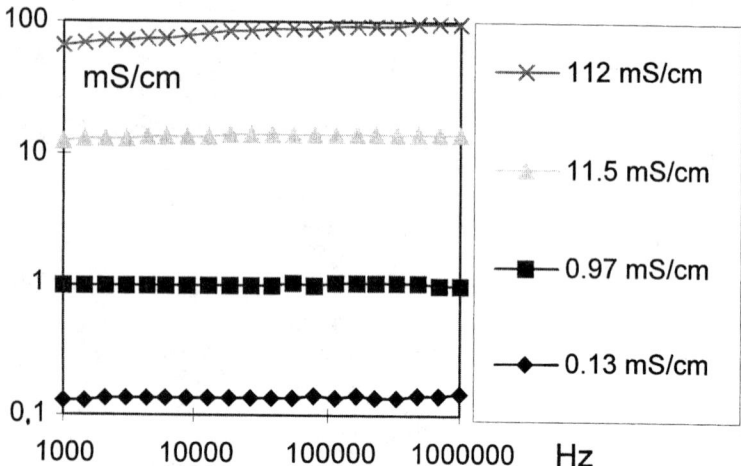

FIGURE 1. Liquid conductivity measurements with the four needle electrode system.

blasts, and nervous and vascular structures. The relative proportion and distribution of those different components vary from place to place and from patient to patient. In addition, vascularization is very present, which has the effect of reducing the measured impedance. In such conditions, one cannot expect to use very acute quantitative reference curves to distinguish between normal and pathological tissues, applicable to a wide population, as reported by Jossinet.[8]

First, we looked at adipose nontumoral mammary tissue far from the tumor (distance greater than 3 cm). The histology control confirmed that it was normal breast tissue. In order to test the reproducibility and heterogeneity of this kind of tissue, different measurements at different places were performed. Typical results are shown in FIGURE 3. The shape of the impedance plots remains quite similar when changing from place to place, even if the absolute values are different.

The behavior of the mammary gland is very specific, with a quite constant real part versus frequency and an increasing imaginary part at high frequency that we did not find in cancerous tissues.

The absolute values of reported data should not be used to compare conductivity between measurements because the geometric factor was not constant. In the mammary gland, electrode contact is not of good quality and we had to insert the needles completely (13 mm) in order to reduce the electrode contact impedance, thus allowing the measurement to be made. In tumors, it is usually impossible to insert needles more than a few millimeters because the tissue is very hard, which is also the case when the tumor is very small.

Invasive ductal carcinomas (IDC) are malignant tumors that develop from the ducts and are composed of variable amounts of carcinomatous epithelial cells and conjunctive reactive cells. The results presented here (FIGURE 4) seem to differ slightly from those reported by Jossinet.[4] For instance, we only observed a break point in the complex loci for those tis-

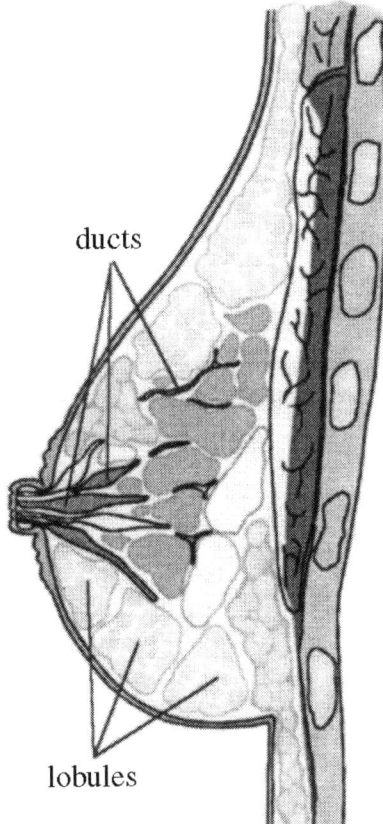

FIGURE 2. Breast anatomy.

sues at high frequency around 1 MHz, that is, in the frequency range where interpretation of the results remains very difficult.

Similar measurements were made in IDC presenting a strong fibrous stromal reaction (FIGURE 5). In this case, the presence of this reaction does not lead to a curve shape very different from that of the former IDC sample, even if the characteristic frequency seems to decrease a bit. This means that the measurements are generally sensitive to IDC, but not so much to stromal reaction. The real part decrease over the frequency range seems to be larger than in simple IDC.

Sometimes, there are some fibrocystic changes in breast tissue. The shape of the impedance plots is different from cancerous tissues (FIGURE 6) with a quite constant real part. A very low imaginary part is measured for those kinds of tissues. The shape of the Cole arc plot clearly demonstrates that in fact the electrical model should contain several poles. The conductivity of fibrosis is much higher than that of carcinoma and this could explain the high current increase that surgeons sometimes observe when using an electric scalpel on those kinds of tissues.

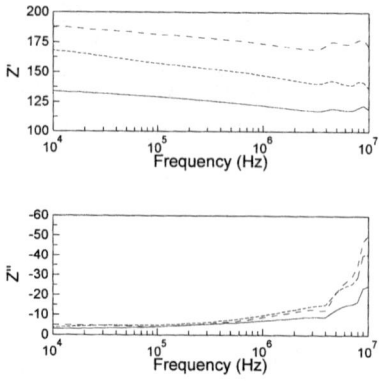
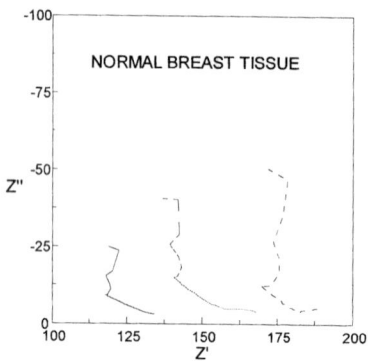

FIGURE 3. Normal breast tissue.

MODELING AND DISCUSSION

We applied the R-S-Z_{cpe} model (FIGURE 7), in which R takes into account the extracellular resistance, S the intracellular resistance, and Z_{cpe} the membrane behavior, similar to a capacitance with depressed phase angle in the complex plane.

Z_{cpe} is a constant phase element (cpe) defined by Macdonald:[9] $Z_{cpe} = 1/(C_\delta \times \omega)^\delta$ is one of the possible expressions, where C_δ is a pseudocapacitance and ω is the angular frequency. For $\delta = 1$, the component is a pure capacitance in which the phase is 90°; for $\delta < 1$, it is a phase constant element of value $\pi/2 \times \delta$. The α dispersion of the relaxation time of the tissue proposed by Cole and Cole[3] is defined as $\alpha = 1 - \delta$ and is the model describing the complex impedance arc depression.

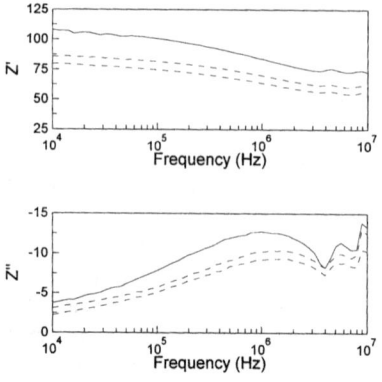
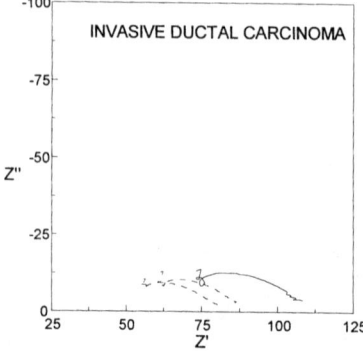

FIGURE 4. Invasive ductal carcinoma.

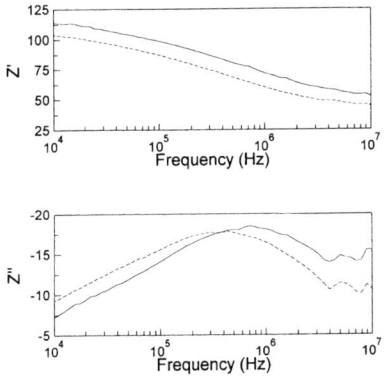
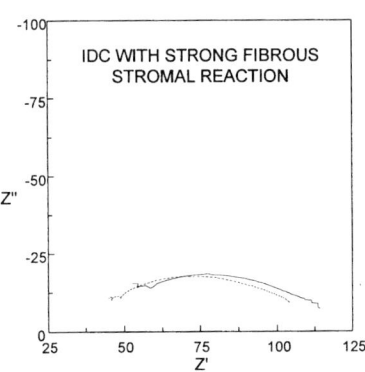

FIGURE 5. IDC with strong stromal reaction.

With the R-S-Z_{cpe} model, four parameters can be extracted from experimental data: R, S, C_δ, and δ. We used this technique in order to identify the previously reported experiments. Results for the four different kinds of tissues are reported in TABLE 1:

(I) normal breast tissue,

(II) invasive ductal carcinoma (IDC),

(III) IDC with strong stromal reaction,

(IV) fibrocystic changes.

In addition to the C_δ parameter, we have also reported the value $C_{\delta=1}$, which is the value of the capacitance without α dispersion. The relation between both values is

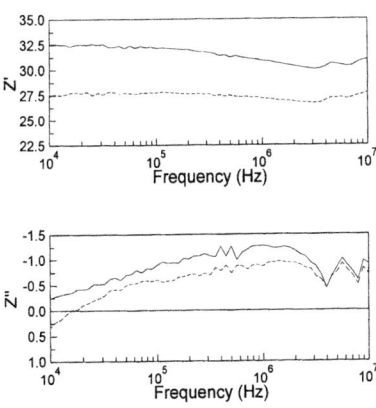
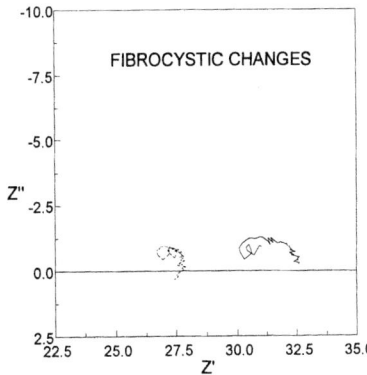

FIGURE 6. Fibrocystic changes.

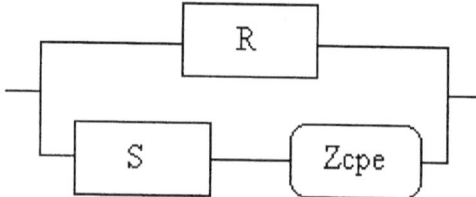

FIGURE 7. R-S-Z_{cpe} model.

$$C_{\delta=1} = C_\delta \times (R + S)^{(1-\delta)/\delta}.$$

The advantage of using $C_{\delta=1}$ is that it facilitates the comparison between measurements. This is not the case when using C and δ, which are tied parameters varying together. C_δ is a fitting parameter, whereas $C_{\delta=1}$ has the physical correspondence of a real capacitance.

In TABLE 1, the values in gray correspond to cancerous tissues. We observe that only normal tissues present $S = 0$ and have lower $C_{\delta=1}$. The $C_{\delta=1}$ values can be separated between cancerous tissues (in gray) and normal tissues, which is not possible for C_δ values.

Ratio indexes are proposed in TABLE 2 to characterize the same tissue categories:

index S/R: the advantage of using a ratio is to lower the effect of absolute measurement value variability;
index $K1 = Z'_{1\,MHz} / Z'_{10\,kHz}$ on the real part;
index $K2 = Z''_{1\,MHz} / Z''_{100\,kHz}$ on the imaginary part.

A two-category classification can be made:

- cancerous tissues: $0.2 < S/R < 2$ or $K1 < 0.85$

TABLE 1. R-S-Z_{cpe} Parameters

category	R (ohms)	S (ohms)	C_δ ($\times 10^{-13}$F)	δ	$C_{\delta=1}$ ($\times 10^{-13}$F)
I	114	0	2	0.5496	1
I	114	0	2	0.5496	1
I	158	0	110	0.8797	2
II	95.9	109	114	0.555	80
II	78	66.2	32	0.4904	56
II	71.3	70.3	75	0.5188	74
III	124	41.9	45	0.4733	133
III	115	45.2	250	0.5148	299
IV	33	160	18	0.4925	40
IV	28	128	17	0.5517	10

TABLE 2. Example of Possible Indexes

category	S/R	K1	K2
I	0	0.91	1.77
I	0	0.88	1.99
I	0	0.93	2.13
II	1.13	0.78	1.61
II	0.85	0.82	1.78
II	0.99	0.80	1.81
III	0.34	0.66	1.29
III	0.39	0.61	1.05
IV	4.83	0.95	1.43
IV	4.56	0.99	1.44

- nonpathological tissue: $S/R < 0.2$ or $S/R > 2$ or $K1 > 0.85$.

The two categories can be described by just one index, S/R or $K1$, or by both together.

A four-category classification gives

- normal tissue: $S/R = 0$ or ($K1 > 0.85$ and $K2 > 1.5$)
- IDC: $0.5 < S/R < 2$ or ($0.7 < K1 < 0.85$ and $K2 > 1.5$)
- IDC with stromal reaction: $S/R < 0.5$ or ($K1 < 0.7$ and $K2 < 1.5$)
- fibrocystic changes: $S/R > 2$ or ($K1 > 0.85$ and $K2 < 1.5$).

CONCLUSIONS

The electrical properties of the breast are quite different between normal and pathological tissues as shown by *ex vivo* measurements carried out with needle electrodes inserted in the samples. Classification based on shape, conductivity, fitting techniques, or special indexes extracted from the curves is possible. However, the interest of direct measurements is limited because they must be achieved either in the operating theater during surgery or after biopsies or surgery and they are invasive. In addition, they will never replace the quality and precision of microscopic examination. The real challenge is to take into account the variations thus defined and try to propose a noninvasive method that could make it possible to sense those changes very early by applying noninvasive measurement on the breast. Such a technique could be of interest in early diagnosis of breast cancer. Thus, the aim is not to compete with existing techniques, but to develop a new prevention technique: are we able or not to detect the changes in the membrane behavior of normal tissues before cancer is diagnosed by conventional methods? That is the challenge for impedance spectroscopy applied to breast cancer detection. Even if, from the results presented here, the possibility of developing a noninvasive method has still to be proven, the idea seems to be realistic according to the recent works presented by Laver-Moskovitz,[10] who developed an impedance spectroscopic technique in Israel, and by Lifen,[11] who recently reported results obtained with a similar technique in China.

REFERENCES

1. SUROWIEC, A. J. *et al.* 1988. Dielectric properties of breast carcinoma and the surrounding tissues. IEEE Trans. Biomed. Eng. **35**(4): 257–262.
2. HEINITZ, J. & O. MINET. 1995. Dielectric properties of female breast tumors. *In* Ninth International Conference on Electrical Bio-Impedance, Heidelberg.
3. COLE, K. S. & R. H. COLE. 1941. Dispersion and absorption in dielectrics. J. Chem. Phys. **9**: 341–351.
4. JOSSINET, J. 1997. Interpretation of complex tissue impedance loci. *In* Fourth European Conference on Engineering and Medicine, Warsaw.
5. BLAD, B. & B. BALDETORP. 1996. Impedance spectra of tumor tissue in comparison with normal tissue: a possible clinical application for electrical impedance tomography. Physiol. Meas. **17**: A105–A115.
6. CHAUVEAU, N. *et al.* 1997. Bioimpédance électrique et inflammation du foie. ITBM **18**(5): 319–326.
7. CHAUVEAU, N. *et al.* 1995. Impedance spectroscopy of MCF-7 tumors in nude mice: measurement problems and examples. *In* Ninth International Conference on Electrical Bio-Impedance, Heidelberg.
8. JOSSINET, J. 1996. Variability of impedivity in normal and pathological breast tissue. Med. Biol. Eng. Comput. **24**: 346–350.
9. MACDONALD, J. R. 1987. Impedance Spectroscopy: Emphasizing Solid Materials and Systems. Wiley. New York.
10. LAVER-MOSKOVITZ, O. 1996. T-scan: a new imaging method for breast cancer detection without X-ray. RSNA '96, Chicago.
11. LIFEN, D. *et al.* 1998. Clinical study on electrical impedance method used in diagnosis of breast diseases. *In* Tenth International Conference on Electrical Bio-Impedance, Barcelona.

In Vivo and In Situ Ischemic Tissue Characterization Using Electrical Impedance Spectroscopy[a]

O. CASAS,[b] R. BRAGÓS,[b] P. J. RIU,[b] J. ROSELL,[b] M. TRESÀNCHEZ,[c]
M. WARREN,[c] A. RODRIGUEZ-SINOVAS,[c] A. CARREÑO,[c] AND J. CINCA[c]

[b]*Divisió d'Instrumentació i Bioenginyeria, Departament d'Enginyeria Electrònica, Universitat Politècnica de Catalunya, 08034 Barcelona, Spain*

[c]*Laboratori de Cardiologia Experimental, Servei de Cardiologia, Hospital General, Universitari Vall d'Hebrón, 08035 Barcelona, Spain*

ABSTRACT: The investigation of processes of ischemia in different organ tissues is very important for the development of methods of protection and preservation during surgical procedures. Electrical impedance spectroscopy was used to distinguish between different tissues and their degree of ischemia. We describe mathematical methods used to adjust experimental data to Cole-Cole models for one-circle and two-circle impedance loci and a study of the main parameters for representing the behavior of ischemia in time. *In vivo* and *in situ* postmortem measurements of different tissues from pigs are shown in the 100 Hz to 1 MHz range. The Cole parameters that best characterize the ischemia are R_0 and f_c.

INTRODUCTION

Investigation of the characterization of tissues and the study of ischemia in different organs is very important for the development of different methods for protecting and preserving human tissues during clinical procedures, such as surgical operations and transplants. The use of a noninvasive technique such as electrical impedance tomography (EIT) would be a great advance in this clinical field. EIT enables us to obtain images of different tissues for characterization. It is possible to obtain dynamic and multifrequency images, and thus to distinguish and characterize tissues by their different behavior in time or in frequency spectrum. A necessary previous step is to study the viability of extracting physical models of tissues from electrical impedance measurements. With this idea, the technique of electrical impedance spectroscopy was used to characterize *in vivo* organ tissues (static measurements) and the level of ischemia (dynamic measurements). Since some of the results published in the literature[1–5] show tissues with a double relaxation, this work considers mathematical methods for fitting the experimental data to Cole models for one-circle and two-circle impedance loci. Based on the experimental data, a study was made of the parameters that best fit the Cole model for characterization of ischemia.

[a]This work was supported by Spanish CICYT Project Nos. SAF 98-0121 and FIS 98/0430.

MATHEMATICAL AND CIRCUIT MODELING

The Cole equation models the behavior of permittivity (ε) or conductivity (σ) with frequency, but it is possible to use a similar expression to characterize the impedance behavior. For tissues with one relaxation, the expression is

$$Z = R_\infty + \frac{R_0 - R_\infty}{1 + \left(j\frac{f}{f_c}\right)^{(1-\alpha)}} = R_\infty + \frac{\Delta R}{1 + \left(j\frac{f}{f_c}\right)^{(1-\alpha)}} \qquad (1)$$

where R_0 and R_∞ are the limiting values of resistance at low and high frequencies, f_C is the characteristic frequency of relaxation, and α, called the angle of depression, is a constant, which has a value between 0 and 1. The plot of the imaginary part of impedance versus the real part is an arc of circumference. The experimental data can be adjusted to this arc and calculations can be made of the parameters R_0, R_∞, and α. This adjustment is made by finding the optimum circumference center (a,b) that minimizes the following error expression for the calculation of the circle:

$$\varepsilon = \frac{1}{n}\sum_{j=1}^{n}\left\{(R_j - a)^2 + (I_j - b)^2 - b^2 - \frac{1}{n}\sum_{i=1}^{n}[(R_i - a)^2 + (I_i - b)^2 - b^2]\right\}^2 \qquad (2)$$

where n is the number of experimental data points with value $R_i + jI_i$. The parameter f_c is obtained by the method of "ln(u/v)" described by Schwan.[6]

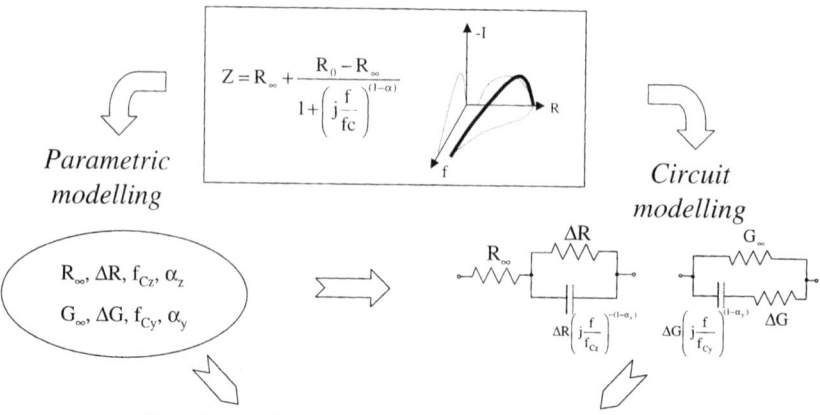

FIGURE 1. Relation between Cole model parameters and elements of two equivalent circuit models.

The "constant phase angle" elements are used to represent mathematical models with a simple equivalent circuit.[7] FIGURE 1 shows one example of two different circuit models and the relations between these circuit elements and the parameters of Cole models.

The process for interpreting the two-circle impedance locus is similar to the procedure for the Cole model with one relaxation. In this case, a simplex method was used to minimize the error involved in calculating the seven independent parameters that characterize the two relaxations. This method is used (i) with the impedance measurements if we must characterize a serial process in the two relaxations or (ii) with the admittance data if we want to fit a parallel double relaxation process (FIGURE 2). These seven parameters are $R_{\infty T} = R_{\infty 1} + R_{\infty 2}$, $\Delta R_1 = R_{01} - R_{\infty 1}$, f_{C1}, α_1, $\Delta R_2 = R_{02} - R_{\infty 2}$, f_{C2}, and α_2. Another interesting parameter is R_{0T}. This is calculated as $R_{0T} = R_{\infty T} + \Delta R_1 + \Delta R_2$. In the same way as in the one-circle impedance locus, it is possible to relate these seven parameters with circuit elements of different circuit models.

In clinical diagnoses, it is more important to obtain a detailed physiological model than an equivalent circuit model. Since it is impossible to find an exact physiological model with our impedance measurements, we apply the simplest model to our data. For this reason, this work only uses the evolution of the Cole parameters (R_0, R_∞, ΔR_1, ΔR_2, f_C, α) to characterize the static and dynamic properties of different tissues.

MATERIALS AND METHODS

Data were obtained from the open chest, α-chloralose anesthetized, artificially ventilated pig model. The sources of ischemia were the occlusion of one artery or the death of the animal. The study was approved by the ethics committee of our institution and complied with international rules for animal care. Tissue impedance was measured with two 4-electrode (5 mm long, 0.4 mm diameter) platinum probes mounted as a linear array sepa-

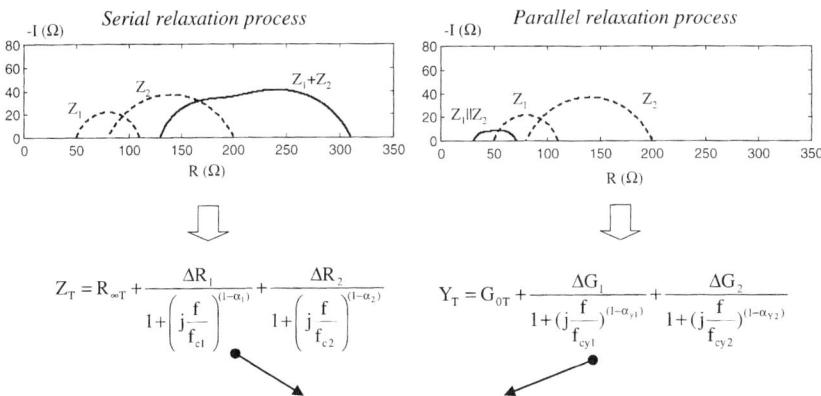

FIGURE 2. Modeling of the serial and parallel double relaxation process.

rated by a distance between electrodes of 2.5 mm. A slight black-platinum deposition was used to reduce the electrode impedance and its effect on the measurements. The measurements were taken with an HP4192A impedance analyzer with a self-designed front end.[8] The front end consists of a differential amplifier that provides a very high common-mode rejection ratio in the measurement range (>90 dB at 1 MHz). Measurements were taken between 100 Hz and 1 MHz. Data acquisition and management used customized software (FIGURES 3 and 4). A three-reference calibration method was used to correct load-dependent errors.[9] Three saline solutions were used to determine a set of coefficients at each frequency. The references were obtained using the same probe to reduce the effects of electrodes, cables, and amplifier response on the measurement.

EXPERIMENTAL RESULTS

Measurements were made *in vivo* over different tissues in 12 pigs to characterize the static behavior of the tissue impedance.

A possible application of the *in vivo* measurement is the differentiation between three states of myocardium (normal, ischemic, and scar).[9,10] In FIGURE 5, we show the spectral behavior in these three tissues. It is possible to see that with electrical impedance spectroscopy we can differentiate the three cases. Normal myocardium has one relaxation in approximately 300 kHz; the ischemic tissue, after one hour of occlusion, shows two relaxations: the same as a normal myocardium, but with a lower central frequency, and a new relaxation at low frequency, 5–10 kHz. In the scar tissue, there is no relaxation process.[11] In this example, it is possible to differentiate the three tissues directly by their different behavior in magnitude or in phase, or by the difference of the parameters in the Cole mod-

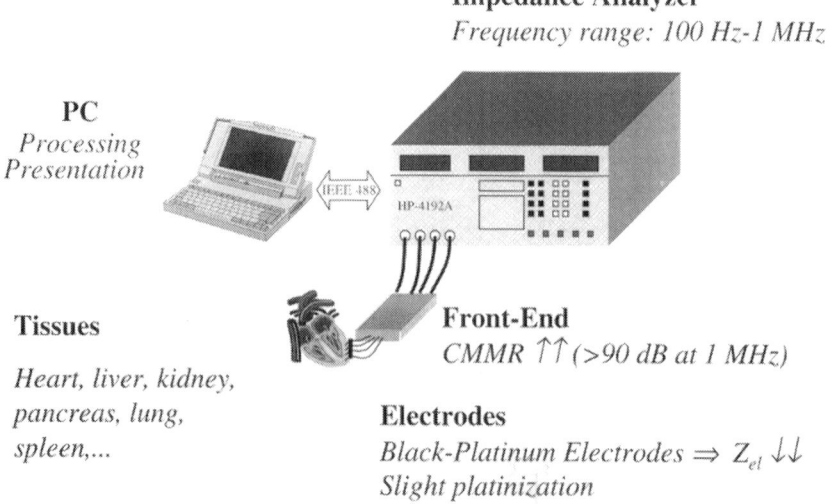

FIGURE 3. Structure of the measurement system.

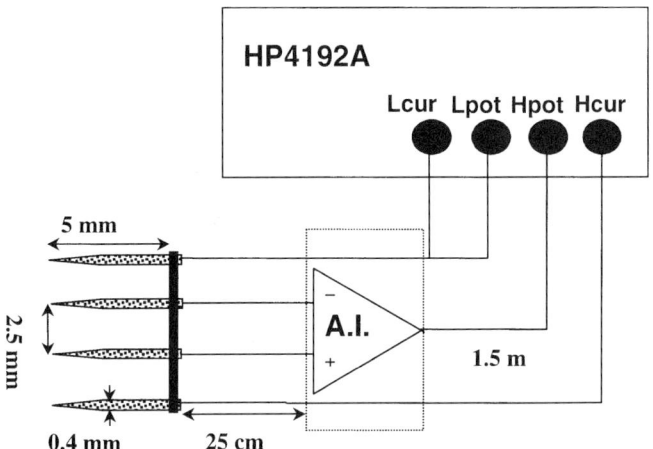

FIGURE 4. Structure of the platinum electrode array.

els. In our measurements of biological tissues, we have used for their characterization the Cole-Cole parameters.[1,12] These results are summarized in TABLE 1. In general with the parameters R_0/R_∞, f_c, and α, it is possible to differentiate all the tissues, and the advantage of these parameters is that they can be obtained by electrical impedance spectroscopy or by parametric images in electrical impedance tomography.

These tissues were also used to obtain measurements of the evolution of the ischemia and to study which parameters of the Cole models could be used for its characterization. The evolution of these parameters shows a similar behavior pattern in all tissues. The two parameters that best characterize the evolution of ischemia are the resistance at low fre-

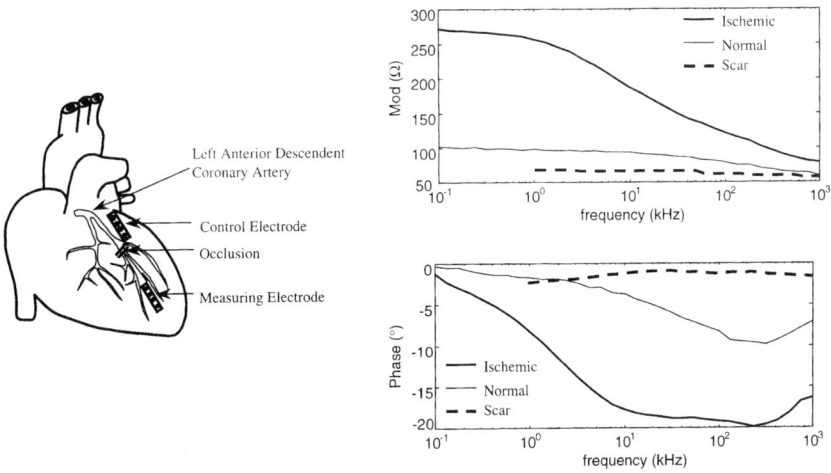

FIGURE 5. Frequency spectrum of normal, infarcted, and scar myocardium.

TABLE 1. *In Vivo* Tissue Impedance Measurements: Cole Model Parameters (Mean ± Standard Deviation)

Tissue	R_0/R_∞	f_C (kHz)	α	Samples	Number of Pigs
myocardium	1.8 ± 0.4	144.2 ± 60.2	0.29 ± 0.04	20	8
scar of myocardium	1.0 ± 0.0	no relaxation	no relaxation	12	5
liver	2.4 ± 0.6	70.9 ± 15.9	0.39 ± 0.05	9	5
pancreas	3.1 ± 0.8	123.0 ± 25.2	0.31 ± 0.05	5	3
kidney	2.5 ± 0.3	24.8 ± 7.8	0.26 ± 0.03	5	3
lung	2.0 ± 0.4	130.6 ± 32.3	0.46 ± 0.13	6	3
spleen	2.4 ± 0.3	230.8 ± 97.3	0.54 ± 0.05	10	5
muscle ∥	3.1 ± 0.3	94.9 ± 17.5	0.20 ± 0.0	9	5
muscle ⊥	3.3 ± 0.4	63.6 ± 10.6	0.19 ± 0.05	9	5
blood	1.9 ± 0.4	2020 ± 420	0.16 ± 0.03	8	4

quency and the characteristic frequency. Measurements have shown that R_0 increases its value after 100 minutes of ischemia. This varies from 20% in longitudinal muscle to 150% in the liver. After the same period of ischemia, f_C reduces its value from 10% in longitudinal muscle to 50% in liver or kidney. R_∞ shows a similar behavior pattern as R_0, but the order of variation is lower (approximately from 5% to 20%). Moreover, in some tissues,

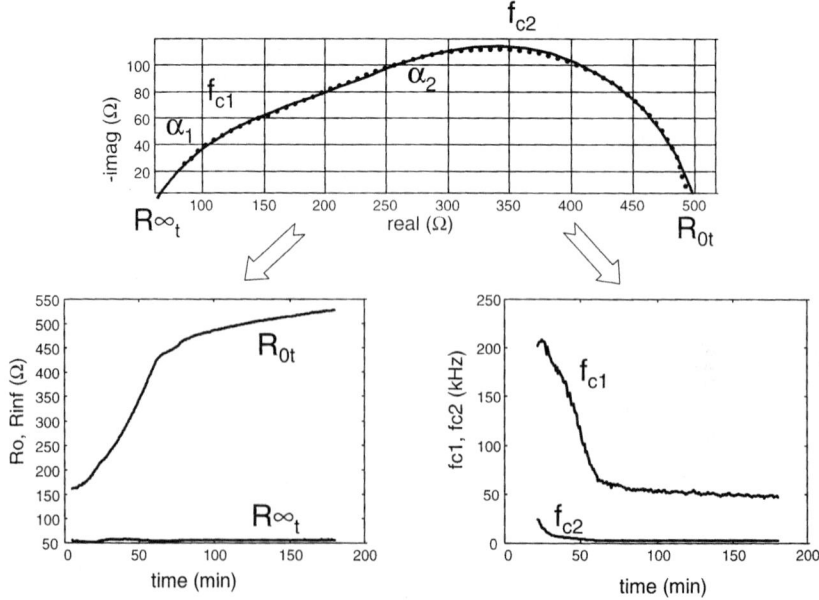

FIGURE 6. Evolution of Cole model parameters with the myocardium ischemia.

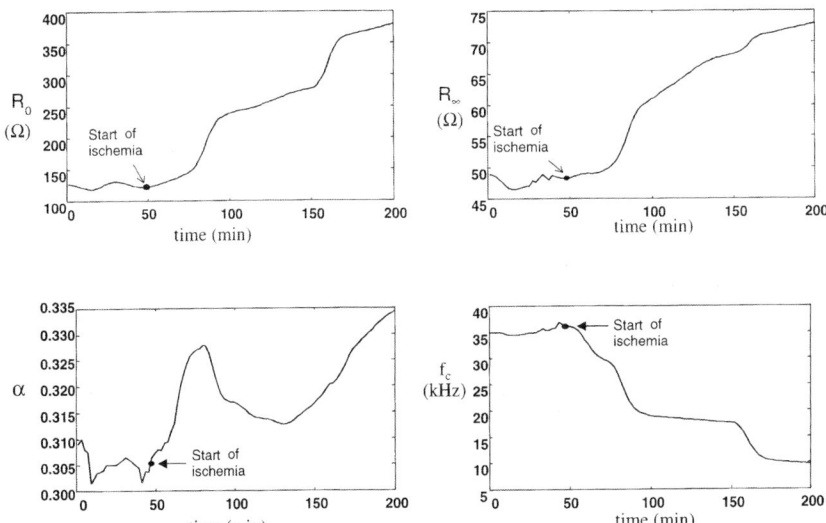

FIGURE 7. Evolution of Cole model parameters with the kidney ischemia.

such as the myocardium,[9,13] a new relaxation appears in the first 20–25 minutes at low frequency, in the range of 10 kHz. This is related to the ischemic process. As an example of these results, FIGURES 6 and 7 show the typical evolution of ischemia in myocardium and in kidney tissues.

The variations between the parameters for normal and ischemic tissues, from 20% to 150% in R_0 or from 10% to 50% in f_c after 100 minutes of ischemia, clearly show the limitations of *in vitro* measurements to characterize *in vivo* tissues.

DISCUSSION AND CONCLUSIONS

We have shown that, according to the literature, impedance spectroscopy is a technique that is capable of characterizing *in vivo* tissues and the evolution of ischemia. Cole parameters for *in vivo* measurements are shown. Our measurements enabled relationships to be established between changes in the parameters of Cole models and the evolution of the ischemia in time. The parameters that best characterize these changes are R_0 and f_C. The differences obtained between the parameters for normal and ischemic tissues clearly show the limitations of *in vitro* measurements for characterizing *in vivo* tissues.

REFERENCES

1. RIGAUD, B., L. HAMZAOUI, M. FRIKHA, N. CHAUVEAU & J. P. MORUCCI. 1995. *In vitro* tissue characterization and modelling using electrical impedance measurements in the 100 Hz–10 MHz frequency range. Physiol. Meas. **16**(Suppl. 3a): 15–28.
2. GABRIEL, C., S. GABRIEL & E. CORTHOUT. 1996. The dielectric properties of biological tissues: I. Literature survey. Phys. Med. Biol. **41**: 2231–2249.

3. GABRIEL, S., R. W. LAU & C. GABRIEL. 1996. The dielectric properties of biological tissues: II. Measurements in the frequency range 10 Hz to 20 GHz. Phys. Med. Biol. **41:** 2251–2269.
4. GABRIEL, S., R. W. LAU & C. GABRIEL. 1996. The dielectric properties of biological tissues: III. Parametric models for the dielectric spectrum of tissues. Phys. Med. Biol. **41:** 2271–2293.
5. GERSING, E., B. HOFMANN, G. KEHRER & R. POTTEL. 1995. Modelling based on tissue structure—the example of porcine liver. Innov. Technol. Biol. Med. **16:** 672–678.
6. SCHWAN, H. P. 1957. Electrical properties of tissue and cell suspensions. Adv. Biol. Med. Phys. **5:** 147–208.
7. MCADAMS, E. T., J. JOSSINET & A. LACKERMEIER. 1995. Modelling the "constant phase angle" behaviour of biological tissues: potential pitfalls. Innov. Technol. Biol. Med. **16:** 662–670.
8. BRAGÓS, R., A. YAÑEZ, P. J. RIU, M. TRESÀNCHEZ, M. WARREN, A. CARREÑO & J. CINCA. 1996. Espectro de la impedancia del miocardio porcino in situ durante la isquemia. Parte I: sistema de medida. *In* XIV Congreso Anual de la Sociedad Española de Ingeniería Biomédica, p. 97–99. Pamplona, Spain.
9. BRAGÓS, R., P. J. RIU, M. WARREN, M. TRESÀNCHEZ, A. CARREÑO & J. CINCA. 1996. Changes in myocardial impedance spectrum during acute ischemia in the *in-situ* pig heart. *In* Eighteenth Annual International Conference of the IEEE Engineering in Medicine and Biology Society, p. 414–415. Amsterdam.
10. TRESÀNCHEZ, M., R. BRAGÓS, O. CASAS, J. ROSELL, M. WARREN, A. CARREÑO, A. RODRÍGUEZ-SINOVAS, P. GÓMEZ & J. CINCA. 1997. Identification of myocardial infarct scar by impedance spectroscopy. Med. Biol. Eng. Comput. **35**(part I): 334.
11. CINCA, J., M. WARREN, A. RODRIGUEZ-SINOVAS, M. TRESÀNCHEZ, A. CARREÑO, R. BRAGÓS, O. CASAS, A. DOMINGO & J. SOLER-SOLER. 1998. Passive transmission of ischemic ST segment changes in low electrical resistance myocardial infarct in the pig. Cardiovasc. Res. In press.
12. LU, L., L. HAMZAOUI, B. H. BROWN, B. RIGAUD, R. H. SMALLWOOD, D. C. BARBER & J. P. MORUCCI. 1996. Parametric modelling for electrical impedance spectroscopy system. Med. Biol. Eng. Comput. **34:** 122–126.
13. LINHART, H. G., E. GERSING, M. SCHÄFER & M. GEBHARD. 1995. The electrical impedance of the ischemic heart at low frequencies. *In* Ninth International Conference on Electrical Bio-Impedance, p. 207–210. Heidelberg.

Dielectric Properties of Skeletal Muscle during Ischemia in the Frequency Range from 50 Hz to 200 MHz

M. SCHÄFER, H-J. KIRLUM, C. SCHLEGEL, AND M. M. GEBHARD

Department of Experimental Surgery, University of Heidelberg, 69120 Heidelberg, Germany

ABSTRACT: The complex dielectric properties of canine skeletal muscles were measured at 25 °C during ischemia in the frequency range from 50 Hz to 200 MHz. The dielectric spectrum of skeletal muscle shows an α-dispersion below 1 kHz and a β-dispersion with a relaxation frequency of about 100 kHz. The α-dispersion disappears between 450 and 500 min of ischemia time, the same time during which mechanical contraction was observed, and was restored later. During ischemia, the β-dispersion is shifted continuously to higher frequencies; and at frequencies above 50 MHz, a decrease of the real part of the dielectric permittivity was measured. The dielectric loss factor decreases during ischemia at frequencies below 500 kHz, only interrupted by a short increase, coinciding with the disappearance of the α-dispersion. The principal processes that happen during ischemia inside the skeletal muscle tissues were studied with the help of a model especially designed to simulate membrane effects on the dielectric spectrum. The disappearance of the α-dispersion is explained by an increase of conductivity in the membrane of the sarcoplasmic reticulum. Shifting β-dispersion to higher frequencies is a result of metabolically produced ions and therefore increasing conductivity of the intracellular medium. Decreasing dielectric permittivity at frequencies above 50 MHz and decreasing dielectric loss factor at low frequencies are caused by the cell edema.

INTRODUCTION

Ischemia of skeletal muscles occurs after arterial embolization, after traumatic interruption of the arterial blood flow, and by using a tourniquet, which is used in several surgical operations to avoid injury of nerves and other small structures or to prevent a loss of blood volume. Ischemia means that there is no blood flow to supply the tissue with oxygen and nutrients and to transport metabolic end products. In order to prevent functional loss, a lot of metabolic processes have to happen inside the muscle tissue. For example, ion pumps have to work in order to stabilize membrane potential—processes that need energy. Energy has to be gained anaerobically, which results in production of lactate, and acidosis occurs. Intraischemic ion production also means changing the osmolarity between the intra- and extracellular compartments—cell edema is the result. After a certain time of ischemia, the biological tissue is damaged irreversibly.

In medicine, there is great interest in atraumatically working diagnostic measurement systems in order to characterize the threshold between reversible and irreversible ischemia damage.

A lot of work was done in order to monitor an organ state by measuring the electrical properties in dependence on ischemia time. In the case of myocardium and liver, characteristic changes were found in the electrical impedance spectrum that show clearly the transition from reversible to irreversible damage.[1,2]

Skeletal muscle tissues, however, show less clearly changes of the electrical properties during ischemia. This work analyzes the dielectric properties of skeletal muscles in a wide frequency range in order to understand the changes occurring during ischemia and in order to discuss the possibility to determine thresholds in the macroscopical electrical properties for characterizing ischemia damage.

METHODS

Experiments were carried out with canine skeletal muscles that were perfused *in situ* with Ringer's solution by a catheter in the arteria iliaca. The Ringer's solution temperature was 8 °C. The muscles were explanted and cut into pieces of 2 cm × 2 cm and incubated in temperature-controlled measuring chambers at 25 °C. Electrical properties of the skeletal muscles were measured in the frequency range from 50 Hz to 10 MHz with a two-electrode probe with fractal-surfaced electrodes[3,4] in order to minimize electrode polarization effects. The impedance spectra were measured with the equipment used in reference 5 consisting of a Solartron 1260 device and a preamplifier. High frequency measurements above 5 MHz up to 200 MHz were performed by measuring HF-wave reflection at an open-ended coaxial line using an HP 3577 A network analyzer.

Saline solutions with different known electrical properties were used for calibration. Measurement errors in the complex dielectric permittivity $\varepsilon = \varepsilon' - i\varepsilon''$ above 100 kHz are <1% and are determined mainly by the accuracy of the used calibration standards. Below 100 kHz, increasing errors occur because of electrode polarization.

RESULTS

FIGURE 1 shows the measured dielectric spectrum of skeletal muscle at three different times during ischemia. The temperature of the skeletal muscle was 25 °C. At 130 min, an α-dispersion below 1 kHz and a β-dispersion with a relaxation frequency of about 100 kHz were found in the dielectric permittivity spectrum ε'. During ischemia, the dielectric loss factor ε'' decreases and the α-dispersion disappears at 480 min and reappears at 630 min.

FIGURES 2 and 3 show the detailed time dependence of the dielectric permittivity ε' and the dielectric loss factor ε'' in the region of the α-dispersion for six different experiments. The decrease of ε' at 230 Hz starts at about 400 min and ε' reaches a minimum between 450 and 500 min. At times greater than 500 min, increasing behavior of ε' was measured. The dielectric loss factor ε'' decreases during the whole time at 230 Hz. This continuous decrease is only interrupted by a short increase, coinciding with the disappearance of the α-dispersion.

Increasing values of ε' at 3 MHz in FIGURE 4 indicate a shift of the β-dispersion to higher frequencies.

At 200 MHz, the dielectric permittivity ε' decreases during ischemia and ε'' shows an increase at about 130 min and a maximum between 400 and 450 min (FIGURE 5).

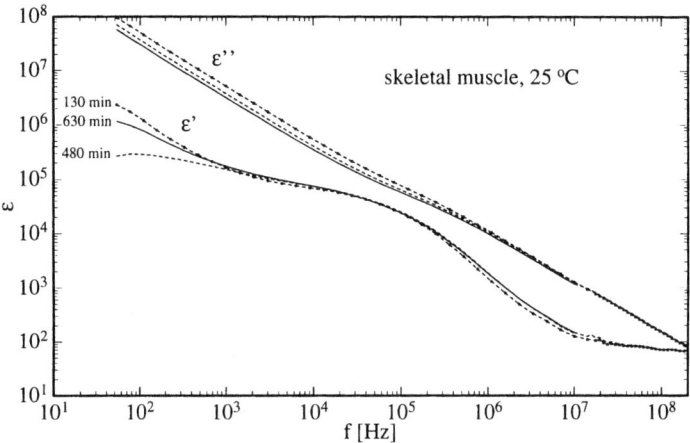

FIGURE 1. Dielectric spectrum of skeletal muscle at three times during ischemia.

DISCUSSION

In order to find out the microscopical reason for the observed alterations of the macroscopical dielectric properties of skeletal muscle during ischemia, a model[6] was used for simulation.

Skeletal muscles have mainly two important membrane types responsible for function. First, an electrical stimulation signal is transmitted in the form of an action potential along the cell membrane. In the cell membrane, there are a lot of potential-dependent ion chan-

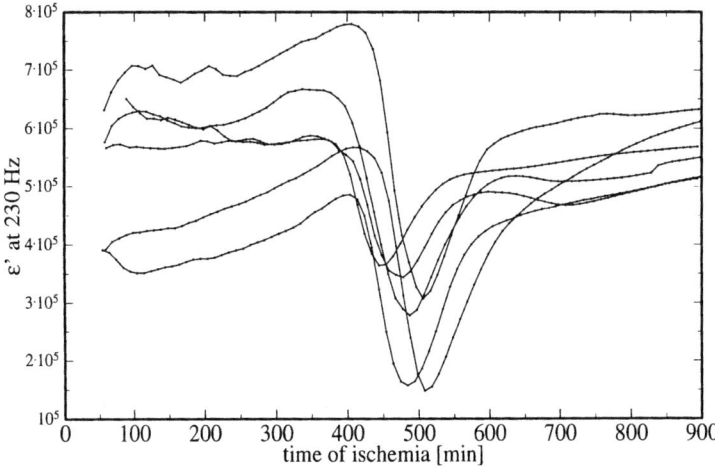

FIGURE 2. Dielectric permittivity ε' at 230 Hz for different experiments.

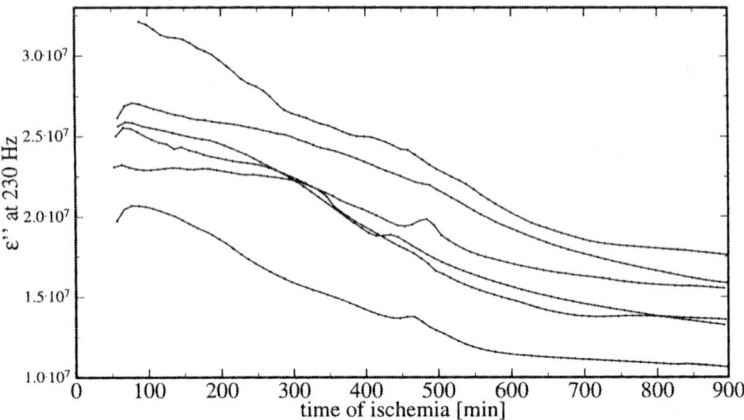

FIGURE 3. Dielectric loss factor ε'' at 230 Hz for different experiments.

nels that are able to reduce membrane resistance instantaneously. The second important membrane type in skeletal muscles is the membrane of the sarcoplasmic reticulum. Opening ion channels in the membrane of the sarcoplasmic reticulum results in a release of Ca^{++} to the actin-myosin filaments and mechanical contraction will occur.[7]

The used model has membrane-shaped cells and, in the intracellular space, there are additional membrane-shaped particles. Simulating an increase of membrane conductivity of the intracellular membranes produces the disappearance of the α-dispersion (situation 1 in FIGURE 6). Because of the observed mechanical contraction of the skeletal muscles at the same time when the α-dispersion disappears, we explain this disappearance with the Ca^{++} release from the sarcoplasmic reticulum.

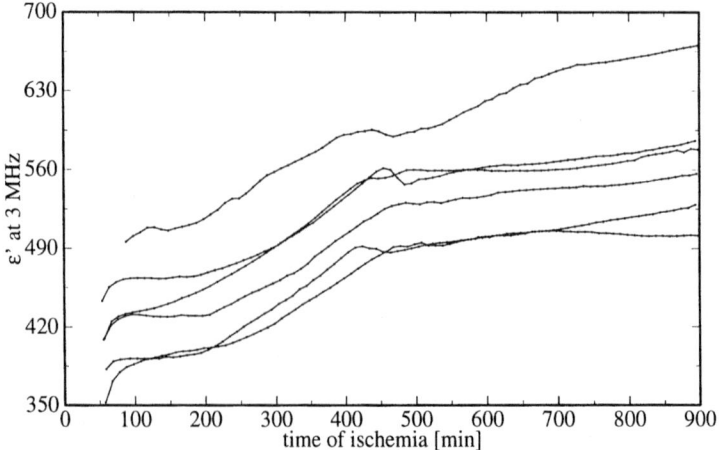

FIGURE 4. Dielectric permittivity ε' at 3 MHz for different experiments.

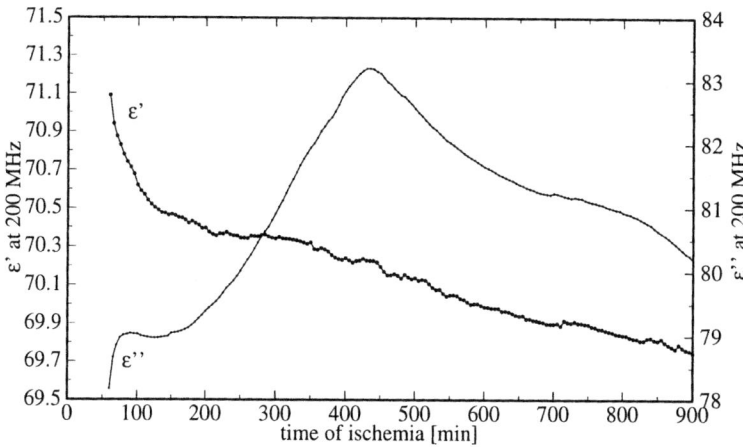

FIGURE 5. Dielectric permittivity ε' and loss factor ε'' at 200 MHz for a single experiment.

Increasing conductivity of the intracellular medium caused by metabolical processes results in a shift of the β-dispersion to higher frequencies (situation 2 in FIGURE 6).

Decreasing dielectric permittivity ε' at 200 MHz and decreasing dielectric loss factor ε'' at low frequencies are produced by the increasing volume fraction of the cellular compartment as an effect of cell edema (situation 3 in FIGURE 6).

What about the possibility of dielectric spectroscopy to be used as a diagnostic system for ischemia damage? So far, we have not performed any reanimation experiments; therefore, we will have to find other parameters characterizing the muscle state. A few experi-

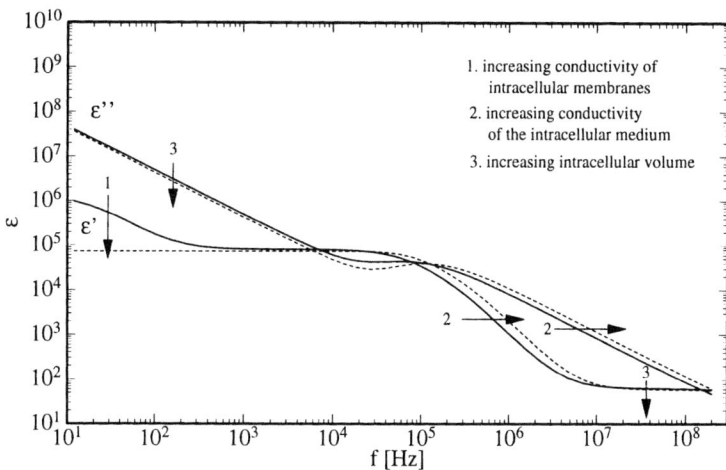

FIGURE 6. Model simulations of the changes of the complex dielectric spectrum, $\varepsilon = \varepsilon' - i\varepsilon''$, measured during ischemia.

ments were performed by measuring membrane signal transmission with an electromyogram (EMG) device at the same time. For the special experiment shown in FIGURE 5, signal transmission of the fast muscle fibers stopped at 135 min. This correlates directly with the starting increase of ε'' at 200 MHz. If interrupted signal transmission along the membranes of the skeletal muscle cells is the threshold between reversible and irreversible damage, then dielectric spectroscopy measurement could be used as a diagnostic tool, especially at high frequencies.

However, we have little experience with skeletal muscle damage during ischemia and have only a small amount of measured data, so a clear statement is not possible at this time.

REFERENCES

1. GEBHARD, M. M. et al. 1987. Impedance spectroscopy: a method for surveillance of ischemia tolerance of the heart. J. Thorac. Cardiovasc. Surg. **35:** 26–32.
2. GERSING, E. et al. 1992. Impedance spectroscopy of tissue structure alterations during organ ischemia. In Proceedings of the Eighth ICEBI, Kuopio, Finland.
3. RIEDMÜLLER, J. et al. 1995. Langzeitstabilität bei elektrischer Belastung von galvanisch abgeschiedenem Iridiumoxyd. Biomed. Tech. **40**(E1): 37–38.
4. RZANY, A. et al. 1995. Elektrochemische Eigenschaften galvanisch abgeschiedener Iridiumoxydschichten im Hinblick auf die Verwendung als elektroaktive Elektrodenbeschichtung. Biomed. Tech. **40**(E1): 399–400.
5. GERSING, E. 1991. Messungen der elektrischen Impedanz von Organen—Apparative Ausrüstung für Forschung und klinische Anwendung. Biomed. Tech. **36:** 6–11.
6. SCHÄFER, M. 1991. Dielektrische Eigenschaften ischämischer Leber- und Nierenproben im Frequenzbereich von 0.3 MHz bis 3000 MHz. Phys. Dissertation, Göttingen.
7. MELZER, W. et al. 1995. The role of Ca^{++} ions in excitation-contraction coupling of skeletal muscle fibers. Biochim. Biophys. Acta **1241:** 59–116.

Quantitative Analysis of Impedance Spectra of Organs during Ischemia

MIHAELA GHEORGHIU,[a] EBERHARD GERSING,[b] AND EUGEN GHEORGHIU[a]

[a]*NIB-UNESCO Center of Biodynamics, Splaiul Unirii 313 (ICPE), Bucharest 4, Romania*
[b]*Department of Anesthesiological Research, University Hospital Göttingen, D-37073 Göttingen, Germany*

> ABSTRACT: We have developed a rapid, quantitative procedure to fit the spectra of the real and imaginary part of tissue impedance, providing characteristic parameters: time constants, their distribution, and the amplitudes of associated dispersions. Based on the time course of tissue impedance during ischemia, we have derived the evolution of characteristic parameters for both myocardial and liver tissue. The similar evolution of the distribution of time constants for myocardial and liver tissue is emphasized and discussed.

INTRODUCTION

Aiming to derive physiological information from impedance spectra, equivalent circuits are frequently used to model the tissue; however, unless they are related with histological information, they fail to reproduce both the electrical properties and the tissue structure. Experiments on ischemic organs in which cells are connected through gap-junctions have shown a characteristic course of the impedance spectra, characterized by a steep increase in impedance at low frequencies, leading to the development of a new model. The model assumes that the closing up of the gap-junctions (as well as cell swelling and accumulation of metabolic products) is responsible for the steep increase in impedance at low frequencies. Unfortunately, only porcine liver tissue exhibits a clear α dispersion; for myocardial muscle, the low frequency dispersion is "hidden" in the β dispersion.

Aiming to characterize the changes of tissue structure underwent during ischemia (e.g., revealed by changes in the distribution of time constants), we were concerned with the development of a fast procedure able to analyze the impedance data and provide time constants and their distribution, as well as amplitudes of the related dispersions.

METHODS

A rapid, quantitative procedure to analyze both the real and imaginary part of the impedance spectra, without considering any a priori model for the tissue, has been developed in the frequency range of 1 Hz to 2 MHz. The Cole-Cole equation (1) with two time constants (or its generalized form: Havriliak-Negami equation)[1] was used for fitting the experimental data. The routine provides the time constants and their distribution as well as the amplitudes of the dispersions:

$$\hat{\varepsilon}(\omega) = \varepsilon_\infty + (\varepsilon - \varepsilon_\infty'') \frac{1}{1+(i\omega\tau_1)^{1-\alpha}} + (\varepsilon_\infty'' - \varepsilon_\infty) \frac{1}{1+(i\omega\tau_2)^{1-\alpha}} \qquad (1)$$

$$\varepsilon'(\omega) = Li + A1\frac{1+(\omega\tau_1)^{1-\alpha}\sin\frac{1}{2}\pi\alpha}{1+2(\omega\tau_1)^{1-\alpha}\sin\frac{1}{2}\pi\alpha+(\omega\tau_1)^{2(1-\alpha)}} + A2\frac{1+(\omega\tau_2)^{1-\beta}\sin\frac{1}{2}\pi\beta}{1+2(\omega\tau_2)^{1-\beta}\sin\frac{1}{2}\pi\beta+(\omega\tau_2)^{2(1-\beta)}}$$

$$\varepsilon''(\omega) = A1\frac{(\omega\tau_1)^{1-\alpha}\cos\frac{1}{2}\pi\alpha}{1+2(\omega\tau_1)^{1-\alpha}\sin\frac{1}{2}\pi\alpha+(\omega\tau_1)^{2(1-\alpha)}} + A2\frac{(\omega\tau_2)^{1-\beta}\cos\frac{1}{2}\pi\beta}{1+2(\omega\tau_2)^{1-\beta}\sin\frac{1}{2}\pi\beta+(\omega\tau_2)^{2(1-\beta)}}$$

where $A1$ and $A2$ are the actual amplitudes of the dispersions, α and β are the Cole parameters, and τ_1 and τ_2 are the two characteristic time constants.

We have investigated data on myocardial and liver tissues perfused with protective solutions during ischemia. The data were measured using a Solartron 1260 Impedance Analyzer and a measurement cell with a four-electrode system[2] at a constant temperature of 25 °C.

RESULTS AND DISCUSSION

The characteristic behavior of the real and imaginary part of impedance spectra of a myocardial tissue (presented in FIGURE 1) displays in the β range a dispersion with an increasing amplitude during ischemia. The additional (small) dispersion at lower frequency might be related with electrode polarization (during ischemia, the tissue is acidified). By applying our procedure, we could follow the time course of the time constant and of the amplitude of the β dispersion. In FIGURES 2A and 2B, the evolution of the time constant and of the related amplitude are presented, showing an increase in the β dispersion amplitude, with a shift toward higher time constants. The amplitude of the high frequency dispersion shows an initial decrease caused by the warming up of the cooled specimen.

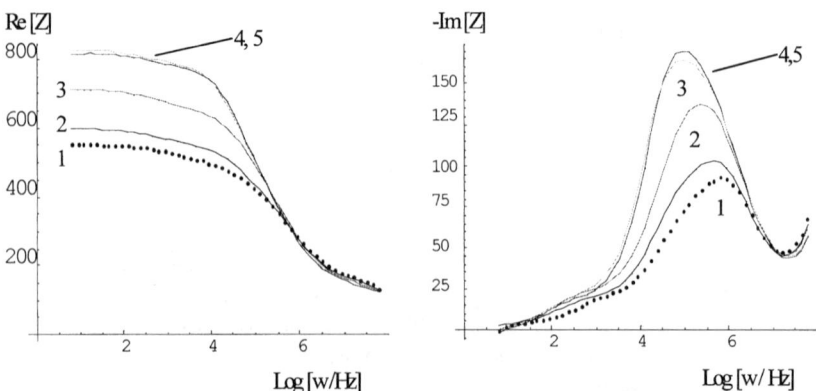

FIGURE 1. Characteristic time evolution of the real and imaginary part of impedance of a heart tissue during ischemia: (1) after 75 min, (2) after 150 min, (3) after 250 min, (4) after 350 min, and (5) after 450 min.

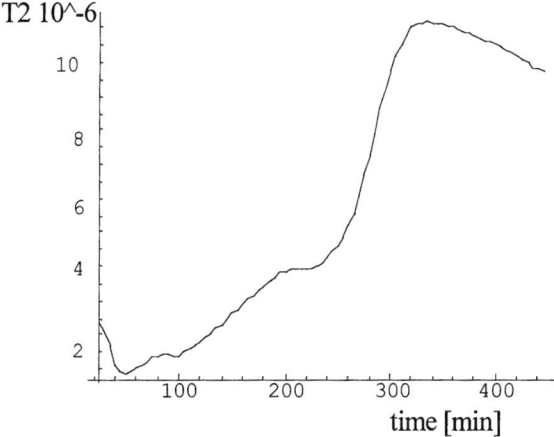

FIGURE 2A. The evolution of the second time constant—heart tissue.

In the first period after the onset of ischemia, the course of the imaginary part of impedance demonstrates a nonsymmetrical distribution of time constants in accordance with the hypothesis of a "hidden" α dispersion. After about 250 minutes, the distribution becomes symmetrical. Further investigations on admittance spectra are in progress.

In the case of a perfused porcine liver, there are two dispersions with a symmetrical distribution of time constants. FIGURE 3 presents the spectra of a perfused porcine liver after 25, 95, 150, 275, and 375 minutes of ischemia duration. In the course of ischemia, the first dispersion disappears (see also FIGURE 4).

The results of the fitting procedure of the experimental data with a Cole-Cole equation (with two time constants) are presented in FIGURE 5 for two moments: 50 minutes and 320

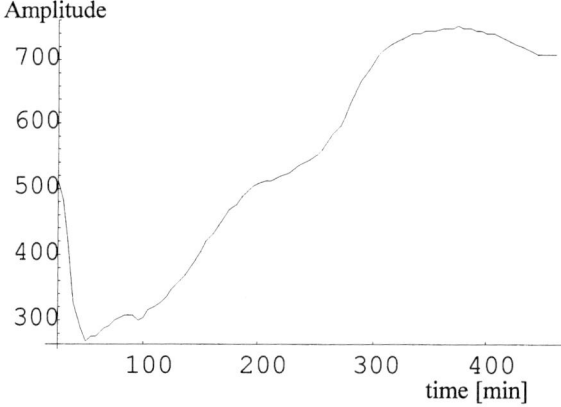

FIGURE 2B. The evolution of the amplitude of the second dispersion—heart tissue.

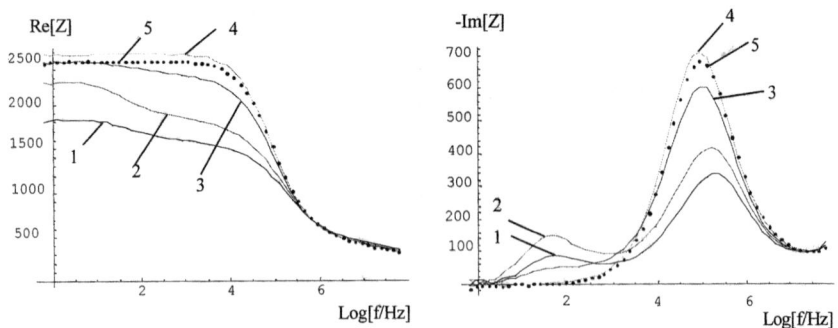

FIGURE 3. The time evolution of the real and imaginary part of a liver tissue impedance during ischemia, after (1) 25 min, (2) 95 min, (3) 150 min, (4) 275 min, and (5) 375 min.

minutes after the onset of ischemia. The Cole-Cole plots show a good agreement between the experimental data and the fitting curve (see also FIGURE 6).

The derived amplitudes (FIGURES 7 and 8B) of the two dispersions show that the amplitude of the α dispersion first increases (up to 120 minutes of ischemia) and then drops rapidly and vanishes completely after 160 minutes of ischemia. After an initial increase, the amplitude of the β dispersion reaches a plateau when the α dispersion disappears. Moreover, both time constants [of α (FIGURE 4) and β (FIGURE 8A) dispersions] shift toward larger values.

FIGURES 9A and 9B present the similar evolution of time constant distributions for the α dispersion, for both heart and liver tissues, respectively. We assume that the peak (indicated with an arrow) in the evolution of the Cole parameter is related to the onset of drastic alteration of the cellular state, while the end of the slope indicates the duration of ischemia

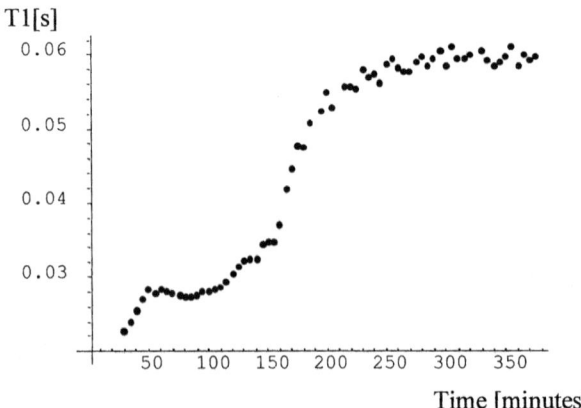

FIGURE 4. The evolution of the first time constant of the impedance spectra of a perfused liver tissue.

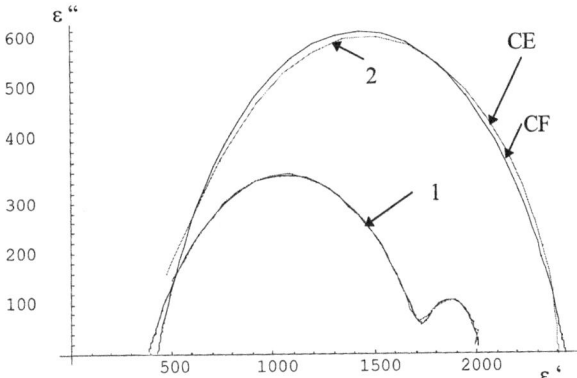

FIGURE 5. The Cole-Cole plots for experimental data (CE) and fitted parameters (CF) after (1) 50 min and (2) 320 min—liver tissue.

after which the organ can no longer be resuscitated[2] due to the irreversible alterations in tissue state.

We emphasize that monitoring the evolution of the distribution parameter of the β dispersion (experimentally more accessible) for both myocardial and liver tissue provides a direct access to the limit of resuscitation of an organ.

CONCLUSIONS

Based on the time course of the real and imaginary part of tissue impedance during ischemia, we have developed a rapid, quantitative procedure to determine the evolution of time constants as well as of the amplitudes of associated dispersions. We pointed out the characteristic time course of the distribution parameter of the β dispersion for both myo-

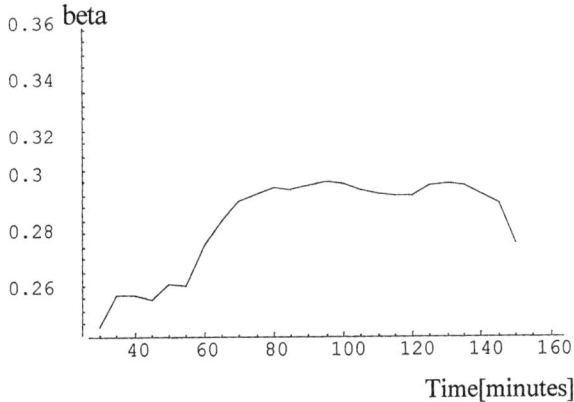

FIGURE 6. The evolution of the distribution of the first time constant—liver tissue.

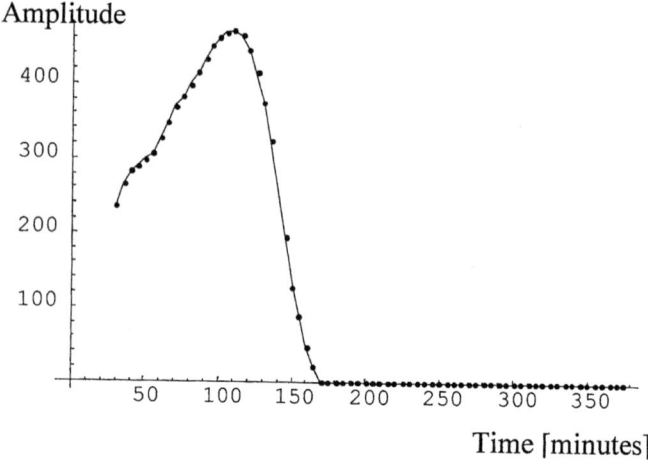

FIGURE 7. The evolution of the amplitude of the first dispersion.

cardial and liver tissue that might provide a direct access to the limit of resuscitation of an organ.

The similar evolution of characteristic parameters related to β dispersion for both liver and myocardial tissue indicates a common process of tissue alteration, during ischemia, able to be quantitatively revealed by impedance spectroscopy.

Measurements on different samples of organ tissues exhibit large variations during ischemia; therefore, single examples are usually reported. A breakthrough might be provided by (non)linear analysis of the evolution of dispersion amplitudes and related time constants of distinct experiments, leading to a "common language" for interpreting the data.

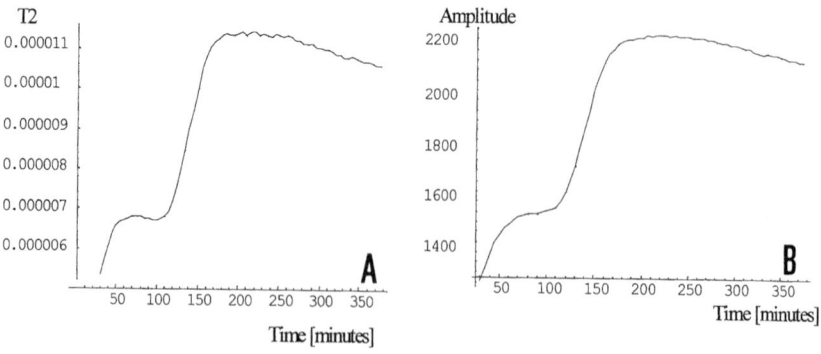

FIGURE 8. The time course of the second time constant (A) and of the amplitude (B)—liver.

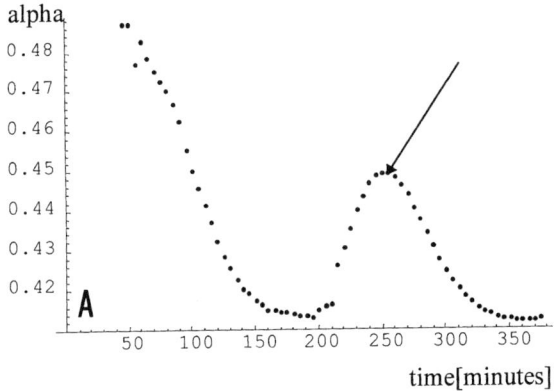

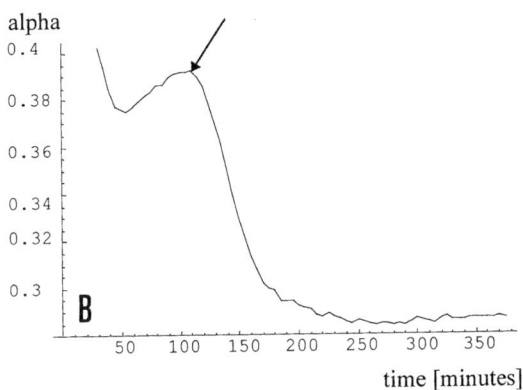

FIGURE 9. The evolution of the Cole parameter for the high frequency dispersion in the case of myocardial tissue (A) and liver tissue (B).

REFERENCES

1. BÖTTCHER, C. F. J. & P. BORDEWIJK. 1978. Theory of Electric Polarization. Volume 2, p. 45–118. Elsevier. Amsterdam/New York.
2. GERSING, E., F. BACH, C. BROCKHOFF, M. M. GEBHARD, G. KEHRER, A. MEISSNER & H. J. BRETSCHNEIDER. 1991. Measurement of electrical impedance in organs. Biomed. Tech. **36:** 70–77.

Requirements for Clinical Use of Bioelectrical Impedance Analysis (BIA)[a]

HENRY C. LUKASKI

United States Department of Agriculture, Agricultural Research Service, Grand Forks Human Nutrition Research Center, Grand Forks, North Dakota 58202-9034

ABSTRACT: The bioelectrical impedance analysis (BIA) method is an attractive tool for use in the clinical assessment of human body composition. Factors such as ease of use, relatively low cost, noninvasive nature, high degree of reproducibility, and safety of operation provide an impetus for the general application of this method. The preponderance of the published applications of BIA focused on applications in healthy populations and indicated a qualitative validity of the method. More recent applications have augmented the quantitative values of the BIA approach and have reported very good specificity and sensitivity. One potential limitation of the BIA approach is the reliance on regression models, derived in restricted samples of human subjects, which restricts the usefulness of the derived model in other patients who differ from the original sample in which the model was developed. Other investigational approaches that use different physical models (bioelectrical impedance spectroscopy and parallel model) have yielded successful and useful measures of human body composition in clinical studies. If BIA is to gain acceptance in clinical diagnosis and evaluation of therapeutic interventions, further efforts will be needed to ascertain more fully the validity, sensitivity, and specificity of biological parameters estimated with the new BIA approaches, and to establish the prognostic values of the BIA estimates of body composition.

INTRODUCTION

The use of electricity in medicine began with the studies of Galvani, who discovered that electrical sparks stimulated muscle contraction. This finding prompted other investigators to examine other biological responses to administered electrical current. Although electricity was originally portrayed as a potential therapeutic modality, the measurement of body impedance was proposed as a useful diagnostic indicator for the physician.[1] This hypothesis led to the identification of physical maladies depicted as "low" impedance illnesses and other conditions characterized as "high" impedance conditions.[1] These early observations stimulated contemporary research to identify altered electrical conductivity as qualitative evidence of disturbed physiological status and to develop mathematical approaches that use BIA measurements to quantitate alterations in body components associated with pathology.

This presentation critically examines the various approaches that have been implemented for the use of BIA in clinical investigations. These approaches center on the development of physical models to translate electrical measurements into biological indexes that can be measured independently and thus used to validate the proposed models. These BIA prediction models also rely on the use of body composition assessment techniques

---

[a]The United States Department of Agriculture (USDA) prohibits discrimination in all its programs and activities on the basis of race, color, national origin, gender, religion, age, disability, political beliefs, sexual orientation, and marital or family status.

that may impact the validity of the BIA estimates. Because research initially focused on applications in healthy individuals, pertinent examples are presented to highlight the strengths and the weaknesses of these approaches when they have been implemented in patients with altered body composition. Where BIA has been shown to be ineffective, reasons for the limitations are described.

BIA MODELS OF BODY COMPOSITION VARIABLES

The impetus for the use of BIA to characterize biological structure and function came from Jan Nyboer,[1] who utilized a tetrapolar BIA method and applied basic physical principles to determine pulsatile blood flow in the body. Hoffer *et al.*[2] extended this pioneering work and showed that impedance was a useful indicator of total body water (TBW) in health and disease. These investigators provided some of the critical findings that fueled the development of BIA as a tool in clinical investigations.

Electrophysical Model: Total Body Water and Fat-Free Mass

Use of BIA to estimate TBW has relied on the electrophysical model, $V = \rho L^2/Z$. Impedance is measured by using a fixed frequency instrument (50 kHz) and stature is accepted as a surrogate for conductor length. This model has been used to develop prediction models for TBW and to cross validate the derived models in independent samples of healthy adults and children. These efforts resulted in excellent correspondence between measured and predicted TBW values, with variability estimates, defined as the standard error of the mean expressed as a percentage of the mean of the sample, ranging from 3% to 10%.[3,4]

Some of these prediction models have been used to estimate changes in TBW in patients with alterations in body water distribution. Studies in obese patients during weight loss or in patients with end stage renal disease have found inaccuracies of 2 to 8 L between BIA predictions and measured TBW values.[5-8] Two important factors contribute to these discrepancies.

The use of the electrophysical model depends on regression analysis to develop a prediction model. This approach, which relies on correlations between TBW and impedance components, is prone to error because of sample specificity. Differences in subject characteristics (i.e., sex, age, body weight, stature, and TBW) between the groups of subjects result in errors in the prediction of the dependent variable. The magnitude of the error depends on the differences between the group in whom the model is developed and the group in whom the model is applied.

A second limitation is the inability of whole body BIA to assess regional accumulation of fluid. Among patients with renal disease and undergoing paracentesis, BIA estimates of TBW are significantly less than values determined by weight change.[9] These differences are attributed to the fact that regions of the body with small diameters (i.e., lower arm and leg) contribute a larger proportion of the impedance while containing a smaller proportion of the whole body conductor, as compared to the torso, which is a low impedance area, but contains the majority of the body conductor.[10]

Other investigators, however, have not reported discrepancies between BIA predictions and reference measurements in obese adults during weight loss and in women during pregnancy and lactation.[11,12] These observations are explained by the use of volunteers with similar physical characteristics in the samples of subjects assigned to the model development and validation groups.

Fat-free mass (FFM) also has been estimated by using the electrophysical model. This approach was implemented because TBW has been shown to be a constant (72–73%) of the FFM in healthy adults.[13] This approach has been shown to yield variability estimates that range from 5% to 10%, which exceeds the errors associated with the methods.[4] This finding indicates that sample specificity limits the general application of the electrophysical model.

Multiple Frequency Models

Recognition of the limitations of the two-component model of body composition and anticipation that the use of more than one signal frequency might provide more precise indexes of body composition (i.e., intra- and extracellular water; ICW and ECW) lead to a modification of the electrophysical model. Jenin et al.[14] used specific low and high frequency current to estimate fluid distribution. They postulated that ECW would be predicted at 5 kHz and TBW at 1 MHz with both measured impedance values corrected for conductor length. Subsequently, other investigators[15,16] were unable to show that specific frequencies were unique predictors of ECW and TBW in healthy adults because correlation coefficients were similar across a broad range of frequencies (5 to 1200 kHz). The failure to identify specific signal frequencies to predict fluid distribution in healthy subjects apparently reflects a constant proportion of ECW to TBW in health.

Bioelectrical Impedance Spectroscopy (BIS)

An alternative to using fixed, multiple frequencies and linear regression modeling to predict conductor volumes is to model impedance data derived from scanning a wide range of frequencies. The impedance data are examined with the Cole model,[17] which permits the determination of ICW and ECW using an iterative procedure. The advantage of this approach is the possible delineation of multiple components of the body for an individual, and thus no reliance on group data for model development. The BIS method has been used in clinical populations and shown to yield estimates of TBW and ECW consistent with isotope dilution methods.[18]

Parallel Model

Recognition that body conductor components (cell membranes, ICW, ECW, and FFM) exist in series and parallel configurations in the body prompted the use of a parallel, as compared to a series, electrical model to estimate body composition. Preliminary studies in which a potato was measured with a 50-kHz BIA device before and after cooking support the use of the parallel model.[19] It was shown that resistance and impedance decreased significantly (70–80%) and reactance decreased to 0, with no change in weight, after cooking the potato. The lack of measurement of reactance after cooking suggested that the cell wall was destroyed. This finding led to the hypothesis that reactance may be an index of ICW, resistance reflects ECW, and impedance indicates TBW. Studies of HIV-infected patients indicate that the parallel transformation of reactance is an accurate and sensitive indicator of body cell mass (BCM).[20,21] This approach also has been used to successfully monitor the nutritional status of patients on chronic hemodialysis.[22]

Regional BIA

Insensitivity of distal electrode placements to detect changes in regional fluid accumulation has promoted the use of regional electrode placements. One interesting application of regional BIA measurements is the determination of upper arm muscle mass.[23] This technique was shown to provide a more accurate determination of muscle mass than anthropometry. Similarly, studies in swine indicate the validity and accuracy of transthoracic impedance measurements to measure extravascular lung water.[24]

SUMMARY AND CONCLUSIONS

The BIA method offers many opportunities for noninvasive assessment of human body composition in clinical investigations and patient care. Initial results with the single frequency, electrophysical model emphasized limitations associated with regression modeling and sample specificity. Similarly, the use of fixed frequency applied current provided no significant advantage for body composition assessment. Recent evidence supports the use of BIS and the parallel model for use in patients with altered fluid distributions (i.e., expanded ECW or decreased BCM). These approaches provide accurate estimates of body composition, in part because they rely on complex body composition models (i.e., three components) that are independent of assumptions regarding body water distribution.

Additional studies are required to further establish the validity, sensitivity, specificity, and accuracy of these approaches. These approaches should be examined in controlled, longitudinal studies of patients with catabolic diseases to establish the prognostic value of these BIA methods.

REFERENCES

1. KING, W. H. 1901. Electricity in Medicine and Surgery. Boericke & Runyon. New York; NYBOER, J. 1970. Electrical Impedance Plethysmography. Second edition. Thomas. Springfield, Illinois.
2. HOFFER, E. C., C. K. MEADOW & D. C. SIMPSON. 1969. Correlation of whole body impedance with total body water volume. J. Appl. Physiol. **27:** 531–534.
3. LUKASKI, H. C. 1991. Assessment of body composition using tetrapolar bioelectrical impedance analysis. *In* New Techniques in Nutritional Research, p. 303–317. Academic Press. New York.
4. BAUMGARTNER, R. N. 1996. Electrical impedance and total body electrical conductivity. *In* Human Body Composition, p. 79–108. Human Kinetics. Champaign, Illinois.
5. DEURENBERG, P., J. A. WESTRATE & K. VAN DER KOY. 1989. Body composition changes by bioelectrical impedance measurements. Am. J. Clin. Nutr. **49:** 401–403.

6. GRAY, D. S. 1988. Changes in bioelectrical impedance during fasting. Am. J. Clin. Nutr. **48:** 1184–1187.
7. GUGLIELMI, F. W., F. CONTENTO, L. LADDAGA, C. PANELLA & A. FRANCAVILLA. 1991. Bioelectric impedance analysis: experience with male patients with cirrhosis. Hepatology **13:** 892–895.
8. MCCULLOUGH, A. J., K. D. MULLEN & S. C. KALHAN. 1991. Measurements of total body water and extracellular water in cirrhotic patients with and without ascites. Hepatology **14:** 1102–1111.
9. ZILLIKENS, M. C., J. W. VAN DEN BERG, J. H. WILSON & G. R. SWART. 1992. Whole body and segmental bioelectrical impedance analysis in patients with cirrhosis of the liver: changes after treatment of ascites. Am. J. Clin. Nutr. **55:** 621–625.
10. LUKASKI, H. C. & M. R. M. SCHELTINGA. 1996. Improved sensitivity of the tetrapolar bioelectrical impedance method to assess fluid status and body composition: use of proximal electrode placements. Age Nutr. **5:** 123–129.
11. KUSHNER, R. F., A. KUNIGK, M. ALSPAUGH, P. T. ANDRONIS, C. A. LEITCH & D. A. SCHOELLER. 1990. Validation of bioelectrical impedance analysis as a measurement of change in body composition in obesity. Am. J. Clin. Nutr. **52:** 219–223.
12. LUKASKI, H. C., W. A. SIDERS, E. J. NIELSEN & C. B. HALL. 1994. Total body water in pregnancy: assessment using bioelectrical impedance. Am. J. Clin. Nutr. **59:** 578–585.
13. LUKASKI, H. C., P. E. JOHNSON, W. W. BOLONCHUK & G. I. LYKKEN. 1985. Assessment of fat-free mass using bioelectrical impedance analysis. Am. J. Clin. Nutr. **41:** 810–817.
14. JENIN, P., J. LENOIR, C. ROULETTE & A. THOMASSET. 1975. Determination of body fluid compartments by electrical impedance measurements. Aviat. Space Environ. Med. **46:** 152–155.
15. VAN LOAN, M. D. & P. L. MAYCLIN. 1992. Use of multifrequency bioelectrical impedance analysis for the estimation of extracellular fluid. Eur. J. Clin. Nutr. **46:** 117–124.
16. DEURENBERG, P. & F. J. M. SCHOUTEN. 1992. Loss of total body water and extracellular water assessed by multifrequency impedance. Eur. J. Clin. Nutr. **46:** 247–255.
17. COLE, K. S. 1972. Membranes, Ions and Impulses: A Chapter of Classical Physics. UCLA Press. Los Angeles.
18. VAN MARKEN LICHTENBELT, W. D., Y. E. M. SNEL, R. J. M. BRUMMER & H. P. F. KOPPESCHAAR. 1997. Deuterium and bromide dilution and bioimpedance spectrometry independently show that growth hormone deficient adults have an enlarged extracellular water compartment related to intracellular water. J. Clin. Endocrinol. Metab. **82:** 907–911.
19. LUKASKI, H. C. 1996. Biological indexes considered in the derivation of the bioelectrical impedance analysis. Am. J. Clin. Nutr. **64**(suppl.): 397S–404S.
20. OTT, M., H. FISCHER, H. POLAT, E. B. HELM, M. FRENZ, W. F. CASPARY & B. LEMBCKE. 1995. Bioelectrical impedance analysis as a predictor of survival in patients with human immunodeficiency virus infection. J. Acquired Immune Defic. Syndr. Hum. Retrovirol. **9:** 20–25.
21. KOTLER, D. P., S. BURASTERO, J. WANG & R. N. PIERSON. 1996. Prediction of body cell mass, fat free mass, and total body water with bioelectrical impedance analysis: effects of race, sex, and disease. Am. J. Clin. Nutr. **64**(suppl.): 489S–497S.
22. CHERTOW, G. M., E. G. LOWRIE, D. W. WILMORE, J. GONZALEZ, N. L. LEW, J. LING, M. S. LEBOFF, M. N. GOTTLIEB, W. HUANG, B. ZEBROWSKI, J. COLLEGE & J. M. LAZARUS. 1995. Nutritional assessment with bioelectrical impedance analysis in maintenance hemodialysis patients. J. Am. Soc. Nephrol. **6:** 75–81.
23. BROWN, B. H., T. KARATZAS, R. NAKIELNY & R. G. CLARKE. 1988. Determination of upper arm muscle mass and fat areas using electrical impedance measurements. Clin. Phys. Physiol. Meas. **9:** 47–55.
24. NIERMAN, D. M., D. I. EISEN, E. D. FEIN, F. HANNON, J. I. MECHANICK & E. BENJAMIN. 1996. Transthoracic bioimpedance can measure extravascular lung water in acute lung injury. J. Surg. Res. **65:** 101–108.

Study of the Relation between Fluid Distribution Change in Tissue and Impedance Change during Hemodialysis by Frequency Characteristics of the Flowing Blood

K. SAKAMOTO,[a] R. SUNAGA,[a] K. NAKAMURA,[a] Y. SATO,[a] M. FUJII,[b] H. KANAI,[b] T. TSUCHIDA,[c] A. UENO,[c] N. KANAI,[d] AND K. HASEGAWA[d]

[a]*Department of Clinical Engineering, School of Allied Sciences, Kitasato University, Kanagawa 228, Japan*

[b]*Department of Electrical and Electronics Engineering, Sophia University, Tokyo 102, Japan*

[c]*Department of Urology*

[d]*Department of Pharmacology, Yamanashi Medical School, Yamanashi, Japan*

ABSTRACT: Erythrocyte orientation and deformation cause differences in impedance between flowing and resting blood. Through theoretical calculation and experimental measurements, we studied the effects of these factors on blood impedance. The size and shape of the erythrocyte and the conductivity of the interior medium of the erythrocyte change when the osmotic pressure of plasma is changed. From experimental results, we obtained the following: when the size of the erythrocyte becomes larger than the normal size due to the osmotic pressure change, the β dispersion frequency decreases and the intra- and extracellular fluid resistance increase. These experimental results corroborate that the change of tissue impedance like muscle impedance during hemodialysis is caused by the change of the fluid distribution and the change of ionic concentration of the electrolyte in tissues during hemodialysis. Also, we could estimate the relative change value of the intra- and extracellular fluid volume by the impedance method, if there were no ionic concentration change in the electrolyte. It would be very difficult to estimate the absolute change value of them because a shadow effect due to the cells depends greatly upon the shape and size of the cells and the cell concentration.

INTRODUCTION

It is very important to monitor the fluid distribution change during artificial dialysis because one of the most likely causes of the symptoms that patients sometimes suffer from (headaches, vomiting, hypotension, etc.) during and after hemodialysis has been that the fluid osmotically shifts from the extracellular to the intracellular compartment. So far, a method of measuring continuously the fluid shifts during hemodialysis has not been available. When the fluid shifts into the intracellular compartment from the extracellular compartment, the intracellular fluid volume resistance decreases and the extracellular fluid volume resistance increases.[1,2] Therefore, the impedance method is expected to measure the fluid shift in tissues. However, this hypothesis has not been corroborated yet. Most erythrocytes rotate and deform themselves in the flow direction when blood (of which the hematocrit is low, like 10) flows in a tube. Deformation is negligible when the shear rate is less than about 200 s^{-1}.[3] When the hematocrit is higher than about 20, the erythrocytes cannot rotate, but they do orient to the flow direction. Therefore, the electrical properties of the flowing blood are anisotropic and can be easily analyzed theoretically.

Here, we tried to corroborate the hypothesis mentioned above theoretically and experimentally by using the flowing blood.

THEORY

From the electrical viewpoint, an erythrocyte can be represented by an ellipsoid with a thin membrane as shown in FIGURE 1.[4] The complex dielectric constant of an erythrocyte with thin membrane is given by equation 1:

$$\varepsilon_\alpha^* = \frac{2\varepsilon_M^* + (\varepsilon^* - \varepsilon_M^*)a_1 b_1 c_1 \left[\int_0^\sigma \frac{d\lambda}{(\lambda + \alpha_1^2) R_1(\lambda)} + \frac{2}{a_2 b_2 c_2} \right]}{2\varepsilon_M^* + (\varepsilon^* - \varepsilon_M^*)a_1 b_1 c_1 \int_0^\sigma \frac{d\lambda}{(\lambda + \alpha_1^2) R_1(\lambda)}} \varepsilon_M^*, \quad (1)$$

$$R_1(\lambda) = \{(\lambda + a_1^2)(\lambda + b_1^2)(\lambda + c_1^2)\}^{\frac{1}{2}},$$

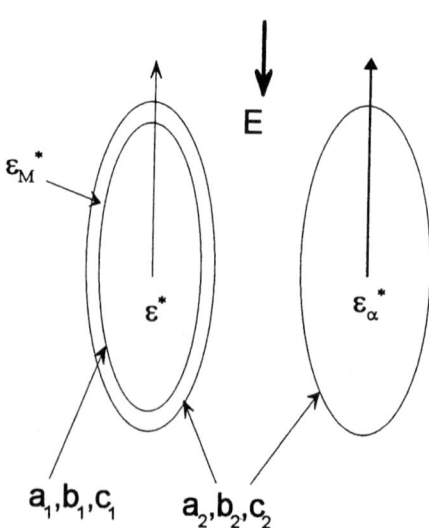

FIGURE 1. Model of the erythrocyte. E: electrical field strength.

$$\alpha_1 = a_1, b_1, c_1,$$

$$\sigma = a_2^2 - a_1^2 = b_2^2 - b_1^2 = c_2^2 - c_1^2,$$

$$b_1 = c_1, \quad b_2 = c_2,$$

where ε^*, ε_α^*, and ε_M^* are the complex dielectric constants of the erythrocyte interior medium, the erythrocyte, and the membrane, respectively; and a, b, and c are the respective half-lengths of the principal axes of the ellipsoid. Even though the conductivity and the dielectric constants ε^* and ε_M^* are constant, they do not depend upon the frequency of the supplied field under a few MHz; thus, ε_α^* has the frequency dependence. Specifically, the complex dielectric constant of the erythrocyte shows a β dispersion phenomenon that is related to the dielectric constant of the membrane, the conductivity of the erythrocyte interior medium, the thickness of the membrane, and the shape and size of the erythrocyte.

In order to obtain the complex dielectric constant ε^* of the erythrocyte interior medium, we should consider the effect of hemoglobin, which can be assumed to be an electrical insulator and spherical suspension. ε^* is given by equation 2:

$$\varepsilon^* = \varepsilon_p^* \left[1 + \frac{2\rho_h \left(\frac{\varepsilon_h^*}{\varepsilon_p^*} - 1 \right)}{2\rho_h + (1 - \rho_h) \left\{ 2 + L \left(\frac{\varepsilon_h^*}{\varepsilon_p^*} - 1 \right) \right\}} \right] \quad (2)$$

$$(L = 0.667)$$

where ε_p^*, ε_h^*, and ρ_h are the complex dielectric constants of saline and hemoglobin and the volume concentration of hemoglobin, respectively. ε^* can be rewritten by the complex conductivity σ^* of the erythrocyte interior medium, as in equation 2':

$$\varepsilon^* = \frac{\sigma^*}{j\omega\varepsilon_0} = \frac{1}{j\omega\varepsilon_0 \rho^*} \quad (2')$$

where ρ^* and ε_0 are the complex resistivity of the erythrocyte interior medium and the dielectric constant, respectively.

If all erythrocytes are oriented to the supplied electrical field direction, the complex dielectric constant of blood ε_B^* is given by equation 3:

$$\varepsilon_{B,\theta}^* = \varepsilon_p^* \left[1 + \frac{2\rho_B \left(\frac{\varepsilon^*}{\varepsilon_p^*} - 1 \right)}{2\rho_B + (1 - \rho_B) \left\{ 2 + L_\theta \left(\frac{\varepsilon^*}{\varepsilon_p^*} - 1 \right) \right\}} \right], \quad (3)$$

$$\theta = a_2, b_2, c_2,$$

$$L_\theta = \int_0^\infty \frac{d\lambda}{(\theta^2 + \lambda)R(\lambda)},$$

where $\varepsilon^*_{B,\theta}$ and ρ_B are the complex dielectric constants of the blood and hematocrit. Note that θ is the axis of the ellipsoid that is parallel to the supplied electrical field. When the axis ratio $a/b = 1, 0.9$, and 0.8, $L_0 = 0.667, 0.638$, and 0.606, respectively. It is experimentally confirmed that equation 3 is available until about a value of 50 of hematocrit.[3]

When the blood of low hematocrit flows steadily and laminarly in a tube, the erythrocytes rotate not at random, but predictably. However, when the hematocrit is high, the long axis of the erythrocytes orients along the stream line without rotation. Therefore, if the supplied electric field is parallel to the stream line of the flowing blood, the complex dielectric constant of the flowing blood is theoretically given by equation 3. When the long axis b of all erythrocytes is parallel to the electric field, the complex dielectric constant of the flowing blood is given by equation 4:

$$\varepsilon^*_{B,b} = \varepsilon_{B,b} + \frac{\sigma_{B,b}}{j\omega\varepsilon_0} \tag{4}$$

where $\varepsilon_{B,b}$ and $\sigma_{B,b}$ are the dielectric constant and conductivity of blood, respectively.

The complex dielectric constant locus of the flowing blood shows a semicircle that cuts diametrically across the real axis of the complex dielectric constant plane in two singular points corresponding respectively to the low and high frequency limit of the β dispersion. The low frequency limit of the dispersion is related to the conductivity of the extracellular medium, and the high frequency limit of the dispersion is related to the conductivity of the intra- and extracellular medium. Therefore, the diameter of the complex dielectric constant locus is related to the conductivity of the intracellular medium. The time constant of the β

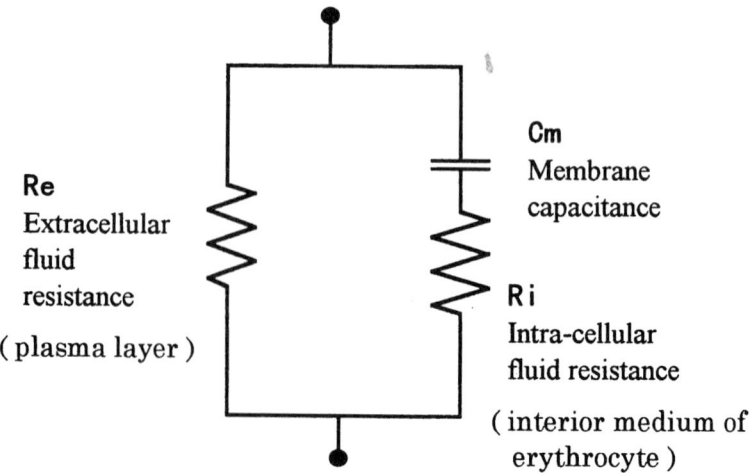

FIGURE 2. Electrical equivalent circuit of the flowing blood (three-element model).

dispersion (structural relaxation), T_0, is single. The value of T_0 is the same as that of the erythrocyte and is determined by the conductivity of the erythrocyte interior medium, the dielectric constant of the erythrocyte membrane, and the shape and size of the erythrocyte. On the other hand, since the erythrocytes in the resting blood randomly orient to the supplied electric field, the time constant of the structural relaxation T_0 is distributed. The characteristic frequency f_0 of the β dispersion is $1/2\pi T_0$.

When blood flows in a circular tube in parallel to the direction of the supplied electrical field, the measured admittance of the flowing blood Y is given by equation 5:

$$Y = j\omega\varepsilon_0 \varepsilon^*_{B,b} \frac{S}{l} = G + j\omega B, \tag{5}$$

$$G = \sigma_{B,b} \frac{S}{l},$$

$$B = \varepsilon_0 \varepsilon_{B,b} \frac{S}{l},$$

where S/l, G, and B show the area/length of the circular tube, the conductance, and the susceptance, respectively. Since the admittance locus shows a semicircle and the time constant of the admittance is single, it can be easily understood that the electrical characteristics of Y are completely shown by the simplified equivalent electrical circuit as in FIGURE 2. Here, Re, Ri, and C_m are the extra- and intracellular fluid volume resistance and the membrane capacitance, respectively. Re and Ri correspond respectively to the reciprocal value of the low and high frequency limit of Y and are given by the following equations:

$$\frac{1}{R_e} = Y_0, \quad \frac{1}{R_e} + \frac{1}{R_i} = Y_\infty; \quad \text{therefore,} \quad \frac{1}{R_i} = Y_\infty - Y_0 \tag{6}$$

where Y_0 and Y_∞ are the admittances when the frequency is zero and infinite, respectively. In this case, the time constant of the structural relaxation T_0 is obtained by multiplying Ri and C_m. At the β dispersion frequency $f_0 \left(\frac{1}{2\pi T_0}\right)$, the imaginary part of the admittance of this circuit becomes maximum.

Furthermore, when the frequency of the supplied current is higher than about 10 MHz, we should take Debye-type dispersion due to hemoglobin into consideration.[5] Equation 7 shows Debye-type dispersion:

$$\rho^* = \rho_\infty + \frac{\rho_0 - \rho_\infty}{1 + j\omega T}, \tag{7}$$

$$\sigma^* = \frac{1}{\rho_\infty} + \frac{\frac{1}{\rho_0} - \frac{1}{\rho_\infty}}{1 + j\omega T\left(\frac{\rho_\infty}{\rho_0}\right)}, \tag{7'}$$

where T is the time constant. In this case, the impedance locus shows a semicircle where the center is on the real axis of the complex impedance. Therefore, it will cut diametrically across the real axis of the complex impedance plane in two singular points corresponding respectively to the low (ρ_0) and high (ρ_∞) frequency limit of the dispersion. The complex conductivity σ^* of the erythrocyte interior medium in equation 2 must be rewritten by σ^* in equation 7′. At low frequency, σ^* in equation 2 is equal to that in equation 7′. Then, by separating the dielectric constant of water, the complex dielectric constant of saline solution ε_p^* in equations 2 and 3 is rewritten by equation 8:

$$\varepsilon_p^* = \varepsilon_w + \frac{\sigma_p}{j\omega\varepsilon_0} \tag{8}$$

where σ_p is the conductivity of the saline solution.

EXPERIMENTAL PROCEDURE

The size and shape of the erythrocyte were measured with a multisizer (Coulter Scientific Instruments) and microscope (Olympus 1X70) as soon as possible after blood was extracted from the donor. At the same time, we produced test blood A, B, and C by centrifuging the blood and pouring a constant amount of erythrocytes into a constant volume of 0.9%, 0.72%, and 0.54% NaCl solutions, respectively. Here, the term "plasma" indicates the NaCl solution, and the term "initial plasma" indicates the plasma before being poured into the erythrocytes. The conductivity of the initial plasma at low frequency and the frequency characteristics of the plasma admittance were measured with a conductance meter (ES-14, 3582, Horiba Co.) and LCR meter (HP Co. 4284A), respectively. After the osmotic pressure came to equilibrium, the erythrocyte size and shape in the test blood were measured again with the multisizer and microscope.

The admittance of the flowing test blood was measured with the LCR meter (HP Co. 4284A). The measurement frequency range is from 75 kHz to 30 MHz. The temperature of blood was 22 ± 0.5 °C. The measurement cell is shown in FIGURE 3. Blood flows in a small channel that is 22 mm in length and 2 mm in diameter. The electrodes were 15 mm in diameter. In the frequency range lower than 100 kHz, the effect of electrode polarization impedance is less than 0.2%. Since the effect of polarization decreases with the increasing of measurement current frequency, the measurement error by the electrode polarization is negligible over the measurement frequency range. The shear rate of the blood flow is about 200/s.

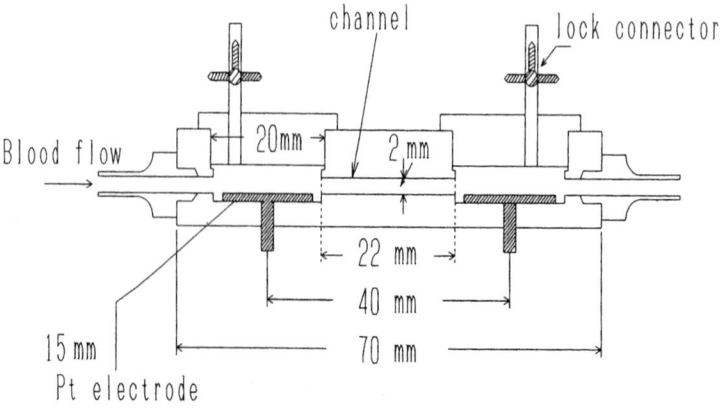

FIGURE 3. Measurement cell.

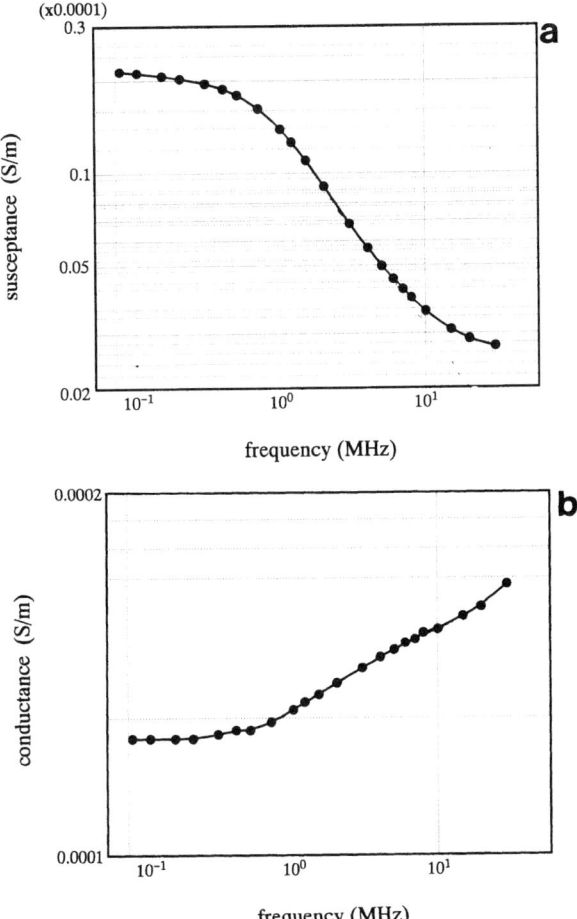

FIGURE 4. Experimental results: (a) frequency characteristics of susceptance of the flowing blood and (b) conductance.

EVALUATION OF Re, Ri, ERYTHROCYTE SIZE, AND HEMATOCRIT

In order to compare the experimental results with the theoretical results, blood impedance and admittance between 75 kHz and 30 MHz were calculated from equations 1 to 8. From the calculated admittance, a Cole-Cole semicircle was obtained. Re and Ri were theoretically determined from the admittance at 50 kHz and 100 MHz without considering the effects of Debye-type dispersion and permittivity of water. The electrical parameters used for calculation are shown in the following paragraph.

The dielectric constant, conductivity, and thickness of membrane are 12, 10^{-3} S/m, and 10 nm, respectively. The dielectric constant of water is 50 and the conductivity of the 0.9%

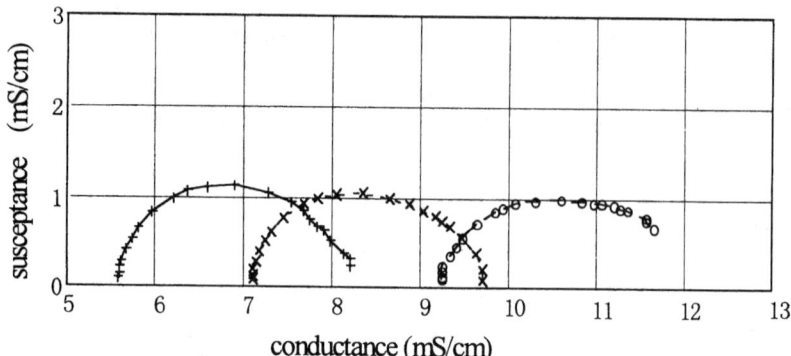

FIGURE 5. The admittance locus obtained experimentally: +, 0.54%; ×, 0.72%; ○; 0.9% NaCl solution.

saline solution is 1.67 S/m. The characteristic frequency of Debye-type dispersion is 190 MHz and ρ_∞ is 0.2 Ω-m.

Since all of the osmotic pressures of test blood A, B, and C came to equilibrium, the following holds true: by making the conductivity of plasma, the size of the erythrocyte, and the hematocrit of test blood A as the standard, erythrocyte size and hematocrit in test blood B and C can be calculated from the equilibrium condition of the osmotic pressure.

RESULTS AND DISCUSSION

FIGURES 4a and 4b show the frequency characteristics of the susceptance and conductance of flowing test blood A. It is obvious that the conductance gradually increases and the susceptance reaches up to some value over 7 MHz. Gradual increasing of conductance is mainly caused by Debye-type dispersion due to hemoglobin. The susceptance of the test blood reaches the susceptance due to the permittivity of water. The effect of the permittivity of water can be easily eliminated from the frequency characteristics of the plasma. However, it is very difficult to eliminate the effect of Debye-type dispersion. FIGURE 5 shows the admittance locus experimentally obtained. These results were obtained by eliminating the effect of the permittivity of water. Over 7 MHz, the admittance loci are distorted because the conductivity is gradually changing due to the effect of Debye-type dispersion. We could find that the effect of Debye-type dispersion on the susceptance is much smaller than that of the permittivity of water. Since all of the admittance loci show a part of the semicircle in the frequency range from 75 kHz to about 7 MHz, we can obtain the β dispersion frequency without any effects of Debye-type dispersion and the permittivity of water mentioned above. The measured β dispersion frequencies for flowing test blood A, B, and C are 3.2 MHz, 2.8 MHz, and 2.6 MHz, respectively. The theoretical β dispersion frequencies for flowing test blood A, B, and C are 3.3 MHz, 2.87 MHz, and 2.5 MHz, respectively. These theoretical results agree well with the experimental results.

From the measurement results of the admittance of the resting blood and the flowing blood, we recognized that the admittance of the resting blood was about 2% less than that

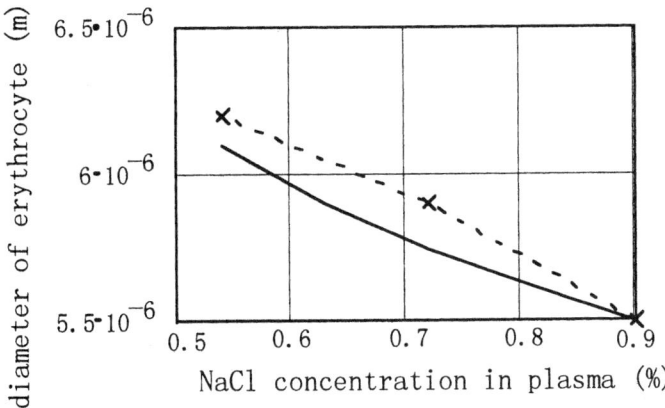

FIGURE 6. Diameter change of the erythrocyte due to the NaCl concentration change in plasma. The solid line shows the theoretical value. The broken line shows the experimental results.

of the flowing blood. This difference of admittance corresponds to the fact that the ratio of the long axis and short axis of the erythrocyte is about 0.9.

FIGURE 6 shows the relation between the NaCl concentration of the initial plasma and the size of the erythrocytes measured with the multisizer and microscope and calculated theoretically. The size of the erythrocytes in test blood C, B, and A is about 6.2 mm, 5.9 mm, and 5.5 mm, respectively. The calculated size of the erythrocytes for test blood C and B is about 6.1 mm and 5.7 mm, respectively. These values agree well with those of the experimental results.

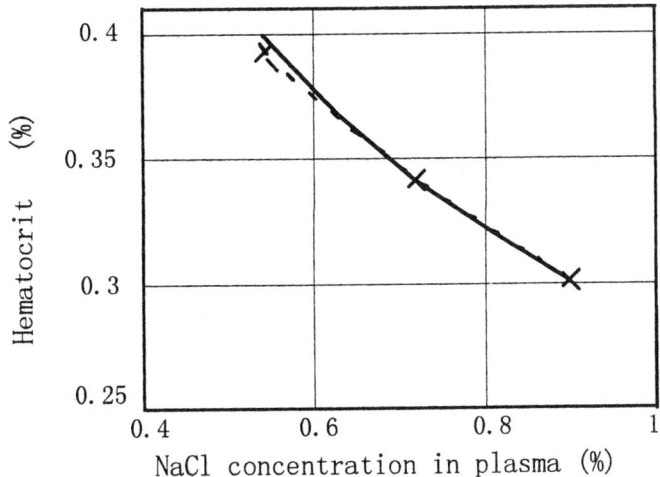

FIGURE 7. Hematocrit change due to the NaCl concentration change in plasma. The solid line shows the theoretical value. The broken line shows the experimental results.

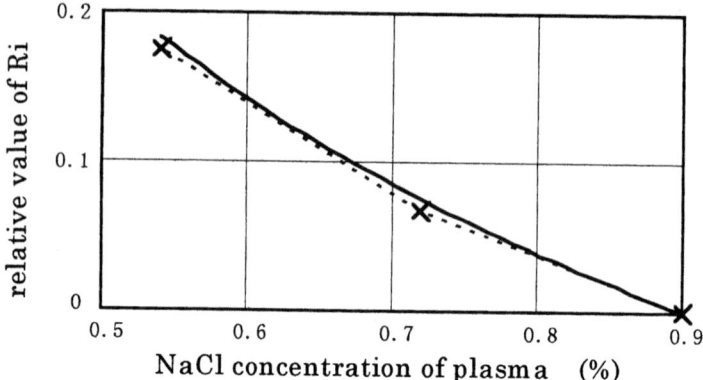

FIGURE 8. Relative change rate of Ri due to the change of NaCl concentration in plasma. The solid line shows the calculated results. The broken line shows the experimental results.

As shown in FIGURE 7, the hematocrit values for test blood C, B, and A were 39%, 34%, and 30%. Under the same assumption, the calculated hematocrit values were 40% and 34% for test blood C and B, respectively. These also agree well with those of the experimental results.

From these theoretical and experimental results, it is obvious that the size of the erythrocyte changes due to the water shifts from the plasma into the erythrocyte in order that osmotic pressure comes to equilibrium. Since the osmotic pressure in all test blood comes to equilibrium after shifting some water in the initial plasma into the erythrocyte, the conductivity of the plasma and the interior medium of the erythrocyte will change.

FIGURE 8 shows the relation between the change rate of Ri of the flowing blood and the NaCl concentration of the initial plasma. Ri increases with the increasing of the erythrocyte size. The theoretical result also agrees well with the experimental result. Since the

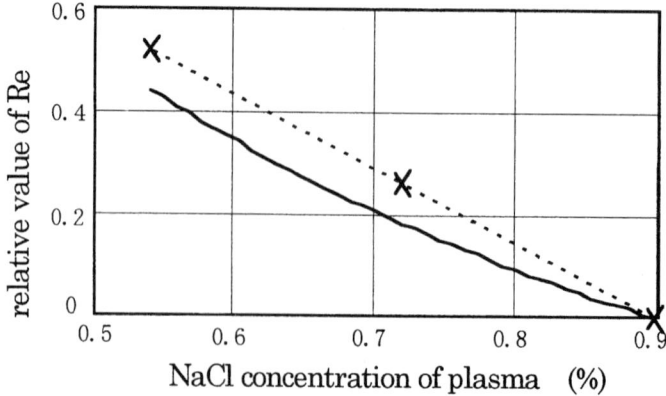

FIGURE 9. Relative change rate of Re due to the change of NaCl concentration in plasma. The solid line shows the calculated results. The broken line shows the experimental results.

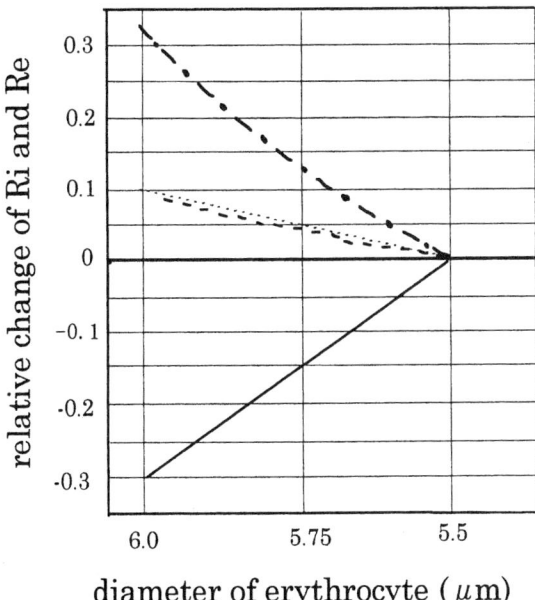

FIGURE 10. Calculated Ri and Re change rates due to the change of erythrocyte diameter (volume change of erythrocyte). There is no change in NaCl concentration in the plasma and interior medium of the erythrocyte: (—) Ri change rate, (···) Re change rate, (---) radius change of erythrocyte, (-·-·-) volume change of erythrocyte.

conductivity of the interior medium of the erythrocyte decreases with the water shifted from plasma, even though the erythrocyte size increases, Ri increases.

FIGURE 9 shows the relation between the change rate of Re of the flowing blood and the NaCl concentration of the initial plasma. Re increases with the increasing of the erythrocyte size. The theoretical result also agrees well with the experimental result. Even though the conductivity of the plasma layer increases due to some water in the plasma shifting into the erythrocyte, Re increases because the hematocrit increases and the plasma layer decreases. From these results, it is obvious that the change of Ri is due to the change of erythrocyte size and ionic concentration of the interior medium and that of Re is due to the change of hematocrit and ionic concentration of the plasma: namely, the changes of Ri and Re are greatly related to the shifted water volume.

In order to discuss the relation between the changes of Re and Ri and the volume changes of plasma and erythrocyte without any ionic concentration change in the plasma and in the interior medium of the erythrocyte, the changes of Ri and Re due to the size change of the erythrocyte, namely, the shifted water volume, were calculated for hematocrit of 30. The relation between the calculated relative changes of Ri and Re and the change of erythrocyte diameter is shown in FIGURE 10. In this figure, the relative changes of the diameter and volume of the erythrocyte are also shown.

We observe that the change rate of Ri corresponds to the change rate of the erythrocyte volume and that the change rate of Re corresponds to the change rate of the erythrocyte diameter. It will be feasible to estimate the relative change of the distribution of intra- and extracellular fluid volume of tissue from the change rate of the tissue impedance.

Since the shadow effect is dependent upon the shape, size, and concentration of cells in the extracellular fluid, it is obvious that the shadow effect for cells such as muscle fiber will be different from that of erythrocyte and spherical cells. In this case, the relation between the change rate of Re and Ri and the diameter change or volume change of cells differs slightly from the results shown in FIGURE 9. Therefore, it would be difficult to estimate the absolute value of the fluid distribution change in tissue by the impedance method.

CONCLUSIONS

We can conclude the following:

(1) the admittance locus of the flowing blood shows a semicircle in the frequency range from 75 kHz to about 7 MHz;

(2) Ri and Re are related not only to the ionic concentration of the electrolyte, but also to the volume of intra- and extracellular fluid;

(3) if there were no change in the ionic concentration of the electrolyte, we could estimate the fluid distribution change in tissue from the tissue impedance change;

(4) it is hard to estimate the absolute change of the fluid distribution in tissue by the impedance method.

ACKNOWLEDGMENT

This work was supported by the National Science Foundation.

REFERENCES

1. KANAI, H. *et al.* 1987. Electrical measurement of fluid distribution in legs and arms. Med. Prog. Tech. **12:** 159–170.
2. MEIJER, J. *et al.* 1989. Measurement of transcellular fluid shift during hemodialysis. Med. Biol. Eng. Comput. **27:** 147.
3. SAKAMOTO, K. *et al.* 1979. Electrical characteristics of flowing blood. IEEE Trans. Biomed. Eng. **BME-26**(12): 686–695.
4. SCHWARZ, G. *et al.* 1965. On the orientation of nonspherical particles in an alternating electrical field. J. Chem. Phys. **43**(10): 3562–3570.
5. JENIN, P. C. *et al.* 1980. Some observations on the dielectric properties of hemoglobin's suspending medium inside human erythrocytes. Biophys. J. **30:** 285–294.

Bioimpedance: Is It a Predictor of True Water Volume?

B. J. THOMAS,[a] B. H. CORNISH,[a] L. C. WARD,[b] AND A. JACOBS[a]

[a]*Center for Medical and Health Physics, Queensland University of Technology, Brisbane, Queensland 4001, Australia*

[b]*Department of Biochemistry, University of Queensland, St. Lucia, Brisbane, Queensland, Australia*

ABSTRACT: Bioelectrical impedance analysis (BIA) has been reported to be insensitive to changes in water volumes in individual subjects. This study was designed to investigate the effect on the intra- and extracellular resistances (Ri and Re) of the segments of subjects for whom body water was changed without significant change to the total amount of electrolyte in the respective fluids. Twelve healthy adult subjects were recruited. Ri and Re of the leg, trunk, and arm of the subjects were determined from BIA measures prior to commencement of two separate studies that involved intervention, resulting in a loss/gain of body water effected either by a sauna followed by water intake (study 1) or by ingestion (study 2). Ri and Re of the segments were also determined at a number of times following these interventions. The mean change in body water, expressed as a percentage of body weight, was 0.9% in study 1 and 1.25% in study 2. For each study, the results for each subject were normalized for each limb to the initial (prestudy) value and then the normalized results for each segment were pooled for all subjects. ANOVA of these pooled results failed to demonstrate any significant differences between the normalized mean values of Ri or Re of the segments measured through the course of each study. The failure to detect a change in Ri or Re is explained in terms of the basic theory of BIA.

INTRODUCTION

One of the basic physical principles supporting the use of bioelectrical impedance analysis (BIA) to measure body water is that the volume of a conducting cylinder is given by

$$V = \rho \times L^2 / R \qquad (1)$$

where L is the length, R is the resistance (or impedance) of the cylinder, and ρ is the resistivity of the conductor. The "conventional" application of BIA, for estimation of body-water volumes, uses equation 1 with substitution of the measured wrist-to-ankle resistance (or impedance) and the height of the subject as the conducting length, L. The constant of proportionality, ρ, is most commonly obtained from calibration of the BIA technique against a gold standard for body-water volume estimation, usually isotope dilution.[1] A less common approach is to insert into equation 1 a value for the resistivity obtained *in vitro*.[2]

Cha and Hill[3] reported that BIA has "limitations for quantifying fluid compartments in the trunk and thus in the whole body." Likewise, others have noted that the wrist-to-ankle methodology is insensitive to changes in the volume of trunk water and postulate that this insensitivity is a result of the fact that the wrist-to-ankle resistance is dominated by the resistance of the limbs, whereas the trunk contains by far the major component of total body water.[4] A modification of the wrist-to-ankle methodology in which the resistances of the leg(s), arm(s), and trunk are measured separately (the segmental methodology) has been proposed to overcome this problem.[5] However, the question still remains as to whether the measurement of bioimpedance can detect changes in body-water volumes when the increase/decrease in water volume is not associated with a corresponding increase/decrease in electrolytes.

The present paper reports the results of a study designed to investigate the efficacy of BIA measurements to detect changes in resistance, and hence body water when the fluid lost/gained is essentially pure water, that is, not containing electrolytes in isotonic concentrations.

THEORY/PHYSICAL PRINCIPLE

The theory of BIA has been well described in the literature (see, for example, reference 6) and hence only a very brief description of aspects relevant to the present study will be provided here.

The equivalent circuit representing biological tissue is considered as parallel branches: the extra- and intracellular pathways. In the last decade, analysis of bioimpedance data obtained at a number of frequencies has been used to obtain the resistances of these pathways (Re and Ri). The values of Re and Ri can be substituted into equation 1 to estimate the extra- and intracellular compartment volumes of body water, respectively.[7]

METHODS

Twelve healthy adult subjects (9 M, 3 F) were recruited for the study. The principal aim of the study was to investigate the effect of water loss/gain on the impedance of the segments (arms, legs, and trunk) of the body. The changes in impedance of the segments of the subjects were measured in two separate aspects of the study that involved loss/gain of (essentially) pure water. The loss/gain resulted from

(1) ingestion of water (1 liter/80 kg body weight);

(2) an extended period (30–45 minutes) in a sauna followed by rehydration by ingestion of water—the quantity of water was equal to the weight lost as a result of the sauna.

The participation of each subject in the two aspects of the study was separated by a minimum of three days.

In both aspects of the study, the impedance and phase of the right leg, right arm, trunk, and total body (wrist-to-ankle) of each subject were measured at 124 logarithmically spaced frequencies between 4 kHz and 1 MHz at the following times:

(1) at the commencement of the study, that is, prior to ingestion of water or to entering the sauna;

(2) 30 minutes after exiting the sauna [study (2) only];

(3) immediately following ingestion of the water;

(4–6) at 20-minute intervals thereafter for a period of 1 hour.

Each BIA measurement set was begun less than 5 minutes after the subject adopted a supine position. Subjects were permitted to move about freely between measurements. The subjects were not permitted to void nor to have food or fluid intake, other than the quantity described above, during the course of each study.

The electrode positions used were those proposed by Organ et al.[5] for the segmental methodology. The data were analyzed using the Cole-Cole approach,[7] and Ri and Re were obtained for each segment at the times indicated above.

Posture has been previously demonstrated to effect segmental and total body bioimpedance.[8] Since the protocol for this study required subjects to repeatedly adopt a supine position, there was some concern that the protocol itself might contribute to changes in fluid redistribution and thus alter the impedance of the segments. Hence, the protocol of the measurement of bioimpedance was repeated for a control group comprising eight subjects, without the concomitant change in body water effected either by ingestion or through a period in a sauna.

Ri and Re measured for each segment were normalized to the initial value for that segment for each subject, and the normalized results for all subjects were pooled to provide mean values at each of the measurement times.

Analysis of variance (ANOVA) was used to test the significance of differences between the (normalized) mean values of the impedance for each segment at times 1 to 6 of the protocol indicated earlier.

RESULTS

The p values resulting from ANOVA of the normalized mean values of Re and Ri determined for each segment at times 1 to 6 indicated in the protocol are presented in TABLE 1.

The Control Group (the Effect of Measurement Protocol)

The analysis of these results showed that there was no significant difference in the mean values of the resistance, Ri, of any of the segments, that is, leg, arm, or trunk at any of the measurement times. Similarly, the mean values of Re of the arm and trunk were not

TABLE 1. Results of ANOVA[a]

	Leg		Trunk		Arm	
	Ri	Re	Ri	Re	Ri	Re
Control study	0.96	0.01	0.66	0.70	0.71	0.31
Effect of water ingestion	0.31	0.98[b]	0.85	0.06	0.62	0.09
Effect of sauna/rehydration	0.26	0.14[b]	0.73	0.63	0.71	0.07

[a]The values are p values resulting from ANOVA applied to the normalized mean values of Re and Ri.
[b]After correction for the effects of posture.

significantly different at any of the measurement times. However, there was a trend for the mean value of Re of the leg to increase significantly from the initial to final measurement time (ΔRe% = +4%, $p = 0.01$). This increase was attributed to the effects of the change in posture due to the protocol and was used to "correct" the values of Re measured for the leg in the subsequent aspects of the study in which a change in body water was effected.

The Effect of Ingestion of Water

There were no significant differences in the mean values of Ri or Re for any of the segments, or total body, after correcting the values of Re measured for the leg for the effects of posture (see TABLE 1).

The Effect of Loss Induced in a Sauna and Rehydration by Ingestion

The mean weight loss as a result of the sauna normalized to body weight was 0.91 ± 0.34% (range 0.33–1.4%). Again, there were no significant differences in the mean values of Ri or Re for any of the segments, or total body, after correcting the values of Re measured for the leg for the effects of posture (see TABLE 1).

DISCUSSION

Theory predicts that the volume of water in a segment of the body is proportional to the reciprocal of the impedance of that segment, or more exactly that the intracellular volume is proportional to 1/Ri and the extracellular volume to 1/Re.

The invariance of Ri in each segment as observed in the control subjects is in keeping with the a priori assumption that the distribution of ICW is not affected by postural changes. Likewise, the increase in the mean value of Re of the leg is indicative of the movement of ECW from the legs to the trunk when a subject becomes supine. Failure to detect a corresponding decrease in the mean value of Re for the trunk is assumed to be due to the fact that the movement of ECW from legs to trunk due to postural changes is relatively small in comparison to the volume of the trunk.

The most important result from the present study is that no significant differences were observed in Re or Ri for any of the segments or total body when actual total body water (TBW) was known to change by approximately 2%. Assuming that this change was initially mainly in the ECW, then the 2% change in TBW would correspond to a 5–6% change in ECW. Changes of these magnitudes—that is, in either TBW or ECW—should have been detectable, given the coefficient of variation measured in the present study, if they had resulted in a similar change in resistance.

This insensitivity can be explained if one considers the effect of a changed water volume on the measured Re (or Ri) while maintaining a constant amount of electrolytes. Since resistivity is inversely proportional to electrolyte concentration, rearrangement of equation 1 yields

$$V = k \times L^2 / CR$$

where k is the constant of proportionality and C is the electrolyte concentration. If the volume, V, contains a mass, M, of electrolyte, then $C = M/V$ and the equation can be further rearranged to

$$V = kV \times L^2/MR$$

or

$$R = kL^2/M.$$

When only the water content of the ICW (or ECW) changes, this final equation indicates that Ri (or Re) is predicted to remain constant since k, L, and M are in this case constants. In practical terms, this means that bioimpedance is only able to accurately detect water volume changes when the electrolyte concentration is maintained constant, which is not always the case in disease states. Indeed, even normal biological variations in the ion concentrations of ICW and ECW may be the cause of some of the relatively large standard errors of the estimate observed in the prediction of these quantities from BIA measures.

ACKNOWLEDGMENTS

We acknowledge the assistance of "The Corporate Health Club," Brisbane, in the conduct of this work.

REFERENCES

1. LUKASKI, H. C. & W. W. BOLUCHUK. 1988. Estimation of body fluid volumes using tetrapolar bioelectrical impedance measurements. Aviat. Space Environ. Med. **59:** 1163–1169.
2. HANAI, T. 1968. Electrical properties of emulsions. *In* Emulsion Science, p. 354–477. Academic Press. New York/London.
3. CHA, K. C. & A. G. HILL. 1995. Multifrequency bioelectrical impedance fails to quantify sequestration of abdominal fluid. J. Appl. Physiol. **78**(2): 736–739.
4. THOMAS, B. J., B. H. CORNISH & L. C. WARD. 1992. Bioelectrical impedance analysis for measurement of body fluid volumes. J. Clin. Eng. **17:** 505–510.
5. ORGAN, L. W. *et al.* 1994. Segmental bioelectrical impedance analysis: theory and application of a new technique. J. Appl. Physiol. **77:** 98.
6. LUKASKI, H. C. 1990. Applications of bioelectrical impedance analysis: a critical review. *In* In Vivo Body Composition Studies: Recent Advances, p. 419–426. Plenum. New York.
7. CORNISH, B. H., B. J. THOMAS & L. C. WARD. 1993. Improved prediction of extracellular and total body water using impedance loci generated by multiple frequency bioelectrical impedance analysis. Phys. Med. Biol. **38:** 337–346.
8. SCHIRREFFS, S. M. & R. J. MAUGHAN. 1994. The effect of posture change on blood volume, serum potassium, and whole body electrical impedance. Eur. J. Appl. Physiol. **69:** 461–463.

Fat-Free Mass Qualitative Assessment with Bioelectric Impedance Analysis (BIA)

T. TALLURI,[a] R. J. LIETDKE,[a] A. EVANGELISTI,[b] J. TALLURI,[a] AND G. MAGGIA[c]

[a]*Akern/RJL Systems R&D, 50127 Florence, Italy*
[b]*Department of Systems and Computer Science, University of Florence, Florence, Italy*
[c]*Department of Human Nutrition, University of Padua, Padua, Italy*

ABSTRACT: Body composition studies, when based on two-compartment volumetric estimates, can hardly assess nutritional states. Phase-sensitive impedance analysis can be used to reflect directly the proportions between intra- and extracellular spaces (ECM/BCM), which is one of the most sensitive indexes of malnutrition. Resistance and reactance values actually measured with BIA are referred to as the series *RC* model; however, due to the morphology of the FFM, which is composed of cells surrounded by interstitial fluids, in reality this should be modeled as a parallel *RC* circuit. A nomogram developed with series-to-parallel transformations of resistance and reactance measured with commercial BIA on controls and patients shows interesting gender and disease sensitivity and specificity.

INTRODUCTION

The human body should be considered as a living system composed of organs, supported and rendered mobile by the muscle-skeleton apparatus. Rather than estimating, as a first option, the mass in excess (fat mass), we believe that it is more clinically relevant to assess the quality of the fat-free mass.

When dealing with body composition, the body is usually modeled in two compartments: fat and fat-free masses, where about 73% of body fluids are assumed to be distributed in the fat-free mass. This approach has given fair results on normal adults, but it is inadequate when dealing with pathology.[1] In abnormal states, the assumption of 73% hydration can be misleading,[2] and a minimum of three-level modeling is necessary to explain weight variations that can take place independently in the extracellular spaces, in the body cell mass, or in the fat mass.

The proportion between the extracellular mass (ECM) and body cell mass (BCM) ratio is used to identify fluid imbalance or malnutrition.[3] In normal subjects, ECM/BCM ratios are recorded between 0.85 and 1.00. Deviations from such figures toward higher values are due either to the erosion of BCM (catabolism) or to fluid expansion in extracellular spaces (edema). In such cases, assessing body fat is unnecessary. A fair analogy can be made with human blood: if, for example, a blood sample test shows a cholesterol level of 300 mg, but at the same time the hematocrit value is only 30%, the urgency will be not to reduce the quantity of lipoproteins, but to increase the amount of blood cells.

The following examples can help to exploit a body composition analysis based on the qualitative approach. The fat-free mass model in normal (healthy) states is shown in FIGURE 1.

In the presence of some pathologies, the correct proportion between ECM and BCM spaces can be modified. For example, the volume of body cell mass lost to the glucogenesis of internal proteins (malnutrition) is replaced by fluids that cannot be accounted as an

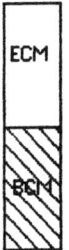

FIGURE 1. ECM/BCM = 1.

overload, even if extracellular water appears expanded as in edematous states (overhydration). In the case of dehydration, we can observe the opposite phenomenon where the ECM/BCM ratio is reduced. The diagrams shown in FIGURE 2 show each single different state.

The lean mass can be composed of either a normal number of cells surrounded by a normal amount of fluids or a depleted quantity of cells surrounded by an expanded amount of fluids, as schematically shown in FIGURE 3.

The two different kinds of tissues can be modeled as circuits, as shown in FIGURE 4.

METHODS

The impedance analyzers most cited in the literature are the BIA series 101–109, manufactured by RJL Systems of Detroit and licensed for Europe to Akern Srl of Florence.[4,5] They are all phase-sensitive devices operating at 800 µA constant sinusoidal current and 50 kHz frequency. Resistance and reactance are readily measured assuming a series RC model that clearly does not match reality. However, equivalent parallel values or resistance and reactance can be mathematically obtained with the following traditional series-to-parallel transforms:

$$Rzp = Rzs + (Xcs^2)/Rzs$$

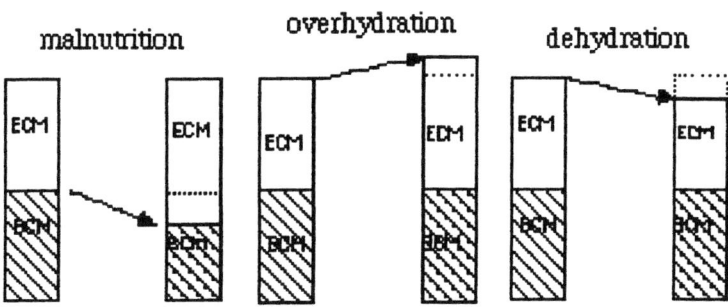

FIGURE 2. Variation of the extracellular compartment induced by overhydration or malnutrition.

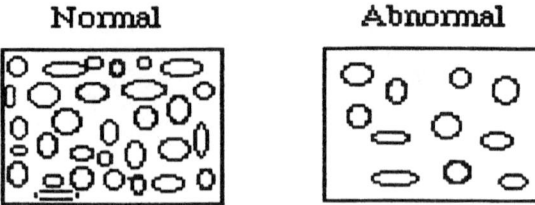

FIGURE 3. Simple schemes of normal and abnormal fat-free tissues.

$$Xcp = Xcs + (Rzs^2)/Xcs$$

where Rzp = parallel resistance, Xcp = parallel reactance, Rzs = series resistance, and Xcs = series reactance.

Such an approach has been validated and appears superior to the series model in assessing the quantity of BCM and ECW.[6]

RESULTS

Utilizing the transformed impedance values recorded on control populations with normal body-mass index, we have constructed a bivariate, 75% confidence graph of normality based on Xcp and Rzp for male and female adults, as shown in FIGURES 5a and 5b.

When the same parameters are measured on female subjects with reduced body-mass index (BMI < 19), the scatterplot distribution falls outside of the nomogram only in the anorexia group. The nonanorexia group is substantially scattered within the nomogram limits, as shown in FIGURE 6.

When bioimpedance measurements are taken just before the treatment on dialysis patients, that is, when the extracellular spaces are expanded, the scatterplots are different from matched and unmatched controls, but are similar between males and females, as shown in FIGURE 7. It appears that overhydration mitigates the significant bioelectrical differences recorded on normal male and female populations.

DISCUSSION

In vivo results are but a confirmation of the validity of series-to-parallel transformation since only 3.2% of the anorectic subjects fall within the 75% confidence area of normality.

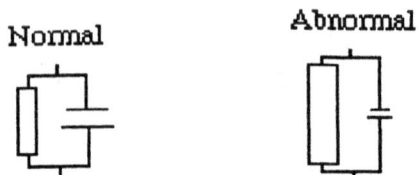

FIGURE 4. Simplified electric models of normal and abnormal fat-free tissues.

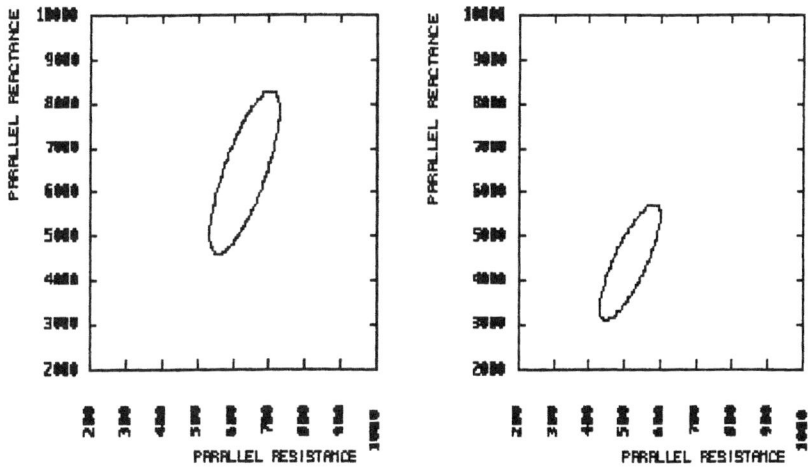

FIGURE 5. Nomograms of female (left) and male (right) controls drawn with 75% confidence limits. The gender-discriminating power of the series-to-parallel transforms is significant.

Also, predialysis patients, irrespective of gender, coherently show lower parallel resistances, with a significant limited presence (3%) within the normal confidence boundaries.

The qualitative analysis that can be performed with parallel modeling deserves further clinical investigation since it might prove practical for clinical use, when the risk of fluid imbalance or malnutrition is high and anthropometry cannot be performed easily, as, for example, in intensive care or surgical theaters.

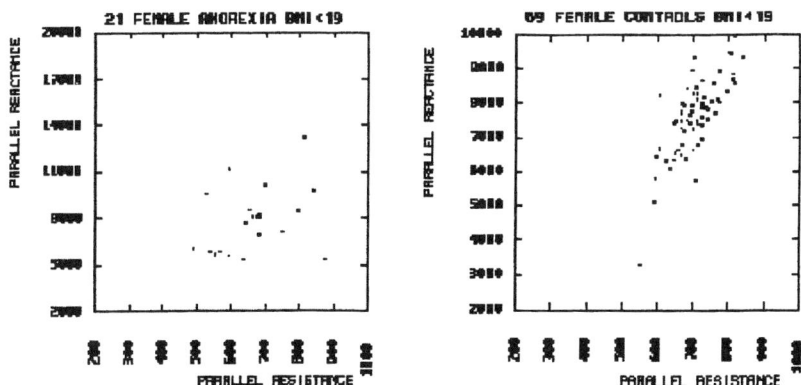

FIGURE 6. Ninety-seven percent of the anorexia nervosa group (left) falls outside of the nomogram; controls (right) are within normal confidence limits.

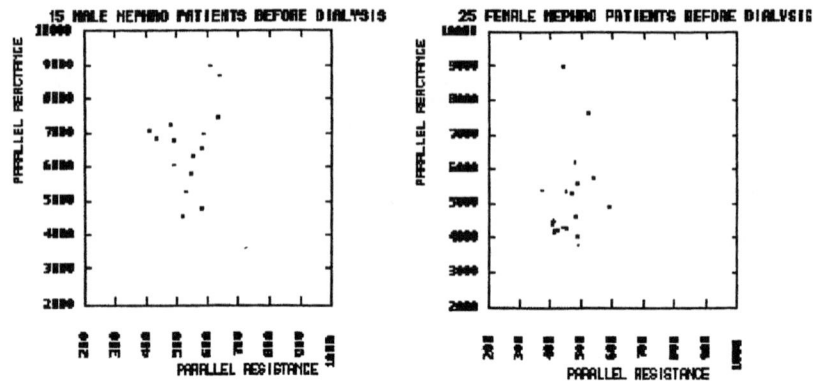

FIGURE 7. Abnormal distribution of impedance values recorded before hemodialysis: males (left); females (right).

REFERENCES

1. SHIZGAL, H. M. 1990. Validation of the measurement of body composition from the whole body bioelectric impedance. Infusionstherapie **3**(suppl. 3): 67–74.
2. MOORE, F. D., K. H. OLESEN, J. D. MCMURREY, H. V. PARKER, M. R. BALL & C. M. BOYDEN. 1963. The body cell mass and its supporting environment. Ediz. Saunders Inc. No. 63-9490.
3. LEMCKE, M., H. FISCHER, R. JAGER, H. POLAT, H. GEIER, M. RECH, S. STASZESWSKI, E. HELM & W. CASPARY. 1993. Early changes of body composition in human immunodeficiency in virus-infected patients: tetrapolar body impedance analysis indicates significant malnutrition. Am. J. Clin. Nutr. **57**: 15–19.
4. PICCOLI, A., B. ROSSI, L. PILLON & G. BUCCIANTE. 1994. A new method for monitoring body fluid variation by bioimpedance analysis: the R-Xc graph. Kidney Int. **46**: 534–539.
5. TALLURI, T. 1996. Assessment of body cell mass and extracellular water without stature height and weight: a new bioimpedance method. International Symposium on Body Composition Studies, Malmö, Sweden.
6. KOTLER, D. P., S. BURASTERO, J. WANG & N. PIERSON, JR. 1996. Prediction of body cell mass, fat-free mass, and total body water with bioelectrical impedance analysis: effects of race, sex, and disease. Am. J. Clin. Nutr. **64**(suppl.): 489S–497S.

Estimation of Extracellular Volume by a Two-Frequency Measurement

H. G. GOOVAERTS,[a] TH. J. C. FAES,[a] G. W. DE VALK–DE ROO,[b]
M. TEN BOLSCHER,[b] J. C. NETELENBOSCH,[b] W. J. F. VAN DER VIJGH,[c]
AND R. M. HEETHAAR[a]

[a]*Department of Clinical Physics and Informatics, Institute of Cardiovascular Research ICarVU*

[b]*Department of Endocrinology*

[c]*Clinical Research Laboratory Internal Medicine, University Hospital Vrije Universiteit, 1007 MB Amsterdam, the Netherlands*

ABSTRACT: An approach to determine intra- and extracellular conduction on the basis of Bode analysis is presented. Estimation of the ratio between intra- and extracellular conduction could be performed by phase measurement only, midrange in the bandwidth of interest. An important feature is that the relation between intra- and extracellular conduction can be continuously monitored by phase measurement and no curve fitting whatsoever is required. Based on a two-frequency measurement determining R_e at 4 kHz and φ_{max} at 64 kHz, it proved possible to estimate extracellular volume (ECV) in 23 patients. Reference values on ECV were determined by sodium bromide. The results show a good correlation ($r = 0.90$) with the reference method. The average error of ECV estimation was –3.6% (SD 8.4).

INTRODUCTION

In the past, several approaches have been presented that describe the conduction of alternating electrical currents along intra- and extracellular pathways. Modeling these currents enables analysis of fluid distribution between both compartments. Equivalent circuits are generally used for convenience to relate measured impedance to tissue structure. One of the most used and simplest models in the β-dispersion region is a circuit composed of three parameters: membrane capacitance, intracellular conduction, and extracellular conduction. This model is known as the Cole-Cole model.

The Cole-Cole Model

The model is based on a function proposed by Cole and Cole[1] describing dielectric relaxation mechanisms. Subsequently, the model has been applied to measurements of the conductivity of suspensions of spherical cells and to impedance measurements on frog eggs.[2] It is commonly implemented by a simple *RC* circuit as given in FIGURE 1a. This circuit would present an impedance locus (FIGURE 1b) according to

$$Z = R_\infty + \frac{R_0 - R_\infty}{1 + j\omega\tau} \qquad (1)$$

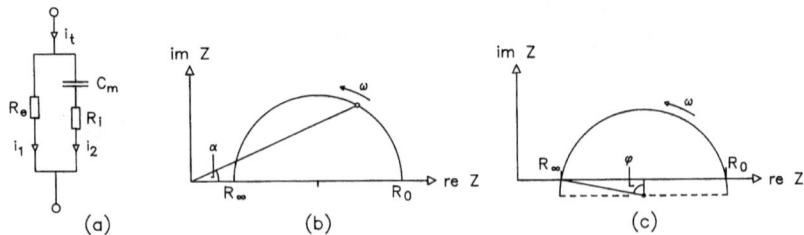

FIGURE 1. *RC* model (a) used to describe intra- and extracellular conduction with root locus diagram (b). The root locus of (c) is based on experimental results.

where R_∞ and R_0 are the high- and low-limit resistances, respectively. The impedance locus obtained by measurements on frog eggs and cell suspensions differs from the one given in FIGURE 1b. The impedance described by the locus of FIGURE 1c is given by

$$Z = R_\infty + \frac{R_0 - R_\infty}{1 + (j\omega\tau)^{\varphi/90°}} \quad (2)$$

where φ is a distribution parameter ($0° < \varphi < 90°$). This is an empirical expression first found by Cole. This equation is one of several that have been suggested to mathematically represent the observed experimental data. It must be pointed out that, in choosing the Cole-Cole equation, one has made an approximation that may significantly affect the accuracy and validity of the subsequent interpretation of data, where R_i and R_e would be obtained by extrapolation from R_∞ and R_0, respectively.[3,4]

Bode Analysis

In order to assess the frequency behavior of *RC* models, we have opted for Bode analysis. In FIGURE 2, the *RC* circuit (a), the vector diagram of currents and voltages (b), as well as the Bode-plot magnitude (c) and phase (d) are shown. It can be seen that two roll-off frequencies are determined by two time constants given by

$$\tau_1 = (R_e + R_i)C_m \quad \text{and} \quad \tau_2 = R_i C_m. \quad (3)$$

Between the roll-off frequencies, a phase maximum occurs at $\omega_{max} = 1/\sqrt{\tau_1 \tau_2}$, the magnitude of which is dependent on the distance between both frequencies as follows:

$$\varphi_{max} = \tan^{-1}\frac{(\tau_2 - \tau_1)}{2\sqrt{\tau_1 \tau_2}}. \quad (4)$$

Hence, measurement of the maximum phase angle contains information regarding the time constants τ_1 and τ_2. It can be shown[5] that equation 4 can be reformulated in terms of τ_2/τ_1, resulting in

$$\varphi_{max} = 90 - 2\tan^{-1}\sqrt{\frac{\tau_2}{\tau_1}} = 90 - 2\tan^{-1}\sqrt{\frac{R_i}{R_e + R_i}}. \quad (5)$$

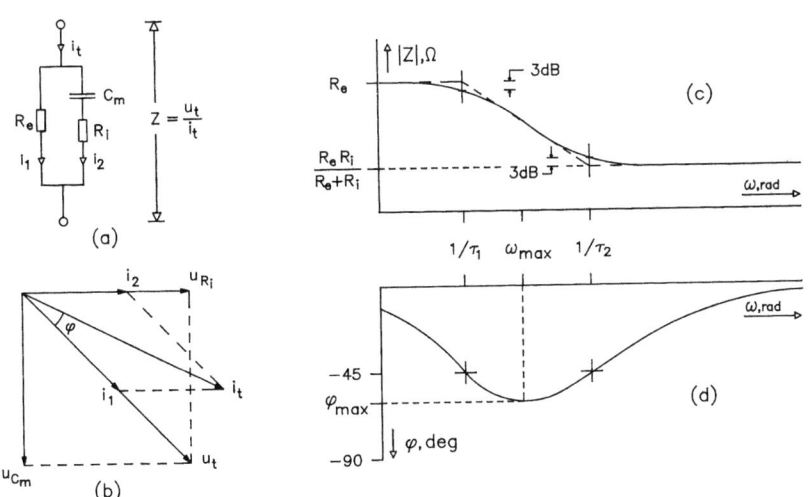

FIGURE 2. Vector diagram (b) and Bode plot (c) and (d) of the *RC* model (a).

Rearranging equation 5 leads to

$$\frac{\tau_2}{\tau_1} = \left[\tan\frac{(90 - \varphi_{max})}{2}\right]^2. \quad (6)$$

This is an important relation, which can be obtained merely by phase measurement at a moderate frequency centered in the bandwidth of interest. Construction of an impedance spectrum would not be necessary and time-consuming curve fitting can be omitted. Phase measurement tends to become inaccurate at relatively high frequencies, which is, among other causes, due to propagation delays occurring in the phase measuring system. Hence, it would be advantageous to derive from the phase maximum a parameter that could be incorporated in the estimation of ECV and that could be measured in an intermediate frequency range.

ECV Estimation

Commonly, ECV is estimated using the following equation based on Hanai's mixture theory:[6]

$$\text{ECV} = k\left(\frac{L^2 W^{1/2}}{R_e}\right)^{2/3} \quad (7)$$

where W is body weight, L is body height, and k is a constant containing factors correcting for whole body measurement, fluid resistivity, and tissue density.[7] This formulation is quite suitable for incorporation of other factors affecting the conduction in the total body volume, such as geometry, conduction through fat tissue, and partial bypassing of current through intracellular pathways in some types of tissues that are not covered by the constant k.

MEASURING SETUP

For the assessment of electrical bioimpedance, a new impedance measuring device, MFI-9404, was developed, capable of measuring electrical impedance at three frequencies: 4 kHz, 64 kHz, and 1024 kHz. The device provides for output of the magnitude of impedance, |Z|, and the phase angle between injected current and measured voltage, φ. The absolute accuracy of the |Z| measurement is within 2%, whereas the repeatability is within 0.1%. The accuracy of phase measurement is 0.1°. We measured |Z| and φ at two frequencies: 4 kHz and 64 kHz. The impedance measured at low frequencies, below a few kHz, should most likely be attributed completely to extracellular conduction. Hence, R_e can be directly measured and needs no estimation based on extrapolation. We added equation 6 as a correction factor in the estimation of ECV according to equation 7. It contains information on both intra- and extracellular conduction and, as such, is suitable for correction with regard to the resistivities in both compartments, body geometry, and leakage pathways. This leads to the following empirical expression:

$$\mathrm{ECV} = k \left(\frac{L^2 \sqrt{W}}{R_e} \right)^{2/3} \frac{\tau_2}{\tau_1} \qquad (8)$$

where R_e is the actually *measured* value at 4 kHz.

The ECV estimates were obtained using data-analysis software (Xitron Technologies, San Diego) containing a set of reference coefficients with respect to extracellular conductivity and tissue density. It should be pointed out that we did not use the algorithm for extrapolation of R_e and R_i based on curve fitting. However, we did use the same constants based on a five-cylinder model[7] that had been applied for ECV estimation on the basis of Cole-Cole extrapolation.

RESULTS

The measurements have been performed within the framework of an investigation of the effect of 17β-estradiol on the extracellular fluid volume, intestinal calcium absorption, and postprandial triglycerides in healthy postmenopausal women. As a reference, the sodium bromide dilution method has been used. Measurements took place between 8:00 and 10:00 A.M. The subjects had been fasting from 10 P.M. of the night before. Each subject was measured twice at an interval of 2 months. The subjects were brought into a horizontal position and two source electrodes were placed in the middle of the dorsal surface of the left hand and foot. Two sensor electrodes were placed 8 cm proximally to the source electrodes. Measurements were done after 10 minutes of rest. Twenty-three subjects were measured twice in different situations, providing a substantial amount of data with regard to ECV estimation. TABLE 1 summarizes the mean values and standard deviation of data obtained from the method. For error calculation, the sodium bromide (NaBr) method is regarded as the "gold standard". In FIGURE 3, the results are shown of ECV estimation based on measurements obtained from the MFI-9404 Bioimpedance System, taken at two

TABLE 1. Summary of Data

	MFI-9404 Bioimpedance Measuring System						Reference Data Subjects		
	4 kHz		64 kHz		ECV (L)	Error (%)	Weight W(kg)	Length L(m)	NaBr ECV (L)
	$|Z|(\Omega)$	$\varphi°$	$|Z|(\Omega)$	$\varphi°$					
Mean	538	2.5	472	6.4	15.9	−3.6	73.0	1.660	16.6
SD	47	0.4	42	0.6	1.5	8.4	11.1	0.077	2.4

frequencies only. The data are obtained by determination of R_e at 4 kHz and phase measurement at 64 kHz. The correlation coefficient is 0.90.

DISCUSSION AND CONCLUSIONS

It appeared from our data that the so-called center frequency where the phase maximum occurs was situated at 68 ± 14 kHz, being the average of all measurements. It is known that there is not such a distinct peak as suggested in FIGURE 2, but a rather flattened maximum. In this study, it was proven that phase measurement at 64 kHz was adequate.

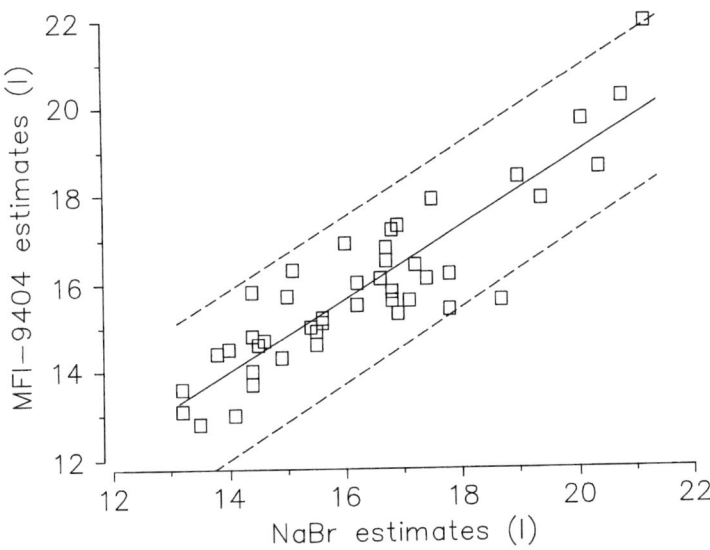

FIGURE 3. Regression of ECV estimation by the MFI-9404 based on phase measurement versus NaBr determination of ECV. The dashed lines indicate the 95% confidence levels.

Automatic determination of φ_{max} by means of a swept-frequency oscillator that is controlled by a maximum-value detecting device would improve the accuracy of ECV estimation.

The correcting factor, k, also contains a term correcting for whole body measurement between the wrist and ankle.[7,8] It is assumed that, in the five cylinders—legs, arms, and trunk—forming the body, a homogeneous electrical current distribution is obtained. This is certainly not true if one measures the impedance of the total body by injecting current at one side only. The electrical current injection into the trunk is not well defined and, subsequently, electrical conduction in that segment will only be partly measured. The impedance will be larger due to inhomogeneities of the electrical field, resulting in an underestimation of the conducting fluid volume. It should be investigated whether improvement can be achieved by current injection in both legs and arms.

To conclude, in order to estimate ECV, simple phase measurement at a center frequency of approximately 64 kHz and determination of the impedance at 4 kHz can replace time-consuming curve fitting according to the Cole-Cole model. The phase measurement can be continuously performed, which makes the described approach very suitable for monitoring purposes.

REFERENCES

1. COLE, K. S. & H. R. COLE. 1941. Dispersion and absorption in dielectrics. J. Chem. Phys. **9:** 341.
2. COLE, K. S. & R. M. GUTTMAN. 1942. Electrical impedance of frog egg. J. Gen. Physiol. **25:** 765.
3. FOSTER, K. R. & H. P. SCHWAN. 1989. Dielectric properties of tissues and biological materials: a critical review. Crit. Rev. Biomed. Eng. **17**(1): 25–104.
4. MCADAMS, E. T., J. JOSSINET & A. LACKERMEIER. 1995. Modelling the "constant phase angle" behaviour of biological tissues: potential pitfalls. Innov. Tech. Biol. Med. **16**(6): 662.
5. DISTEFANO, J. J., III, A. R. STUBBERUD & I. J. WILLIAMS. 1967. Theory and Problems of Feedback and Control Systems. McGraw–Hill. New York.
6. HANAI, T. 1968. Electrical properties of emulsions. In Emulsion Science, p. 354–477. Academic Press. New York.
7. MATTHIE, J. R., P. O. WITHERS, M. D. VAN LOAN & P. L. MAYCLIN. 1992. Development of a commercial complex bio-impedance spectroscopy (CBIS) system for determining intracellular water (ICW) and extracellular water (ECW) volumes. In Proc. Eighth Int. Conf. on Electrical Bio-Impedance (Kuopio, Finland).
8. WITHERS, P. 1995. Multi-frequency impedance measurements of extracellular fluid volume. Physiol. Meas. **16:** 71–76.

The RXc Graph in Evaluating and Monitoring Fluid Balance in Patients with Liver Cirrhosis

FRANCESCO WILLIAM GUGLIELMI, TECLA MASTRONUZZI,
LORENA PIETRINI, ALBA PANARESE, CARMINE PANELLA, AND
ANTONIO FRANCAVILLA

Department of Gastroenterology, University of Bari, 70124 Bari, Italy

ABSTRACT: A recent study, using height-standardized resistance (R/H) and reactance (Xc/H) and assuming a bivariate distribution, has proposed the "RXc graph". We applied this new approach for patients with chronic liver disease in differentiating various degrees of fluid unbalance. Our data showed that a 95% confidence ellipse of patients with chronic hepatitis (CH) overlapped that of healthy control subjects (CONTR), while those of patients with liver cirrhosis (CIR), patients with cirrhosis and ascites (ACIR), and patients with cirrhosis, edemas, and ascites (AECIR) were clearly different for both genders. A progressively shorter mean impedance vector proportional to the stage of liver disease and to the degree of fluid unbalance was found. The lower half of the 50% tolerance ellipse for the healthy population proved to be a threshold for cirrhotics, while almost all the subjects with clinically detectable edema fell outside this limit. The RXc graph was shown to be useful in monitoring the treatment of fluid unbalance and for the immediate selection of patients in whom BIA can precisely assess body composition.

INTRODUCTION

The BIA-derived equations currently available for assessing body composition have been shown to be reliable when used for normal subjects. Their limits clearly emerge in patients with diseases associated with fluid overloading or dehydration; as we have shown, total body[1] and segmental[2] BIA measurements never produced precise estimates of total body water volumes. Recently,[3] impedance measurements were utilized in a new approach to evaluate the hydration state of subjects without making any assumptions on body composition. It assumes a bivariate distribution of impedance measurements standardized by height (H) expressed in ohm/m as R/H and Xc/H plotted on a diagram called the RXc graph. This method was able to (i) calculate a specific 95% confidence ellipse qualified to distinguish controls from obese and renal patients, but not nephrotics from patients with chronic renal failure; (ii) directly assess the state of hydration of individual patients by plotting their values on the 75% and 95% tolerance ellipses for the healthy population; and (iii) demonstrate the utility of this method even in dynamic situations when fluid is either removed or infused. We validated clinically the RXc graph method in patients with varying degrees of liver disease associated with fluid unbalance. Our aim was to verify whether it was possible to (a) identify a specific impedance vector for the different phases of liver disease; (b) establish hydration of individual patients by just plotting their R/H and Xc/H values as an RXc graph on the reference distribution for the healthy population; (c) define a bioelectric cutoff for the identification of visible edema; and (d) monitor body fluid variations produced in these patients by treatment with diuretics or paracentesis.

METHODS

Patients

We studied 810 subjects with liver disease (481 males and 329 females, ages 13 to 82 years) who had been hospitalized at the Department of Gastroenterology of the University of Bari. Patients were divided into four groups: 272 males and 166 females with chronic hepatitis (CH); 144 males and 116 females with cirrhosis (CIR); 33 males and 24 females with cirrhosis and ascites (ACIR); 32 males and 23 females with cirrhosis, ascites, and edemas of the lower limbs (EACIR). These were compared with a group of 208 healthy subjects (88 males and 120 females, ages 15 to 92 years).

Anthropometry

Weight (W) and height (H) were measured in all the subjects by using the same scale and meter. The body mass index (BMI) was computed as W/H^2.

Bioelectrical Impedance

Whole body BIA at 50-kHz frequency was performed with an impedance plethysmograph that emitted 800 mA (model BIA-101, RJL System–Akern, Florence, Italy). We strictly followed the tetrapolar method reported in the literature.[2]

Statistics

The main effect of each variable and the interactions between variables were assessed by a 2×5 analysis of variance (ANOVA) considering gender and disease groups as classification criteria, and the Bonferroni t test was used for multiple comparisons. Hotelling's T^2 test was used for vector analysis and $p < 0.05$ was considered to be the significance level.

Definitions and calculations for confidence and tolerance ellipses are reported elsewhere.[3] Since the lower pole of the reference gender-specific 75% tolerance ellipse was found to be a threshold for apparent edemas in renal patients, we calculated the frequency distribution of vectors from patients with chronic liver disease falling outside of the lower half of the reference 95%, 75%, and 50% tolerance ellipses.

RESULTS

Characteristics of the subjects are reported in TABLE 1. With the exception of age, which did not differ by gender, all other variables considered differed (significant "main effect") by gender and disease grade. A significant interaction between sex and disease group was documented for phase angle. By ANOVA on individual variables, we found that only Xc/H and phase angle were useful in discriminating among the four groups of liver

TABLE 1. Anthropometric and Impedance Parameters[a]

	CONTR		CH		CIR		ACIR		EACIR		p_s	p_d	p_{sxd}
	M = 88	F = 120	M = 272	F = 166	M = 144	F = 116	M = 33	F = 24	M = 32	F = 23			
Age (years)	43 ± 16	44 ± 18	48 ± 12	50 ± 11	55 ± 10	58 ± 8	58 ± 10	56 ± 11	57 ± 13	58 ± 13	NS	<0.001	NS
	0.8		0.4	0.4	0.5	0.5	1.2	1.2	1.4	1.5			
Height (cm)	168 ± 8	156 ± 7	168 ± 7	155 ± 5	164 ± 7	152 ± 5	165 ± 7	155 ± 6	168 ± 8	153 ± 17	<0.001	<0.001	NS
	1.07	0.6	0.4	0.4	0.5	0.5	1.2	1.2	1.4	1.5			
Weight (kg)	67 ± 10	58 ± 11	71 ± 10	64 ± 10	69 ± 10	63 ± 10	67 ± 10	58 ± 8	77 ± 13	65 ± 12	<0.001	<0.001	NS
	1.07	1.07	0.6	0.8	0.8	1.0	1.7	1.7	2.3	2.6			
BMI	23 ± 3	23 ± 5	25 ± 3	26 ± 4	25 ± 3	27 ± 4	24 ± 3	24 ± 3	27 ± 3	27 ± 4	<0.05	<0.001	NS
	0.3	0.4	0.2	0.3	0.3	0.3	0.5	0.7	0.6	0.9			
R/H (ohm/m)	300 ± 44	386 ± 55	289 ± 35	366 ± 44	290 ± 42	361 ± 50	301 ± 58	366 ± 51	248 ± 47	313 ± 80	<0.001	<0.001	NS
	4.6	5.04	2.2	3.4	3.5	4.7	10.2	10.5	8.4	16.6			
Xc/H (ohm/m)	34 ± 6	38 ± 7	33 ± 5	38 ± 7	30 ± 6	34 ± 7	27 ± 9	29 ± 6	17 ± 5	23 ± 8	<0.001	<0.001	NS
	0.7	0.7	0.3	0.5	0.5	0.6	1.5	1.3	1.05	1.8			
Phase angle (°)	6.5 ± 1.1	5.6 ± 1.1	6.7 ± 1.0	5.9 ± 1.1	6.0 ± 1.1	5.4 ± 1.0	5.2 ± 1.4	4.6 ± 1.1	4.0 ± 1.1	4.2 ± 1.0	<0.001	<0.001	<0.05
	0.1	0.1	0.06	0.09	0.09	0.09	0.2	0.2	0.2	0.2			
r(R, Xc)	0.3	0.4	0.4	0.3	0.4	0.4	0.5	0.2	0.6	0.8			

[a] Anthropometric and impedance measurements (mean ± SD, SEM = standard error of the mean) by gender and disease group: CONTR = healthy population; CH = chronic hepatitis; CIR = cirrhosis; ACIR = cirrhosis with ascites; EACIR = cirrhosis with ascites and edemas; R = resistance; Xc = reactance; H = height; r(R, Xc) = correlation coefficient between R and Xc; p_s, p_d, p_{sxd} = significance level for s = gender, d = diagnosis, s × d = gender × diagnosis; NS = not significant.

patients due to a progressive and significant decrease from CIR to ACIR. No variable significantly differed between the CH and CONTR groups. The gender-specific 50%, 75%, and 95% tolerance ellipses for the control group and the mean vectors with 95% confidence ellipses of healthy and disease groups were depicted by gender and are shown in FIGURE 1. Mean vectors in women were longer and had smaller phase angle than in men. CIR, ACIR, and AECIR groups had down-sloping and shorter mean vectors than either healthy or CH groups, indicating progressive fluid overload. However, in patients with

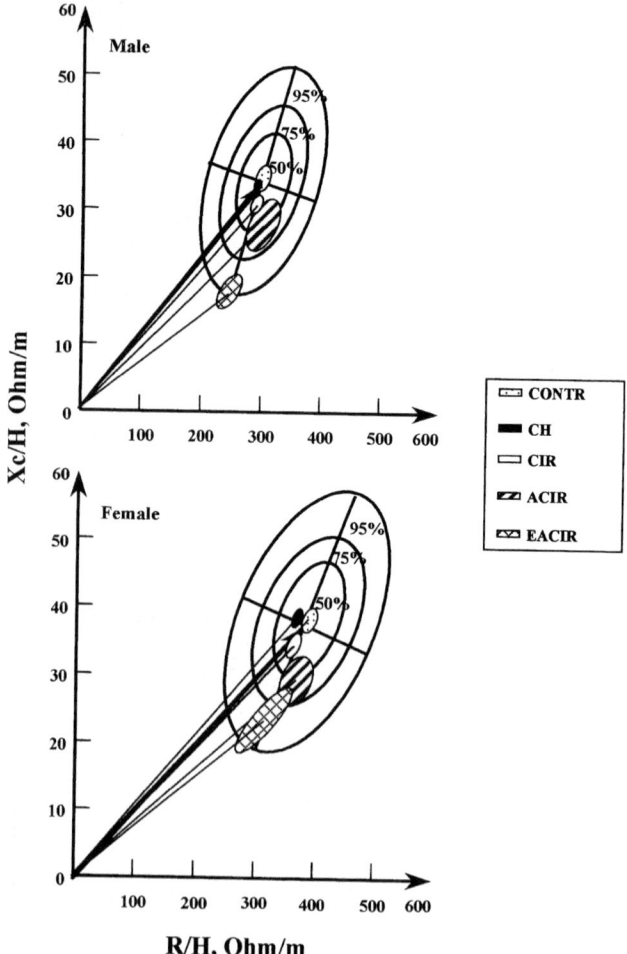

FIGURE 1. Gender-specific 95%, 75%, and 50% tolerance ellipses of the control population. R/H = resistance normalized by height; Xc/H = reactance normalized by height. Gender-specific "mean RXc graphs": 95% confidence ellipse of the control group plotted with the groups of liver patients—CONTR = healthy population, CH = chronic hepatitis, CIR = cirrhosis, ACIR = cirrhosis with ascites, EACIR = cirrhosis with ascites and edemas.

liver disease, significant vector displacements (i.e., separated 95% confidence ellipses) were observed between EACIR, ACIR, and CH groups in men, and between EACIR, CIR, and CH groups in women. TABLE 2 contains the distribution of subjects in each group who fell outside of the lower half of the 50%, 75%, and 95% reference tolerance ellipses. The distribution of CH patients falling outside of the three halves of the ellipses was close to the expected amount (i.e., 1.5%, 4.8%, and 28.5% versus 2.5%, 12.5%, and 25%, respectively). The percentages of cirrhotic vectors falling outside of the ellipses were progressively higher in each of the three groups considered, and almost all the subjects with detectable edema fell outside of the lower half of the 50% ellipse, proving that the 50% ellipse behaved as a threshold for apparent edemas with 96% and 87% sensitivity and 67% and 68% specificity, respectively, in male and female patients.

FIGURE 2 shows the effects of paracentesis and therapy with diuretics in two groups of patients with altered fluid balance: 11 cirrhotics with ascites and 5 cirrhotics with edemas. Removal of ascitic fluid did not cause a great change in the mean impedance vector, which remained below the lower half of the 75% tolerance ellipse. Conversely, although Hotelling's T^2 test was not significant, treatment with diuretics produced a considerable lengthening and steepening of the mean impedance vector, bringing vectors of these patients back to the lower half of the reference 50% tolerance ellipse.

DISCUSSION

Our reference sex-specific 50%, 75%, and 95% tolerance ellipses were very close to those reported by Piccoli from a different Italian region.[3] We found that in our patients the 50% tolerance ellipse for the healthy population served as a cutoff by which to identify patients with detectable edemas (with 96% and 87% sensitivity and 67% and 68% specificity, respectively, in males and females), whereas in the nephropathics the 75% ellipses identified 97% of the patients with edemas.

Our results clearly show that CH patients, as expected, have a normal fluid balance, as revealed by their normal distribution on the three reference ellipses considered, while almost all the cirrhotics with edemas fell outside of the lower half of the 50% tolerance

TABLE 2. Percentage of Subjects Who Fell Outside of the Lower Half of the Reference 95%, 75%, and 50% Tolerance Ellipses[a]

	Expected Values (%)	CH		CIR		ACIR		EACIR	
		M	F	M	F	M	F	M	F
total N		272	166	144	116	33	24	32	23
95% half-ellipse	2.5	1.5	2.4	6.9	2.6	27.3	8.3	59.4	39.1
75% half-ellipse	12.5	4.8	7.2	22.9	15.5	39.4	45.8	84.4	73.9
50% half-ellipse	25.0	26.5	19.3	36.8	40.5	57.6	70.8	96.6	87.0

[a]Evaluation of the percentage of patients who fell outside of the sex-specific 95%, 75%, and 50% lower half tolerance ellipses divided by disease group: CONTR = healthy population; CH = chronic hepatitis; CIR = cirrhosis; ACIR = cirrhosis with ascites; EACIR = cirrhosis with ascites and edemas; M = male; F = female.

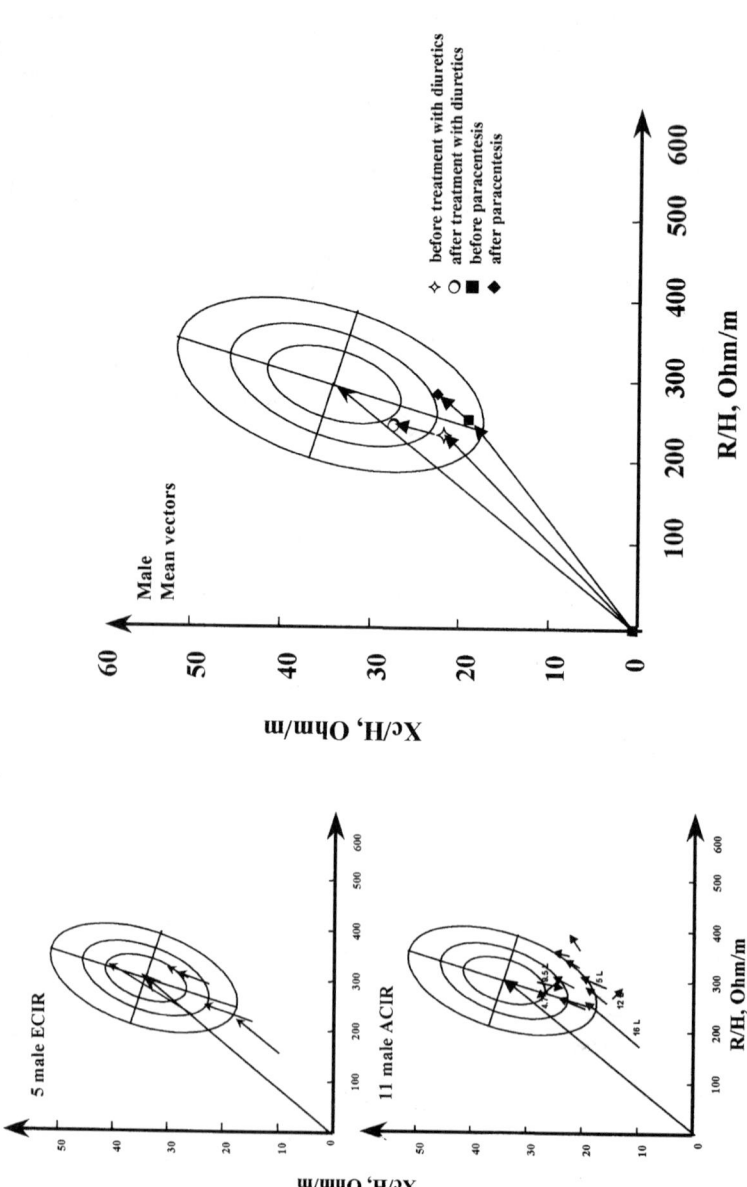

FIGURE 2. Evaluation of individual patients: 11 male cirrhotics with ascites (ACIR) who underwent paracentesis; 5 male cirrhotics with edemas, but without ascites (ECIR), treated with diuretics.

ellipse (CIR: 36.8% M, 40.5% F; ACIR: 57.6% M, 70.8% F). This observation substantiates the idea that, by using this method, it is also possible to differentiate patients with an initial increase in the extracellular compartment, even in the absence of evident clinical signs.

The clinical impact of this was verified when we examined the results obtained in the patients with ascites and those with edemas and no ascites who underwent paracentesis and treatment with diuretics, respectively. In fact, removal of ascitic fluid produced a mean impedance vector that fell outside of the lower pole of the 75% tolerance ellipse, thus confirming that cirrhotics with ascites have a peripheral fluid retention that is not clinically apparent, while therapy with diuretics in patients with edemas, but without ascites, normalized their fluid balance, as well as their bioelectrical parameters. After the complete regression of the edema, we documented a longer mean impedance vector that closely approximated the threshold of detectable edemas (i.e., lower half of the 50% tolerance ellipse). All these results are perfectly understandable considering our previous findings,[1,2] which demonstrated that the acute removal of ascitic fluid led to only slight variations in BIA values, both in total body and in trunk measurements.

The data reported in this paper are useful for practical purposes because by using this new approach of BIA we can distinguish patients with a normal state of hydration (as their bioelectrical parameters fall within the 50% ellipses) and in whom BIA may be used for a precise evaluation of their body composition from those in whom this is not feasible because they are outside of the lower half of the 50% tolerance ellipse for an abnormal state of hydration.

REFERENCES

1. GUGLIELMI, F. W., F. CONTENTO, L. LADDAGA, C. PANELLA & A. FRANCAVILLA. 1991. Bioelectric impedance analysis: experience with male patients with cirrhosis. Hepatology **13**: 892–895.
2. PANELLA, C., F. W. GUGLIELMI, T. MASTRONUZZI & A. FRANCAVILLA. 1995. Whole body and segmental bioelectrical parameters in chronic liver disease: effect of gender and disease stages. Hepatology **21**: 1–5.
3. PICCOLI, A., B. ROSSI, L. PILLON & G. BUCCIANTE. 1994. A new method for monitoring body fluid variation by bioimpedance analysis: the RXc graph. Kidney Int. **46**: 534–539.

Measurement of Leg Arterial Compliance of Normal Subjects and Diabetics Using Impedance Plethysmography

DEOK WON KIM AND SOO CHAN KIM

Department of Biomedical Engineering, College of Medicine, Yonsei University, Seoul, Korea

ABSTRACT: In this study, compliance, a mechanical characteristic of the lower leg arteries, was measured noninvasively. Changes in blood volume and pressure were measured using impedance plethysmography and a mercury sphygmomanometer, respectively. Compliance was calculated by dividing the change in blood volume by the change in pulse pressure (systolic-diastolic pressure). Subjects were 24 asymptomatic persons ranging from 30 to 58 years and 14 diabetics ranging from 41 to 59 years. Peak compliance, mean pressure, and systolic pressure were statistically analyzed using a t test between the asymptomatic and diabetic groups. The average peak compliance of the asymptomatic and diabetic groups was measured as 2.79 and 1.82 µL/mmHg/cm, respectively, and these were significantly different ($p < 0.01$). It was also found that compliance is a better parameter in differentiating vascular disease than the mean or systolic blood pressure.

INTRODUCTION

As people's incomes and intakes of animal fat have rapidly increased, so has the cholesterol concentration in the blood of Koreans. Thus, diseases such as non-insulin-dependent diabetes mellitus (NIDDM), myocardial infarction, high blood pressure, and cerebral stroke resulting from atherosclerosis have recently increased.[1] However, it is very difficult to diagnose atherosclerosis early because its progress is so slow and there are no symptoms in the early stage of disease.

Angiography has been widely used for detecting vascular diseases. However, it has disadvantages such as the extended time required, high cost, some risk, and low sensitivity at the early stage of the diseases. Although B-mode ultrasonography[2,3] and fluoroscopy[4] have been used to diagnose various arterial diseases, these methods are useful only in such cases as occluded or considerably narrowed arteries. Imura and colleagues[3] found that E_p, the pressure-strain elastic modulus, was significantly higher in subjects older than 60 years. Shankar and Bond[5,6] have conducted a pertinent pathologic validation study on the upper thigh of 15 monkeys and found a good correlation (LOS of 0.01) of the peak compliance with morphometric data from iliac and carotid arteries.

A noninvasive technique measuring arterial compliance has also been developed to diagnose atherosclerosis by Shankar and Webster.[7] In their study, maximal compliance (C_p) of the human leg artery was found to correlate well with known cardiovascular risk factors. For example, C_p decreased on average from 3.08 to 1.92 µL/mmHg/cm in groups of subjects of increasing age from 22 to 70 years. Subjects on a regular exercise program had an average value of 3.86, while those with proven peripheral vascular disease had a value of 0.70. In this study, we used our own impedance plethysmograph[8] and a pressure cuff to determine the peak or maximal arterial compliance in the lower legs of 24 asymptomatic subjects and 14 diabetics. We found that peak compliance was a better parameter for differentiating vascular disease than the mean or systolic blood pressure.

METHODS

FIGURE 1 shows a typical volume-pressure curve and compliance-pressure curve derived from the volume-pressure curve.[7] The volume-pressure curve has the well-known shape of decreasing slope at increasing transmural pressures. We assume that the internal arterial pressure is maintained at 110 mmHg and a pressure cuff has been wrapped around the artery. Then, as the pressure in the cuff is increased, the transmural pressure would decrease, and the arterial volume would decrease along the curve (FIGURE 1a). If the artery were perfused from a pulsatile pump with a 35-mmHg pulse, we would record a pulsatile change in arterial volume. The amplitude of this pulsatile change in arterial volume would be maximal when the transmural pressure was near zero. FIGURE 1a shows this case for a subject with a blood pressure of 110/75 mmHg. A cuff pressure of 80 mmHg results in the maximal arterial volume change of 155 µL/cm, yielding peak compliance C_p as 4.4 µL/mmHg/cm (FIGURE 1b).

FIGURE 2 shows an experimental setup measuring the arterial compliance of legs. With the subject supine, both systolic and diastolic pressures for each lower leg artery were measured using a mercury sphygmomanometer and stethoscope. Since measurement of these pressures was not easy, particularly for diabetics, it was determined three times by a doctor and averaged. Then, the mean blood pressure and arterial pulse pressure (ΔP) were calculated. With the mean blood pressure applied to the cuff, arterial pulse volume (ΔV) was measured by our own impedance plethysmograph. Disposable aluminum tape (3M, M6001) was used for the current electrodes, I_1 and I_2, while meshed brass 7 cm apart inside the cuff was used for the voltage electrodes, V_1 and V_2, as shown in FIGURE 2.

Compliance was defined as a ratio of blood volume change (ΔV) to blood pressure change (ΔP):

$$C = \Delta V / \Delta P \ [\mu L/mmHg/cm].$$

Maximal compliance was measured when the internal pressure of an artery and the cuff pressure were equal.[7] In other words, it was measured when the cuff pressure was the same as the mean blood pressure. ΔV values were measured twice more with the cuff pressure decreased by 5 mmHg each time, and thus three compliance values were obtained for each leg. Among these compliances, the largest value was chosen and assigned as C_p.

FIGURE 3 shows a typical set of recordings at selected cuff pressures. At low cuff pressure, arterial compliance is low. Thus, ΔV recorded is also low. As the cuff pressure is increased, pressure across the arterial wall decreases. Arterial compliance and hence ΔV increase, reaching a maximum at 85 mmHg of the cuff pressure. At higher cuff pressure, the artery is collapsed for part of the cycle, resulting in a lower ΔV.

FIGURE 4 shows a block diagram of the real-time digital plethysmograph built in this study. It consists of analog and digital parts. The analog part basically consists of a 100-kHz, 1-mA constant current source, demodulator, filter, and amplifier. The digital part consists of an 80C196KC microcontroller, 8 kbytes ROM, 32 kbytes RAM, keypad, and LCD (liquid crystal display). The keypad was used for entering the distance (L) between

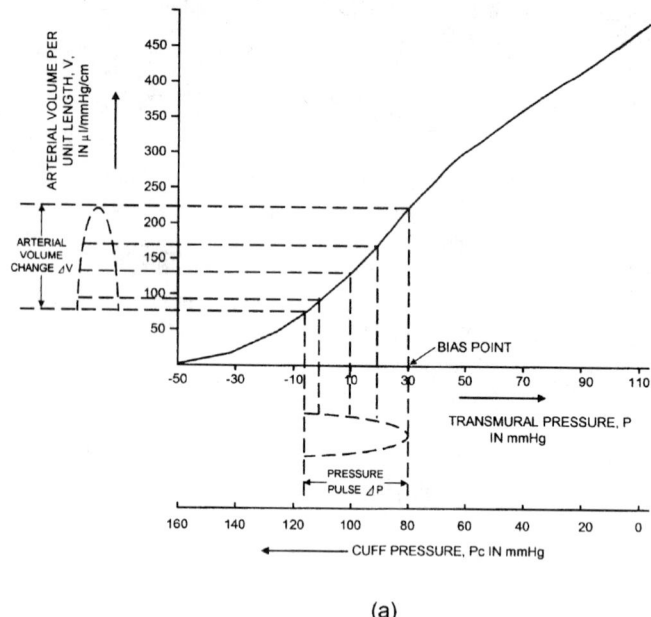

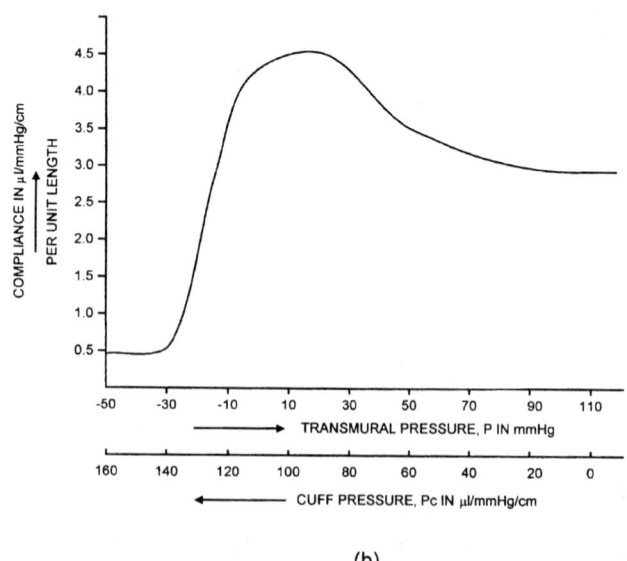

FIGURE 1. (a) Typical volume-pressure curve. (b) Compliance-pressure curve derived from (a). From Shankar and Webster.[7]

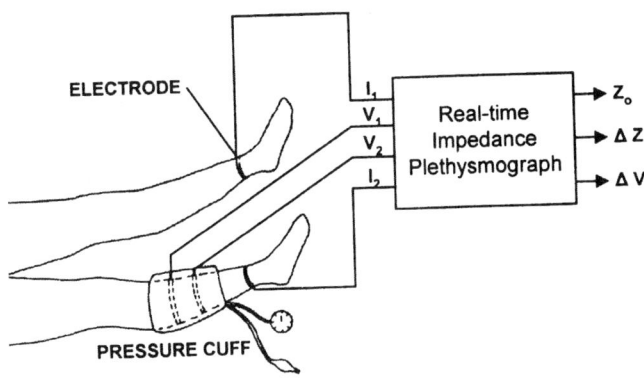

FIGURE 2. Experimental setup for measuring compliance.

the voltage-sensing electrodes in cm and the blood resistivity (ρ) in Ω-cm. The LCD displays arterial pulse volume (ΔV) in μL and basal impedance (Z_o) in Ω.

FIGURE 5a shows a typical impedance change (ΔZ) and its derivative waveform (dZ/dt) recorded from the analog part, and FIGURE 5b shows the three-period ensemble-averaged ΔZ and dZ/dt waveforms. The impedance plethysmograph built in this study displays digi-

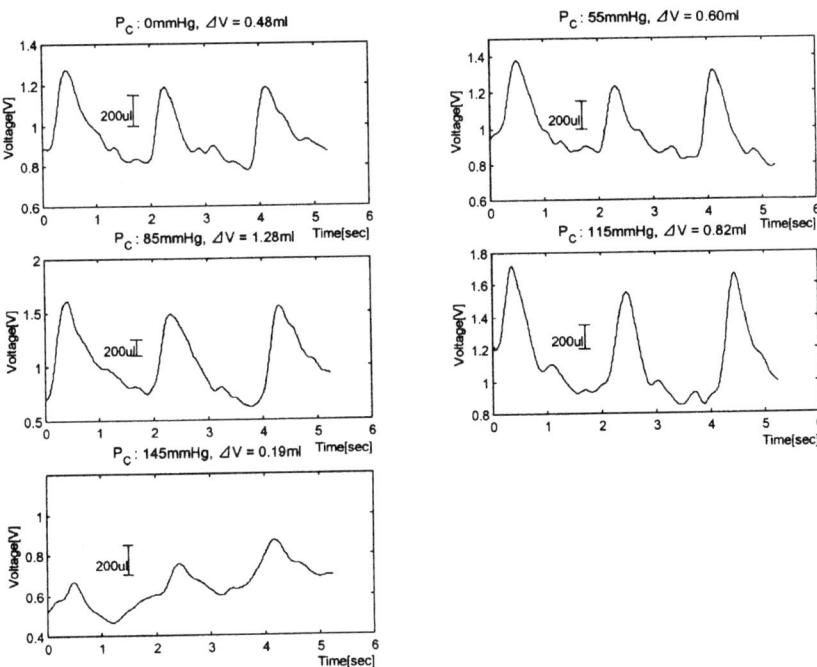

FIGURE 3. Typical set of recordings for various cuff pressures. P_c = cuff pressure, ΔV = arterial volume change. Blood pressure = 120/60 mmHg.

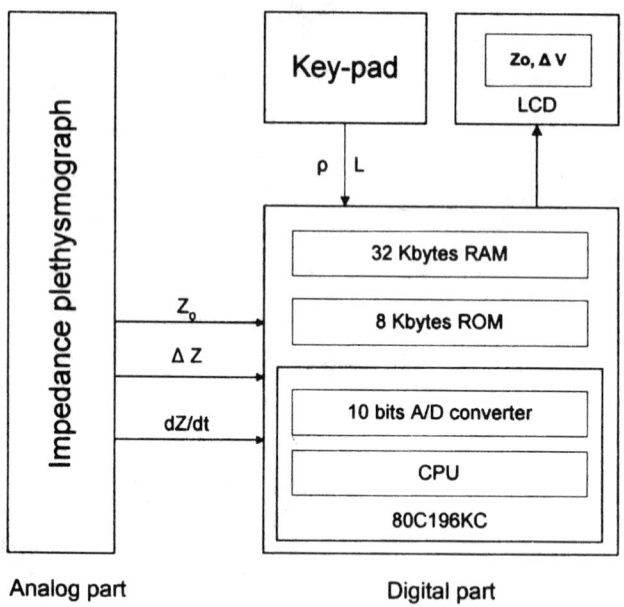

FIGURE 4. Block diagram of the real-time digital plethysmograph built in this study.

tal arterial pulse volume every five seconds. In order to display digital arterial pulse volume, the magnitude of ΔV should be determined. However, the ΔV signal itself drifts, resulting in inaccurate determination of its magnitude due to respiration, motion artifact, etc.[9] Therefore, the dZ/dt_{max} was used as a reference for the ensemble average to obtain the magnitude of ΔZ.

The procedure for ensemble averaging to determine the magnitude of ΔZ is as follows:[9]

(1) Z_o, ΔZ, and dZ/dt signals are digitized with 10-bit resolution at a 100-Hz sampling rate using the A/D converter embedded in the microcontroller for five seconds.

(2) The dZ/dt_{max} points are searched within the five-second interval.

(3) Three periods of the dZ/dt and ΔZ signals are ensemble-averaged with the dZ/dt_{max} point as a reference during the EAI (ensemble average interval).

(4) In the ensemble-averaged dZ/dt signal as shown in FIGURE 5b, a zero-crossing point A is searched backward from point B.

(5) Another zero-crossing point C is searched forward from point B.

(6) Point A′ of the ΔZ signal corresponding to point A of the dZ/dt signal is found, and point C′ is found in the same way.

(7) The magnitude of the ΔZ is the vertical difference between point A′ and C′ as shown in FIGURE 5b.

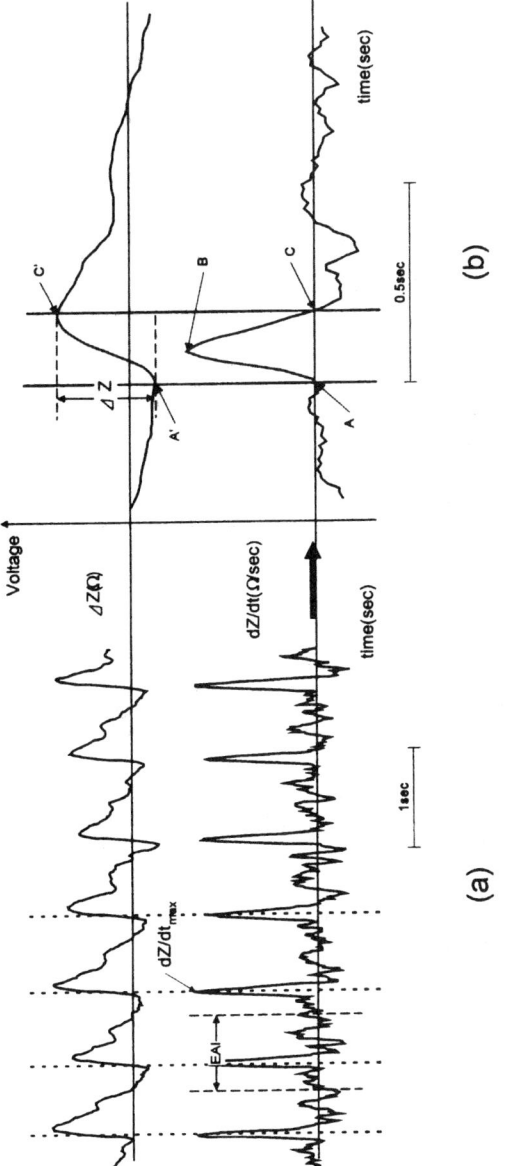

FIGURE 5. (a) Analog ΔZ and dZ/dt signals. (b) The three-period ensemble-averaged ΔZ and dZ/dt signals.

We collected data from a total of 38 subjects at Yonsei University Medical Center. We divided these subjects into two groups. There were 24 asymptomatic subjects ranging from 30 to 58 years and 14 diabetics in the hospital ranging from 41 to 59 years.

RESULTS

TABLE 1 shows the results for five groups: normal 30s, 40s, and 50s; and diabetic 40s and 50s. The columns list age, mean pressure, systolic pressure, and C_p. There was almost no difference in the mean pressure for normal groups between the 30s, 40s, and 50s probably due to the insufficient number of subjects. Also, both the mean and systolic pressures did not increase with age among the normal and diabetic groups. However, C_p decreased with age for both the normal and the diabetic groups on average, and the C_p values of diabetics were lower than those of normal subjects for both age groups, as in Shankar and Webster.[7] FIGURE 6 plots the same data against age. The dashed line is the regression line for normal 30s, normal 40s, and normal 50s. It is evident that the combined diabetic 40s and 50s lie under this dashed line.

In their study, the average C_p values for normal white males with an average age of 30 and for normal Asian males with an average age of 45 were 2.87 and 2.94 µL/mmHg/cm, respectively. In TABLE 1, the C_p of normal 40s with an average age of 45 was 3.18 µL/mmHg/cm, which correlated well with the value of Shankar and Webster.[7] They also found that C_p correlated well with known cardiovascular risk factors. In their study, C_p decreased on average from 3.08 to 1.92 µL/mmHg/cm in groups of subjects of increasing age from 22 to 70 years. From TABLE 1, C_p decreased from 3.98 to 2.40 µL/mmHg/cm in groups of subjects of increasing age from 33 to 53 years. Comparing the two results of the above C_p values, our values of the mean C_p are quite higher than theirs. However, these values should be higher because of the low incidence of atherosclerosis in Asians.

TABLE 2 shows the results for two groups—the normal and the diabetic, with combined 40s and 50s for each group. These two groups were chosen from TABLE 1 in order that the normal and patient groups would be of approximately the same age for comparison. We analyzed data with the unpaired, one-tail t test to compare mean pressure, systolic pressure, and C_p between normal subjects and diabetics in their 40s and 50s using STATVIEW II for Macintosh.

The ages of both groups were not significantly different ($p = 0.10$). Mean blood pressures of the normal and diabetic groups were 100.6 ± 11.9 and 112.0 ± 16.0 mmHg, respectively, and they were significantly different ($p = 0.017$). Systolic pressures of the

TABLE 1. Data on Different Groups of Normal Subjects and Diabetics (Mean ± SD)

Group (n)	Age (years)	Mean Pressure (mmHg)	Systolic Pressure (mmHg)	C_p (µL/mmHg/cm)
normal 30s (8)	32.8 ± 3.2	100.5 ± 14.4	128.2 ± 15.8	3.98 ± 1.79
normal 40s (10)	45.3 ± 3.0	101.5 ± 12.3	143.0 ± 20.6	3.18 ± 1.16
normal 50s (6)	53.0 ± 2.9	100.3 ± 11.4	135.7 ± 22.8	2.40 ± 0.55
diabetic 40s (6)	45.7 ± 2.9	117.3 ± 21.5	160.0 ± 28.1	1.89 ± 0.87
diabetic 50s (8)	55.8 ± 2.8	108.0 ± 10.1	149.4 ± 16.6	1.76 ± 1.04

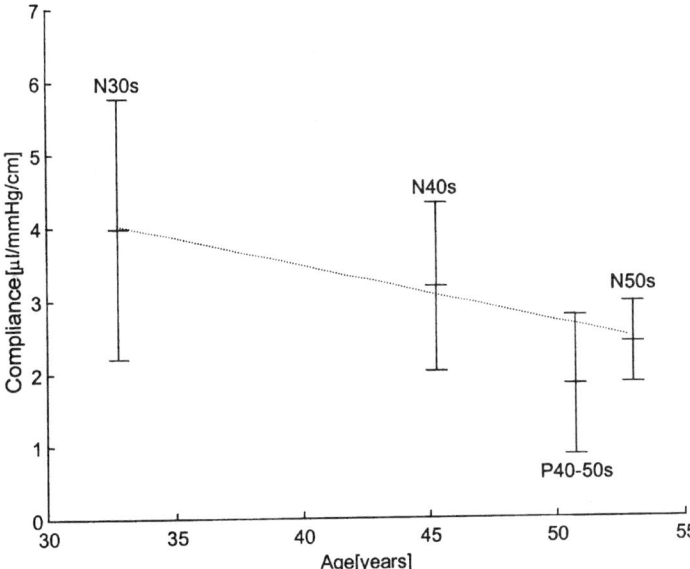

FIGURE 6. Plot of peak compliance versus age for all subjects. The vertical bars represent ±1 SD with respect to the mean value.

normal and diabetic groups were 139.4 ± 21.7 and 153.9 ± 21.9 mmHg, respectively, and they were also significantly different ($p = 0.039$). Peak compliances of normal and diabetic groups were 2.79 ± 1.00 and 1.82 ± 0.94 µL/mmHg/cm, respectively, and they were the most significantly different ($p = 0.005$). The correlation coefficients of C_p with mean pressure, systolic pressure, and age were −0.31, −0.33, and −0.21, respectively.

The results of this study suggest the following:

(1) The peak compliance decreased significantly with increases in age, even though the mean or systolic pressure did not increase for normal subjects as shown in TABLE 1.

(2) Peak compliance is a better parameter for differentiating vascular disease in diabetics than the mean or systolic blood pressure.

TABLE 2. Data on Normal Subjects and Diabetics in 40s and 50s (Mean ± SD)

Group (n)	Age (years)	Mean Pressure (mmHg)	Systolic Pressure (mmHg)	C_p (µL/mmHg/cm)
normal (16)	49.0 ± 4.5	100.6 ± 11.9	139.4 ± 21.7	2.79 ± 1.00
diabetics (14)	51.4 ± 5.9	112.0 ± 16.0[a]	153.9 ± 21.9[a]	1.82 ± 0.94[b]

[a] $p < 0.05$.
[b] $p < 0.01$.

DISCUSSION

Milio et al.[10] suggested that stable hypertensive patients developed principally arterial structural changes, while borderline hypertensive patients had only functional modifications, such as reduced compliance. Examination of the peripheral arteries is a useful screening procedure for the identification of individuals prone to coronary heart disease.[11] Therefore, measurement of compliance of human leg arteries can be useful as a screening procedure for the diagnosis of coronary heart disease, as well as diabetes.

For our method to be clinically useful, the following variables have to be reduced: day-to-day repeatability, position of the cuff on the leg, blood resistivity change, etc.[7] However, this study showed that compliance can be a better index than mean or systolic blood pressure in the diagnosis of vascular diseases, even though the number of samples was insufficient. In conclusion, measurement of leg arterial compliance could be simple, quick, noninvasive, and inexpensive for assessing diabetes.

REFERENCES

1. HUH, K. B. 1990. Exercise cure for diabetics. Diabetes **9:** 5–9.
2. BOND, M. G., W. A. RILEY, R. W. BARNES, J. M. KADUCK & M. R. BALL. 1982. Validation studies of a noninvasive real time B-scan imaging system. *In* Noninvasive Techniques for Assessment of Atherosclerosis in Peripheral, Carotid, and Coronary Arteries, p. 197–203. Raven Press. New York.
3. IMURA, T., K. YAMAMOTO, K. KANAMORI, T. MIKAMI & H. YASUDA. 1984. Noninvasive ultrasonic measurement of the elastic properties of the human abdominal aorta. Cardiovasc. Res. **20:** 208–214.
4. MISTRETTA, C. A., R. A. KRUGER, D. E. ERGUN, C. G. SHAW *et al.* 1982. Intravenous angiography using fluoroscopy techniques. *In* Noninvasive Techniques for Assessment of Atherosclerosis in Peripheral, Carotid, and Coronary Arteries, p. 71–77. Raven Press. New York.
5. SHANKAR, R. & M. G. BOND. 1988. Correlation of noninvasive arterial compliance with anatomic pathology of atherosclerotic nonhuman primates. Eighth. Int. Symp. Atherosclerosis, poster paper no. 237.
6. SHANKAR, R. & M. G. BOND. 1990. Correlation of noninvasive compliance data with morphologic data in a controlled study of cholesterol fed monkeys. Atherosclerosis **85:** 33–46.
7. SHANKAR, R. & J. WEBSTER. 1991. Noninvasive measurement of compliance of human leg arteries. IEEE Trans. Biomed. Eng. **38:** 62–67.
8. KIM, D. W., C. G. SONG, W. K. KIM & M. H. LEE. 1991. Development of impedance plethysmograph and measurement of digital blood flow. J. Korean Soc. Med. Biol. Eng. **12:** 23–28.
9. KIM, D. W., C. G. SONG & M. H. LEE. 1992. A new ensemble averaging technique in impedance cardiography for estimation of stroke volume during treadmill exercise. Front. Med. Biol. Eng. **4:** 179–188.
10. MILIO, G., V. COSPITE & M. COSPITE. 1995. Hypertension and peripheral arterial hemodynamics. Angiology **46:** 1069–1074.
11. FRIEDMAN, S. A., M. PANDYA & E. GRIEF. 1973. Peripheral arterial occlusion in patients with acute coronary heart disease. Am. Heart J. **86:** 415–419.

A Meta-analysis of Published Studies Concerning the Validity of Thoracic Impedance Cardiography

E. RAAIJMAKERS,[a] TH. J. C. FAES,[b] R. J. P. M. SCHOLTEN,[c] H. G. GOOVAERTS,[b] AND R. M. HEETHAAR[b]

[a]*Dr. B. Verbeeten Institute, 5000 LA Tilburg, the Netherlands*
[b]*Department of Medical Physics and Informatics, Institute of Cardiovascular Research VU*
[c]*Institute for Research in Extramural Medicine, Vrije Universiteit, Amsterdam, the Netherlands*

> ABSTRACT: Our aim was to provide a meta-analysis of the literature concerning the validation of thoracic impedance cardiography (TIC) and to explain variations in reported results from differences in the studies. One hundred fifty-four studies (164 Fisher's Z-transformed correlation coefficients) comparing measurements of cardiac output or related parameters from TIC and a reference method were analyzed. Papers were classified according to differences in TIC methodology, reference method, and subject characteristics. Pooling using the random-effects method yielded an overall correlation of $r = 0.82$ (95% confidence interval: 0.80–0.84). ANOVA revealed a significant influence of the reference method and the subject characteristics on the correlation coefficient. In cardiac patients, the correlation was significantly decreased. No influence of the applied TIC methodology was found. Conclusion: TIC might be useful for trend analysis of different groups of patients. However, since the reference method was of significant influence, differences between TIC and the reference method are incorrectly attributed to TIC alone.

INTRODUCTION

In the last three decades, thoracic impedance cardiography (TIC) has received relatively much attention in the literature as it is a noninvasive, easy to use method for measuring stroke volume (SV) or related parameters. In order to investigate the validity of TIC, many authors have compared the results obtained from TIC to values obtained from a number of alternative methods, in different research settings. These studies have reported both very good and very bad correlations between TIC and the reference method.

The aim of this study was to explain the variations in correlation coefficients between TIC and a reference method from the differences in the studies. Therefore, we conducted a meta-analysis of the current literature concerning the validation of SV (or CO) measurements using TIC. The studies were classified according to differences in (i) methodology (i.e., use of the Kubicek or Sramek-Bernstein equation), (ii) reference method (being the technique to which TIC was compared), and (iii) subject characteristics (differences in illness); they were then treated in a subgroup analysis.

METHODS

Search Strategy

In order to collect the majority of the literature concerning the validation of TIC, a MEDLINE search was performed over the period from January 1966 to April 1997. A combination of MeSH headings was used to represent TIC and to restrict the search to validation studies. The headings, (a) impedance cardiography, (b) impedance plethysmography, (c) electric impedance, (d) electric conductivity, (e) comparative study, (f) cardiac output, (g) stroke volume, and (h) cardiac volume, were combined as (a or b or c or d) and e and (f or g or h). In addition, the text words, (A) impedance, (B) conductance, (C) plethysmography, (D) stroke volume, (E) stroke index, (F) cardiac output, (G) cardiac index, (H) thermodilution, (J) dye dilution, (K) echocardiography, (L) Fick, and (M) electromagnetic flow, were combined as (A or B or C) and (D or E or F or G) and (H or J or K or L or M). Only papers published in English, German, or Dutch were included. Finally, studies from references of review papers were retrieved.[1–6]

Inclusion and Exclusion Criteria

Studies were included in the analysis if they reported a correlation coefficient between the results of TIC and a single reference method. Studies were excluded if different reference methods were used for the calculation of a single correlation coefficient or if only mean differences[7] were reported. In addition, studies were excluded if the applied TIC method or the subject characteristics were not specified.

Data Extraction

The studies were classified with respect to three main aspects: the applied TIC method, the applied reference method, and the characteristics of the subjects studied. For the applied TIC method, we distinguished between two equations to determine SV: the so-called Kubicek and Sramek-Bernstein equations. Studies using the Kubicek equation[8] determined SV according to

$$SV = \frac{\rho L^2}{Z_0^2}\left(\frac{dZ}{dt}\right)_{MIN} T_{LVE}$$

and studies using the Sramek-Bernstein equation[9,10] determined SV according to

$$SV = \frac{\delta}{4.25}\frac{(0.17H)^3}{Z_0}\left(\frac{dZ}{dt}\right)_{MIN} T_{LVE}$$

where SV = stroke volume (mL), δ = a weight correction factor obtained from a nomogram, L = distance between measuring electrodes (cm), H = total body height (cm), Z_0 = mean thoracic impedance (Ω), T_{LVE} = left ventricular ejection time (s), and $(dZ/dt)_{MIN}$ = minimum value of the first derivative of $Z(t)$ to time (Ω/s).

To investigate the influence of the "gold standard," the reference method to which TIC was compared was noted. Rebreathing methods were combined in a group labeled "indirect Fick."

To investigate the influence of subject characteristics, the studies were divided into six groups: (i) healthy subjects, (ii) cardiac patients, (iii) critically ill patients, (iv) pregnant women, (v) animal studies, and (vi) a group called "other," which included other diseases as well as studies with a combination of the above-mentioned patient groups. Finally, if mentioned, the number of subjects and the mean age of the subjects included in the study were noted, as well as the number of measurements on which the correlation coefficient was determined.

Statistical Methods

From each study, the reported Pearson's correlation coefficient, r, was noted. Because a normal distribution is mandatory for the pooling of data, Fisher's Z-transformation (Z) was applied[11] according to

$$Z = \text{arctanh}(r) = \frac{1}{2}\ln\frac{(1+r)}{(1-r)}$$

where arctanh(r) = the arc-hyperbolic tangent.

Next, the Z values were pooled according to a general parametric statistical model[12] based on the random-effects method as described by DerSimonian and Laird.[13] In that method, the studies are weighted by the variance of the Fisher transformed correlation coefficients, s_z. Since the variance is not reported in general, it is estimated from the number of measurements according to[14]

$$s_z^2 \approx \frac{1}{n-1} + \frac{4-r}{2(n-1)^2}.$$

Subsequently, 95% confidence intervals (95% ci) were calculated according to $Z \pm 1.96\, s_z$. Finally, the pooled r and 95% ci were calculated by applying Fisher's back-transformation:

$$r = \tanh(Z).$$

In the results, differences were reported as being statistically significant if the 95% ci did not coincide.

A three-way analysis of variance (ANOVA) was performed on Z to explore the possible sources of heterogeneity. Subgroup analysis was performed on the main effects having a statistically significant influence. One-way ANOVA was performed using Duncan's multiple range test to compare the mean values.

RESULTS

With a MEDLINE search, 372 articles were found, of which many were concerned with EKG impedance and vascular impedance. After reading the titles and abstracts of the articles, and tracking references of review papers, we found a total number of 154 references concerning the validation of TIC, of which 46 were not previously described in review papers.[1-6] A summary of the reviewed literature can be obtained from the authors upon request.

Pooling the 164 correlation coefficients of 112 studies yielded an overall correlation coefficient of $r = 0.82$ (95% ci: 0.80–0.84). In two-thirds of the studies, repeated measurements were performed in the same subject (repeated measurement design). In this measurement design, data might not be completely independent, which is a presumption of correlation analysis. This effect might yield an overestimation of the correlation coefficient.[15] Only 31 studies (50 correlation coefficients) satisfied the criteria of single measurement design (i.e., one measurement per subject). Fifty-five percent of these studies involved correlation coefficients obtained from cardiac patients. Pooling of the latter studies revealed a significantly lower correlation coefficient of $r = 0.73$ (0.66–0.79). FIGURE 1 shows the Fisher-transformed correlation coefficients and 95% confidence intervals of the individual studies using single measurement design. Also indicated is the pooled correlation with its 95% ci.

One-way ANOVA revealed a significant difference in mean age in the various patient groups. Healthy subjects (22 years average) and pregnant women (29 years average) were significantly younger than cardiac patients (49 years average), critically ill patients (57 years average), and "other" patients (46 years average). However, correlation analysis revealed no relation between age and Fisher-transformed correlation coefficients ($r = 0.19$, $p = 0.11$) (see FIGURE 2).

Three-way ANOVA on the Fisher-transformed correlation coefficients (Z values) revealed $p = 0.06$ for the subject characteristics, $p = 0.03$ for the reference method, and $p = 0.85$ for the TIC method. One-way ANOVA revealed a significant influence of the reference method in healthy subjects ($p = 0.04$).

Subgroup analyses were performed on subsets of subject characteristics (TABLE 1) and the reference method. Cardiac patients showed a lower pooled correlation coefficient ($r = 0.77$), whereas healthy subjects and animal studies, as well as critically ill patients and pregnant women, showed correlation coefficients in the same range (see TABLE 1). In healthy subjects, studies using indirect Fick [$r = 0.91$ (0.87–0.93)] yielded significantly higher correlation coefficients than studies using dye dilution [$r = 0.82$ (0.75–0.87)] and echocardiography [$r = 0.69$ (0.48–0.82)].

CONCLUSIONS

An overall correlation between CO measurements using TIC and a reference method of 0.82 was found. No evidence of publication bias was found in the data; hence, the overall correlation is unlikely to be overestimated by the influence of unpublished data. However, the pooled value can be overestimated due to repeated measurement design. In our data of single measurement design, the correlation coefficient is significantly lower (0.73).

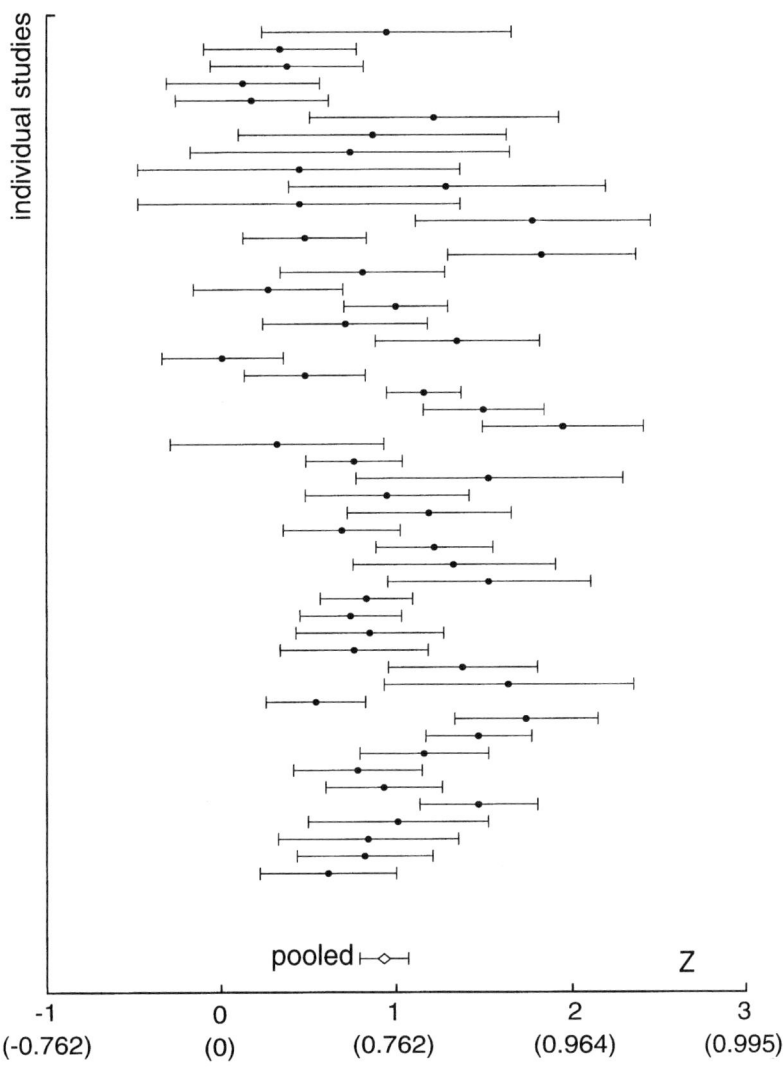

FIGURE 1. Individual Z values and 95% confidence intervals of the separate studies using a single measurement design. The pooled Z is also indicated. The related correlation coefficients are indicated between parentheses.

To compare TIC, several reference methods have been used due to the lack of an overall accepted "gold standard." The reported correlation coefficients proved to be influenced by the applied reference method. As it seems highly unlikely that the performance of TIC is influenced by the applied reference method, this finding represents the inaccuracy of the reference methods themselves. However, by using the reference method as the gold stan-

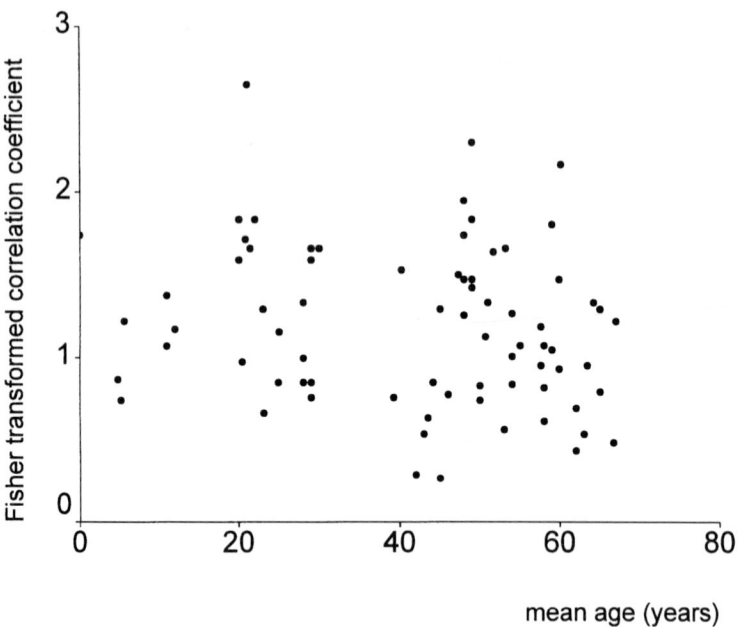

FIGURE 2. Correlation between Fisher-transformed correlation coefficients (Z) and mean ages as reported in the studies ($r = 0.19$, $p = 0.11$).

dard, the inaccuracies are erroneously attributed to TIC exclusively. Thus, the overall correlation coefficient underestimates the actual accuracy of TIC.

We found that the Sramek-Bernstein equation showed no improvement in the correlation as compared to the Kubicek equation. The basic difference between both equations is the applied volume conduction model relating an impedance change to stroke volume. As the model of Sramek-Bernstein incorporates more assumptions, we slightly prefer the Kubicek equation. The finding that both equations have equal performance needs further physical-physiological investigation.

TABLE 1. Pooled Correlation Coefficients in Subgroups of Population with 95% Confidence Intervals

Subjects	Repeated Measurement	Single Measurement
healthy	0.84 (0.80–0.88)	0.86 (0.70–0.93)
cardiac	0.77 (0.71–0.82)	0.66 (0.53–0.75)
critically ill	0.82 (0.77–0.86)	0.86 (0.73–0.93)
pregnant	0.80 (0.68–0.88)	0.80 (0.47–0.93)
animal	0.86 (0.83–0.89)	0.81 (0.64–0.91)
other	0.79 (0.73–0.84)	0.83 (0.76–0.88)
overall	0.82 (0.80–0.84)	0.73 (0.66–0.79)

The performance of TIC was similar in various groups of patients with different diseases, with the exception of cardiac patients, in which group the correlation was decreased. Note that relatively many of the published studies (33% of the total number of studies and 55% of the single measurement design studies) were performed in these cardiac ill patients. Consequently, a superficial investigation of the published literature leads to a misleading overestimation of disappointing results in these cardiac ill patients, suggesting a controversy of TIC on possibly misinterpreted findings. Moreover, in our results, the pooled estimate of the single measurement design studies will also be largely determined by these poor results.

In conclusion, this meta-analysis of published literature on the validity of TIC showed a pooled correlation coefficient of 0.82 (95% ci: 0.80–0.84) for repeated measurements and 0.73 (95% ci: 0.66–0.79) for single measurements. From these findings, we draw the conclusion that TIC is a useful method for measuring cardiac output for research (comparing groups of subjects) and for monitoring in noncardiac ill subjects. For diagnosis, the performance of TIC needs further improvement.

REFERENCES

1. FULLER, H. D. 1992. The validity of cardiac output measurement by thoracic impedance: a meta-analysis. Clin. Invest. Med. **15:** 103–112.
2. JENSEN, L. et al. 1995. A review of impedance cardiography. Heart & Lung **24:** 183–193.
3. MILLER, J. C. & S. M. HORVATH. 1978. Methodology/impedance cardiography. Psychophysiology **5:** 80–90.
4. LAMBERTS, R. et al. 1984. Impedance cardiography. Van Gorcum. Assen, the Netherlands.
5. SHERWOOD, A. et al. 1990. Committee report/methodological guidelines for impedance cardiography. Psychophysiology **27:** 1–23.
6. SCHUSTER, C. J. & H. P. SCHUSTER. 1984. Application of impedance cardiography in critical care medicine. Resuscitation **11:** 255–274.
7. BLAND, J. M. & D. G. ALTMAN. 1986. Statistical methods for assessing agreement between two methods of clinical measurement. Lancet **8:** 307–310.
8. KUBICEK, W. G. et al. 1966. Development and evaluation of an impedance cardiac output system. Aerosp. Med. **37:** 1208–1212.
9. SRAMEK, B. B. et al. 1983. Stroke volume equation with a linear base impedance model and its accuracy, as compared to thermodilution and magnetic flowmeter techniques in humans and animals. *In* Proceedings of the Sixth International Conference on Electrical Bioimpedance (Zadar, Yugoslavia), p. 38–41.
10. BERNSTEIN, D. P. 1986. A new stroke volume equation for thoracic electrical bioimpedance: theory and rationale. Crit. Care Med. **14:** 904–909.
11. COOPER, H. & L. V. HEDGES. 1994. The Handbook of Research Synthesis. Russell Sage Foundation. New York.
12. WHITEHEAD, A. & J. WHITEHEAD. 1991. A general parametric approach to the meta-analysis of randomized clinical trials. Stat. Med. **10:** 1665–1677.
13. DERSIMONIAN, R. & N. LAIRD. 1986. Meta-analysis in clinical trials. Controlled Clin. Trials **7:** 177–188.
14. KENDALL, M. & A. STUART. 1977. The Advanced Theory of Statistics. Volume 1. Griffin. London.
15. BLAND, J. M. & D. G. ALTMAN. 1994. Correlation, regression, and repeated data. Br. Med. J. **308:** 896.

Towards a Theoretical Understanding of Stroke Volume Estimation with Impedance Cardiography[a]

TH. J. C. FAES, E. RAAIJMAKERS, J. H. MEIJER, H. G. GOOVAERTS, AND R. M. HEETHAAR

Department of Clinical Physics and Informatics, Institute for Cardiovascular Research, University Hospital Vrije Universiteit, 1007 MB Amsterdam, the Netherlands

ABSTRACT: In electrical impedance cardiography, Kubicek's formula is often used to measure stroke volume from thoracic impedance variations synchronously to heart activity. To calculate stroke volume from impedance variations, the so-called outflow problem should be adequately solved. This outflow problem refers to the joint causes of impedance change due to blood entering the aorta from the heart, as well as blood leaving the aorta due to arterial runoff. The *aim* of this study was to investigate the Kubicek formula as a solution of the outflow problem. Kubicek's formula was theoretically investigated using a simple model of the volume-conducting properties of the thorax (two-cylinder model), as well as the hemodynamics of the systemic circulation (three-element "windkessel" model). The mathematical analysis showed that the outflow problem was not solved by the Kubicek formula. Moreover, this theoretical result was experimentally confirmed.

INTRODUCTION

In the late sixties, Patterson, Kubicek, and coworkers developed a formula for the estimation of cardiac stroke volume from thoracic impedance variations synchronously to heart activity. The formula reads

$$V_K = \rho_B \frac{L^2}{Z_0^2} \left(\frac{dZ_0(t)}{dt}\right)_{MAX} T_{LVE} \tag{1}$$

where V_K (mL) is "Kubicek's estimate" of stroke volume, ρ_B (Ω-cm) is the specific resistivity of blood, L (cm) is the length of the thorax segment considered, Z_0 (Ω) is the mean value of the measured thoracic impedance, and $[dZ_0(t)/dt]_{MAX}$ is the maximum value of the first derivative of $Z(t)$ to time (Ω/s).

Although Kubicek's formula was used in many clinical studies,[1] some mathematical aspects remain obscure: in particular, the rationale of the first derivative of the impedance signal [i.e., $(dZ_0/dt)_{MAX}$] in connection with the so-called outflow problem.[2] The outflow problem refers to the joint causes of the measured impedance change during the cardiac cycle. This impedance change is considered to be the combined result of blood entering the aorta from the heart, as well as blood leaving the aorta due to arterial runoff. To calculate stroke volume from impedance changes, impedance cardiography should adequately deal with the arterial runoff (outflow problem). Kubicek's formula is frequently inter-

---

[a] Financial support was provided by the Dutch Department of Economic Affairs (Grant No. ITU 950340).

preted as a solution of the outflow problem by the following reasoning: At the beginning of systole, the inflow of blood into the aorta is maximal, while the outflow is still minimal. Therefore, forward extrapolation of the steepest part of the impedance signal to the end of systole would provide an estimate of the impedance change as if the arterial runoff is absent.[3,4] In Kubicek's formula, this extrapolation is implemented by taking the maximum value of the first derivative to time of the impedance change and multiplying this value with the ventricular ejection period. According to this reasoning, the term $(dZ_0/dt)_{MAX} \cdot T_{LVE}$ in the Kubicek formula is a solution to the outflow problem.

The *aim* of this study was to investigate Kubicek's formula as a solution of the outflow problem. A simple model was used to study the properties of the Kubicek formula from a theoretical point of view. Moreover, empirical results will be discussed to test the theoretical findings.

THEORY

Approach

The rationale of Kubicek's formula is found in the following sequence of processes: In the k-th heartbeat, an amount of blood is ejected from the heart into the aorta; the amount of blood ejected is called stroke volume $V_S[k]$ (mL). This ejection leads to an inflow $F_I(t)$ (mL/s) of blood into the aorta, an increased volume $V_A(t)$ (mL) of the aorta, and an increased outflow $F_O(t)$ (mL/s) of blood from the aorta (arterial runoff). The volume increase of the relatively good conducting blood in the aorta results in a decreased impedance $Z_A(t)$ (Ω) of the aorta and, in turn, to a decreased measured thoracic impedance $Z_0(t)$ (Ω). Visualization of the sequence of processes leads to

$$V_S[k] \to F_I(t) \to V_A(t) \to F_O(t) \to Z_A(t) \to Z_0(t). \qquad (2)$$

Going from stroke volume $V_S[k]$ to measured impedance change $Z_0(t)$ may be looked upon as a forward problem.

Kubicek's formula claims implicitly to be a solution of the inverse problem, that is, going backward from thoracic impedance change $Z_0(t)$ to stroke volume $V_K[k]$. In mathematical terms,

$$Z_0(t) \to \text{Kubicek's formula} \to V_K[k] \qquad (3)$$

where the subscript K was used to distinguish Kubicek's estimate V_K from the actual stroke volume V_S.

The accuracy of Kubicek's formula can be studied theoretically by comparing V_S and V_K. For that purpose, the forward problem needs to be modeled to obtain $Z_0(t)$ as a function of $V_S[k]$, that is, $Z_0(t) = f(V_S[k])$. Substitution of this $Z_0(t)$ into Kubicek's equation yields the required relation between $V_S[k]$ and $V_K[k]$.

Forward Problem

Cardiovascular System

The electrical analogy of the cardiovascular system is shown in FIGURE 1.

The heart was modeled as a blood volume source (current source) with a high source resistance (R_H). The inflow into the aorta $F_I(t)$ was defined as a rectangularly pulsatile flow

$$F_I(t) = \begin{cases} F_M & \text{for } T_D[k] \leq t \leq T_S[k] \quad \text{(systole)} \\ 0 & \text{for } T_S[k] \leq t \leq T_D[k+1] \quad \text{(diastole)} \end{cases} \quad (4)$$

where $T_D[k]$ and $T_S[k]$ are the time moments of end-diastole and end-systole of the k-th beat, respectively. By definition, left ventricular ejection time is $T_{LVE}[k] = T_S[k] - T_D[k]$ and stroke volume is $V_S[k] = F_M T_{LVE}[k]$. For a stroke volume of 100 mL and a left ventricular ejection time of 0.2 s, F_M is 500 mL/s.

A three-element windkessel model was used to model the hemodynamical properties of the systemic circulation.[5] The resistance of the peripheral blood vessels is pooled into a single resistor with a constant resistance R_P (typically, 0.95 mmHg • s/mL), to which Ohm's law applies. The compliance of the aorta is pooled into a single capacitor with a constant capacitance C_A (typically, 1.5 mL/mmHg). The Z, representing a hemodynamic impedance, appears irrelevant in our application.

From Kirchhoff's law, it follows that $F_I(t) = F_0(t) + F_A(t)$; from Ohm's law, it follows that $F_0(t) = P_A(t)/R_P$, with $P_A(t)$ being the blood pressure (mmHg); and for constant compliance, it follows that $F_A(t) = dV_A(t)/dt = CdP_A(t)/dt$. Hence, the ordinary differential equation for $V_A(t)$ is

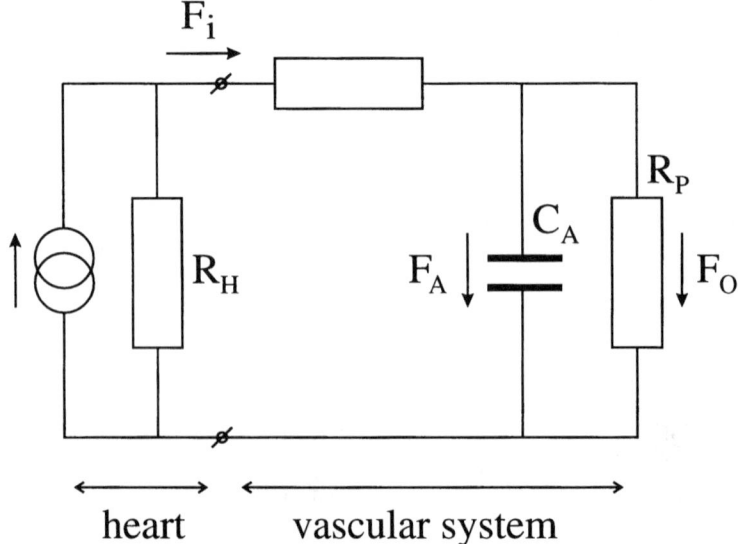

FIGURE 1. Electric analogy of the cardiovascular system (consult text for details).

$$\frac{dV_A(t)}{dt} + \frac{1}{R_P C_A} V_A(t) = F_1(t) \tag{5}$$

with the initial condition $V_A(T_D[k])$ at $t = T_D[k]$. For systole, $T_D[k] \leq t \leq T_S[k]$, the solution is

$$V_A(t) = F_M R_P C_A \left(1 - e^{-\frac{(t-T_D[k])}{R_P C_A}}\right) + V_A(T_D[k]) e^{-\frac{(t-T_D[k])}{R_P C_A}}. \tag{6}$$

Electrical Volume Conductor

In Kubicek's original approach, the electrical properties of the thorax were modeled using a cylinder with specific resistivity ρ_B, length L, time-dependent cross-sectional surface $A_A(t)$, and volume $V_A(t) = LA_A(t)$. The time-dependent impedance of the aorta is

$$Z_A(t) = \rho_B \frac{L}{A_A(t)} = \rho_B \frac{L^2}{V_A(t)}. \tag{7}$$

We follow Geddes and Baker in using a two-compartment model with a second cylinder, enclosing Kubicek's cylinder, with specific resistivity ρ_T, length L, and time-independent cross-sectional surface A_T.[3] In this model, the inner cylinder represents the aorta and the outer cylinder represents the remaining thoracic tissue. Since both cylinders are electrically connected in parallel, the (longitudinal) impedance $Z_0(t)$ is

$$Z_0(t) = Z_A(t) | \, | Z_T = \frac{Z_A(t) Z_T}{Z_A(t) + Z_T}. \tag{8}$$

The appropriateness of a cylinder model in modeling the volume-conducting properties of the thorax has been questioned by Wang and Patterson.[6] Nevertheless, we used a two-cylinder model to stick close to Kubicek's original approach.

The Inverse Problem

Applying the chain rule for differentiation of composite functions to equation 2 yields

$$\frac{dZ_0(t)}{dt} = \frac{dZ_0(t)}{dZ_A(t)} \frac{dZ_A(t)}{dV_A(t)} \frac{dV_A(t)}{dt}. \tag{9}$$

To obtain $dZ_0(t)/dt$, substitute the derivatives of equation 6, 7, and 8 into equation 9 and take the limit $t \downarrow T_D[k]$ to obtain $(dZ_0/dt)_{MAX}$. Hence, it appears that

$$\left(\frac{dZ_0(t)}{dt}\right)_{MAX} = \frac{Z_0^2}{\rho_B L^2} \left\{ F_M - \frac{V_A(T_D[k])}{R_P C_A} \right\}. \tag{10}$$

Substitution of $(dZ_0/dt)_{MAX}$ into Kubicek's formula (equation 1), using $T_{LVE}[k] = T_S[k] - T_D[k]$ and $V_S[k] = F_M T_{LVE}[k]$, yields the required relation between the actual $V_S[k]$ and the estimated $V_K[k]$:

$$V_K = V_S - V_A(T_D[k])\frac{T_{LVE}[k]}{R_P C_A}. \tag{11}$$

This result shows that Kubicek's estimate of stroke volume $V_K[k]$ differs from the actual $V_S[k]$ by a nonzero bias term ($V_A T_{LVE}/R_P C_A$).

The bias term is strongly connected to the outflow problem because the bias term $V_A T_{LVE}/R_P C_A$ is equal to $F_0(T_D[k]) \cdot T_{LVE}[k]$, which directly follows from $C_A = V_A(t)/P_A(t)$ (constant compliance) and $F_0(t) = P_A(t)/R_P$ (Ohm's law). Thus, stroke volume is overestimated by a quantity equal to the flow from the considered aorta at end-diastole, $F_0(T_D[k])$, times the left ventricular ejection time, $T_{LVE}[k]$. Hence, Kubicek's formula leaves the outflow problem unsolved.

Although some parameters of the bias term are unknown, equation 11 predicts that the relative difference $(V_S - V_K)/V_S$ is proportionally related to the quotient T_{LVE}/V_S: that is,

$$\frac{V_S - V_K}{V_S} = \frac{V_A(T_D[k]) T_{LVE}[k]}{R_P C_A \ V_S} \propto \frac{T_{LVE}[k]}{V_S}. \tag{12}$$

Actually, the proportionality is positive because the parameters V_A, R_P, and C_A are positive by nature. This positive proportionality is a prediction testable empirically by measuring V_K and T_{LVE} with impedance cardiography and V_S with a thermodilution technique.

EMPIRICAL RESULTS

Subjects

In 12 critically ill patients (intensive care unit), stroke volume was measured with a thermodilution method and with an impedance cardiograph applying Kubicek's formula. In these patients, a total of 30 measurements were made. Measurements were performed every 24 hours on two to four consecutive days, with the actual number of measurements depending upon the recovery of the patients or upon catheter breakdown. The patients (9 males and 3 females) suffered from acute lung injury (7) or acute respiratory distress syndrome (6). The cause of lung injury and acute respiratory distress syndrome was sepsis [abdominal (6), pulmonary (5), urogenital (1), trauma (1)]. All patients were mechanically ventilated with PEEP and an inspiratory oxygen level chosen according to clinical requirements. The patients' ages were 50 ± 17 years (mean ± SD) (range, 24–57 years), and their weights were 76 ± 22 kg (range, 40–120 kg). The protocol was approved by the institutional ethics committee.

Methods

Impedance recordings were made using a nine-spot electrode (Ag/AgCl) array developed at our hospital.[7] Voltage-recording electrodes were placed on the neck (two connected parallel) and on the thorax at 0.17 times the body height from the neck electrodes (two connected parallel). Current-injecting electrodes were placed on the forehead (one) and 12 cm below the lower voltage-measuring electrodes (four connected parallel). Impedance recordings (impedance and first derivative to time) were obtained with a cardiograph developed in our laboratory,[8] using a sinusoidal current of 1 mA (rms) at a frequency of 64 kHz. To reduce the breathing effect, the impedance signals were coherently averaged (off-line) over 30 heartbeats, using the peak of the first derivative as a trigger reference. This averaged signal was used to determine the mean thoracic impedance (Z_0 in ohms), the maximum value of the first derivative [$(dZ/dt)_{MAX}$ in ohms/s], and the left ventricular ejection time (T_{LVE} in s). Stroke volume was calculated using Kubicek's formula with ρ_B taken as 150 Ω-cm for males and 135 Ω-cm for females.

Cardiac output was simultaneously measured with a thermodilution method: measurements were made by injection of 10 mL saline bolus (room temperature) into the right atrium at the end-expiratory phase of the respiratory cycle. The average of five measurements was determined.

Statistical Analysis

A correlation coefficient was used to measure the strength of the theoretically predicted relationship between the relative difference $(V_S - V_K)/V_S$ and T_{LVE}/V_S. Spearman's correlation coefficient was used because binormality of the empirical data could not be demonstrated.

Results

A total number of 30 measurements of the relative difference and T_{LVE}/V_S were available. FIGURE 2 shows a scatterplot of the results with the relative difference $(V_S - V_K)/V_S$ (%) on the ordinate and T_{LVE}/V_S on the abscissa. As predicted by our theoretical model analysis, a positive correlation, weak, but statistically significantly different from zero, was found (Spearman: $r = 0.5$, $p < 0.02$). The correlation was presumably weak because the unknown parameters V_A, R_P, and C_A interfered, but could not be taken into account. Moreover, only 3 measurements out of a total of 30 showed a negative value of the relative difference, which indicated that Kubicek's formula indeed overestimates stroke volume. Thus, these experimental results confirmed the predictions derived from the model.

CONCLUSIONS

Kubicek's formula was found to be biased in a mathematical analysis concerning a simple model of the volume-conducting properties of the thorax and the hemodynamics of the systemic circulation. The bias was shown to depend on several cardiovascular parameters, such as left ventricular ejection time T_{LVE}, the "windkessel" time constant $R_P C_A$, and the end-diastolic aorta volume V_A. Moreover, this bias was shown to be directly related to the outflow of blood from the considered aorta. The existence of this bias term was experimentally confirmed.

Our theoretical analysis showed that Kubicek's formula overestimated stroke volume. Moreover, our experimental results, obtained in a group of critically ill patients, showed that the overestimation was considerable. Hence, it appears that the outflow problem might be one of the major error sources in impedance cardiography. The inappropriateness

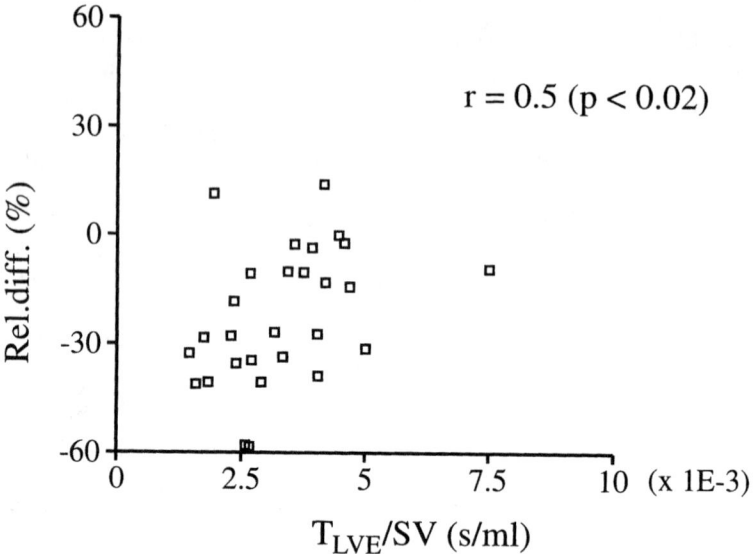

FIGURE 2. Scatterplot between the relative difference $(V_S - V_K)/V_S$ (%) on the ordinate and T_{LVE}/V_S (s/mL) on the abscissa (consult text for details). Spearman's correlation coefficient was $r = 0.5$ ($p < 0.02$).

of a cylinder model in modeling the volume-conducting properties of the thorax has been identified by Wang and Patterson as another major error source.[6]

In conclusion, the outflow problem is not solved by the Kubicek formula. To save impedance cardiographic measurements of stroke volume from obscurity, the outflow problem is one of the problems to be solved.

REFERENCES

1. RAAIJMAKERS, E. *et al.* 1999. A meta-analysis of published studies concerning the validity of thoracic impedance cardiography. This volume.
2. FAES, TH. J. C. *et al.* 1995. Mathematical analysis of impedance cardiography. *In* Proceedings of the Ninth International Conference on Electrical Bio-Impedance (Heidelberg), p. 480–483.
3. GEDDES, L. A. & L. E. BAKER. 1989. Principles of Applied Biomedical Instrumentation, p. 591–639. Wiley. New York.
4. SHERWOOD, A. *et al.* 1990. Methodological guideline for impedance cardiography. Psychophysiology **27:** 1–23.
5. WESTERHOF, N. 1993. Arterial haemodynamics. *In* The Physics of Heart and Circulation, p. 355–382. Inst. Phys. Pub. Bristol/Philadelphia.
6. WANG, L. & R. PATTERSON. 1995. Multiple sources of the impedance cardiogram based on 3-D finite difference human thorax models. IEEE Trans. Biomed. Eng. **BME-42:** 141–148.
7. WOLTJER, H. H. *et al.* 1996. Optimalization of the spot electrodes array in impedance cardiography. Med. Biol. Eng. Comput. **34:** 84–87.
8. GOOVAERTS, H. G. *et al.* 1999. Some design concepts for electrical impedance measurement. This volume.

Lead Field Theoretical Approach in Bioimpedance Measurements: Towards More Controlled Measurement Sensitivity[a]

PASI K. KAUPPINEN,[b] JARI A. HYTTINEN,[b] TIIT KÖÖBI,[c] AND JAAKKO MALMIVUO[b]

[b]*Ragnar Granit Institute, Tampere University of Technology, Fin-33101 Tampere, Finland*
[c]*Department of Clinical Physiology, Tampere University Hospital, Fin-33521 Tampere, Finland*

ABSTRACT: This study was conducted to demonstrate the potentiality of lead field theoretical approach in analyzing bioimpedance (BI) measurements. Anatomically accurate computer models and the lead field theory were used to develop BI measurement configurations capable of detecting more localized BI changes in the human body. The methods were applied to assess the measurement properties of conventional impedance cardiography (ICG) and such BI measurement configurations as can be derived using (i) the 12-lead electrocardiography (ECG) and (ii) the international 10–20 electroencephalography (EEG) electrode systems. Information as to how various electrode configurations are sensitive to detecting conductivity changes in different tissues and organs was thus obtained. Theoretical results with the 12-lead system suggested that, compared to conventional ICGs, significantly more selective ICG configurations can be derived for cardiovascular structures. In addition to theoretical investigations, clinical test measurements were made with the 12-lead system to establish whether characteristic waveforms are available. Sensitivity distributions obtained with the 10–20 electrode system give promise of the possibility of monitoring noninvasively cerebrospinal fluid (CSF) impedance changes related to impending epileptic seizures.

INTRODUCTION

Measurement of tissue BI is a well-known technique that can be applied for various physiological investigations. Measuring BI variations on the thorax surface provides an interesting possibility of obtaining valuable information regarding the status of the heart and the vascular system. In ICG, the pumping actions of the heart and other mechanical events in the cardiovascular system, and not the electrical functioning of the heart as in ECG, give rise to the measured signal. Another attractive application of BI measurement is an attempt to measure noninvasively the CSF impedance changes on the surface of the scalp. It has been found that epileptic seizures, at least those induced with an intramuscular injection of penicillin in cats, elevate the invasively measured CSF impedance at 5–15 minutes prior to seizure activity.[1]

The origin of the ICG signal has been investigated in a number of studies using physiological manipulations or computer modeling.[2–8] The applied electrode configuration

[a]This work was supported financially by the Academy of Finland, the Ragnar Granit Foundation, the Medical Research Fund of Tampere University Hospital, and the Tampere City Science Foundation.

should offer high sensitivity to record changes in the organ or region of interest, giving detectable and reliable BI data originating mostly in that region. According to a study by Wang and Patterson, multiple sources contribute to the ICG signal.[2] These authors conclude that ICG should not be used for determining cardiac output with any of the ICG methods currently employed. However, in addition to cardiac output, there are many situations where clearly defined BI measurements of living tissue and especially cardiac tissue could possibly be used. Since noninvasive BI techniques are indirect methods, particular care must be taken in selecting the electrode configurations for the measurements.

Modeling and simulating ICG or other BI signal formation is a tedious and time-consuming task involving many uncertainties and assumptions. The main objective of this study was to demonstrate the potentiality of the lead field and reciprocity theoretical approach in analyzing and developing BI measurements. Useful information can be obtained from BI measurements provided that relationships between the waveforms and changes occurring in the measured volume are understood. Sensitivity distributions afford an approximation of these relationships. This paper explains how the measurement sensitivity distribution of any impedance measurement configuration could be obtained with the modern numerical computer modeling utilizing the lead field and reciprocity concepts. The methods were applied to investigate the sensitivity distributions of (a) conventional ICGs recorded with band or spot electrodes, (b) regional measurements using the 12-lead ECG electrode locations, and (c) measurements using the international 10–20 EEG electrode system for detecting CSF impedance changes related to epileptic activity. Information as to how different BI measurements are able to detect conductivity changes occurring in different tissues and organs in the human thorax and head was obtained, providing theoretical knowledge in terms of measurement sensitivity distributions.

METHODS

Sensitivity Distribution of BI Measurement: Lead Field and Reciprocity

Each cell, organ, and tissue makes its contribution to the formation of the BI signal. With the lead field method, all these contributions to the signal can be taken into account and simulated simultaneously. According to Geselowitz,[9] the measured impedance Z and its change ΔZ resulting from the conductivity σ and its change $\Delta \sigma$ within a volume conductor can be evaluated by

$$(\Delta)Z = \int_v \frac{1}{(\Delta)\sigma} S \, dv \qquad (1)$$

where S is the measurement sensitivity distribution associated with the electrode configuration. Sensitivity S is obtained by first determining the current field generated by a unit current applied to the current injection electrodes. This current field in the volume conductor forms the lead field of the current injection electrodes. The second lead field associated with voltage measurement is then obtained by calculating the current field produced by a reciprocally injected unit current between the voltage measurement electrodes. By taking the dot product of the two fields, a scalar field S is obtained, which describes how a conductivity change in a certain location affects the measured potential at the measurement leads. The combined sensitivity field of the BI measurement is then

$$S = J_{LE} \bullet J_{LI} \qquad (2)$$

where J_{LI} is the lead field produced by current excitation electrodes and J_{LE} is the lead field produced by the reciprocal energization of voltage measurement leads.[10] Depending on the angle of the two fields, there can be (according to the dot product) regions where the sensitivity is zero, positive, or negative to measure conductivity changes. For example, in a region of null sensitivity, slight changes in conductivity are not sensed, while increasing conductivity in a region of negative sensitivity will result in increasing impedance. A time-varying impedance signal is produced by anything altering the lead fields of current and voltage leads, including complex simultaneous variations in tissue electrical, geometrical, and physiological properties. These changes will also evidently alter the sensitivity distribution; however, in analysis of the sensitivity distribution it can be approximated to remain constant under slight variations in volume conductor properties. A substantial advantage of the lead field theoretical approach is that approximations of quantitative conductivity changes occurring in different regions are not needed to obtain the sensitivity distribution. Moreover, the method allows rapid simulation of a large number of different measurement configurations. By appropriately changing or selecting the location of the electrodes forming J_{LI} and J_{LE}, the resulting combined sensitivity field can be controlled to a considerable extent. This opens up a novel possibility in the search for a BI configuration suitable for detecting certain desired locations with appropriate, more precisely directed measurement sensitivity. If the lead fields of a certain electrode configuration are obtained by model simulation, various sensitivity fields can be derived simply by linear combination of the original lead fields. The sensitivity field may then be used to assess the relative contribution of each elementary volume source to the composition of the basal and time-varying impedance signal. Finite-difference method (FDM) modeling provides a solution at all hexahedral volumetric elements in the model, being thus useful in detailed field analysis.

Simulation of BI Measurement Configurations Using Thorax and Head Models

Methods to construct and solve accurate volume conductor computer models based on the FDM have been previously developed and validated.[11–13] The lead fields generated by BI measurements can be obtained by applying the methods developed. For ICG analysis, an anatomically highly detailed 3-D model of the thorax and neck was constructed based on the United States National Library of Medicine's Visible Human Man digital anatomy data.[14] Thirty-two distinct organs and tissue types were segmented from the data, resulting in 3,176,872 volume elements. For computational reasons, the accuracy of the model was reduced to 477,611 and 83,987 elements in the present study. A realistic, 3-D head model of a male epilepsy patient was constructed based on an MR image set for simulating noninvasive measurement of CSF impedance changes. The scalp, skull, CSF, white matter, and gray matter were segmented and classified from the image set. The total number of identified voxels was 1,670,000, which was downscaled by a factor of 4 with a uniform rectangular grid to reduce solution time.

Electrode locations of the conventional ICG electrode configurations and the 12-lead system were set on the surface of the thorax model. For the head model, the 10–20 EEG electrode locations were obtained directly from the MR images since the electrode positions were marked with oil-filled capsules prior to the MR imaging session. FIGURE 1 shows the appearance of the models and the placement of various electrodes on the surface of the models.

Applying the FDM, simulations were conducted for the conventional ICGs to obtain the basal impedance, the lead fields in the thorax generated by the current and the measurement leads J_{LI} and J_{LE}, and the resulting measurement sensitivity distributions given by equation 2. Reciprocal energization of all electrode pairs was carried out individually by applying constant voltages at the electrode nodes in the model, which produced a current injection through the nodes. The currents were then adjusted after the simulation to obtain equal unit current strengths for the lead fields. The overall sensitivity of any tissue type (or group of tissues considered as one target volume) contributing to the measured signal was obtained by integrating the sensitivity value of the tissue over the FDM volume elements that it occupied according to equation 1. This sensitivity value was compared with the total sensitivity of the electrode setup to obtain a quantitative measure of partial contributions from each organ and tissue to the basal and time-varying impedance.

For more specifically regional impedance measurements, lead fields of the 12-lead ECG and 10–20 EEG electrode systems were simulated similarly, one electrode at a time. Since the system is assumed to be linear (at any given frequency), lead fields once calculated may be utilized in various combinations to obtain new BI measurement setups. By selecting two to four lead fields of either electrode system at a time for the measurement, several thousand sensitivity distributions were established according to equation 2. The resulting measurement configurations utilize altogether two to four precalculated lead fields, one or two for current injection and similarly one or two for voltage measurement. A computer algorithm was implemented to automatically combine various BI configurations and to assess the partial contributions to basal impedance and measurement sensitivity from each tissue and organ for further investigations. Several 12-lead-based BI

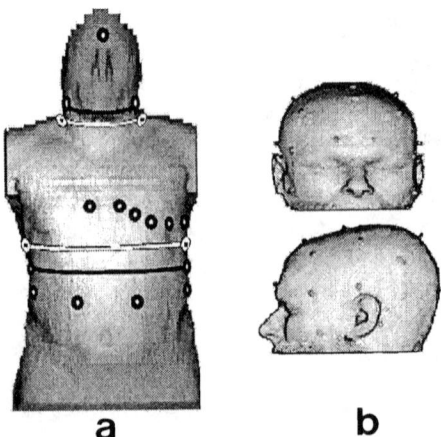

FIGURE 1. Placement of electrodes on the surface of the FDM models: (a) the Visible Human Man thorax model with the conventional ICGs and the 12-lead ECG electrodes; (b) the head model with the international 10–20 EEG electrode system.

measurement configurations sensitive in the heart, blood, and lung tissues were selected for clinical test measurements for comparison with the theoretical expectations. For the 10–20 BI configurations, those with the highest sensitivity to the CSF were included in additional simulations, with 20% decreased conductivity for the CSF.

RESULTS

Sensitivity Distributions of Conventional ICGs

The lead field analysis indicated that none of the conventional ICG setups was specifically sensitive to detect conductivity changes in the region of the blood masses, heart muscle, or lungs. More than 50% of the measurement sensitivity was concentrated in the skeletal muscle, which also occupied the largest volume in the model. The lungs contributed more than all the heart and blood masses together. The total contribution from the ventricles, aortas, carotid artery, and jugular vein was less than 5% in each case. The sensitivity distributions obtained clearly emphasized the multiregional sampling sensitivity and information content of the measured impedance signal. Conventional ICG techniques provide a single waveform in which regional information on impedance changes associated with the function of the heart is not clearly retrieved. The relative proportion of basal impedance caused by all the blood masses, heart muscle, and lungs was approximately 15% in simulated conventional ICGs.

Sensitivity Distributions of ICGs Using 12-Lead ECG Electrode Locations

The results obtained with the lead fields of the 12-lead ECG electrode system showed that the selection of electrode configuration has a significant effect on the established measurement sensitivity. Simulated electrode configurations indicated markedly different sensitivity distributions as compared to the conventional ICGs. Sensitivity to cardiovascular structures with certain configurations was increased tenfold. Since the sensitivity field may also exhibit negative values, the contribution from, for example, skeletal muscle was reduced to less than 5% with some configurations. Nevertheless, the general trend observable in regional configurations suggested that it is not possible to separate definitively the contribution from any single organ or blood mass from the measurement using the configurations obtained with the 12-lead electrode system selected. It is especially difficult to obtain configurations selective between the left and right side of the heart.

Clinical test measurements revealed the richness of the signal patterns of regional impedance recordings. Clinical recordings also showed significantly differing waveforms between the selected configurations. As predicted by computer simulations, some configurations showed almost no changes in signal tracing due to ventilation, while other configurations with high sensitivity to the lung region were especially sensitive to breathing. FIGURE 2 shows an example of a regional BI recording sensitive to the blood masses and cardiac tissue. This waveform bears a resemblance to the aortic blood pressure and flow curves shown in the same figure.

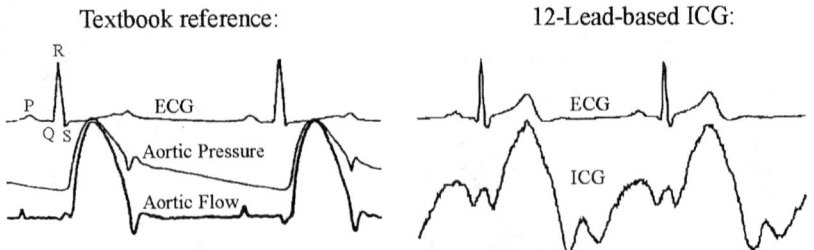

FIGURE 2. Cardiac-sensitive impedance measurement recorded with a configuration using the electrode locations of the 12-lead ECG. Aortic measurements on the left are taken from a textbook for reference.

Sensitivity of 10–20 Derived Measurements in Recording CSF Impedance Changes

The key point was to observe whether such BI measurement configurations existed that could monitor the CSF impedance changes noninvasively from the surface of the scalp with sufficient sensitivity. The average absolute contribution to the measured impedance from the CSF was 4.2%, with a standard deviation of 5.2% among all the 97,273 combined and analyzed electrode configurations. The proportional contribution from the CSF with the most selective configuration was as much as 69%, which in theory provides sufficiently high selectivity for successful measurement. The contribution from the skull was 15.7%; from the brain (gray and white matter together), it was 12.9% with the same configuration. With a single measurement, it is impossible to conclude which tissue or tissues cause the change in measured impedance. The reliability of CSF impedance measurement may be improved by making multiple measurements using, for example, configurations expressing negative sensitivity to the brain, while keeping positive sensitivity to CSF impedance changes. Combining several measurements with known properties may provide reliable data for determining whether the impedance of the CSF is actually changing. According to the simulations, several such configurations are derivable using the 10–20 EEG electrode system. Simulations with 20% decreased conductivity of the CSF produced expected changes in the simulated impedance, following the proportional sensitivity values obtained with the analyzing algorithm within a few percent variation.

DISCUSSION

While BI techniques have been proposed for a variety of purposes, the theoretical bases for the procedure have seldom been satisfactorily established. The potential of a BI measurement to detect conductivity changes in the volume conductor has previously been investigated with computer modeling by changing the conductivity values of the constructed model and then calculating the subsequent difference in the resulting basal impedance. With this procedure, the capacity of a lead setup to detect the total conductivity changes generated in specific regions (where conductivity is altered) can be calculated. To obtain a wider view in the measurement, the total system should be carefully investigated, each tissue type and organ at a time. This requires a large amount of computing time and work. Even so, the distribution of measurement sensitivity remains unknown, and a special limitation is that one cannot decide what quantitative changes in conductivities are brought about in the volume conductor as a result of, for example, cardiac function. The lead field theoretical approach has been proved to provide a more useful and powerful means of analyzing and developing BI measurements. It yields direct evidence regarding the ability of a measurement configuration to monitor impedance changes occurring in various regions of the modeled system; that is, it provides the sensitivity of the measurement in all modeled tissues with a single simulation.

The data obtained here suggested that conventional ICG configurations do not deliver selective information related to any part of the cardiovascular structure. Using the lead fields of 12-lead ECG offers better possibilities in forming measurement configurations with more localized sensitivity properties, implying a potential for providing additional information on physiological factors related to cardiac function. The ratio of signals from desired sources to undesired ones with selected 12-lead configurations should be higher as the measured signal contains more information from the appropriate area, and not from the whole volume between the leads as in conventional ICGs. Clinical experiments with the 12-lead configurations confirmed more regional information content; the configurations selected produced the waveforms intimately related to cardiovascular function. However, the differences in signal waveforms between the individuals subjected to clinical tests were significant and probably largely affected by differences in body shape, size, and cardiovascular function. The limitations of the existing standard BI instrumentation introduce further variations in 12-lead measurements, especially when the sensitivity field is obtained using several electrode locations simultaneously. If the skin-electrode contacts are not electrically identical, they function as unbalanced current or voltage dividers directing the lead fields differently from what was intended. The same problem is present in all BI measurements utilizing multielectrode terminals. Several simultaneous BI measurements should be made with known recording properties to obtain enough independent information for a reliable estimation of the cardiac condition.

As another example of lead field analysis, the methods were used to determine the sensitivity of 10–20 EEG electrode system-based BI measurements in detecting regional conductivity changes occurring in the CSF. Numerical experiments indicated that it should be possible to estimate changes in CSF impedance noninvasively. Several BI combinations based on the 10–20 EEG electrode system provided more than 50% sensitivity to measure the CSF. This result implies a possibility of noninvasive BI measurement to detect oncoming seizures, but again the existing bioimpedance instrumentation needs further development to accommodate the developed electrode configurations utilizing several electrode locations for each terminal of the measurement device. It should also be noted that the idea of detecting impending seizure activity by BI relies on one major assumption: the conductivity of CSF changes due to an oncoming seizure. Thus, clinical relevance and potential remain to be established.

Computer modeling based on accurate anatomical data and the lead field theoretical simulation and analyzing approach can provide an alternative and promising means of analyzing and developing various BI measurements. The method improves the understanding of the relationships between changes in the body and the BI signals measured, providing a theoretical basis for the development of multiple, more reliable BI measurements.

REFERENCES

1. MILLER, G. E. & T. L. GERBER. 1986. Cerebrospinal impedance response to induced epileptic activity. IEEE Trans. Biomed. Eng. **33:** 626–632.
2. WANG, L. & R. PATTERSON. 1995. Multiple sources of the impedance cardiogram based on 3-D finite difference human thorax models. IEEE Trans. Biomed. Eng. **42:** 141–148.
3. KIM, D. W. *et al.* 1988. Origins of the impedance change in impedance cardiography by a three-dimensional finite element model. IEEE Trans. Biomed. Eng. **35:** 993–1000.
4. WTOREK, J. & A. POLINSKI. 1995. Examination of impedance cardiography properties—FEM model studies. Biomed. Sci. Instrum. **31:** 77–82.
5. VISSER, K. R., R. LAMBERTS & W. G. ZIJLSTRA. 1990. Investigation of the origin of the impedance cardiogram by means of exchange transfusion with stroma free haemoglobin solution in the dog. Cardiovasc. Res. **24:** 24–32.
6. NOPP, P. *et al.* 1995. Electric field plethysmography signals of the human thorax as determined by a 2-D FE-model. Med. Prog. Technol. **21:** 135–145.
7. BROWN, B. H., *et al.* 1994. Cardiac and respiratory related electrical impedance changes in the human thorax. IEEE Trans. Biomed. Eng. **41:** 729–734.
8. LAMBERTS, R., K. R. VISSER & W. G. ZIJLSTRA. 1984. Impedance Cardiography. Van Gorcum. Assen, the Netherlands.
9. GESELOWITZ, D. B. 1971. An application of electrocardiographic lead theory to impedance plethysmography. IEEE Trans. Biomed. Eng. **18:** 38–41.
10. MALMIVUO, J. & R. PLONSEY. 1995. Bioelectromagnetism: Principles and Application of Bioelectric and Biomagnetic Fields. Oxford University Press. London/New York.
11. HYTTINEN, J. 1994. Development of regional aimed ECG leads especially for myocardial ischemia diagnosis. Ph.D. thesis, Tampere University of Technology, Tampere, Finland.
12. LAARNE, P. *et al.* 1995. Validation of a detailed computer model for the electric fields in the brain. J. Med. Eng. Technol. **19:** 84–87.
13. KAUPPINEN, P. *et al.* 1999. A software implementation for detailed volume conductor modeling in electrophysiology using finite difference method. Comput. Methods Programs Biomed. **58:** 191–203.
14. KAUPPINEN, P. *et al.* 1998. Detailed model of the thorax as a volume conductor based on the Visible Human Man data. J. Med. Eng. Technol. **22:** 126–133.

Impedance Stroke Volume Compared with Dye and Electromagnetic Flowmeter Values during Drug-Induced Inotropic and Vascular Changes in Dogs

ROBERT P. PATTERSON, DAVID A. WITSOE, AND ARTHUR FROM

University of Minnesota, Minneapolis, Minnesota 55455

ABSTRACT: Stroke volumes measured by impedance were compared with values obtained by dye dilution and an electromagnetic flowmeter (EMF) on 14 dogs during drug-induced changes in cardiac contraction strength and peripheral resistance changes. Grouping all data for a total of 305 points showed correlations between dye and EMF, dye and impedance, and EMF and impedance of 0.89, 0.68, and 0.72, respectively. Correlations for individual dogs between dye and EMF, dye and impedance, and EMF and impedance ranged from 0.60 to 0.99, −0.39 to 0.96, and −0.26 to 0.89, respectively. These data suggest that the use of impedance cardiac output measurements to make treatment decisions about individual patients could result in serious error.

INTRODUCTION

Impedance cardiography continues to be a controversial method for measuring cardiac stroke volume.[1] Although many studies report good correlation of impedance-determined stroke volume compared to other standard methods, some studies, particularly in very sick patients, show poor agreement.[1-6] It is generally agreed that the relative change in stroke volume is more accurate than the absolute value. The waveform used to make the calculations appears to have multiple sources, which may lead to varying results as different regions in the thorax change their influence.[7]

The standard of comparison for most studies has been thermo- or indication-dilution cardiac output, which has been criticized because it has its own possible source of error. In some past reported comparison studies, the change in cardiac output was small and/or the physiological status of the subject was unknown. Changes in cardiac output due to peripheral resistance changes may influence the impedance values differently than changes caused directly by cardiac action.

To answer some of these questions, a study in dogs was undertaken that used two independent methods for measuring cardiac output under drug-induced conditions that somewhat independently changed the peripheral resistance and the strength of heart contractions.

METHODS

The study was conducted on 14 mongrel dogs. A left thoracotomy was performed and an electromagnetic flow transducer (Biotronex model 410) was placed around the ascending aorta. While the chest was opened, catheters were placed in either the right atrium or pulmonary artery for dye injection and in the ascending aorta for sampling and pressure. The thoracotomy was then closed and the air evacuated by continuous suction. Dye for the indicator dilution studies was injected into either the right atrium or main pulmonary artery and sampled from the ascending aorta. Four electrode bands for impedance measurements, using a Minnesota Impedance Cardiograph model 303, were placed on the neck and lower thorax in the standard positions. The impedance values were calculated using the standard method as first described in reference 8.

For each experimental condition, a minimum of two dye dilution curves with simultaneous impedance and electromagnetic flowmeter (EMF) recordings were obtained. All measurements were taken during periods of end-expiration apnea to eliminate respiration artifacts from the impedance signals.

To obtain an increase in peripheral resistance with a minimal effect on contractility, methoxamine was infused at a constant rate by a pump. The levels of methoxamine infusion depended primarily upon the response of the particular animal as measured by ascending aortic blood pressure. Infusion rates ranged from 0.25 mg/min to 1.0 mg/min.

Decreased peripheral resistance, increased contractility, and increased heart rate were produced by infusion of isoproterenol at constant rates over several levels ranging from 0.25 to 10.0 micrograms.

To lower the heart rate and decrease contractility, propranolol was given intravenously in one bolus at the rate of 0.25 mg/kg of body weight.

Although the electromagnetic flowmeter was calibrated, only the relative changes from the initial control measurements are reported.

RESULTS

A total of 305 comparisons were made on 14 dogs. The range of cardiac output was from 1 to 10 L/min. Using the entire data set, the correlation coefficients for stroke volume comparing dye and EMF, dye and impedance, and EMF and impedance were 0.89, 0.68, and 0.72, respectively. Graphs comparing the percent change in stroke volume from the initial control period for dye versus EMF and dye versus impedance are shown in FIGURES 1 and 2, respectively.

FIGURE 3 shows the individual correlation coefficients comparing dye-EMF, dye-impedance, and EMF-impedance for each dog.

FIGURES 4, 5, and 6 show typical responses due to the induced stroke volume change for three of the dogs. FIGURE 4 is an example of an experiment (dog 8 in FIGURE 3) in which the agreements between the three methods are good. FIGURE 5 (dog 4 in FIGURE 3) and FIGURE 6 (dog 12 in FIGURE 3) show large differences in the measured stroke volume changes compared to either the dye dilution or EMF.

DISCUSSION

When the data from all the experiments are considered as one data set, the agreement between dye and the electromagnetic flowmeter ($r = 0.89$) is considerably better than between impedance and either of the other two techniques ($r = 0.68$ and 0.72). The most serious difficulty occurs when individual experiments are considered. Comparing the cor-

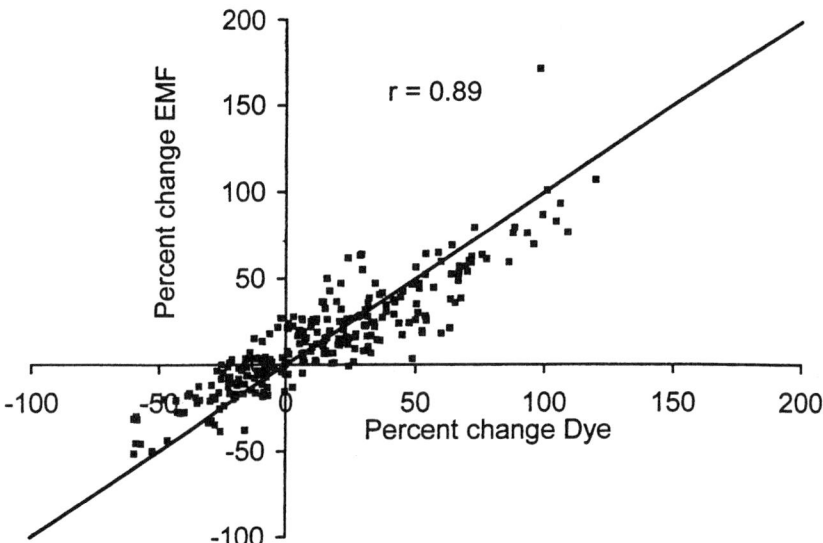

FIGURE 1. Comparison of the change in stroke volume measured by dye dilution and electromagnetic flowmeter (EMF) combining all experiments.

relation coefficients of impedance to dye and impedance to EMF for individual dogs shows that only 8 of 14 and 7 of 14, respectively, are above 0.6. In some cases, the correlation is negative, indicating changes in the opposite direction. This markedly contrasts with the correlation coefficients comparing dye to EMF, which are all above 0.6, and 8 of 14 are

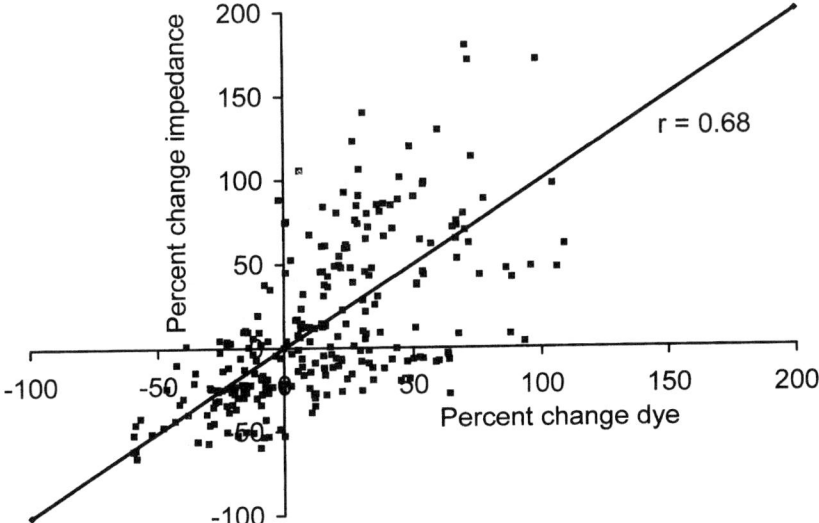

FIGURE 2. Comparison of the change in stroke volume measured by dye dilution and impedance for all experiments.

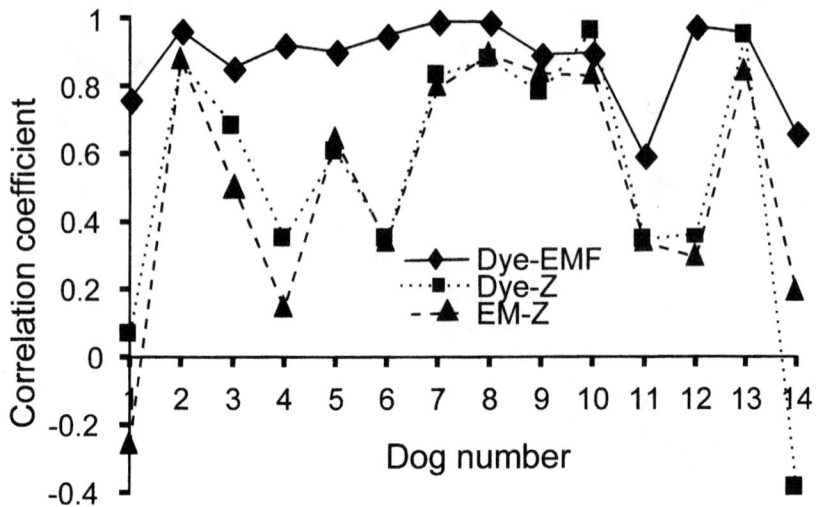

FIGURE 3. Correlation coefficients between dye dilution, EMF, and impedance for each of the 14 dogs.

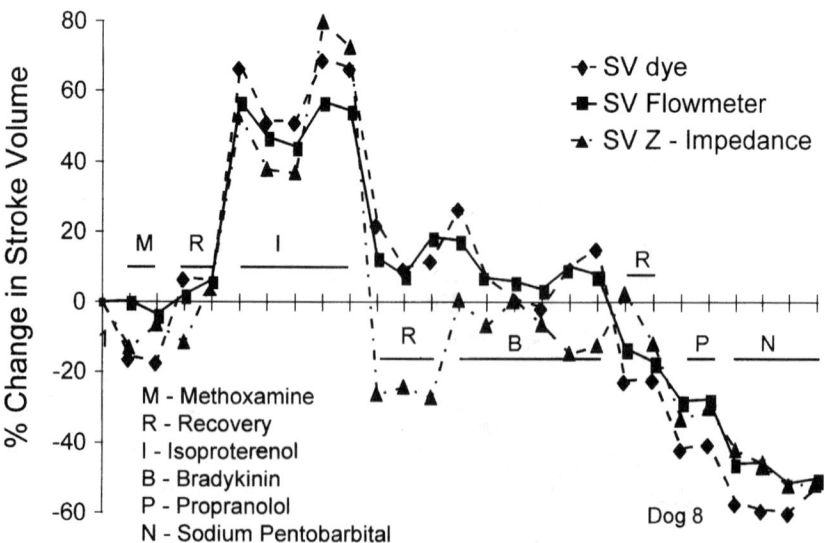

FIGURE 4. The percentage change in stroke volume from control due to the drug-induced alterations for dog 8. The horizontal lines show the response to the type of drug indicated by the letter label. These data show one of the best agreements obtained between the three methods.

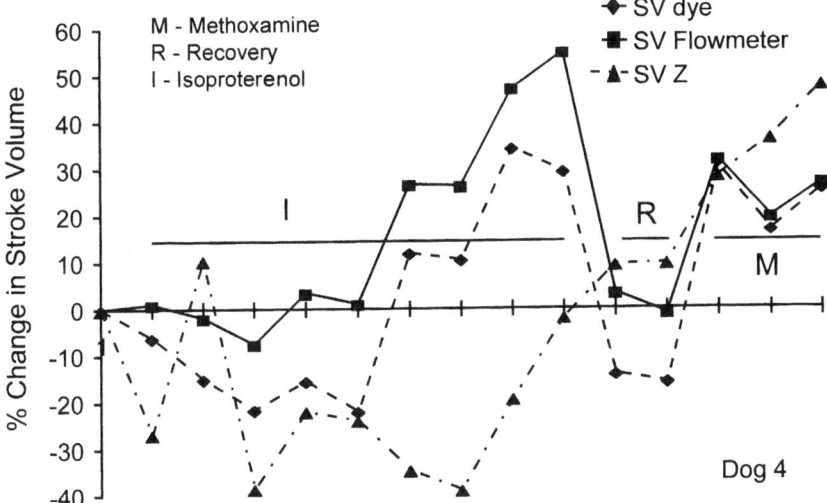

FIGURE 5. The percentage change in stroke volume from control due to the drug-induced alterations for dog 4. The horizontal lines show the response to the type of drug indicated by the letter label. These data are an example of the poor agreement between the three methods.

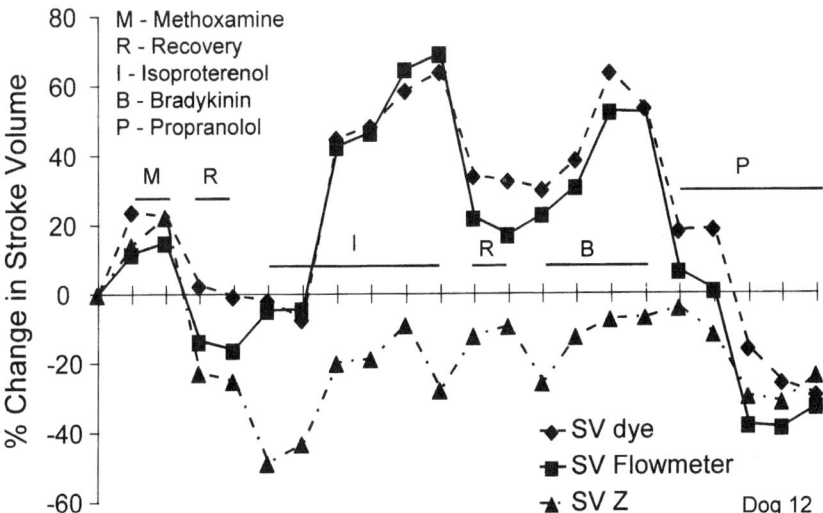

FIGURE 6. The percentage change in stroke volume from control due to the drug-induced alterations for dog 12. The horizontal lines show the response to the type of drug indicated by the letter label. These data are an example of the poor agreement between the three methods.

above 0.9. Comparing impedance with dye showed that 42 out of 305 measurements were more than 50% different, whereas none of the dye-EMF measurements showed such a difference.

Examination of the data did not reveal any unique drug-induced state or condition that resulted in a poorer lack of agreement between impedance and dye dilution or EMF measurements.

Studies have indicated that repeated impedance measurements show close agreement,[4] which appears at first to be a good result. However, in the case of using impedance in clinical medicine, repeatability can be a serious problem. If a given impedance measurement displays a significant difference from the truth, repeated measurements will continue to show error. Indicator or dye dilution measurements appear to have more true random error. If repeated dye measurements are averaged, they will tend to approach the truth.[9]

These data suggest that the use of impedance cardiac output measurements to make treatment decisions about individual patients with critical circulatory problems could result in serious error.

REFERENCES

1. JENSEN, L., J. YAKIMETS & K. K. TEO. 1995. A review of impedance cardiography. Heart & Lung **24:** 183–193.
2. ATALLAH, M. M. & A. D. DEMAIN. 1995. Cardiac output measurements: lack of agreement between thermodilution and thoracic electric bioimpedance in two clinical settings. J. Clin. Anesth. **7:** 182–185.
3. DONOVAN, K. D., G. J. DOBB, W. P. W. WOODS & B. E. HOCKINGS. 1986. Comparison of transthoracic electrical impedance and thermodilution methods of measuring cardiac output. Crit. Care Med. **12:** 1038–1044.
4. TEO, K. K., M. D. HETHERINGTON, R. G. HAENNEL, P. V. GREENWOOD, R. E. ROSSALL & R. G. KAPPAGODA. 1985. Cardiac output measured by impedance cardiography during maximal exercise tests. Cardiovasc. Res. **19:** 737–743.
5. PATTERSON, R. P., L. WANG & B. RAZA. 1991. Impedance cardiography using band and regional electrodes in supine, sitting, and during exercise. IEEE Trans. Biomed. Eng. **38:** 393–400.
6. PATTERSON, R., L. WANG, G. MCVEIGH, R. BURNS & J. COHN. 1993. Impedance cardiography: the failure of sternal electrodes to predict changes in stroke volume. Biol. Psychol. **36:** 33–41.
7. WANG, L. & R. PATTERSON. 1995. Multiple sources of the impedance cardiogram based on 3D finite difference human thorax models. IEEE Trans. Biomed. Eng. **42:** 393–400.
8. PATTERSON, R. P., W. G. KUBICEK, E. KINNEN, D. WITSOE & G. NOREN. 1964. Development of an electrical impedance plethysmograph system to monitor cardiac output. *In* First Annual Rocky Mountain Bioengineering Symposium, p. 56–71. U.S. Air Force Academy.
9. KIESS, E. & J. MERSCH. 1987. Thermodilution cardiac outputs using room and ice temperature injectate: comparison with the Fick. Heart & Lung **16:** 294–300.

A Comparison of Bioimpedance and Echocardiography in Measuring Systolic Heart Function in Cardiac Patients

H. J. JURN KERKKAMP[a] AND ROB M. HEETHAAR

Department of Clinical Physics and Informatics, Institute of Cardiovascular Research VU, Vrije Universiteit, Amsterdam, the Netherlands

ABSTRACT: To investigate the ability of bioimpedance cardiography to assess left ventricular systolic function in comparison with known echocardiographic parameters and to establish the most informative bioimpedance parameter, 28 cardiac patients were submitted to simultaneous echocardiography and bioimpedance cardiography. Bioimpedance systolic time ratio, Heather index, acceleration index, and index of contractility were compared with echocardiographically obtained left ventricular dimensions, 2D left ventricular ejection fraction, fractional shortening, and mean velocity of circumferential shortening. The systolic time ratio and Heather index correlated significantly well with, respectively, 2D ejection fraction ($r = -0.73$) and, respectively, fractional shortening ($r = 0.69$). The systolic time ratio was the best parameter in recognizing impaired left ventricular systolic function ($F = 12.6$) in comparison with the Heather index ($F = 6.5$). This study demonstrates the applicability of bioimpedance cardiography in assessing left ventricular systolic function similar to echocardiography in clinical cardiology.

INTRODUCTION

It is a major request in clinical cardiology to assess systolic heart function noninvasively and continuously; however, appropriate devices are still lacking. In clinical practice, systolic heart function is mainly assessed by echocardiography, but it cannot be done on a continuous basis. Thoracic electrical bioimpedance is known for its noninvasive and continuous nature and is applied to measure cardiac output. Several authors reported on the results of assessing the systolic heart function by measuring the systolic time ratio (ratio of the preejection period and left ventricular ejection time), Heather index (ratio of minimum systolic dZ/dt and time from the electrocardiographic R wave to this minimum), index of contractility, and acceleration index.[1–3] Comparisons were made between the systolic time ratio and left ventricular ejection fraction by a gated blood pool scan. In daily practice, left ventricular systolic function is assessed by measuring the two-dimensional left ventricular ejection fraction, the left ventricular end diastolic diameter, the fractional shortening (percent change in left ventricular dimension), and the mean velocity of circumferential fiber shortening.[4,5] Previous studies did not compare the four mentioned bioimpedance parameters of systolic function with these echocardiographic parameters.

[a]Address for correspondence: Department of Cardiology, Bronovo Ziekenhuis, Bronovolaan 5, 2597 AX The Hague, the Netherlands.

The aim of this study was to investigate the ability of bioimpedance cardiography to assess left ventricular systolic function in comparison with known echocardiographic parameters and to establish the most informative bioimpedance parameter.

METHODS

Patients

Twenty-eight patients (15 men and 13 women) with heart disease underwent simultaneous echocardiography and bioimpedance cardiography. The mean age was 65.4, with a range of 39 to 86 years. Five had uncomplicated coronary artery disease, 9 had a myocardial infarction, and 14 had a cardiomyopathy. Six patients were classified as New York Heart Association class I, 12 were class II, 8 were between classes II and III, and another 2 were in class III.

Methodology

Echocardiography was performed using Toshiba Sonolayers SSH 140A. Internal dimensions of the left ventricle were measured according to the standard, and left ventricular ejection fraction was measured by the single plane area length method.[5] Fractional shortening was defined as the percent change in left ventricular diameter between end diastole and end systole. The mean velocity of circumferential fiber shortening was calculated by dividing the fractional shortening by the left ventricular ejection time. The mean from three consecutive measurements was taken.

A BoMeds NCCOM3-R7 was used to measure bioimpedance parameters. Ten skin electrodes were placed according to the manufacturer's specifications. Parameters were defined as follows: systolic time ratio (STR) is the ratio of the preejection period and left ventricular ejection time; index of contractility (IC) is the maximum value of bioimpedance change $-dZ$ normalized by total impedance of the thorax; acceleration index (ACI) is the maximum value of $-d^2Z/dt^2$ normalized by total impedance of the thorax; and Heather index is the ratio of maximum systolic $-dZ/dt$ and time from the electrocardiographic R wave to this maximum (FIGURE 1). Systolic time ratio, index of contractility, and acceleration index were displayed by the device directly; the Heather index was calculated from the preejection period, acceleration index, total impedance of the thorax (transthoracic fluid index), and maximum $-dZ/dt$ amplitude during systole. The mean from 50 consecutive heartbeats was taken.

Statistics

Data are expressed as the mean ± standard deviation. Pearson's correlation coefficient, t-test statistics, and linear regression with F-statistics were used for the analysis. The SPSS-PC package was used for the statistics.

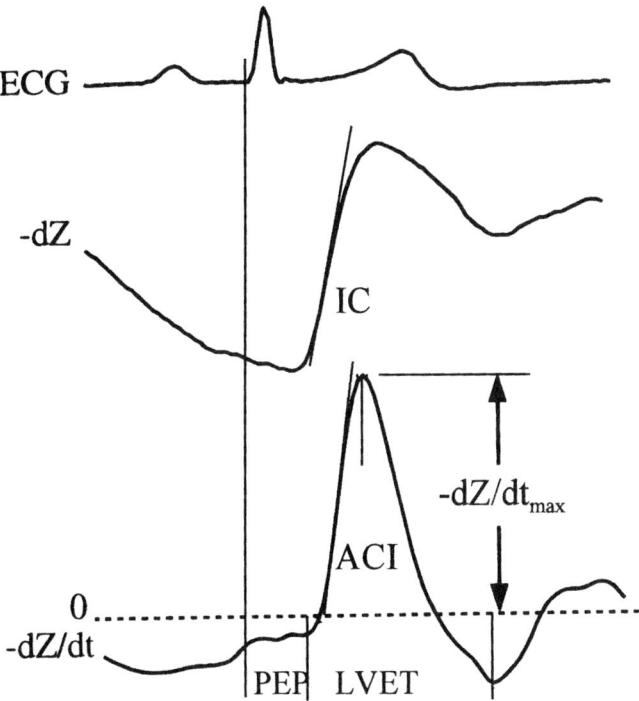

FIGURE 1. Left ventricle function parameters on bioimpedance curves.

RESULTS

The best correlations with echocardiographically obtained parameters of left ventricular systolic function were found to be the systolic time ratio and the Heather index (TABLE 1). The acceleration index and index of contractility correlated poorly with the fractional shortening and mean velocity of circumferential shortening and not at all with the other echocardiographic parameters of left ventricular function. The systolic time ratio corresponded more to the two-dimensional ejection fraction (FIGURE 2), while the Heather index inclined towards the end diastolic dimension, fractional shortening (FIGURE 3), and mean velocity of circumferential shortening.

If impaired left ventricular function was defined by an ejection fraction of 35% or less and/or an end diastolic diameter of 60 mm or more, then differences in systolic time ratio and Heather index would be significant (TABLE 2). In the regression analysis, the systolic time ratio performed better ($F = 12.6$; $p = 0.002$) than the Heather index ($F = 6.5$; $p = 0.01$) in discriminating between a normal and impaired left ventricular function.

TABLE 1. Correlations between Echocardiographic and Bioimpedance Parameters of Left Ventricular Function[a]

	EDD	ESD	FS	Vcf	LAD	LVEF	EDV
STR	0.46^b	0.52^c	−0.39	0.04	0.45^b	$−0.73^c$	0.37
HI	$−0.52^c$	$−0.63^c$	0.69^c	0.65^c	0.50^b	0.26	−0.26
ACI	−0.22	−0.36	$−0.46^b$	0.45^b	−0.33	0.18	−0.09
IC	−0.18	0.28	0.44^b	0.43^b	−0.30	0.17	−0.04

[a]EDD = end diastolic diameter; ESD = end systolic diameter; FS = fractional shortening; Vcf = mean velocity of circumferential shortening; LAD = left atrial diameter; LVEF = 2D left ventricular ejection fraction; EDV = 2D end diastolic volume; STR = systolic time ratio; HI = Heather index; ACI = acceleration index; IC = index of contractility.
[b]$p < 0.05$.
[c]$p < 0.01$ (Pearson's correlation coefficient).

DISCUSSION

Measuring the left ventricular systolic function is an important feature in clinical cardiology since it is related to survival in coronary artery disease and cardiomyopathy and to cardiac complications, morbidity and mortality in surgery, acute myocardial infarction, and other serious diseases. A noninvasive and simple to use monitor is the best to implement and, in situations where sequential monitoring is required, other aspects like real-

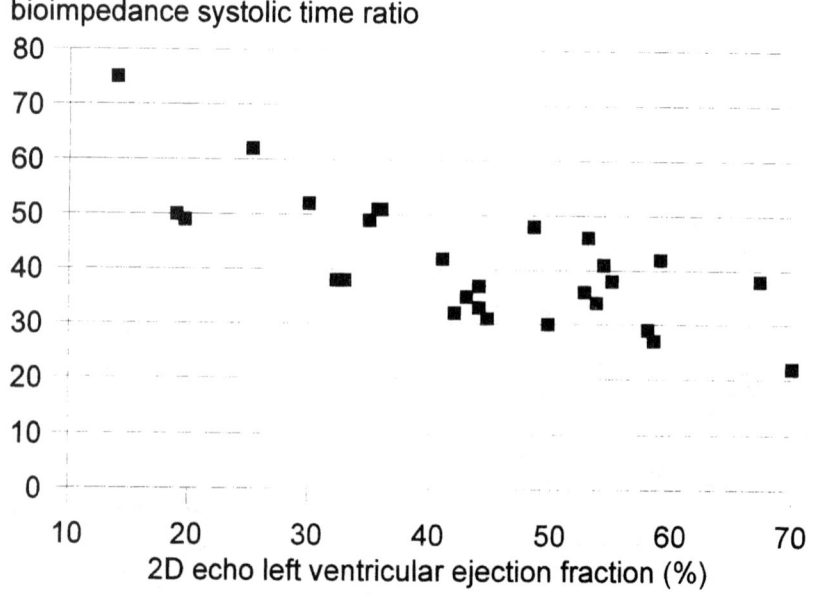

FIGURE 2. Systolic time ratio versus ejection fraction.

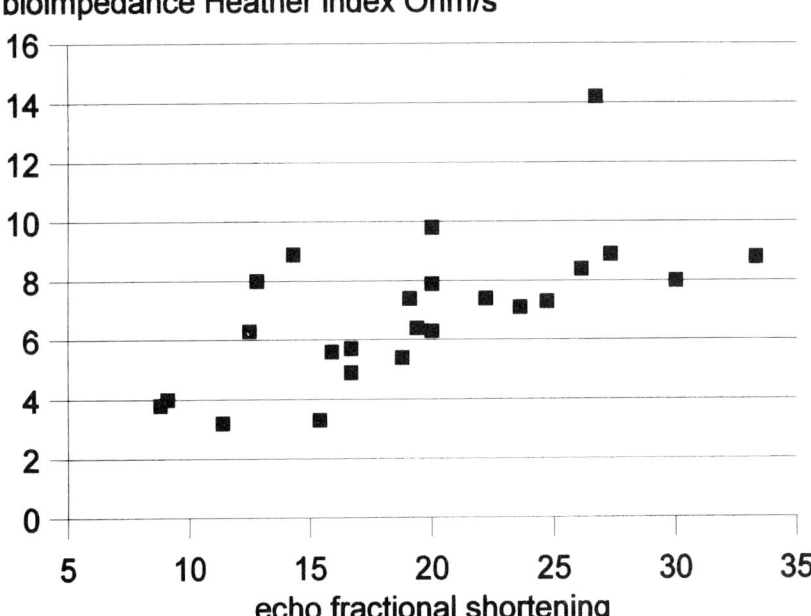

FIGURE 3. Heather index versus fractional shortening.

time mode and continuity are prerequisites. It is clear that the commonly used techniques, that is, echocardiography and nuclear angiography of the left ventricle, do not fulfill these requirements, but bioimpedance cardiography does.

Four bioimpedance parameters of left ventricular systolic function are recognized today. To our knowledge, this study is the first to compare these four parameters with commonly used echocardiographic ones. Temporal bioimpedance parameters such as systolic time ratio and Heather index showed better correlations with standard echocardiographically obtained parameters than the direct bioimpedance amplitude–related ones like acceleration index and index of contractility. The mentioned amplitude-related parameters are more dependent on the flow and rate of left ventricular contraction than on the degree of

TABLE 2. Differences of STR and HI according to Left Ventricular Function Class[a]

	n	STR	HI
normal	13	35.5 ± 7.0	9.1 ± 2.6
impaired	15	47.1 ± 11.9[b]	6.2 ± 2.1[c]

[a]STR = systolic time ratio; HI = Heather index; n = number of patients.

[b]p = 0.004.

[c]p = 0.01 (t test).

contraction.[2] Since in clinical cardiology contraction parameters are used more in practice than velocity and flow rates, it is logical to use the systolic time ratio and Heather index in bioimpedance cardiography in order to assess left ventricular systolic function.

This study demonstrates the comparability of the bioimpedance cardiography–derived systolic time ratio and Heather index in assessing left ventricular systolic function and in recognizing impaired function. Clinical studies should be undertaken to assess the applicability in clinical cardiology.

REFERENCES

1. HEATHER, L. W. 1969. A comparison of cardiac output values by the impedance cardiograph and dye dilution techniques in cardiac patients. Progress Report No. Na 594500. National Aeronautics and Space Administration, Manned Spacecraft Center, Houston.
2. SRAMEK, B. 1989. Hemodynamic and pump-performance monitoring by electrical bioimpedance. Probl. Respir. Care **2:** 274–290.
3. FULLER, H. D. 1994. Evaluation of left ventricular function by impedance cardiography: a review. Prog. Cardiovasc. Dis. **36:** 267–273.
4. BOROW, K. M., R. H. MARCUS, A. NEUMANN & R. M. LANG. 1992. Modern noninvasive techniques for the assessment of left ventricular systolic performance. *In* Heart Disease, p. 389–398. Saunders. Philadelphia.
5. FEIGENBAUM, H. 1994. Echocardiography, p. 135–180. Lea & Febiger. Philadelphia.

Thoracic Bioimpedance as a Basis for Pacing Control[a]

MART MIN,[b] TOOMAS PARVE,[b] AND ANDRES KINK[c]

[b]*Department of Electronics, Tallinn Technical University, EE-0026 Tallinn, Estonia*
[c]*Department of Thoracic Surgery, Hospital of the University of Tartu, EE-2400 Tartu, Estonia*

ABSTRACT: Periodic variations of the thoracic bioimpedance due to breathing and heartbeating carry confidential information that is used for pacing rate control in rate-adaptive pacemakers. The respiratory parameters—the respiration rate and tidal volume—are detected from the filtered breathing signal component (0.1 to 1.0 Hz), and are used for fuzzy feed-forward adaptive control of the pacing rate to meet the needs of the organism. The cardiac parameters—the actual heart rate and stroke volume—are measured from the heartbeating signal component (1.0 to 3.0 Hz) and are proposed for feedback correction of the feed-forward control to meet the heart's ability. The problems of electrical bioimpedance measurement and design of the rate-adaptive pacemaker, wherein the intracardiac impedance is used as the main information source for pacing control, are discussed in this paper.

INTRODUCTION

Almost all periodical variations of the thoracic electrical impedance are related with the physiological processes, breathing and heartbeating, which have different frequencies, typically 0.1 to 1.0 Hz and 1.0 to 3.0 Hz. This matter gives a possibility to extract and separate both the respiratory and cardiac components of the complex bioimpedance signal using more or less complicated filtering in the frequency domain.

The respiration component of the bioimpedance signal has been found to relate to changes in the respiratory rate and volume. This relationship has been used in rate-adaptive pacemakers, which monitor changes in thoracic impedance, measured between the electrodes and metal housing of the pacemaker (FIGURE 1), to match the pacing rate with the patient's physical and emotional needs.

The minute volume (MV), the product of the respiratory rate (RR) and tidal volume (TV), reflects closely the metabolic demands of physical exercise.[1] Therefore, both the frequency and amplitude of the respiratory component of the thoracic impedance (in accordance with the rate and depth of breathing) are of interest. Experiments confirm an excellent adequacy between the MV and heartbeating rate in the case of dynamic physical work.[2] However, despite the long-term use in commercially available pacemakers (e.g., META MV pacemakers of Telectronics, Limited), the MV does not reflect adequately the static physical efforts.

During almost all static efforts, the inspiration is rather deep, but the breathing rate is low. Such a situation takes place in everyday life during pushing, pulling, and carrying heavy loads. Breathing can even stop temporarily. This means that the RR falls down and also the value MV = RR × TV reduces steeply during heavy static exercises. However, the

---

[a]This work was supported by the Estonian Science Foundation under Grant No. 2123 and by EC Copernicus JEP 94-0202.

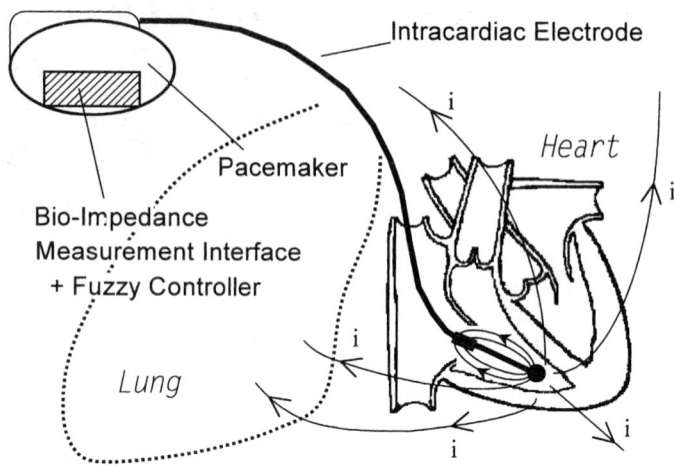

FIGURE 1. Measurement of the bioimpedance between the tip of the intracardiac electrode and the metal housing of the pacemaker.

pacing rate should rise greatly at the same time. Thus, the MV responses are inadequate in this case and, for that reason, it cannot serve as an entirely satisfactory parameter for pacing control.

To obtain a better response, an attempt was made to use the RR and TV separately as two independent inputs for fuzzy logic control of the pacing rate since the fuzzy logic control algorithms could operate more adequately than the traditional crisp control methods in the case of irregular loads.

Use of only the feed-forward (fuzzy or crisp) control based on respiratory parameters cannot give highly confident results in rather different life situations without taking into account the final result of the control, the actual cardiac output. The actual cardiac output, defined as the product of the heart rate (HR) and stroke volume (SV), can be determined from the cardiac component of the bioimpedance signal. The actual cardiac output can be used for the feedback or supervisory control introduced for correction of the results or algorithms of the feed-forward control. Several additional precautions must be taken to avoid overpacing and other dangerous situations for the unhealthy heart working in rather different everyday conditions. Therefore, more complicated neurofuzzy control algorithms containing supervisory functions must be taken into use.

To develop effective control algorithms, numerous noninvasive experiments have to be carried out with patients. Simple and convenient means based on lock-in measurement of bioimpedance have been developed and are taken into use for this purpose.

CONCEPT OF LIMITATIONS TO THE PACING RATE

One idea is to keep the heart rate in the physiologically acceptable range, between the minimal and maximal allowable values for a patient. These limit values for the heart rate can be calculated continuously by using stroke volume SV and diastole duration t_d.

Minimal Heart Rate (Bradycardia)

Dangerous ventricle overloading may occur as a result of too long filling time (low heart rate). We proposed to set a "maximal stroke volume" (MSV) for the pace rate control algorithm. If the measured stroke volume is more than the MSV, then the heart rate will be increased automatically.

Maximal Heart Rate (Tachycardia)

Myocardial ischemia appears when an imbalance exists between the cardiac oxygen supply and demand, or "demand ischemia", in which the coronary reserve is insufficient to cope with raised requirements (e.g., during tachycardia). The maximal heart rate is calculated using the cardiac oxygen supply/demand ratios in resting conditions.

Oxygen demand S_{dem} of the left ventricle is well correlated with the ventricle pressure-volume loop area,[3] and oxygen supply S_{supp} is correlated with diastole duration and mean arterioventricular pressure differences in diastole.

In normal conditions, energy demand E_{dem} and energy supply E_{supp} must be in balance:

$$E_{dem} = E_{supp}, \qquad (1)$$

where

$$E_{dem} = \Delta P \cdot \Delta V = \Delta P_{dem} \cdot SV = S_{dem}, \qquad (2)$$

$$\Delta P_{dem} = [(P_{as} - P_{ves}) + (P_{ad} - P_{ved})]/2,$$

as follows from FIGURE 2a, and

$$E_{supp} = Co_2 \cdot K \cdot F_{cor} \cdot t_d = Co_2 \cdot K \cdot \Delta P_{supp}/R \cdot t_d = Co_2 \cdot K \cdot S_{supp}/R, \qquad (3)$$

$$\Delta P_{supp} = [(P_{as} - P_{ves}) + (P_{ad} - P_{ved})]/2,$$

as follows from FIGURE 2b. Here, Co_2 is the concentration of oxygen in blood, K is the energy productivity of blood oxygen, and F_{cor} is the blood flow in coronary arteries.

Inserting equations 2 and 3 into equation 1 gives

$$\Delta P_{dem} \cdot SV = Co_2 \cdot K \cdot (\Delta P_{supp}/R) \cdot t_d.$$

Here, $\Delta P_{dem} = \Delta P_{supp}$ and we can obtain the coronary arteries' energy influx resistance:

$$R = Co_2 \cdot K \cdot t_d/SV.$$

From this, we can turn to the coronary reserve:

$$CR = R/R_{rest}.$$

If Co_2 and K are constant, then

$$CR = (SV_{rest} \cdot t_d)/(t_{d_{rest}} \cdot SV).$$

If the CR is higher than the set maximum allowable value, then the heart rate should be decreased.

Thus, this calculation has been carried out for the left ventricle, where pressures are higher than in the right ventricle, but the stroke volumes SV and diastole duration t_d are the same.

CR varies in healthy hearts from 4 to 6, but in coronary atherosclerosis it is lower, from 1 to 2. This is important when we are pacing damaged heart with coronary insufficiency.

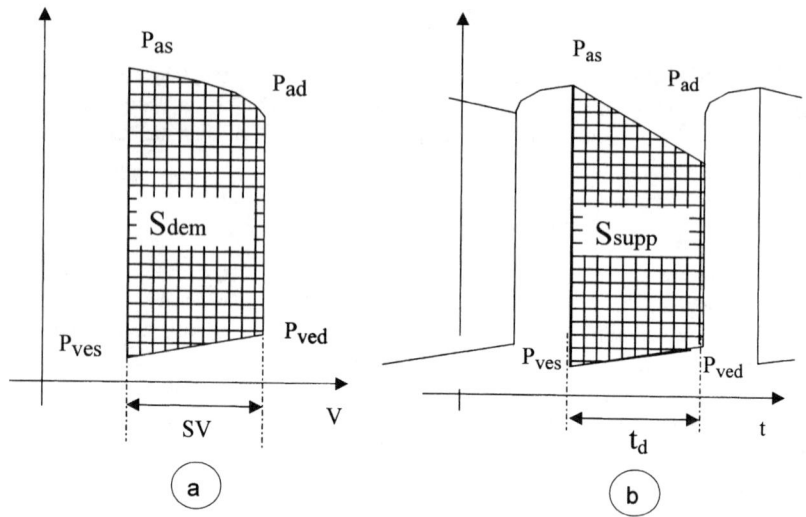

FIGURE 2. Ventricular pressure-volume loop (a) and variation of arterial pressure (b).

BIOIMPEDANCE IN RATE-ADAPTIVE PACEMAKERS

Electrical bioimpedance can be effectively used to determine cardiac and respiratory parameters.[1,2,4] A diagram of a typical bioimpedance signal measurement system is given in FIGURE 3. This enables one to use bioimpedance measurement as a source of information for pacing rate control in fuzzy-logic-controlled rate-adaptive pacemakers. The information about the respiratory rate and tidal volume, and about the heartbeat rate and stroke volume, can be obtained from the time variation of the bioimpedance measured between the tip of the intracardiac electrode and the housing of the pacemaker (FIGURE 1), when the excitation current proceeds from the electrode tip.

The thoracic bioimpedance measured in the aforementioned way varies slightly with breathing and significantly with contractions of the heart. These variations of the bioimpedance are considered to be relatively regular during a short time interval. The main harmonic of the signal component that reflects breathing (the breathing component) is assumed to reside in the frequency range of 0.2–1 Hz. The main harmonic of the signal component reflecting the beating of the heart (the heartbeat component) is assumed to reside in the range of 1–3 Hz, or 60–180 beats per minute. Values exceeding these limits are possible, but the probability of their occurrence is small in the case of pacemaker patients.

One cannot assume that waveforms of the intracardiac bioimpedance signals have harmonic shape. Thus, the higher harmonics of the breathing component can reside in the frequency range of (the main harmonic of) the heartbeat component. This complicates the separation of the components.

The magnitude of the relatively strong heartbeat component has a good correlation with the stroke volume of the heart. By multiplying the magnitude with the heart rate, one can obtain a parameter characterizing the blood circulation volume or the cardiac output. Combining it with the difference of oxygen (or carbon dioxide) concentration in the blood in

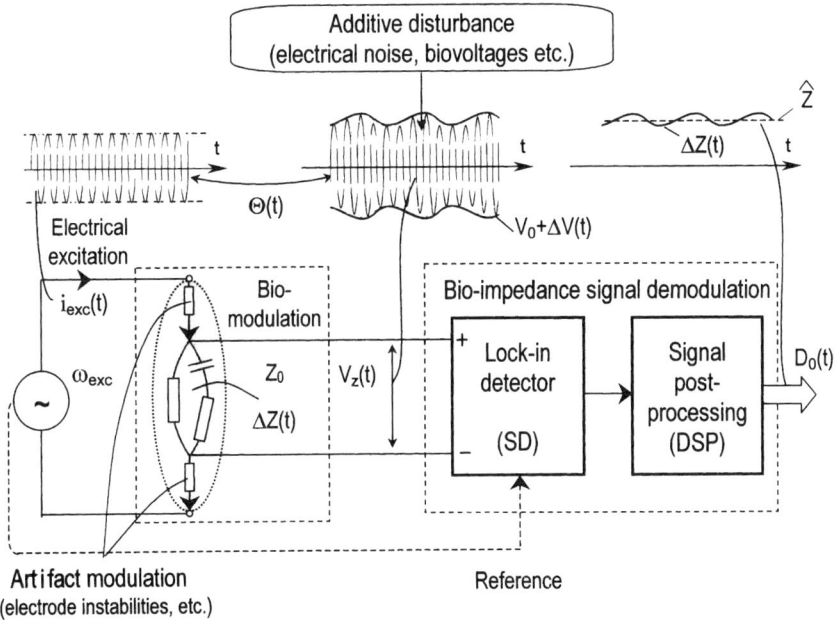

FIGURE 3. Bioimpedance measurement system.

certain points of the blood circulation system would yield a good estimation of the physical load rate. Unfortunately, at present, the available gas concentration sensors do not provide long-term stability and reliability high enough for the case of implanted pacemakers.

The respiratory parameters, particularly minute ventilation, are also the physiological variables, which reflect closely the metabolic demands during physical loads both for normal subjects and for those with heart problems.[2] Measurement of these parameters together with signals from other sensors (e.g., an activity sensor), and the ECG signal as well,[5] can be of value in the context of rate-responsive pacing.

Employment of a fuzzy logic controller in addition to the conventional control system would further improve the physiological compatibility of rate-adaptive pacemakers. Fuzzy control enables one to match the control facilities very closely to the personal demands of the individual for different kinds of physical loads.

LOCK-IN MEASUREMENT OF BIOIMPEDANCE

The electrical bioimpedance as a complex (vector) measurand can be represented by its real part I (in instrumentation known as the in-phase component) and imaginary part Q (the quadrature component), or can be described by modulus M and phase θ, where I = M•cos θ and Q = M•sin θ.

The block diagram of an analog interface for measuring the electrical bioimpedance through measurement of the real part I (or the imaginary part Q) of the response V_i to the excitation current I_e is shown in FIGURE 4.

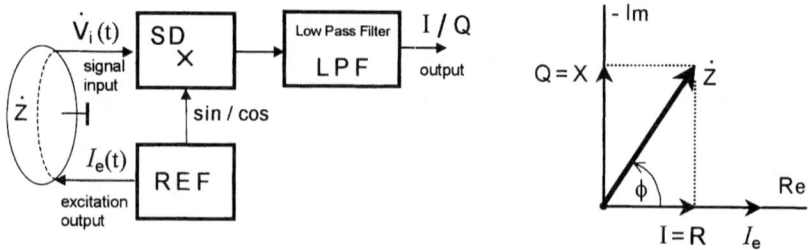

FIGURE 4. Block diagram of the analog interface of the bioimpedance measurement system.

Knowing the values of the components I and Q, one can determine the value of the bioimpedance using the predetermined value of the current I_e through the impedance:

$$Z = (I + jQ)/I_e = R + jX. \quad (4)$$

After obtaining the values of R and X, the modulus (magnitude) and phase of the bioimpedance can also be calculated if they are of interest.

However, measuring of the real part I (or the imaginary part Q) of the electrical impedance at a relatively high frequency (near to 100 kHz) and with good resolution from the other vector component Q (or I) cannot be easily performed in the case of very limited power consumption requirements. In this situation, application of current mode techniques[5] enables one to improve substantially the high-frequency behavior of the lock-in instrument.

The widely used technique of primary analog-to-digital conversion combined with further digital signal processing is complicated and is not applicable at all frequencies above 10 kHz due to the increase of power consumption. Employing analog synchronous detection of the in-phase and quadrature components I and Q of the input signal vector V_i can remove a lot of the problems.[6,7]

Modern current mode components, like transconductance amplifiers, current mode amplifiers (diamond transistors), and current switches, realized in high-speed CMOS technology, make it possible to create on-chip measurement units for different applications of electrical bioimpedance measurement. Of course, the specific requirements of bioimpedance measurement must be taken into account when designing a pacemaker, with a limited supply voltage level and low power consumption (single 2.5-V Li-battery-powered operation).

The simplest first-order low-pass filter is used to separate the breathing signal, and a high-pass filter is used to separate the heartbeat signal. Due to the low cutoff frequency (about 1 Hz) of both filters, the needed time constant is rather great. For an implantable device, this causes problems, which are difficult to overcome without using active elements (e.g., capacitance multipliers) or the SC technique.

MEASUREMENT INTERFACE

As electrical bioimpedance (EBI) measurement devices must be designed to meet some specific needs like being limited to the 10-μA value of the excitation current, etc., the level of interference is relatively high and varies greatly with the environment. The basic value of the bioimpedance at higher frequencies, where it is of interest, is usually less than 1 kΩ (at the excitation signal frequency on the order of 100 kHz) and can vary significantly (even 10 times) during a measurement session. Of course, one is interested only in those small time-domain variations of the impedance, which correspond to certain physiological processes (heartbeating, breathing). In the case of noninvasive experiments, like the hand-to-hand measurement, these variations are in the limits of 0.1%. The accuracy of the measurement unit is allowed to be modest, but it must be guaranteed (for repeatability of the measurements).

The EBI measurements are not always well determined: some bio-objects can be significantly nonlinear. Effects from the electrodes' instability are not well defined. In addition, several phenomena of straight biophysical nature (e.g., the artifacts caused by muscular contractions) can affect the measurements. In different conditions (in hospitals, in everyday life), different artifacts can be met.

Analog Measurement Interface Circuit for Bioimpedance Measurement

The limitations characterizing digital techniques do not enable one to minimize the analog part to consist of a good enough A/D converter only. Thus, some analog interfacing parts are still needed to convert the signal that is obtained from the object under test into the form that is suitable for the digital (post)processing part. To illustrate the situation, one can calculate that the voltage drop from the allowable excitation current of 10 μA at the bioimpedance of about 1 kΩ is of the order of 10 mV. The variation of the component of interest is approximately 0.1% of it, that is, 10 μV.

This is just nearly the LSB value for a 100-mV full-scale 14-bit (including sign bit) ADC. To measure quadrature components at 50 kHz, the sample rate must be at least 200 kHz. This is not impossible, but it is not very suitable for battery operating biomedical devices with low power consumption. Thus, amplification of the picked-up signal is needed. Also, some prefiltering of the detected signal is needed to prevent strong aliasing effects in analog-to-digital converting. This prefiltering causes some distortion of the signal of interest and this distortion should be compensated afterwards during digital processing as much as possible.

To provide information about changes of the thoracic bioimpedance, the pacemaker in FIGURE 1 contains a measurement interface. This chip delivers about 10 μA of current ($f > 10$ kHz), which returns back to the pacemaker's metal housing through the heart muscles and lungs. About 5-Ω pulsation of the thoracic impedance due to breathing causes the microvolt range and 0.1 to 1.0 Hz frequency band voltage response. This breathing response is filtered out from the disturbing noise and higher band (1 to 3 Hz) heartbeating component after the lock-in (synchronous) detection.[6,8] Then, the frequency of inspiration pulses (RR) is measured and the area of every inspiration/expiration pulse (TV) is determined using integration. The measurement results are converted into the DC current level and will be directed to the inputs of the pacing rate fuzzy controller in the form of averaged currents I_i.

Circuit Design Concepts

The lock-in interface for electrical bioimpedance measurement is accomplished on the basis of current mode components using low-power CMOS technology (2.5 V, 5 μA). (See FIGURE 5.)

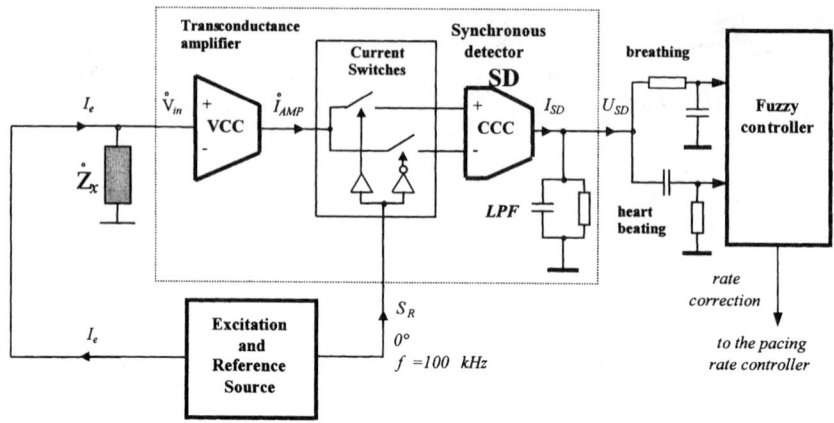

FIGURE 5. Simplified circuit diagram of an electrical bioimpedance measurement interface.

The availability of the current mode integrated circuits, such as transconductance amplifiers, current-feedback amplifiers (diamond transistors), current switches, and also high-speed CMOS digital circuits, has opened a possibility to develop simple PC-card format lock-in instruments covering the frequency band up to the MHz range. However, even then, a lot of difficulties will appear when an on-chip solution for the pacemaker is needed, and mainly because of the low power consumption requirement.

Bipolar transconductance amplifiers seem to be very suitable elements for the voltage-to-current converter VCC for wide band conversion of the input voltage into the current I_{AMP}, but the current consumption is too big. CMOS circuits consume much less power at the frequencies below 100 kHz.

In order to minimize several electrode problems, a current source is used for excitation. The Howland current pump circuit is often used to accomplish the current source, but unfortunately this circuit can be effectively used only at low frequencies. Moreover, this circuit is not well suited at low current values (10 μA in our case).

The problem was solved by using resistor matrices (or a set of weighting resistors) controlled by a CMOS sequential trigger circuit, which generates the stepwise approximated sine-wave excitation current I_e.[6,7,9]

The 1% calibration accuracy of the whole analog interface and a 100-kHz operating frequency are assumed to be reachable. A quadrature component separation better than 100 times has been achieved at these frequencies.

FUZZY CONTROLLER

Experiments

The noninvasive hand-to-hand impedance measurements were carried out with five healthy persons using lock-in signal demodulation and digital filtering methods.[10] Both

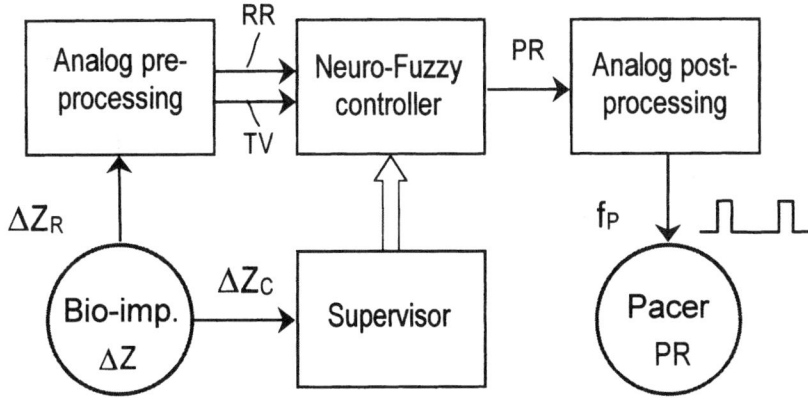

FIGURE 6. Structure of a fuzzy logic pacing rate controller.

dynamic and static physical loads were applied. The results obtained have been used as an input basis for design of the fuzzy logic pacing rate controller.

Fuzzification

The fuzzy controller in FIGURE 6 enables one to obtain complicated control algorithms without accurate mathematical description. The first step in fuzzy design is identifying and naming of the fuzzy inputs and outputs, and their linguistic description (TABLE 1), on the basis of experimental results and other knowledge. The next step is forming of membership functions. This procedure can be fulfilled almost automatically using some software package, for example, fuzzyTECH products. The following fuzzy inferencing and defuzzification process can be done fully automatically.

The current mode mixed-signal analog/digital low-power CMOS fuzzy processor is recommended for pacemaker application because of the lowest power consumption.[11]

TABLE 1. Identifying and Naming the Fuzzy Inputs and Outputs

Respiratory Rate (RR) [breaths/minute]		Tidal Volume (TV) [liters/breath]		Pacing Rate (PR) [beats/minute]	
Name	Range	Name	Range	Name	Range
very slow	0–10	small	0–0.45	very slow	40–60
slow	9–15	medium	0.4–0.6	slow	55–65
pretty fast	12–30	big	0.45–0.8	medium	60–70
very fast	23–60	real big	0.6–1.0	fast	65–160

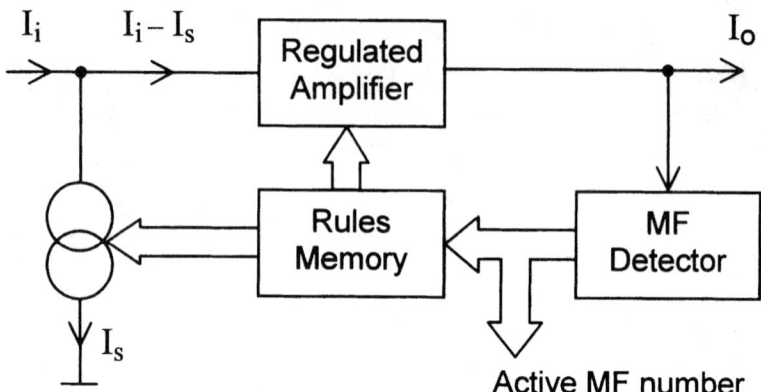

FIGURE 7. The current mode fuzzification cell.

The current mode fuzzification cell in FIGURE 7 is used for shaping of membership functions (MF). The cell contains a regulated amplifier with the code-controlled gain. The gain depends on the code from a rules memory, which defines the ascending and descending parts of the trapezoidal MF. The code-controlled sink current I_s regulates the core level $I_i - I_0$ of the MF.

Results

The input/output relationship of the designed fuzzy-controlled pacer is given in FIGURE 8. The two inputs are the respiratory rate RR and the tidal volume TV, and the only output is the pacing rate. The performance of the controller remains adequate in the case of both dynamic and static physical loads.

SUMMARY

The results of this work confirm the efficiency of using bioimpedance-based information for fuzzy logic control of the pacing rate in rate-adaptive pacemakers. An attempt has been made to use the respiration rate and tidal volume in the role of fuzzy control inputs. The good provisional results encourage us to continue the research in this field for improving the control rules and introducing additional inputs. The results of noninvasive measurements, an example of which is given in FIGURE 9, can also be useful for experimental studies.

The current mode lock-in technology for signal processing makes it possible to realize the bioimpedance measurement interface as a part of a low-voltage and very-low-power CMOS integrated circuit for implantable cardiac pacemakers. The circuit design concepts of the considered instrument can be used as the basis for further development towards the design of a complex bioimpedance analysis system for implantable pacemakers, which will accomplish more complicated functions like determination of cardiac ischemia.[12,13]

MIN et al.: PACING CONTROL

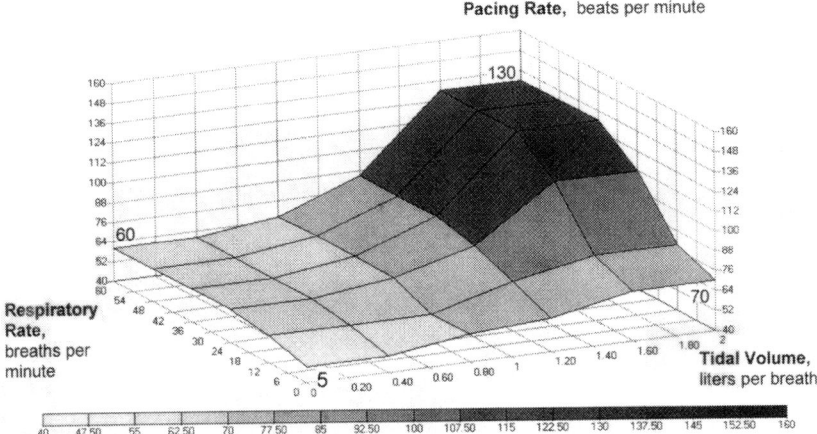

FIGURE 8. Input/output relationship of the fuzzy-controlled pacer.

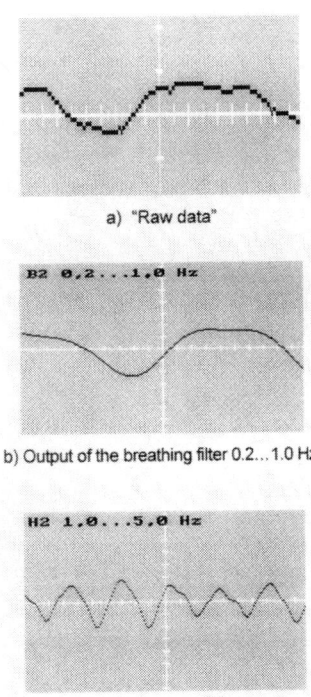

FIGURE 9. Example of signals during rest.

SUMMARY

The results of this work confirm the efficiency of using bioimpedance-based information for fuzzy logic control of the pacing rate in rate-adaptive pacemakers. An attempt has been made to use the respiration rate and tidal volume in the role of fuzzy control inputs. The good provisional results encourage us to continue the research in this field for improving the control rules and introducing additional inputs. The results of noninvasive measurements, an example of which is given in FIGURE 9, can also be useful for experimental studies.

The current mode lock-in technology for signal processing makes it possible to realize the bioimpedance measurement interface as a part of a low-voltage and very-low-power CMOS integrated circuit for implantable cardiac pacemakers. The circuit design concepts of the considered instrument can be used as the basis for further development towards the design of a complex bioimpedance analysis system for implantable pacemakers, which will accomplish more complicated functions like determination of cardiac ischemia.[12,13]

REFERENCES

1. MOND, H., N. STRATMORE, P. KERTES, D. HUNT & G. BAKER. 1988. Rate responsive pacing using a minute ventilation sensor. PACE **11**(suppl. II): 1866–1874.
2. WEBSTER, J. G. 1995. Rate adaption by minute ventilation. In Design of Cardiac Pacemakers. Chapter 17, p. 397–404. IEEE Press. Piscataway, New Jersey.
3. SUGA, H. 1979. Total mechanical energy of a ventricular model and cardiac oxygen consumption. Am. J. Physiol. **236**: H498–H505.
4. SCHALDACH, M. & A. URBASZEK. 1995. Unipolar intracardiac impedance—an optimal biosensor for closed loop rate-responsive cardiac pacing. In Proceedings of the Ninth International Conference on Electrical Bio-Impedance, p. 137–140. Heidelberg, Germany.
5. DE VRIES, P. M. J. M., H. H. WOLTJER, B. J. M. VAN DER MEER, A. VONK NOORDEGRAAF & H. J. BOGAARD. 1995. Impedance cardiography gives a complete picture of cardiac performance. In Proceedings of the Ninth International Conference on Electrical Bio-Impedance, p. 189–191. Heidelberg, Germany.
6. MIN, M., T. PARVE, A. EEK & H. MÄRTIN. 1995. An instrument for measurement of vector parameters of electrical bio-impedance. In Proceedings of the Ninth International Conference on Electrical Bio-Impedance, p. 40–43. Heidelberg, Germany.
7. MIN, M. & T. PARVE. 1997. Current mode signal processing as a challenge for improvement of lock-in measuring instruments. In Proceedings of the Fourteenth IMEKO World Congress "New Measurements—Challenges and Visions." Vol. VII, p. 186–191. Tampere, Finland.
8. MIN, M. & T. PARVE. 1996. Current mode signal processing in lock-in instruments for bioimpedance measurement. In Proceedings of the First International Conference on Bioelectromagnetism, p. 167–168. Tampere, Finland.
9. MIN, M., T. PARVE & A. RONK. 1992. Design concepts of instruments for vector parameter identification. IEEE Trans. Instrum. Meas. **IM-41**: 50–53.
10. MÄRTENS, O., H. MÄRTIN, M. MIN, T. PARVE & A. RONK. 1998. Digital post-processing of the bio-impedance signal. In Proceedings of the Tenth International Conference on Electrical Bio-Impedance, p. 445–448. Barcelona, Spain.
11. GUO, S., L. PETERS & H. SURMANN. 1996. Design and application of an analog fuzzy logic controller. IEEE Trans. Fuzzy Syst. **4**(no. 4): 429–438.
12. GHEORGHIU, M., E. GERSING & E. GHEORGHIU. 1999. Quantitative analysis of impedance spectra of organs during ischemia. This volume.
13. WARREN, M., O. CASAS, R. BRAGÓS, M. TRESÀNCHEZ, A. CARREÑO, A. RODRÍGUEZ-SINOVAS, A. YÁÑEZ, J. ROSELL, P. RIU & J. CINCA. 1998. Time course of myocardial tissue electrical impedance during ischemia and reperfusion in in vivo pig hearts. In Proceedings of the Tenth International Conference on Electrical Bio-Impedance, p. 81–84. Barcelona, Spain.

Evaluation of Systolic Performance by Automated Impedance Cardiography

ARMIN W. SCHERHAG,[a] JANA STASTNY,[a] STEFAN PFLEGER,[b] WOLFRAM VOELKER,[b] AND DIETER L. HEENE[a]

[a]*I. Medical Clinic*
[b]*II. Medical Clinic, Universitätsklinikum Mannheim, Faculty for Clinical Medicine Mannheim, University of Heidelberg, 68135 Mannheim, Germany*

ABSTRACT: Impedance cardiography (ICG) is a noninvasive method for evaluating cardiac function. Left ventricular stroke volume (SV) is the basic hemodynamic parameter derived from thoracic bioimpedance curves. Issues of our study were to investigate the diagnostic value of other indices of left ventricular systolic performance, such as ejection fraction (EF), index of contractility (IC), peak flow index (PFI), and acceleration index (ACI), which can also be calculated by ICG. Forty patients (PTS) with suspected coronary artery disease (CAD) were monitored by automated ICG during pharmacologic stress testing with dobutamine. All PTS underwent subsequent cardiac catheterization. In PTS with single vessel disease, the dobutamine-induced changes of SV, EF, IC, PFI, and ACI were comparable to those of PTS without CAD. In PTS with multivessel disease, the impaired systolic performance during dobutamine stimulation could be clearly demonstrated. We conclude that automated ICG is a useful method for monitoring SV and other indices of left ventricular systolic performance for detecting PTS with ischemic left ventricular dysfunction during cardiovascular stress.

INTRODUCTION

Left ventricular ejection fraction (EF) is an important indicator of global left ventricular systolic function and influences the outcome in patients (PTS) with various cardiac diseases. However, in clinical cardiology, the EF is routinely described only by semiquantitative estimation from two-dimensional echocardiograms in terms of "good", "fair", "impaired", or "severely reduced". For more quantitative assessment of systolic performance, calculations of the EF by echocardiographic techniques (planimetry, modified Simpson's rule) or (if performed) by cineventriculography are used.

Impedance cardiography (ICG) is a noninvasive method for evaluating cardiac function. By automated analysis of thoracic bioimpedance curves (ICG curves), quantitative data of many parameters of left ventricular systolic function can be obtained in a simple and time effective way. In recent reviews, good correlations (mean $r = 0.81$–0.88) of ICG-derived measurements of left ventricular stroke volume (SV) and cardiac output (CO) in comparison to invasive standard techniques have been reported.[1–3] Besides the evaluation of systolic time intervals in the early 1970s for noninvasive characterization of left ventricular systolic function[4–7] and the evaluation of the Capan formula[8] and Judy formula[9] for calculation of the EF, the diagnostic value of other impedance-derived parameters of systolic function derived from the ICG curves like the index of contractility (IC), acceleration index (ACI), and peak flow index (PFI) has not been extensively studied. Furthermore, no studies exist in which the clinical value of these parameters has been determined during cardiovascular stress testing. Pharmacologic cardiovascular stress testing by dobutamine stress echocardiography (DSE) has become an established alternative method for the noninvasive evaluation of PTS with suspected coronary artery disease who are unable to perform physical exercise.[10–12]

Issues of our study were therefore (a) to investigate whether automated ICG could be used for evaluating systolic performance during pharmacologic stress testing with dobutamine and (b) to evaluate the potential diagnostic value of the above-mentioned indices of left ventricular systolic performance calculated by automated ICG.

METHODS

Study Patients

Forty PTS (26 males, 14 females, mean age 61.4 ± 7.3 years) referred for dobutamine stress testing because of suspected coronary artery disease (CAD) were continuously monitored by automated impedance cardiography (ICG). The standard infusion protocol for performing DSE was used (see below). All PTS underwent cardiac catheterization within the following 2–6 days after the echocardiographic study and had given informed consent for participation in the study. The study protocol was approved by the appropriate ethics committee. PTS with poor echocardiographic image quality, valvular regurgitation, intracardiac shunts, low cardiac output, or extreme obesity were not included in the study. Coronary angiography (Judkin's technique) was performed in all 40 PTS. Significant CAD was defined as ≥50% reduction in luminal diameter of at least one major coronary vessel or its main branches.

Dobutamine Stress Echocardiography

Dobutamine stress echocardiography (DSE) has been demonstrated to be a valuable method for the noninvasive diagnosis of PTS with suspected CAD.[10–12] Stress-induced left ventricular wall-motion abnormalities have been shown to be a more sensitive marker of functional relevant myocardial ischemia than stress-induced ECG abnormalities.[13–15]

After completion of a baseline echocardiogram at rest, stepwise infusion of dobutamine by an infusion pump was initiated starting at 10 µg/kg/min up to 20/30/40 µg/kg/min in 3-min intervals. Rhythm and heart rate were continuously monitored, and blood pressure was measured every 3 min (Riva-Rocci method). Criteria for the termination of the DSE test were the detection of stress-induced wall-motion abnormalities (WMA) as echocardiographic indicators of ischemic left ventricular dysfunction, severe angina pectoris, significant arrhythmias, hypertension (blood pressure ≥ 220 mmHg), and achievement of the age-predicted target heart rate (85% of 220 minus age).

Echocardiographic images in standard views were digitally stored at baseline and at each stage of pharmacologic stress. In the absence of stress-induced WMA or adverse events, the DSE test was stopped after a maximum of 40 µg/kg/min by the injection of a short-acting beta-blocker (esmololhydrochloride, 50–100 mg). All DSE studies were reviewed by two experienced echocardiographers blinded to the angiographic results. A DSE test was defined as pathologic if dobutamine-induced new left ventricular WMA occurred during the test or if a worsening of preexisting WMA could be observed compared to baseline recordings at rest.

Automated Impedance Cardiography

An automated ICG system (cardioscreen professional, Medis GmbH, Ilmenau, Germany) was used for hemodynamic monitoring. The thoracic bioimpedance field was recorded by the four-pair electrode method. Two pairs of electrodes were placed above the sternocleidomastoid region of the patient's right and left neck; two more pairs of electrodes were placed in the medioclavicular line at each side at the lower thoracic aperture at the xiphoid level. The distance between one pair of electrodes was 5 cm. Correct identification of points B (opening of the aortic valve), P (maximum systolic flow), and X (closure of the aortic valve) on the ICG curves was automatically confirmed by marker channels. The modified Bernstein formula[15] was used for calculation of SV.

The following formulas were used for calculating the systolic functional indices: (1) index of contractility, IC = $(dz/dt)_{max}/z_0$; (2) peak flow index, PFI = dz/dt_{max}; (3) acceleration index, ACI = $(dz^2/dt^2)_{max}$/TFI [TFI = thoracic fluid index]. The software was programmed to average all hemodynamic parameters (HR, EF, IC, PFI, ACI) automatically every 10 consecutive beats.

Statistical Analysis

The Mann-Whitney u test was used for comparisons of hemodynamic variables between the patient groups. The Wilcoxon test was used for comparisons within the groups. A value of $p \leq 0.05$ was regarded as significant. All continuous data are expressed as mean values ± standard deviations (SD). Sensitivity and specificity of the DSE test were calculated according to the standard definitions.

RESULTS

Depending on the results of coronary angiography, patients were divided into three groups: no significant CAD ($n = 10$), single vessel disease ($n = 10$), or multivessel disease ($n = 20$). Mean values of all parameters were compared both within and between the patient groups at baseline and at peak stress with dobutamine. The detailed hemodynamic data are listed in TABLE 1. The mean dose of dobutamine until termination of the test was 32.6 ± 5.3 µg/kg/min. Sensitivity of the DSE test for detection of patients with significant CAD was 80% (24 of 30 PTS), and specificity was 90% (9 of 10 PTS). The stroke volume index (SI) was used to minimize the effects of body size and weight on SV.

Baseline values of all parameters did not significantly differ between PTS with and without CAD. The infusion of dobutamine resulted in a significant increase of HR, SI, IC, PFI, and ACI in all three patient groups ($p < 0.001$). There were no significant differences in peak stress values of all parameters between PTS without CAD and PTS with single vessel disease. Significant differences at peak stress (indicated by * or **) could be found for SI, IC, PFI, and ACI between PTS with single vessel disease and PTS with multivessel

TABLE 1. Measurements of Systolic Functional Parameters by Automated Impedance Cardiography[a]

	No CAD (n = 10)		Single Vessel Disease (n = 10)		Multivessel Disease (n = 20)	
	Baseline	Peak	Baseline	Peak	Baseline	Peak
HR	72.3 ± 10.5	120.9 ± 14.8	73.1 ± 6.5	117.1 ± 12.1	74.9 ± 14.7	122.7 ± 16.0
SI	36.3 ± 7.0	54.1 ± 10.9	36.7 ± 9.5	53.6 ± 8.7*	33.4 ± 7.7	41.3 ± 8.2*
EF	61.1 ± 5.5	72.3 ± 2.9	59.4 ± 8.2	69.9 ± 1.3	63.7 ± 5.1	69.8 ± 5.1
IC	0.04 ± 0.007	0.07 ± 0.014	0.04 ± 0.006	0.07 ± 0.014**	0.037 ± 0.009	0.05 ± 0.013**
PFI	130.7 ± 18.4	254.4 ± 44.0	136.8 ± 21.4	241.3 ± 33.7**	116.8 ± 20.5	166.2 ± 45.4**
ACI	0.92 ± 0.24	2.18 ± 0.48	1.05 ± 0.25	2.06 ± 0.45*	0.91 ± 0.32	1.66 ± 0.36*

[a]Mean values of stroke index (SI), ejection fraction (EF), index of contractility (IC), peak flow index (PFI), and acceleration index (ACI) are compared at baseline and at peak stress. Baseline values do not significantly differ between the three patient groups. Significant differences between peak stress values are indicated by $p \leq 0.05$ (*) or $p \leq 0.01$ (**) (normal values at rest: HR 60–80 bpm, SI 35–60 mL/m^2, EF 50–70%, IC 0.045–0.075 s^{-1}, PFI 170–270 mL/s/m^2, ACI 0.9–1.6 s^{-2}).

disease (TABLE 1). Comparison of peak values for EF failed to reach any statistical difference between the groups, but the mean increase of EF from baseline to peak stress in PTS with no CAD or single vessel disease (11.1 ± 4.7% and 9.7 ± 4.8%, respectively) was significantly higher when compared to PTS with multivessel disease (4.2 ± 3.6%, $p \leq 0.05$).

DISCUSSION

The results of our study show that impedance-derived indices of left ventricular systolic performance can be monitored by automated ICG not only at rest, but also during cardiovascular stress with dobutamine. Furthermore, we demonstrated the clinical value of the Bernstein formula and Capan formula for calculations of SV and EF to discriminate between PTS with normal or abnormal left ventricular responses to cardiovascular stress.

Three other impedance-derived parameters of left ventricular systolic function—the index of contractility (IC), the acceleration index (ACI), and the peak flow index (PFI)—were evaluated in the present study. Statistically significant differences could be found for all three parameters between PTS with no CAD or single vessel disease and PTS with multivessel disease. These functional results provided by ICG are in concordance with the clinical concept that, in most PTS with single vessel disease, left ventricular function during cardiovascular stress is close to normal, except in PTS with tight proximal stenosis of the left coronary artery.

Comparison to Previous Studies

Only a few studies exist in which EF and SV have been investigated during DSE. The findings of our study are supported by the results of other groups who performed hemodynamic studies during DSE by the thermodilution method[16] or Doppler-echocardiography.[17–19] In the study of Pierard and coworkers[16] SV and CO were measured invasively during various stages of pharmacological stress with dobutamine (10–40 µg/kg/min) by right heart Swan-Ganz catheterization. Patients with an ischemic response to dobutamine showed a significantly smaller increase of SV and CO at maximum doses compared to PTS without CAD, reflecting left ventricular dysfunction during cardiovascular stress similar to the results in our study. In the echocardiographic studies of Pellikka et al.[17] and Tanimoto et al.[18] SV (resp. SI) was calculated by the Doppler method in PTS without echocardiographic signs of ischemia (negative DSE test). The results of these Doppler-echocardiographic studies confirmed our hemodynamic findings in PTS without CAD. The stress-induced changes of EF during DSE have been studied by two other groups.[19,20] The impedance-derived calculations of EF at baseline and at peak stress with dobutamine in our study correspond well to the findings of Nixdorff[19] and Reiss,[20] who tried to define normal values for the increase of EF during DSE using two-dimensional echocardiography and the planimetric method for calculating EF. Concerning evaluation of IC, PFI, and ACI during pharmacologic stress, to our knowledge no comparable studies have been published in which these parameters have been investigated in PTS with or without CAD.

Study Limitations

The present study confirms the high sensitivity of automated ICG for detecting dobutamine-induced changes of left ventricular systolic pump function. However, the use of the impedance method for hemodynamic measurements during pharmacologic stimulation with catecholamines is not established and has so far been reported only by two authors who used much lower doses than those used in the present study.[21,22]

Furthermore, automated analysis of ICG curves by signal-averaging algorithms has been controversial because automated analysis can produce results that may considerably differ from values obtained by the conventional (manual) method.[22] However, a cost- and time-effective analysis of various parameters of systolic performance during cardiovascular stress testing is, in our opinion, only possible by using an automated approach. In addition, this guarantees user-independent results and better reproducibility of the hemodynamic measurements.

Another frequent point of criticism often brought up against ICG is that all parameters resulting from impedance-derived measurements are dependent on the formula used for calculation of SV and on the electrode configuration. The use of other formulas instead of the Bernstein formula for calculation of SI and the Capan formula for calculation of EF (e.g., Kubicek's formula[23] or Sramek's formula[24] for calculation of SI and Judy's formula[9] for calculation of EF) could result in different findings.[25,26]

CONCLUSIONS

The findings of our study demonstrate that monitoring of left ventricular systolic function by automated ICG is possible not only at rest, but also during pharmacological stress echocardiography with dobutamine. Compared to echocardiographic evaluation of left ventricular function, monitoring by ICG is a simple and feasible method that can provide quantitative information on many systolic functional parameters. Besides using stroke index, cardiac index, systolic time intervals, and EF provided by automated ICG, our results show that other impedance-derived parameters such as IC, ACI, and PFI might also be useful in characterizing left ventricular systolic performance at rest and during cardiovascular stress testing.[27,28] Further studies are needed to investigate whether the measuring of these additional systolic parameters by automated ICG can contribute to a better and possibly earlier identification of ischemic left ventricular dysfunction.

REFERENCES

1. FULLER, H. D. 1992. The validity of cardiac output measurement by thoracic impedance: a meta-analysis. Clin. Invest. Med. **15:** 103–112.
2. JENSEN, L., J. YAKIMETS & K. K. TEO. 1995. Issues in cardiovascular care: a review of impedance cardiography. Heart & Lung **24:** 183–193.
3. WOLTJER, H. H., H. J. BOGAARD & P. M. J. M. DE VRIES. 1997. The technique of impedance cardiography. Eur. Heart J. **18:** 1396–1403.
4. WEISSLER, A. M. D. & C. L. GARRAD. 1971. Systolic time intervals in cardiac disease. Mod. Concepts Cardiovasc. Dis. **1:** 1–4.
5. AHMED, S. S., G. E. LEWINSON, C. J. SCHWARTZ & P. O. ETTINGER. 1972. Systolic time intervals as measures of the contractile state of the left myocardium in man. Circulation **46:** 559–564.
6. GARRAD, C. L., A. M. D. WEISSLER & H. T. DODGE. 1970. The relationship of alterations in systolic time intervals to ejection fraction in patients with cardiac disease. Circulation **42:** 455–462.
7. CARDUS, D. & L. VERA. 1974. Systolic time intervals at rest and during exercise. Cardiology **59:** 133–153.
8. CAPAN, L. M., D. P. BERNSTEIN, K. P. PATEL, J. SANGER & H. TURNDORF. 1987. Measurement of ejection fraction by the bioimpedance method. Crit. Care Med. **15:** 402.
9. JUDY, W. V., J. H. HALL & W. C. ELLIOT. 1983. Left ventricular ejection fraction measured by the impedance cardiography method [abstract]. Fed. Proc. **41:** 1006.
10. COHEN, J., T. GREENE, J. OTTENWELLER, S. BINENBAUM, S. WILCHFORT, C. KIM & J. ALSTON. 1991. Dobutamine digital echocardiography for detecting coronary artery disease. Am. J. Cardiol. **67:** 1311–1318.
11. SAWADA, S. G., D. S. SEGAR, T. RYAN, S. E. BROWN, A. M. DOHAN, R. WILLIAMS, N. S. FINEBERG, W. F. ARMSTRONG & H. FEIGENBAUM. 1991. Echocardiographic detection of coronary artery disease during dobutamine infusion. Circulation **83:** 1605–1614.
12. SALUSTRI, A., P. FIORETTI, A. MCNEILL, A. POZZOLI & J. R. T. C. ROELANDT. 1992. Pharmacological stress echocardiography in the diagnosis of coronary artery disease and myocardial ischemia. Eur. Heart J. **13:** 1356–1362.
13. NESTO, R. & G. KOWALCHUK. 1987. The ischemic cascade: temporal sequence of hemodynamic, electrocardiographic, and symptomatic expressions of ischemia. Am. J. Cardiol. **57:** 23C–30C.
14. L'ABBATE, A. 1991. Pathophysiological basis for non-invasive functional evaluation of coronary stenosis. Circulation **83**(suppl. III): 2–7.
15. BERNSTEIN, D. P. 1986. Continuous noninvasive real-time monitoring of stroke volume and cardiac output by thoracic electrical bioimpedance. Crit. Care Med. **14:** 898.
16. PIERARD, L. A., C. BERTHE, A. ALBERT, J. CARLIER & H. E. KULBERTUS. 1989. Haemodynamic alterations during ischaemia induced by dobutamine stress echocardiography. Eur. Heart J. **10:** 783–790.
17. PELLIKKA, A. P., V. L. ROGER, R. B. MCCULLY, D. W. MAHONEY, K. R. BAILEY, J. B. SEWARD & A. J. TAJIK. 1995. Normal response during dobutamine stress echocardiography in subjects without left ventricular wall motion abnormalities. Am. J. Cardiol. **76:** 881–886.
18. TANIMOTO, M., R. G. PAI & W. JINTAPAKORN. 1995. Normal changes in left ventricular filling and hemodynamics during dobutamine stress echocardiography. J. Am. Soc. Echocardiogr. **8:** 488–493.
19. NIXDORFF, U., S. WAGNER, R. ERBEL, P. WEITZEL, S. MOHR-KAHALY & J. MEYER. 1995. Normalwerte für die Dobutamin-Streßechoakardiographie. DMW **120:** 1761–1767.

20. Reiss, G., P. A. Marcovitz, A. B. Leichtman, R. M. Merion, W. P. Fay, S. W. Werns & W. F. Armstrong. 1995. Usefulness of dobutamine stress echocardiography in detecting coronary artery disease in end-stage renal disease. Am. J. Cardiol. **75:** 707–710.
21. Acton, G. & C. Broom. 1990. A comparison of attenuation compensated volume flow based Doppler echocardiography and impedance cardiography in healthy volunteers. Am. J. Noninvasive Cardiol. **4:** 290–297.
22. De Mey, C. & D. Enterling. 1993. Disagreement between standard transthoracic impedance cardiography and the automated transthoracic electrical bioimpedance method in estimating the cardiovascular responses to phenylephrine and isoprenaline in healthy men. Br. J. Clin. Pharmacol. **35:** 349–355.
23. Kubicek, W. G., J. N. Karnegies, R. P. Patterson, D. A. Witsoe & R. H. Mattson. 1966. Development and evaluation of an impedance cardiac output system. Aerosp. Med. **17:** 1208–1212.
24. Sramek, B. B. 1983. Stroke volume equation with linear base impedance model and its accuracy, as compared to thermodilution and magnetic flowmeter techniques in humans and animals. *In* Proceedings of the Sixth International Conference on Electrical Bioimpedance, Zadar, Yugoslavia, p. 38–41.
25. Van De Meer, B. J. M., H. H. Woltjer, A. M. Sousman, W. O. Schreuder, E. R. Bulder, M. A. J. M. Huybregts & P. M. J. M. de Vries. 1996. Impedance cardiography: importance of the equotation and electrode configuration. Intensive Care Med. **22:** 1120–1124.
26. De Mey, C. & D. Enterling. 1988. Non-invasive assessment of cardiac performance by impedance cardiography: disagreement between two equations to estimate stroke volume. Aviat. Space Environ. Med. **59:** 57–62.
27. Scherhag, A., S. Pfleger, C. De Mey, A. B. Schreckenberger, U. Staedt & D. L. Heene. 1997. Continuous measurement of hemodynamic alterations during pharmacological cardiovascular stress by automated impedance cardiography. J. Clin. Pharmacol. **37:** 21S–28S.
28. Scherhag, A., S. Pfleger, U. Staedt, A. B. Schreckenberger, C. Ceconi, W. Voelker & D. L. Heene. 1997. Automated impedance cardiography for the measurement of systolic time intervals and ejection fraction during dobutamine infusion [abstract]. Eur. J. Clin. Pharmacol. **52:** A3.

Impact of Cardiovascular Reactions Using the Impedance Cardiography Method in Borderline Hypertension

T. NAWARYCZ,[a] L. OSTROWSKA-NAWARYCZ,[b] AND J. KACZMAREK[c]

[a]*Department of Biophysics, Military Medical Academy, 90-647 Lodz, Poland*
[b]*Department of Pediatrics, Military Medical Academy, 90-329 Lodz, Poland*
[c]*Department of Informatics, Military Medical Academy, 90-647 Lodz, Poland*

ABSTRACT: This paper evaluates the hemodynamics of 30 young men, aged 17–19 years, with borderline hypertension (BHT) and 29 normotensive (NT) patients within the same age range. The study has been carried out using the impedance cardiography method at rest and under passive orthostatic test, cold test, and hyperventilation test. In the BHT patients, the following features have been observed: increased values of the cardiac index (CI), stroke volume index (SVI), mean blood pressure (MBP), and left ventricle work index (LVWI), as well as the accompanying normal values of the total peripheral resistance index (TPRI). The reactions of the cardiovascular systems during the functional tests are similar in both tested groups; however, they are most clearly distinct in the BHT patients, where the differences are statistically significant. This may support the argument that the activity of the adrenergic system in this group is intensified.

INTRODUCTION

Hemodynamic disturbances at the early stages of hypertension, including borderline hypertension (BHT), are diversified and less known in comparison with fixed hypertension. During the early phase, the raised pressure is not a permanent state and secondary organ changes are not observed. An important role in cardiovascular disturbances is played by irregularities in the functions of the autonomic nervous system. Numerous studies have shown that the young patient with borderline or early established hypertension is hemodynamically characterized by an elevation of cardiac output (CO) and a numerically normal total peripheral resistance (TPR).[1–3] With increasing severity of hypertension and progressive age, the levels of CO revert to normal and TPR becomes elevated.

The aim of the present paper was to estimate the hemodynamic state of the nervous system of young male patients suffering from BHT with the use of the impedance cardiography method and to review vegetative regulatory mechanisms on the basis of the impact that tone changes in the autonomic system caused by passive tilt, local cold, and hyperventilation may exert upon the hemodynamics of patients with BHT.

MATERIALS AND METHODS

The research was conducted on the sample of 30 young male patients at the age of 17–19 (average age, 17.9 ± 0.7) suffering from BHT and on 29 boys at the same age (average age, 17.8 ± 0.8) with normal blood pressure. The first group was selected according to

WHO criteria[4] on the basis of arterial blood pressure values—systolic blood pressure (SBP), diastolic blood pressure (DBP), or both—of the boys measured in three independent takings with the use of centile charts within the range of the 90th to 95th percentile. Medium rest pressure values have been calculated from three independent measurements of SBP, DBP, and mean blood pressure (MBP). In both groups, the level of sexual development has been checked and all the boys defined as being at the juvenile stage. In the BHT group, secondary causes for it or organ changes have been excluded.

The hemodynamic state of all the young men tested has been estimated with the use of impedance cardiography techniques and arterial blood pressure measurements.[5–7] The following parameters and hemodynamic indexes have been defined: heart (rhythm) rate HR in (1/min), mean blood pressure MBP in (mmHg), stroke volume index SVI in (mL/m^2), cardiac index CI in (L/min/m^2), total peripheral resistance index TPRI in (dyn·s·cm^{-5}·m^2), and left ventricle work index LVWI in (J/min/m^2). The TPRI and LVWI were calculated from the following approximate equations: TPRI ≈ 80 · MBP/CI and LVWI ≈ 0.133 · MBP · CI, where TPRI is in [dyn·s·cm^{-5}·m^2], LVWI is in [J/min/m^2], MBP is in [mmHg] [MBP = DBP + (SBP − DBP)/3], and CI is in [L/min/m^2] (CI = CO/BSA, where BSA is the body surface area in [m^2]).

In order to estimate the impact of the vegetative system on the tested hemodynamic parameters, the following investigations were carried out in the NT subjects and the BHT patients: (1) hemodynamic state under the conditions of rest, (2) passive orthostatic test (3 min of head-up tilting with a 70° elevation), (3) cold pressor test after Hines (immersion of left hand and distal half of the forearm in ice water for 1 min), and (4) hyperventilation test (deeply breathing for 30 s). The hemodynamic state was presented graphically in orthogonal MBP-CI coordinates according to Sramek.[8] Statistical analyses were performed by Student's *t* test or Wilcoxon's ranking test for paired data.

RESULTS

In the BHT group, under the conditions of rest, significantly higher medium SBP, DBP, and MBP values as well as SVI, CI, and LVWI have been observed (TABLE 1). However, there are not any relevant differences between both groups as far as the HR values and the TPRI are concerned. Both groups are characterized by different "areas of hemodynamic state" defined in the MBP-CI coordinates as ellipses whose main axes are standard deviations of the examined parameters (FIGURE 1). The medium values of the four basic hemodynamic parameters of the group with normal blood pressure—MBP = 91.26 mmHg, CI = 3.31 L/min/m^2, TPRI = 2410 dyn·s·m^2·cm^{-5}, and LVWI = 40.18 J/min/m^2—constitute the reference parameters. The characteristic features of the BHT group are bigger dispersion of the resting cardiac indexes and significantly increased heart work.

Under the conditions of the orthostatic provocation, the characteristic changes of the hemodynamic parameters have been observed in both groups; however, they have been more distinct in the group with BHT (FIGURE 2). In this group, both the HR increase and the MBP decrease at tilting were of significant character and lasted longer after tilting. The decreases of both blood flow parameters, SVI and CI, during the process of passive tilt were better marked in the NT group of boys. In both groups, the hemodynamic parameters showed a similar tendency of changes, but at a different level. The TPRI was more dis-

TABLE 1. Resting Values of Hemodynamic Variables in Normotensive (NT) and Borderline Hypertensive (BHT) Patients[a]

Parameter	NT ($n = 29$)	BHT ($n = 30$)	Significance of Difference
HR [1/min]	76.3 ± 13.5	67.9 ± 11.5	ns
SBP [mmHg]	126.0 ± 6.2	135.3 ± 5.6	$p < 0.001$
DBP [mmHg]	78.9 ± 2.4	85.5 ± 4.0	$p < 0.001$
MBP [mmHg]	91.3 ± 4.0	102.4 ± 5.2	$p < 0.001$
SVI [mL/m^2]	44.5 ± 13.4	58.6 ± 22.9	$p < 0.01$
CI [L/min/m^2]	3.31 ± 0.96	3.9 ± 1.5	$p < 0.05$
TPRI [dyn·s·cm^{-5}·m^2]	2410.4 ± 813.4	2398.3 ± 877.8	ns
LVWI [J/min/m^2]	40.2 ± 11.9	52.6 ± 18.9	$p < 0.05$

[a]HR = heart rhythm; SBP, DBP, MBP = systolic, diastolic, and mean blood pressure, respectively; SVI, CI = stroke volume and cardiac index, respectively; TPRI = total peripheral resistance index; LVWI = left ventricle work index; ns = not significant between groups.

tinctly increasing in BHT patients (FIGURE 2), which is graphically illustrated by a shift of "the hemodynamic area" to the left side in the MBP-CI coordinate system.

Under the cold test, in the cooling phase, a slight increase of the HR and SVI, and consequently the CI as well, has been observed in both groups (FIGURE 3). However, the percentage increments of these parameters were higher in the BHT group. The cold stimulus significantly increased the LVWI, with the changes of the TPRI being relatively small. In the group of boys with BHT, we observed hyperreactions (pressure increase > 20 mmHg) to the cold pressor in 23.4% and 6.4% of the cases as regards DBP and SBP, respectively. The percentage of hyperreactions in the NT group was lower (8% and 3.5%, respectively).

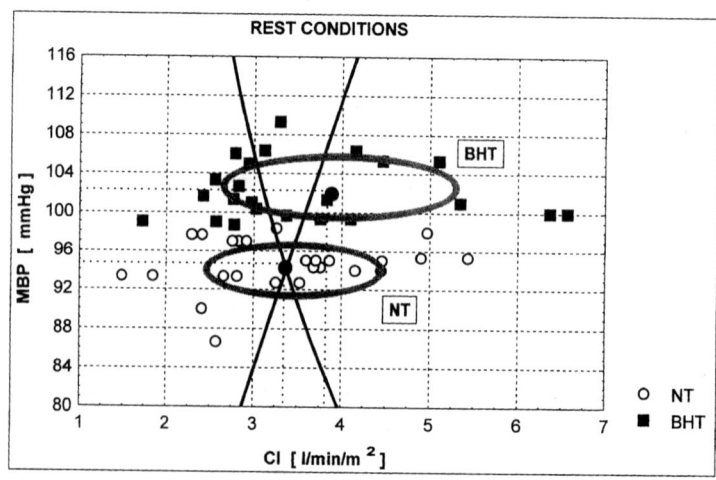

FIGURE 1. Hemodynamic states of the normotensive (NT) and the borderline hypertension (BHT) groups in rest conditions.

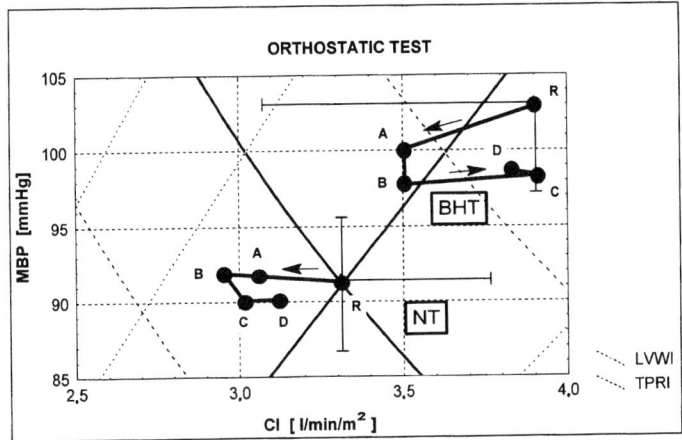

FIGURE 2. Hemodynamic changes during the orthostatic test in the normotensive (NT) and the borderline hypertension (BHT) groups; R: rest; A,B: 10 s and 3 min of orthostatic provocation; C,D: 10 s and 3 min after provocation.

The bigger pressure increase in BHT patients at the cooling stage resulted mainly from the higher share of the peripheral resistance and the stroke volume increase. Directly after the cooling process, the increased pressure lasted longer in the BHT group.

Under the conditions of hyperventilation (FIGURE 4), the changes of the hemodynamic state parameters were more distinct and longer lasting in the BHT group and mainly amounted to the significant HR increase and the decrease of MBP and TPRI. In the MBP-

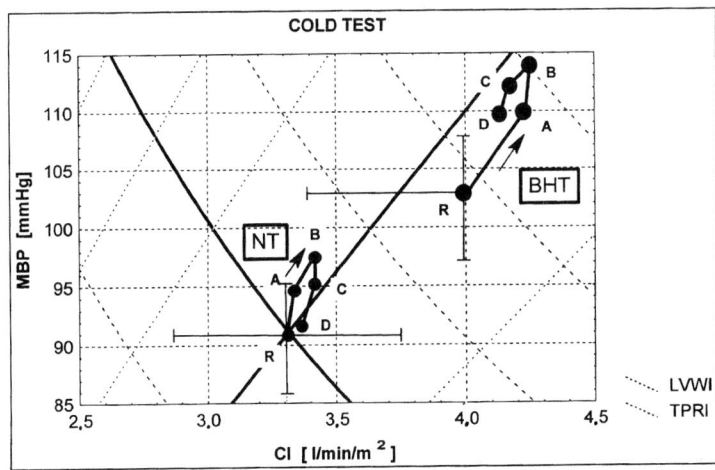

FIGURE 3. Hemodynamic changes during the cold test in the normotensive (NT) and the borderline hypertension (BHT) groups; R: rest; A,B: 10 s and 60 s of cold provocation; C,D: 10 s and 60 s after provocation.

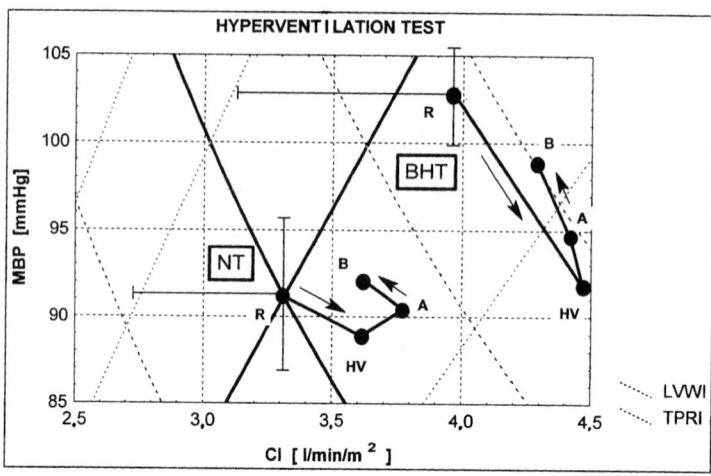

FIGURE 4. Hemodynamic changes during the hyperventilation test in the normotensive (NT) and the borderline hypertension (BHT) groups; R: rest; HV: 30 s of hyperventilation; A,B: 10 s and 60 s after provocation.

CI coordinate system, "hemodynamic trajectories" were similar in both groups, but more distinct and changed in the BHT group.

DISCUSSION

The results of the research proved that significant differences of the hemodynamic parameters characteristic for both groups tested can already be observed under the conditions of rest. The research conducted by the authors did not give evidence of the dominant impact of the rest tachycardia on the CO volume and CI values in the BHT group. The raised resting value of the CI in this group resulted from the significantly higher SVI ($p < 0.01$) as compared with the NT group.

The role of the raised CO or CI in the pathogenesis of hypertension has not been fully explained yet. In recent years, the papers published on that topic have represented views both for and against the hypothesis that the raised flow plays some role in the blood pressure increase.[9,10] Comparison between medium values of the TPRI in both groups has not shown any significant differences. It has been found in the BHT group that the resting mean value of LVWI is significantly higher ($p < 0.05$). According to some authors,[10,11] the increased heart work in BHT with normal arteriovenous oxygen difference results from the increased metabolic requirement. Thus, the hypertension patients are not characterized by "wasteful heart work" as is, for example, the case with hyperkinetic patients whose arteriovenous oxygen difference is low. It should be emphasized that the characteristics of the circulatory hyperkinesis in the group with BHT were mainly significantly higher indexes of stroke volume and heart work accompanied by slightly lower values of the HR.

In order to estimate the influence of the vegetative system upon the hemodynamic parameters, the following functional tests have been used: passive orthostatic test, cold pressor test after Hines, and hyperventilation test. Frohlich and coauthors[12] proved that patients who developed a serious course of hypertension and were highly resistant to medical treatment showed excessive susceptibility to orthostatic hypotension. This fact has been explained by most authors as resulting from the lower activity of baroreceptors in hypertension patients.[11,13–15] The phenomena of this kind are also considered to be the result of the aging processes, especially those of atherosclerotic changes and nerve degenerations. The increased orthostatic hypotension has been observed in hypertension patients pharmacologically treated. Tuckman and coauthors[16] noted that even a small tilt (about 20%) results in relatively big changes of the CO. The blood pressure decrease in hypertension patients, clearly marked at the tilt stage, continued during the stages of returning to the lying position. The tilt adrenergic stimulation of the patients suffering from BHT was mainly reflected in bigger MBP falls, higher percentage increases of the HR, and lower percentage decreases of the cardiac and stroke volume indexes.[15] We observed similar reactions in our investigations. The resting mean value of LVWI in the BHT patients was significantly higher and, in both groups, it was parallel decreasing during elevation. The graphic presentation of the hemodynamics during the tilt process indicated in an integrated way that the hemodynamic parameters change in the same direction in both groups; however, a wider range of those changes can be observed in the BHT patients. Summing up, the results obtained under the conditions of the passive orthostatic test proved that each group possesses a distinct cardiovascular reflex regulation. The boys suffering from BHT can be characterized by bigger and longer lasting decreases of the MBP, normal values of the TPRI, and higher increments of the HR.

The influence of cold upon the cardiovascular system has been an important area of interest for cardiologists. A lot of attention has been paid to the problem of how to use the influence of cold in order to diagnose the early stages of hypertensive disease and angina pectoris (stenocardia). The sympathetic system of a healthy human is subject to a reflex agitation under the influence of the cold stimulus affecting skin thermoreceptors. The agitation of the sympathetic system supplying the cardiovascular system results in vascular stenosis, tachycardia, and the CO increase. Hines and Brown[17] introduced a simple cold pressor test, which is still in use, for example, to diagnose the early stages of hypertension. The above-mentioned authors assumed that the excessive pressure increase of healthy people could reflect their constitutional proneness to hypertension.[18,19] The views on that, though, are not consistent. Rostrup et al.[20] indicated that a psychological factor played an important role in the process of the cold pressor test. People who had been previously informed about their hypertensive disease showed an increased vascular reactiveness to the cold provocation. The results of our own research showed that the reactions occurring in both groups analyzed were partially described by other authors.[6] In the cooling phase, a slight increase of the HR and SVI, and consequently the CI as well, has been observed in both groups. However, the percentage increments of these parameters were higher in BHT patients. The bigger pressure increase in BHT patients at the cooling stage resulted mainly from the stroke volume increase. Directly after the cooling process, the increased pressure lasted longer in the BHT group. Also, under the conditions of the hyperventilation provocation, the hemodynamic parameters in both groups changed in the same directions, but were more distinct in BHT patients.

The results obtained under all the analyzed tests demonstrated a strong neurogenic component in young BHT patients.

CONCLUSIONS

(1) The characteristic features of the hypertension patients were the increased values of the cardiac index, stroke volume index, medium blood pressure, and left ventricle work index, accompanied by the normal total peripheral resistance index values.

(2) The reactions of the cardiovascular system during the functional tests were similar in both groups; however, in the group with BHT, they were most clearly distinct, which may speak in favor of the increased activity of the adrenergic system.

(3) The use of impedance cardiography and graphic presentation of the hemodynamic state in the system of coordinates—medium blood pressure–cardiac index—provides a clear method for the evaluation of the cardiovascular system reactions under the conditions of vegetative provocation.

REFERENCES

1. JULIUS, S. *et al.* 1991. Hyperkinetic borderline hypertension in Tecumseh, Michigan. J. Hypertens. **9:** 77–84.
2. CULPEPPER, W. S. *et al.* 1983. Cardiac status in juvenile borderline hypertension. Ann. Intern. Med. **98:** 1–12.
3. PALATINI, P. & S. JULIUS. 1997. Heart rate and the cardiovascular risk. J. Hypertens. **15:** 3–17.
4. NATIONAL HEART, LUNG, AND BLOOD INSTITUTE. 1987. Report of the second task force on blood pressure control in children. Pediatrics **79:** 1–25.
5. KUBICEK, W. G., R. P. PATTERSON & D. A. WITSOE. 1970. Impedance cardiography as a noninvasive method of monitoring cardiac function and other parameters of the cardiovascular system. Ann. N.Y. Acad. Sci. **170:** 724–732.
6. BUELL, J. C. & M. D. LUBBOCK. 1988. A practical cost-effective, noninvasive system for cardiac output and hemodynamic analysis. Am. Heart J. **116:** 657–664.
7. MUZI, M. *et al.* 1985. Determination of cardiac output using ensemble-averaged impedance cardiograms. J. Appl. Physiol. **58:** 200–205.
8. SRAMEK, B. B. 1989. Hemodynamic and pump performance monitoring by electrical impedance: new concepts. Probl. Respir. Care **2:** 271–289.
9. JULIUS, S. 1988. Transition from high cardiac output to elevated vascular resistance in hypertension. Am. Heart J. **116:** 600–606.
10. PAGE, I. H. 1987. Hypertension Mechanisms. Grune & Stratton. New York.
11. WEBER, M. A. 1992. The hypertension syndrome and the sympathetic nervous system. Cardiovasc. Rev. Rep. **13:** 14–27.
12. FROHLICH, E. D. *et al.* 1967. Tilt test for investigating a neural component in hypertension. Circulation **36:** 387–393.
13. SMITH, J. J. & T. J. EBERT. 1990. General response to orthostatic stress. *In* Circulatory Response to the Upright Posture, p. 1–46. CRC Press. Boca Raton, Florida.
14. BESTLER, M. *et al.* 1989. Cardiodynamic response to passive tilt into the supine position—impedance cardiographic measurements. Z. Kardiol. **78:** 519–522.
15. BOER, P. *et al.* 1979. Measurement of cardiac output by impedance cardiography under various conditions. Am. J. Physiol. **237:** H491–H496.
16. TUCKMAN, J. & J. SHILINGFORD. 1966. Effect of different degrees of tilt on cardiac output, heart rate, and blood pressure in normal men. Br. Heart J. **28:** 32–39.
17. HINES, E. A. & G. E. BROWN. 1936. The cold pressor test for measuring the reactibility of blood pressure: data concerning 571 normal and hypertensive subjects. Am. Heart J. **11:** 1–9.

18. JULIUS, S. 1993. Syphatetic hyperactivity and coronary risk in hypertension: coronary lecture. Hypertension **21:** 886–893.
19. MANTYSAARI, M., K. ANTILA & T. PELTONEN. 1985. Rapid changes in rate-corrected and uncorrected systolic time intervals during cold pressor test. Aviat. Space Environ. Med. **56:** 165–170.
20. ROSTRUP, M., S. E. KJELDSEN & I. K. EIDE. 1990. Awareness of hypertension increases blood pressure and sympathetic responses to cold pressor test. Am. J. Hypertens. **3:** 912–917.

Stroke Volume Variability— Cardiovascular Response to Orthostatic Maneuver in Patients with Coronary Artery Diseases

JANUSZ SIEBERT,[a] JERZY WTOREK,[b] AND JAN ROGOWSKI[a]

[a]*First Department of Cardiology and Cardiosurgery, Institute of Cardiology, Medical University of Gdańsk, 80-211 Gdańsk, Poland*

[b]*Department of Medical and Ecological Electronics, Technical University of Gdańsk, 80-952 Gdańsk, Poland*

ABSTRACT: The dynamics of cardiovascular responses to postural stress have not been fully recognized. To determine whether coronary artery bypass grafting (CABG) has any effect on stroke volume variability (SVV), the power spectrum components of SVV were measured in 60 patients before and at 6 weeks after CABG. Stroke volume was assessed by means of the thoracic bioimpedance method. The thoracic impedance cardiogram and ECG were recorded in the supine and standing positions with controlled breathing rate (0.25 Hz) during 10-minute periods. The analysis of SVV was done by means of the autoregressive method. The total power, the power in the low-frequency band LFSV (0.05–0.15 Hz), the power in the high-frequency band HFSV (0.15–0.5 Hz), and the LFSV/HFSV ratio were analyzed. Before CABG, we did not notice any significant changes in the stroke volume spectral power indices. After CABG, all spectral indices were significantly decreased in the standing position.

INTRODUCTION

An assessment of myocardial function and autonomic control of the cardiovascular system is an important aspect when making a decision about a patient's functional status and medication. Impedance cardiography (ICG) is a method helpful in diagnosis of cardiac failure.[1,2] In patients with myocardial ischemia, a regional loss of myocardial contractile activity depresses the overall left ventricular function, producing reductions of stroke volume, stroke work, cardiac output, and ejection fraction while elevating the ventricular end-diastolic volume and pressure. Ischemia thus causes an impairment of cardiac contraction and an incomplete ventricular emptying (systolic failure). In addition, it impairs the ventricular relaxation and shifts the diastolic pressure-volume curve upward (diastolic failure). The compensatory hyperfunction of the uninvolved normal myocardium is mediated in part by adrenergic stimulation, operation of the Frank-Starling mechanism, activation of the renin-angiotensin-aldosterone system, and other neurohormonal adjustments. Except for the terminal stages of heart failure, the augmented ventricular end-diastolic volume must be regarded as helping to maintain the cardiac output. Elevation of the ventricular end-diastolic volume and pressure, in accordance with the Frank-Starling mechanism, increases ventricular performance.[3] In those cases, the heart rate variability is decreased.[4-6] The performance of the Valsalva maneuver—a forced expiration against the closed glottis—is helpful in diagnosis of heart failure. During this maneuver, the intrathoracic pressure rises, the venous return to the heart diminishes, the stroke volume falls, and the venous pressure rises. Arterial pressure tracings normally show four distinct phases. In heart failure, phases 1 and 3 are normal; that is, there is a normal transmission of the elevated intrathoracic pressure into the arterial tree during phase 1 and a sudden loss with a release of strain during phase 3. As the heart operates on the flat portion of its Starling curve, the impedance of venous return during phase 2 does not affect the stroke volume. Therefore, the baroreceptor reflex is not activated and there is no overshoot on release of the strain. The changes of stroke volume are rather small.[7] The effect of coronary artery bypass grafting (CABG) on standard cardiovascular reflex tests and pupillometry was studied in patients with coronary artery disease without previous infarction. The heart rate responses to the deep breathing test and Valsalva maneuver were attenuated after CABG, whereas CABG had no effect on beat-to-beat measured blood pressure responses.[8] The dynamics of the cardiovascular responses to changes in venous return to the heart have not been fully recognized in patients with coronary artery disease (CAD). There have been several studies on cardiovascular changes following a change of the position from the supine to the upright one in controls and patients.[9–13] Abnormal cardiovascular responses to orthostatic stress have been reported in patients with congestive heart failure.[14]

There is little information on short-term power spectral analysis of stroke volume variability (SVV) in cardiovascular diseases.[6,15–17] Spectral analysis of the SVV could be an estimator of the cardiovascular adaptation process following the postural change.

Impedance cardiography (ICG) is based on measurement of the thoracic electrical impedance and allows noninvasive real-time monitoring of stroke volume (SV) trends by analyzing the thoracic electrical bioimpedance beat-by-beat. This feature can be used to estimate other descriptions or presentations of SV, like histograms or SVV. The value of thoracic impedance is modified by respiration and by the volume of blood inside the thorax. This volume is subject to change as a result of heart contractions. Blood conductivity is greater than that of tissues involved in the measurement and, typically, the increase in blood volume reduces the electrical impedance of the thorax. This reduction is about 0.1% of the impedance modulus.[1,2]

The aim of our study is to determine whether coronary artery bypass grafting has any effect on SVV.

MATERIALS

The study group consisted of 60 male patients with three-vessel coronary diseases (CAD) (mean age, 57 ± 8 years). The mean ejection fraction was 47 ± 12%. Consecutive CAD patients admitted to the Cardiosurgery Department were included in the study. Twenty-four of them had a history of prior myocardial infarction and 10 had a history of hypertension. Patients with ejection fraction < 35%, diabetes mellitus, atrial fibrillation, frequent premature ectopic beats, or a coexisting valvular heart disease were excluded from the study. Preoperative therapeutic regimens included nitrates and β-blockers or calcium antagonists. No patients were treated with antiarrhythmic drugs. The drug regimen was kept constant until the ambulatory follow-up visit at 6 weeks after CABG. None of the patients suffered from the postoperative myocardial infarction.

METHODS

Analysis of SV, HR, and SVV

In order to obtain the main aim of the study, estimation of SVV is crucial. SV was calculated from ICG under the assumption that the characteristic points were recognized properly. The process of recognition was automatic, yet with some possibility of correction. The value of SV was excluded from the analysis when the recognition failed. A sequence of events in the recognition process was accepted. It was assumed that the "R" wave in the ECG preceded the systolic waves ("B", "E", etc.) in the ICG. The detection of the "R" wave was a relatively easy task and was done by using a "monitoring lead". An ECG, one-channel measurement module was developed for this purpose. A three-electrode measurement system was used. The additional third electrode was to reduce artifacts, especially those caused by the mains. This solution was known from the literature and was called a *driven-right-leg* circuit. Detailed analysis of this circuit was done by Winter and Webster.[18] The averaged common voltage created on the subject by power lines was sensed with a differential electrode pair. Then, it was amplified, inverted, and fed back to the body via a third electrode. Such a connection reduced the effective resistance to common and thus reduced common voltage appeared at the inputs of the differential amplifier. An additional reduction of influence of common voltage resulted from the application of a floating (isolated) input ECG amplifier. The signal via an isolation circuit was passed to the amplifier of a programmable gain and then to a filter circuit. The interpersonal signal input dynamics was assumed to be 20 dB. The filter was used in order to avoid aliasing effects and its cutoff frequency was 100 Hz. The ECG signal was sampled at 250 Hz.

There are many methods devoted to impedance measurement. The choice of appropriate methods depends on such factors as the frequency range, the amplitudes of real and imaginary parts, and the assumed measurement accuracy. In order to avoid the influence of electrode polarization effects on measurement accuracy, a four-electrode technique was used. Two electrodes were used to pass the current through the examined part of the body (thorax), while the other two were used to measure the voltage drop created by this current. Application (current) band electrodes were placed on the neck and below the sternum. Measurement (voltage) spot electrodes were attached to both ends of the sternum. A 1 mA_{p-p} current of 50 kHz was used. In order to minimize the influence of electrode impedances on the current magnitude, the actual amplitude of current was monitored and compared with the referential value in the feedback circuit. The resulting error signal modified the value of the output current to the desired level. It was achieved by using two multipliers (one as a demodulator) in the feedback loop. The amplitude of the voltage signal proportional to the measured impedance was registered using the synchronous detector. The output signal from the synchronous detector was filtered to obtain the so-called basal impedance (low-pass filter cutoff frequency of 1 Hz) and a time-varying signal (band-pass filter from 0.01 Hz to 50 Hz) synchronous with heart contractions. It was assumed that the interpersonal dynamics of the impedance signals was 20 dB. The ICG signal was sampled at 250 Hz.

Both ECG and ICG signals are shown in FIGURE 1. The digitized forms of the signals were sent to a PC computer where postprocessing was done. First, signals were filtered in order to remove the noise and other artifacts (50 Hz, etc.). Some IIR and morphological filters were used. Then, the ECG signal was processed to obtain information on "R" wave positions and "R-R" intervals. This information could be used as input data for detection of ICG waves and for calculating an "R-R" histogram or HRV. SV was calculated according to Kubicek's formula modified by individual blood resistivity. Having calculated the SV for each heartbeat, an interpolation procedure was applied. It allowed the SV to be obtained as a continuous function of time, which was necessary in further calculations (FIGURE 2). The SV values were spaced nonuniformly in the time domain according to a nonuniform frequency of heart contractions. In order to obtain SVV, the SV signal had to be spaced uniformly. This was obtained by uniformly sampling the continuous version of the SV signal. An autoregressive method was used to estimate the spectral density of the SVV (FIGURE 3). Before applying this procedure, the constant value was removed from the signal. The total power (PSSV), the power in the low-frequency band (LFSV: 0.05–0.15 Hz), the power in the high-frequency band (HFSV: 0.15–0.5 Hz), and the LFSV/HFSV ratio were analyzed.[19]

Procedures

All subjects underwent an investigation by the same procedure. Power spectrum components of SVV and ECG were measured beat-by-beat on the day before CABG and at 6 weeks after. The thoracic impedance cardiogram and ECG were recorded in the supine and standing positions with the controlled breathing rate (0.25 Hz) during 10-minute periods. The procedure was called an active orthostatic load test. Adaptation for the position was done during 10 minutes before collecting the data.

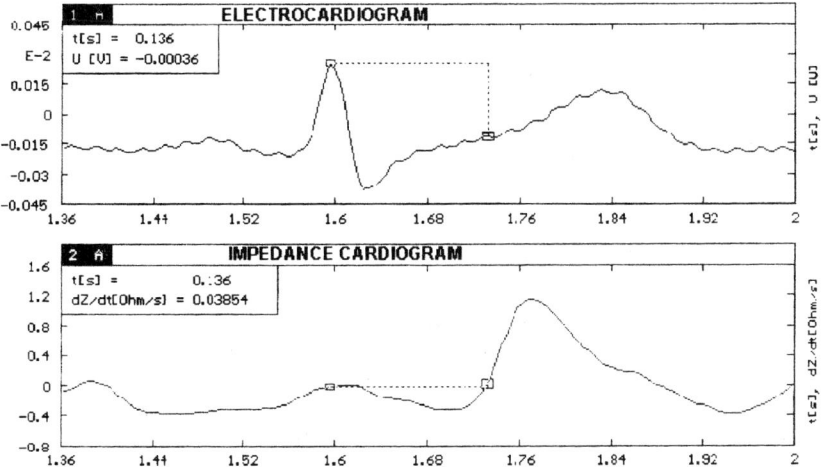

FIGURE 1. Simultaneous records of electrocardiogram and impedance cardiogram waveforms.

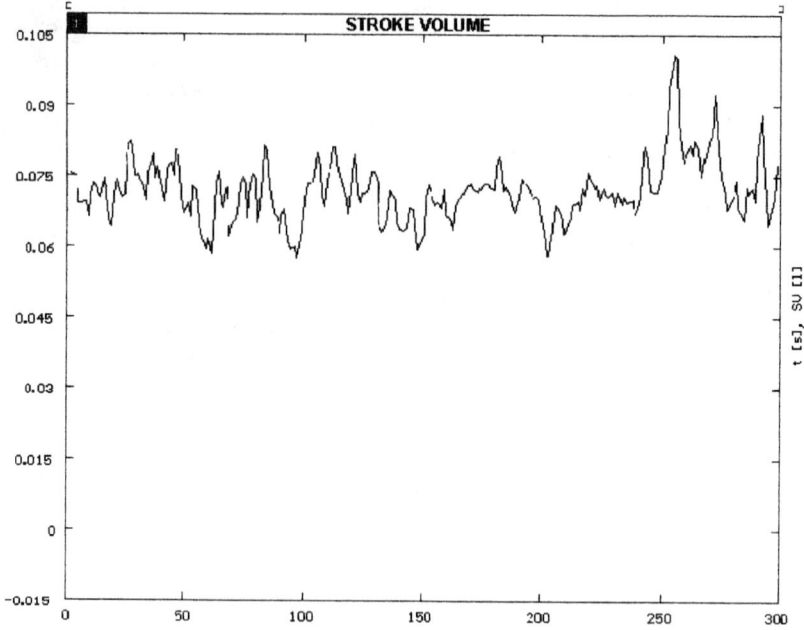

FIGURE 2. Continuous function of SV obtained by using spline function interpolation.

Statistics

The power spectral measures of SVV were logarithmically transformed because their distribution was positively skewed. The data were summarized as the mean ± SD of the log-transformed data. The differences between the supine and standing data were evaluated using a paired t test on the log-transformed data. $p < 0.05$ was considered significant.

RESULTS

Comparison of the Mean Values of SV and Heart Rate Calculated for 10-Minute Segments of ICG and ECG Recordings in Supine and Standing Positions

TABLE 1 lists the values of heart rate and stroke volume in the supine and standing positions before and 6 weeks after CABG. The upright position resulted in a significant decrease in the average RR intervals in both groups. Heart rate levels were significantly increased before and after CABG to a similar degree. The changes in heart rate were associated with changes in stroke volume. Stroke volume levels were decreased significantly in response to the active orthostatic load test to a similar degree before and after CABG. This was an effect of blood redistribution.

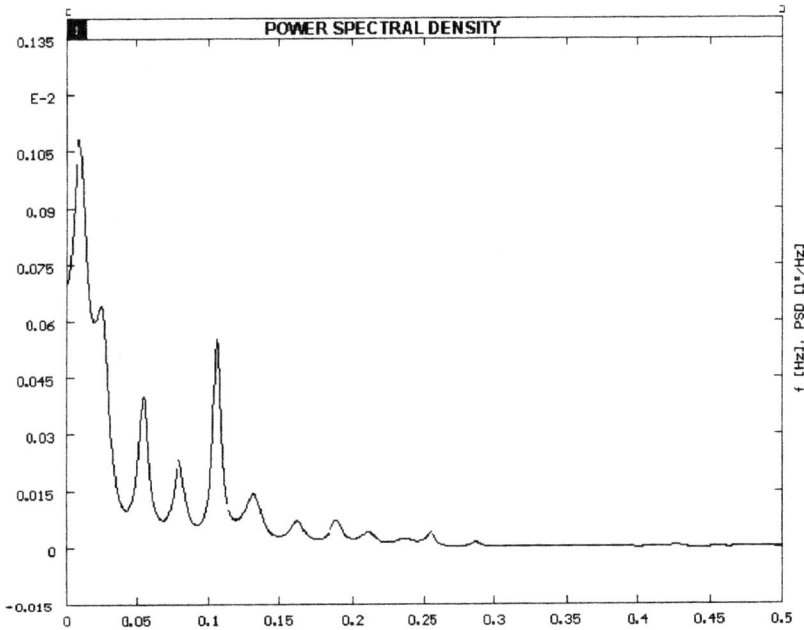

FIGURE 3. Power spectral density of SV estimated by an autoregressive model.

Comparison of the Mean Values for Power Spectral Measures of SVV Calculated for 10-Minute Segments of ICG Recordings in Supine and Standing Positions

TABLE 2 shows the means and standard deviations (SD) for the log-transformed values for 60 power spectral measures of SVV in the supine and standing positions before CABG. The mean logarithms for PSSV, LFSV, and the LFSV/HFSV ratio calculated from the supine records were bigger than the values calculated for the standing records. Conversely, HFSV power values calculated from the supine records were smaller than the val-

TABLE 1. Stroke Volume and Heart Rate Expressed as RR Intervals during the Active Orthostatic Load Test in 60 Male Patients with CAD before and after CABG[a]

	Position		
	Supine	Standing	*p*
RR (s) before CABG	0.954 ± 0.115	0.811 ± 0.129	0.001
RR (s) after CABG	0.915 ± 0.118	0.708 ± 0.132	0.001
SV (mL) before CABG	100 ± 38	77.1 ± 34	0.01
SV (mL) after CABG	104 ± 39	83 ± 18	0.05

[a]SV = stroke volume in mL; RR = intervals between consecutive R waves in the ECG in s.

TABLE 2. Stroke Volume Power Analysis in 60 Male Patients with CAD before CABG during the Active Orthostatic Load Test[a]

	Position		
	Supine	Standing	p
PSSV (mL$^2 \times 10^{-3}$)	1.11 ± 1.02	0.81 ± 0.8	0.2 (NS)
LFSV (mL$^2 \times 10^{-3}$)	0.39 ± 0.37	0.26 ± 0.26	0.1 (NS)
HFSV (mL$^2 \times 10^{-5}$)	9.2 ± 8.7	11.5 ± 10.8	0.3 (NS)
LFSV/HFSV	6.92 ± 6.2	5.81 ± 4.96	0.2 (NS)

[a]PSSV indicates the total power, LFSV indicates the low-frequency power, and HFSV indicates the high-frequency power. Values were log-transformed as the data were positively skewed. NS = not significant.

ues calculated from the records in the standing position. Resting supine and standing SVV did not change significantly.

TABLE 3 shows the data obtained during active orthostatic tests at 6 weeks after CABG. The values were collected in the supine and upright postures. Analysis of the components of SVV revealed that subjects after CABG had a significant lower level of component power. The total power stroke volume variability, the power in the LFSV, the power in the HFSV, and the LFSV/HFSV ratio decreased significantly in the standing position. In patients with CAD at 6 weeks after CABG, significant changes of stroke volume power indices were noticed in response to the orthostatic load test.

TABLE 3. Stroke Volume Power Analysis in 60 Male Patients with CAD after CABG during the Active Orthostatic Load Test[a]

	Position		
	Supine	Standing	p
PSSV (mL$^2 \times 10^{-3}$)	0.895 ± 0.575	0.459 ± 0.338	0.03
LFSV (mL$^2 \times 10^{-3}$)	0.492 ± 0.337	0.181 ± 0.114	0.01
HFSV (mL$^2 \times 10^{-5}$)	10.807 ± 8.98	5.348 ± 3.343	0.05
LFSV/HFSV	6.993 ± 5.13	3.825 ± 1.94	0.04

[a]PSSV indicates the total frequency power, LFSV indicates the low-frequency power, and HFSV indicates the high-frequency power. Values were log-transformed as the data were positively skewed.

DISCUSSION

Manifestations of heart failure are common in patients with CAD, but they can be a dominant feature in some patients, especially in those with prior myocardial infarction. Ischemic focus may have become a fibrous scar, with disappearance or reduction of the angina. The three most common causes of heart failure are left ventricular aneurysm, mitral regurgitation due to papillary muscle dysfunction, and an inadequate mass of properly contracting myocardium. The latter can be secondary to extensive myocardial infarction; a large quantity of viable, but "hibernating", "stunning" myocardium; or a combination of these two.[3] Cardiac surgery appears to be the treatment of choice for patients with extensive CAD and abnormal left ventricular function. An improvement in the left ventricular function has been reported in survivors at 3 months to 3 years after a complete revascularization. Regional wall-motion abnormalities have also been diminished after revascularization surgery. Our data suggest that the patients with CAD have had the same level of stroke volume variability in the supine and standing position and that was because of cardiac performance impairment. The baroreceptor reflex is not activated during the redistribution of blood. Delayed recovery of ventricular function following successful coronary artery bypass graft surgery may be explained by the disappearance of myocardial stunning. The systolic or diastolic dysfunction is reversible and the myocardium exhibits some contractile reserve. The baroreceptor reflex is activated by the blood redistribution. In this case, significant changes are observed in stroke volume variability indices during the active orthostatic load test.

CONCLUSIONS

Before CABG, we did not observe any significant changes in the stroke volume variability indices during the active orthostatic load test. After CABG, the total, low-, and high-frequency power of stroke volume variability significantly decreased in response to the active orthostatic load test.

REFERENCES

1. EBERT, T. J., D. L. ECKBERG, G. M. VETROVEC & M. J. COWLEY. 1984. Impedance cardiograms reliably estimate beat-by-beat changes of left ventricular stroke volume in humans. Cardiovasc. Res. **18:** 354–360.
2. KUBICEK, W. G., J. N. KARNEGIS, R. P. PATTERSON, D. A. WITSOE & R. H. MATTSON. 1966. Development and evaluation of an impedance cardiac output system. Aviat. Space Environ. Med. **37**(10): 1208–1212.
3. BRAUNWALD, E., Ed. 1992. Heart Disease. Saunders. Philadelphia.
4. NIEMELA, M. J., K. E. J. AIRAKSINEN, K. U. O. TAHVANAINEN, M. K. LINNALUOTO & J. T. TAKKUNEN. 1992. Effect of coronary bypass grafting on cardiac parasympathetic nervous function. Eur. Heart J. **13:** 932–935.
5. BIGGER, J. T., J. L. FLEISS, L. M. ROLNITZKY & R. C. STEINMAN. 1993. The ability of short-term measures of RR variability to predict mortality after myocardial infarction. Circulation **88:** 927–934.
6. SIEBERT, J., J. WTOREK, J. BELLWON & M. SMIETAŃSKI. 1995. Stroke volume and heart rate power spectral analysis in the patients before and 6 weeks after coronary artery bypass grafting. *In* Proceedings of the Ninth International Conference on Bio-impedance and European Community Concerted Action on Impedance Tomography (Heidelberg), p. 287–290.

7. BELLWON, J., J. SIEBERT, J. ROGOWSKI, J. SZULC, D. CIEĆWIERZ, T. DEPTULSKI, M. NARKIEWICZ & A. RYNKIEWICZ. 1996. Heart rate power spectral analysis in patients before and 6 weeks after coronary artery bypass grafting. Clin. Sci. **91**(suppl.): 19–21.
8. NISHIMURA, R. A. & A. J. TAJIK. 1986. The Valsalva maneuver and response revisited. Mayo Clin. Proc. **61:** 211.
9. BORST, C., W. WIELING, J. F. M. VAN BREDERODE, A. HOND, L. G. DE RIJK & A. J. DUNNING. 1982. Mechanism of initial heart rate response to postural change. Am. J. Physiol. **243:** 676–681.
10. BORST, C., J. F. M. VAN BREDERODE, W. WIELING, G. A. VAN MONTFRANS & A. J. DUNNING. 1984. Mechanism of initial blood pressure response to postural change. Clin. Sci. **67:** 321–327.
11. EWING, D. J., L. HUME, I. W. CAMPBELL, A. MURRAY, J. M. M. NEILSON & B. F. CLARKE. 1978. Immediate heart rate response to standing: simple test for autonomic neuropathy in diabetes. BMJ **I**(6106): 145–147.
12. EWING, D. J., L. HUME, I. W. CAMPBELL, A. MURRAY, J. M. M. NEILSON & B. F. CLARKE. 1980. Autonomic mechanisms in the initial heart rate response to standing. J. Appl. Physiol. **49:** 809–814.
13. CYBULSKI, G. 1996. Influence of age on the immediate cardiovascular response to orthostatic manoeuvre. Eur. J. Appl. Physiol. **73:** 563–572.
14. KASSIS, E. 1987. Cardiovascular response to orthostatic tilt in patients with severe congestive heart failure. Cardiovasc. Res. **21:** 362–368.
15. PIHA, S. J. & H. HAMALAINEN. 1993. Effect of coronary bypass grafting on autonomic cardiovascular reflexes. Ann. Med. **26:** 53–56.
16. SIEBERT, J., J. BELLWON, A. RYNKIEWICZ, J. ROGOWSKI, D. CIEĆWIERZ & M. NARKIEWICZ. 1996. Stroke volume power spectral analysis in the patients before and 6 weeks after coronary artery bypass grafting [abstract]. Noninvasive Electrocardiol. **1**(2): 214.
17. SIEBERT, J., J. ROGOWSKI, M. BRZEZIŃSKI, J. WTOREK, K. ROSZAK & M. NARKIEWICZ. 1997. Heart rate variability and stroke volume power spectral analysis during postural changes before and after coronary artery bypass grafting [abstract]. J. Cardiovasc. Diagnosis Procedures **14**(2): 102.
18. WINTER, B. B. & J. G. WEBSTER. 1983. Driven-right-leg circuit design. IEEE Trans. Biomed. Eng. **30**(1): 62–66.
19. WANG, X., H. H. SUN & J. M. VAN DE WATER. 1995. An advanced signal processing technique for impedance cardiography. IEEE Trans. Biomed. Eng. **42**(2): 224–230.

Assessment of Left Ventricular Systolic Function and Diastolic Time Intervals by the Bioimpedance Polyrheocardiographic System

MICHAIL ZUBAREV, ANDREY DUMLER, VLADIMIR SHUTOV, AND NICOLAY POPOV

Department of Introduction into Internal Diseases, Perm Medical Academy, City Clinical Hospital 4, Perm 614107, Russia

ABSTRACT: In order to detect left ventricular systolic function and diastolic time intervals using a new improved bioimpedance polyrheocardiographic system (BPCS), 110 healthy subjects and 128 patients with myocardial infarction were examined. Twenty-four simultaneous measurements of cardiac output by thermodilution and BPCS were performed in 11 patients with complicated acute left ventricular failure. Studies demonstrated a high degree of correlation ($r = 0.91$, $p < 0.001$). The correlation between the methods of using signals of the second derivative and the subtracted first derivative waveform of BPCS and continuous-wave Doppler echocardiography of systolic and diastolic time intervals was studied in 51 patients. The methods were closely correlated, especially with respect to left ventricular ejection time ($r = 0.95$), isovolumic relaxation time ($r = 0.85$), time to peak filling ($r = 0.90$), and deceleration of rapid filling time ($r = 0.91$). New bioimpedance hemodynamic parameters such as peak volume acceleration of ejection (PVAE) and peak power ejection (PPE) in patients with heart failure (NYHA Class I–III) were studied. Significant reductions of PVAE and PPE in groups of patients with marked progression of heart failure were noted. These results have demonstrated that BPCS is a noninvasive, simple accurate method of assessment of left ventricular systolic function and diastolic time intervals.

INTRODUCTION

Tetrapolar transthoracic impedance cardiography[1,2] and its modifications[3,4] are widely used to estimate the parameters of cardiac output and systolic time intervals. Despite the advantages over noninvasive methods of hemodynamics research, there are some limitations:

(1) 15% originally assumed conditionality in determination of the left ventricular ejection time (LVET) and difficulty in finding the end of ejection on the first derivative waveform of the impedance cardiogram (ICG) give errors in determination of stroke volume (SV);

(2) extremely approximate estimation of cardiac contractility, which is performed without taking into consideration the velocity and power components of the left ventricular blood output;

(3) impossibility of estimating left ventricular diastolic function.

The purpose of this study was to elaborate a computer modification of the transthoracic bioelectrical impedance method for assessment of left ventricular function with high-accuracy determination of left ventricular ejection acceleration, LVET, and diastolic time intervals.

METHODS

BPCS

The computer diagnostic bioimpedance polyrheocardiography system (BPCS) has been elaborated on the basis of the method of transthoracic bioelectrical impedance.[1] The system is able to synchronously register waveforms of signals (FIGURE 1): the first derivative (FD), the second derivative (SD) of thoracic ICG, the subtracted first derivative (SFD) of ICG, the phonocardiogram (PCG), and the electrocardiogram (ECG).

The technical decision is based on the use of two ICG channels in blocks of subtraction, addition, and repeated differentiation. An improved tetrapolar technique of electrode location is used, in which current electrodes are placed traditionally[1] and potential electrodes are partitioned and located at opposite sides of the thorax (FIGURE 2). A partition of electrodes allows receiving of waveform signals of the subtracted first derivative on sym-

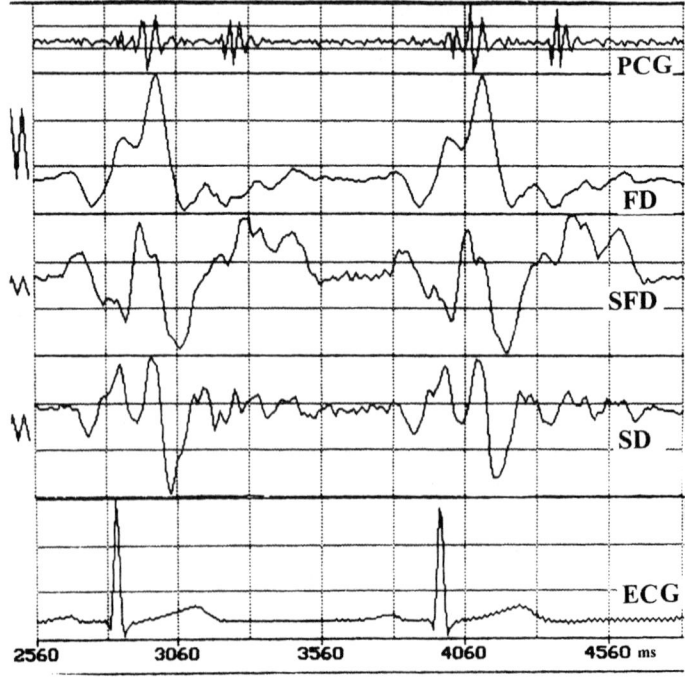

FIGURE 1. Polyrheocardiogram: PCG, phonocardiogram; FD, first derivative signal; SFD, subtracted first derivative signal; SD, second derivative signal; ECG, electrocardiogram.

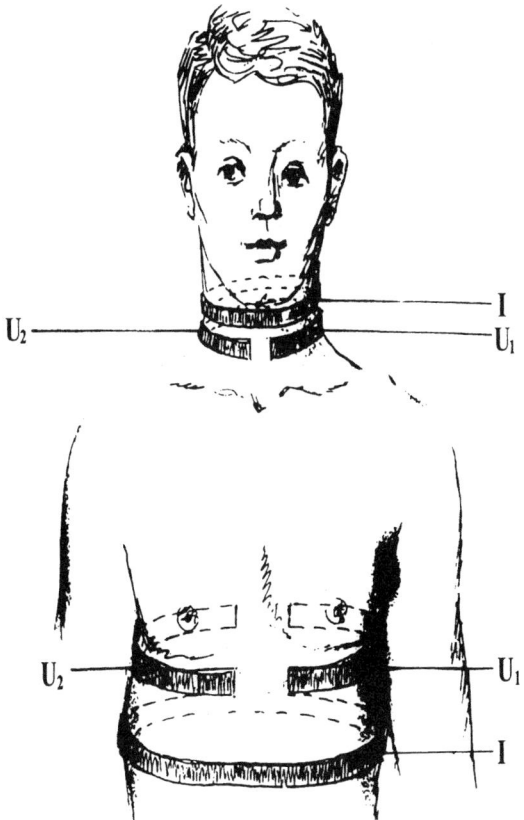

FIGURE 2. Schematic representation of the bioimpedance polyrheocardiographic system (BPCS). Electrode placement: I = constant current electrodes; U_1 and U_2 = detecting (potential) electrodes.

metrical areas of the right and left chest. The medical aspect of the technology has been patented.

Calculation of Hemodynamic Parameters

Stroke volume of blood is determined by the equation for the heterogeneous model of the thorax:[3]

$$SV = 0.9 \cdot K \cdot \rho \cdot Q^2 \cdot L \cdot \text{Ad} \cdot \text{LVET}/Z_0^2 \cdot 1000 \qquad (1)$$

where SV = stroke volume (L), 0.9 = correction coefficient, K = Gundarov's constant,[3] ρ = blood resistivity (ohm • cm), Q = circumference of the thorax (cm), L = distance between the electrodes (cm), Ad = maximum rate of change in the impedance signal (ohm/s), LVET = left ventricular ejection time (s), Z_0 = base impedance (ohm), and 1000 = coefficient for conversion into liters. LVET is determined on the SD waveform as an interval from the beginning of the sudden deviation of a systolic wave up to peak negative oscillation, which directly precedes the ascending part of the early diastolic FD wave coincident with S_2 PCG.

$$PVAE = 0.9 \cdot K \cdot \rho \cdot Q^2 \cdot L \cdot AEA/Z_0^2 \cdot 1000 \qquad (2)$$

where PVAE = peak volume acceleration ejection (L/s), and AEA = acceleration of ejection amplitude (ohm/s^2), which is determined on an SD waveform from the baseline to the peak of the systolic ejection wave. Other parameters of the formula correspond to equation 1. Also,

$$PPE = SBP \cdot PVAE \qquad (3)$$

where PPE = peak power of ejection (W/s) and SBP = systolic blood pressure (kPa).

The hemodynamic parameters such as preejection period, cardiac output, systemic vascular resistance, and cardiac index are counted on the basis of the standard formulas.[5]

The structure of the diastolic intervals of the left ventricle was determined by markers of the SFD waveform. The isovolumic relaxation time (IRT) interval goes from the beginning of the ascending knee of the early diastolic wave coincident with S_2 PCG to the incisure on its ascending knee or to the sharp oscillation on the top. Rapid filling time (RFT) phase begins from the IRT top and proceeds to the end of the downward-directed knee of the wave. The duration of this knee corresponds to the deceleration of rapid filling time (DRFT). The period from IRT up to the peak of the positive RFT wave is the time to peak filling (TPF). The left atrial systolic time (LAST) phase corresponds to the duration of the SFD wave coincident with the P-Q interval on ECG. The slow filling time (SFT) phase is the time from the PFT end to LAST.

RESULTS

Twenty-four simultaneous measurements of CO by thermodilution and BPCS were performed in 11 patients with myocardial infarction complicated by acute left ventricular failure. The methods correlated closely ($r = 0.91$, $p < 0.001$). BPCS methodology had better reproducibility than thermodilution in serial measurements of the same patients.

LVET determination and diastolic time interval measurements made by BPCS and continuous-wave Doppler echocardiography were performed in 21 normal subjects and 30 cardiac patients. The correlation of the methods was high—LVET ($r = 0.95$), IRT ($r = 0.85$), TPF ($r = 0.90$), RFT ($r = 0.80$), DRFT ($r = 0.91$), and LAST ($r = 0.71$).

One hundred ten healthy subjects and 128 patients with myocardial infarction complicated by heart failure (HF) (NYHA Class I–III) (aged 30 to 60 years) were studied. In normal subjects, the mean values ($M \pm m$) were PVAE 7.5 ± 0.27 L/s^2 and PPE 114 ± 3.2 W/s. In patients with HF Class I, they were significantly lower: PVAE 6.3 ± 0.4 L/s^2 ($p < 0.01$) and PPE 97 ± 5.5 W/s. Patients with HF Class II had PVAE 5.0 ± 0.39 L/s^2 and PPE 77 ± 6.0 W/s. These values were significantly lower ($p < 0.05$) than those of the group with HF Class I. Patients with HF Class III had even lower values: PVAE 3.1 ± 0.41 L/s^2 and PPE 58 ± 7.7 W/s ($p < 0.05$ as compared to the group with HF Class II).

DISCUSSION

The impedance cardiogram has been in clinical use for 30 years as the method of SV measuring[1]. Many attempts have since been made to enter a correction coefficient into Kubicek's formula for increasing the accuracy of the SV measurement. We use a modified formula with correction coefficients connected with peculiarities of the structure of the human thorax as a frustum of a cone,[3] not that of a cylinder as is supposed in Kubicek's formula. The error in SV determination depends on the correctness of the LVET on the FD waveform of the ICG, on which it is very difficult or even impossible to find markers of the beginning and end of ejection. During blood ejection, the increase of velocity on its entrance into the aorta (the acceleration) is absolutely abrupt.[2,5] This is represented by a sudden, sharp increase of acceleration of varying impedance and causes a precise labeling of the beginning of ejection on an SD waveform. During aortic valve closure, the blood inflow into the aorta is stopped; thus, the thoracic impedance suddenly increases with acceleration. This gives the second precise marker of the LVET ending on an SD waveform. Therefore, the SD waveform has more precise markers for LVET measurement.[6]

It is established that a varying thoracic impedance reflects pulsatile aortic blood flow;[2] therefore, it is possible to suggest that the amplitude of the systolic SD wave reflects volume blood ejection acceleration into the aorta. As the blood is practically not compressed, the volumetric velocity parameters of the blood flow in the aorta are functions of two components: first is the acceleration effect of the volumetric output of the left ventricle and preload; second is the effect of afterload, which interferes with the velocity parameters of volumetric output of the left ventricle and should be taken into account during contractility assessment of the left ventricle.[7] Calibrated SD with respect to the size of the systolic wave amplitude allows the determination of PVAE, reflecting the peak value of ejection acceleration. The product of PVAE and SBP is a rather sensitive contractility parameter taking into account the processes of cardiac preload and afterload simultaneously.

The ideas of markers of diastolic time intervals on an FD waveform were assumed before.[8,9] These assumptions did not have practical use because of significant morphological wave variabilities in the diastolic phase. Variability is due to the peculiarity of the blood flow in the thorax. It has two basic independent components: the first is caused by central blood flow from the veins into the atriums and ventricles; the second is caused by the blood flow in the walls of the thorax. For the left and right chests, blood flows in the thoracic wall are symmetric and identical to a greater degree than the central blood flow. Central blood flow in the left and right chest halves is nonsymmetric and asynchronous, which is connected with the anatomical structure of the heart and major vessel location and with asynchronous blood flows in halves of the heart.

Subtraction of symmetric signals of the first derivative of the ICG of the left and right chest halves of the second component allows the strengthening of asymmetric signals of the central blood flow, including those caused by pulsatile blood flow of pulmonary veins during diastole (markers of diastolic time intervals).

The present report on clinical BPCS use is preliminary. In further work, we shall summarize the results of BPCS application obtained by monitoring hemodynamics and thoracic fluid volume of patients with acute myocardial infarction and with subsequent control during the period of a month and longer. We shall also monitor diagnostic stress tests and hemodynamic assessment in patients with different pacemaker programs.[10,11]

REFERENCES

1. KUBICEK, W. G. *et al.* 1966. Development of an evaluation of an impedance cardiac output system. Aerosp. Med. **37:** 1208–1212.
2. KUBICEK, W. G. *et al.* 1974. The Minnesota impedance cardiograph: theory and applications. IEEE Trans. Biomed. Eng. **9:** 410–416.
3. GUNDAROV, I. A. *et al.* 1983. Standards of the central hemodynamics derived by tetrapolar chest rheography. Ter. Arkh. **55:** 26–28.
4. SRAMEK, B. B. *et al.* 1993. Stroke volume equation with a linear impedance model and its accuracy as compared to thermodilution and magnetic flowmeter techniques in animals and humans. *In* Proceedings of the Sixth International Conference on Electrical Bioimpedance (Yugoslavia), p. 38–41.
5. SRAMEK, B. B. *et al.* 1995. Biomechanics of the Cardiovascular System. Prague.
6. ZUBAREV, M. A. & A. A. DUMLER. 1995. New method of blood expulsion determination according to the second derivative thoracic tetrapolar rheogram. Perm Med. J. **12:** 41–43.
7. BRYG, R. J. *et al.* 1989. Effects of isometric handgrip exercise on Doppler-derived parameters of aortic flow in normal subjects. Am. J. Cardiol. **63:** 1410–1412.
8. BUELL, J. C. 1988. A practical cost-effective, noninvasive system for cardiac output and hemodynamic analysis. Am. Heart J. **116:** 657–664.
9. PATTERSON, R. P. *et al.* 1991. Impedance cardiography using band and regional electrodes in supine, sitting, and during exercise. IEEE Trans. Biomed. Eng. **38:** 393–400.
10. ZUBAREV, M. A. *et al.* 1994. Evaluation of the functional state of the left ventricle with the use of second derivative thoracic rheogram during graded isometric leg exercise. Kardiologiya **34:** 156–158.
11. ZUBAREV, M. A. *et al.* 1991. Rheographic technique for determining the length of diastole phases. Kardiologiya **31:** 36–38.

In Vivo ac Impedance Spectroscopy of Human Skin

Theory and Problems in Monitoring of Passive Percutaneous Drug Delivery

A. H. LACKERMEIER,[a] E. T. McADAMS,[a,b] G. P. MOSS,[c] AND A. D. WOOLFSON[c]

[a]*Northern Ireland Bio-Engineering Center, University of Ulster at Jordanstown, County Antrim BT37 OQB, United Kingdom*

[c]*School of Pharmacy, The Queen's University of Belfast, Belfast BT7 1NN, United Kingdom*

ABSTRACT: The use of impedance spectroscopy to evaluate transdermal drug delivery is discussed and new techniques and protocols are suggested to avoid or minimize potential problems. A novel multichannel impedance analyzer, exploiting the advantages of the "three-electrode" configuration, was employed to measure the effects of differing topically applied concentrations of the percutaneous local anesthetic amethocaine on the electrical properties of the treated skin sites. Each measured impedance spectrum was modeled by an equivalent circuit consisting of a resistor in series with the parallel combination of a pseudocapacitance and a resistor. Due to differences in skin sites and to the finite times taken to apply each electrode, it was difficult to satisfactorily compare and contrast the results obtained from adjacent skin sites. Normalization of data highlighted differences in relative impedance changes and aided the meaningful comparison of treated skin sites.

INTRODUCTION

Electrical impedance spectroscopy (EIS) has been recently applied in the field of transdermal drug delivery[1–8] to monitor the electrical properties of treated skin sites in an effort to monitor changes resulting from transdermal drug diffusion. At present, there is no acceptable method of accurately assessing how much drug has crossed, is crossing, or will cross the skin barrier and of establishing the presence and degree of skin damage occurring under occlusive, drug-containing patches. Researchers therefore hope that it will be possible to use EIS to detect at a latent stage and to quantify the extent of tissue damage caused rather than relying on (i) subjective statements from patients as to the amount of discomfort they experience or (ii) subsequent clinical observation based on the degree of induced erythema.[2] This is particularly important during the delivery of a local anesthetic.

It is common in biomedical engineering circles to model the electrical properties of biological tissues by means of equivalent electrical circuits. With the appropriate choice of model, it may be possible to relate the circuit elements to underlying physical processes. For example, it appears that there is a correlation between drug permeability of the skin and the measured value of the skin's low-frequency impedance, in particular the value of the skin's dc resistance.[2] Burnette and Bagniefski[1] showed that there was a linear correla-

---

[b]To whom all correspondence should be addressed.

tion between the inverse of the impedance at 0.2 Hz and skin permeability to Na^+ ions. The capacitance of the skin appears to reflect the condition of the stratum corneum. For example, although Foley et al.[3] found that the skin's capacitance was not significantly affected during drug delivery through the stratum corneum, they reported however that the use of penetration enhancers or the application of high current densities (during iontophoretic delivery) altered the skin's capacitance, indicating changes in the structure of the stratum corneum or its destruction.

It is anticipated that the measurement of the skin's ac impedance over an adequately wide frequency range and with a sufficiently large number of frequencies will enable the choice of a suitable model that in turn will, prior to treatment, provide useful information on (i) the integrity of the skin, (ii) the quality of the electrode-skin contact, and (iii) the magnitude of the epidermal impedance and its likely permeability. Monitoring the ac impedance of the skin during delivery is expected to give information on (i) the penetration of the drug through the skin, (ii) the quality of the electrode contact, and (iii) the onset of skin damage. Monitoring the ac impedance of the skin following drug treatment may provide information on (i) the skin's storage of drug (reservoir effect) and (ii) the recovery of the skin following treatment.

It is the intention of this review to outline the potential of EIS in investigating *in vivo* the effects of transdermal drug delivery on the skin. The potential pitfalls associated with the use of ac impedance techniques, equivalent circuits, and the graphical presentations of data will be discussed. Improved techniques and protocols will be suggested.

THE APPLICATION OF IMPEDANCE SPECTROSCOPY TO SKIN IMPEDANCE MEASUREMENT

The outer layer of the epidermis, the stratum corneum, is relatively nonconductive and presents a high impedance to the transmission of electrical current. It can be considered as a membrane that is semipermeable to ions.[9] This membrane limits the flow of ionic current, but (due to its thinness and dielectric properties) permits the capacitive coupling between a metal electrode placed on the skin and the underlying conductive tissues.[9] These capacitive properties are due to the lipid-protein matrix of the skin. Some ions do manage to traverse the stratum corneum via the paracellular pathways and through the skin's appendages, and this flow of ionic current has been represented in an equivalent circuit model by a large resistance, R_p, shunting the skin's capacitance, C_p.[10]

This "classical" model has one essential drawback. The impedance locus of this model in a complex impedance plane plot should consist of a semicircular arc whose center is located exactly on the real axis. This unfortunately does not agree with experimental loci whose centers tend to be located below the resistive axis. A typical impedance locus of the electrode-skin interface is schematically shown in FIGURE 1. R_∞ and R_0, the intercepts with the real axis at high and low frequencies, respectively, are the high- and low-frequency limit resistances. The "depression" of the center of the arc below the real axis is expressed in terms of the angle ϕ. ω_0 ($=2\pi f_0$) is the angular velocity of the "peak" of the arc, that is, the point with the largest value of reactance, X_s.

Such impedance loci have been found to be well modeled by the following empirical expression proposed by Cole in 1940[11] to describe the complex impedance of certain biological tissues:

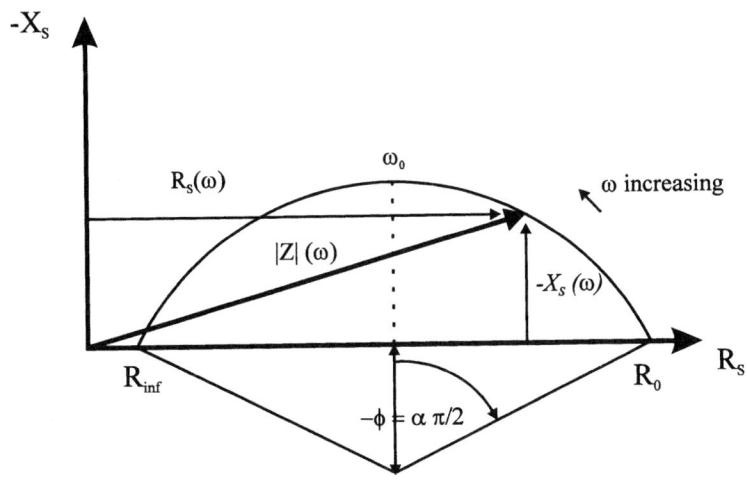

FIGURE 1. A typical impedance locus in the complex impedance plane.

$$Z = R + (R_0 - R_\infty)/[1 + (j\omega/\omega_0)^\alpha] \tag{1}$$

where α is dimensionless and has a value between 0 and 1. It is found to be related to ϕ such that $\phi = \alpha\pi/2$. If $\alpha = 1$, the impedance locus is a semicircular arc whose center lies on the real axis. In this case, the high-frequency intercept angle ϕ will be equal to 90°. If $\alpha < 1$, the locus has the form of a "depressed" semicircular arc whose center lies below the real axis. In this case, the intercept angle ϕ is less than 90°.

A potential problem arises due to the fact that equivalent circuits are rarely unique and several circuit models can have identical or very similar impedances. The choice of the equivalent circuit will depend on the system under investigation and on the physical intuition of the researcher.[12] The complex impedance described by the Cole equation corresponds to that of either one of the two simple circuits shown in FIGURE 2. More complex circuits incorporating large numbers of elements can enable excellent fits with experimental data; however, the relevance of such circuits is difficult to establish. We prefer circuit A, which consists of a resistance R_∞ in series to a parallel configuration of a "constant phase angle" impedance, Z_{CPA}, shunting a resistance R_p, where

$$Z_{CPA} = K(j\omega)^{-\alpha}. \tag{2}$$

K is a measure of the magnitude of Z_{CPA} (i.e., $K = |Z_{CPA}|_{\omega=1}$) and has units of $\Omega s^{-\alpha}$. These circuit elements can be expressed in terms of the Cole parameters, R_∞, R_0, ω_0, and α, as follows:

$$R_p = (R_0 - R_\infty) \tag{3}$$

$$K = (R_0 - R_\infty)/T_0^\alpha = R_p/T^\alpha. \tag{4}$$

Equation 1 can therefore be rewritten as

$$Z = R_\infty + R_p/[1 + (R_p/K)(j\omega)^\alpha] = R_\infty + R_p \parallel Z_{CPA}. \tag{5}$$

In the literature, various alternative and equally valid expressions for Z_{CPA} have been used and some examples are listed below:

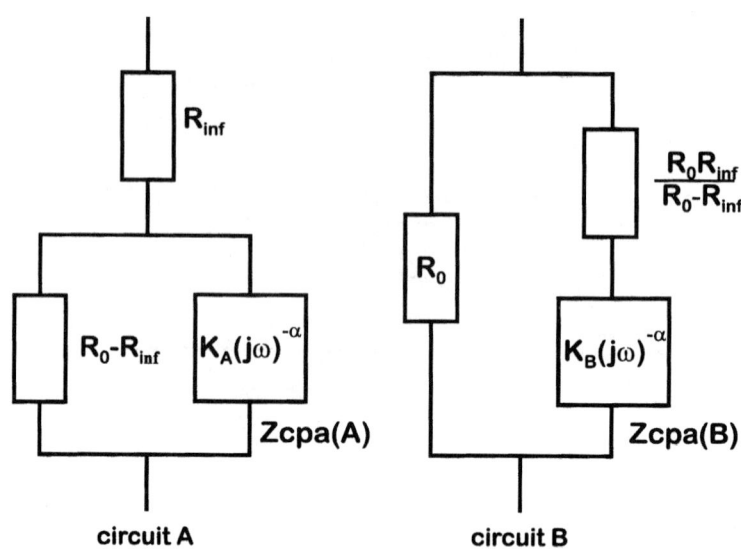

FIGURE 2. Equivalent circuits A and B to describe the Cole equation.

$$Z_{CPA} = K(j\omega)^{-\alpha} \tag{6}$$

$$Z_{CPA} = R_1(j\omega T)^{-\alpha} \tag{7}$$

$$Z_{CPA} = (j\omega C_{eff})^{-\alpha} \tag{8}$$

where $K = R_1 T^{-\alpha} = C_{eff}^{-\alpha}$.

K and R_1 tend to be used in more empirical approaches where no detailed physical significance is attributed to Z_{CPA}. Some researchers prefer the use of R_1 to K because the former has units of Ω, whereas the latter has units of $\Omega s^{-\alpha}$.[13] C_{eff} tends to be preferred by researchers who wish to derive a simple capacitance value from the experimental data and compare this with the prediction from their theoretical model of the system, which generally does not account for the nonideal behavior of the "capacitance". However, it must be pointed out that a Z_{CPA} impedance cannot be accurately represented by a simple capacitor and that C_{eff} is only the "effective capacitance" at $\omega = 1$. The magnitude of the measured value of capacitance C of the system will vary significantly with frequency (if $\alpha \neq 1$) such that [using $1/\omega C = |Z_{CPA}| = K(\omega)^{-\alpha}$]

$$C = 1/K\omega^{-(1-\alpha)}. \tag{9}$$

A further problem arises when Z_{CPA} is arbitrarily subdivided into either its series or parallel equivalent resistance and capacitance. Using the equation $j^{-\alpha} = \exp(-j\alpha\pi/2) = \cos(\alpha\pi/2) - j\sin(\alpha\pi/2)$, Z_{CPA} can be rewritten in terms of its series components:

$$Z_{CPA} = R_i - jX_i \tag{10}$$

$$R_i = K\omega^{-\alpha}\cos(\alpha\pi/2) \tag{11}$$

$$X_i = -K\omega^{-\alpha}\sin(\alpha\pi/2) \tag{12}$$

$$C_i = (1/K)\omega^{\alpha-1}\operatorname{cosec}(\alpha\pi/2). \tag{13}$$

The phase angle ϕ of the impedance is given by

$$\phi = \tan^{-1}(X_i/R_i) = -\alpha\pi/2 \text{ rad}. \tag{14}$$

Use of the Cole equation generally evokes the concept of a "distribution of relaxation times".[14] If an impedance cannot be characterized by a simple time constant, it can be thought of as being composed of a series of time constants with a particular statistical distribution. Such a probability distribution is often termed a "distribution of relaxation times". In such an approach, T (where $T = 1/\omega_0$) is considered to be the average relaxation time and α is a distribution parameter related to the width of the particular distribution. However, the mere possibility of such a description does not in itself prove the physical existence of a particular distribution of relaxation times. Cole and Cole[14] therefore concluded that, "in the absence of any satisfactory explanation of these features, the distribution is nothing more than a means of modeling the experimental data".

The graphical presentation of data is often very confusing as the electrical properties of biological tissue can be presented in several different plots. In a complex impedance plot, such as that shown in FIGURE 1, the negative equivalent series reactance, $-X_s$, is plotted against the equivalent series resistance, R_s, over a range of frequencies. As biological tissues, including the skin, are capacitive in nature, it is convenient to plot such data in the first quadrant of the complex impedance plane. Complex impedance plots are often referred to by a variety of names, such as "Argand diagram", "Nyquist plot", and "Cole-Cole plot". A plot of a complex number using real and imaginary axes is termed an Argand diagram, an expression sometimes used to describe the complex impedance plot in FIGURE 1. A term widely used to describe complex plane plots is the Nyquist diagram. MacDonald and Johnson[15] claim that this term is a misnomer in the present context as it traditionally refers to transfer function (three- or four-terminal) response, while conventional complex plane plots involve only two-terminal input immittances. A Cole-Cole plot originated from Cole and Cole's pioneering work[14] on the complex permittivities of various materials. They obtained semicircular arcs whose centers lie below the real axis, similar to that shown in the complex impedance plane. Since then, the term Cole-Cole is used indiscriminately to describe any complex impedance plot regardless of the form of the locus.[16]

It must be appreciated that simply choosing the form of plot on which to present the experimental data can in itself influence the subsequent description, modeling, and interpretation of the observed electrical behavior.[16] A Bode plot, which is a plot of the logarithm of the modulus of the measured impedance against the logarithm of frequency, will highlight the frequency dependence of the Z_{CPA} impedance (the $\omega^{-\alpha}$ term in equation 2), and terms such as "frequency-dependent capacitance" and "pseudocapacitance" have been used in the literature. The complex impedance plot of the same Z_{CPA} impedance emphasizes the phase angle (the $j^{-\alpha}$ term in equation 2), and terms such as "constant phase angle" impedance and "constant phase element" are used.

Although the above equivalent circuit model (FIGURE 2A) has been derived empirically, the parameters R_∞, R_p, α, and K can be attributed some physical significance. For example, the sum of the impedances of the leads, the gel pad, the conductive underlying tissues (dermis and subcutaneous layer), and the electrode-gel interface are represented by the high-frequency resistance R_∞.

The value of R_p is closely associated with the flow of ionic current and hence with the passive ion permeability of the skin.[1,3] R_p is the parameter most often used in transdermal drug delivery to evaluate the effects of hydration, passive diffusion, and iontophoresis on the skin. When comparing the R_p values of hydrated skin and iontophoresed skin, it was found that the iontophoresed skin had much lower R_p values, indicating that iontophoretically induced charge had increased the permeability of skin to passive ion transport.[1,3] R_p depends on inter- and intrahuman variabilities such as the presence and activity of sweat glands.[10] It depends further on psychological events; on the thickness, permeability, and integrity of the epidermis; on the electrode application time; and on the composition of the electrode gel, drug, or bathing solution.[10]

The fractional power α of the pseudocapacitive impedance is a measure of the deviation from pure capacitive behavior. If the epidermal layer behaved as a simple capacitance, α would equal unity. Salter[13] related the fractional power α to the hydration of the stratum corneum.

Very little of the published research has involved monitoring changes in the fractional power α during *in vivo* drug diffusion and iontophoresis. In reference 6, when observing the effects of different application times for the local anesthetic amethocaine as compared to a placebo, we found significantly smaller values of α at all drug-treated sites as compared to placebo-treated areas. In the latter cases, the observed decrease in α with time was thought to be due to increased skin hydration as a result of the aqueous placebo gel. In the former cases, the more marked decrease in α may additionally reflect a change in the structure of the epidermal layer due to the diffusion of drug into the skin. Kontturi *et al.*,[5] presumably noting the similarities between the electrical properties of the skin and those of the electrode-electrolyte interface, suggested that the value of α is related to the fractal dimension of the skin's surface and that it can be considered as a measure of the surface roughness of the skin. Unfortunately, little information was given on this intriguing concept.

K is a measure of the magnitude of the high-frequency gel-skin interface impedance. As this impedance is largely capacitive, it depends on the area of the gelled portion of the skin, on the thickness and permittivities of the epidermal and gel layers, on the quality of contact between the gel and the skin surface, and on the physical condition of the epidermis.[17] The capacitive properties have been used to study the integrity of the skin. For example, in experiments involving heating of the skin,[7,8] the capacitance was found to increase with increasing temperature. At temperatures beyond the phase transition of the stratum corneum lipids (60 °C), Oh *et al.*[8] reported that the total impedance became independent of the frequency (i.e., purely resistive), suggesting that the capacitive properties of the barrier had been lost.

IMPEDANCE TECHNIQUE

The ac impedance can be determined in two ways: (i) the injection of a constant current and the measurement of the voltage dropped across the skin and (ii) the application of a constant voltage and the measurement of the resulting current through the skin. As the electrode-skin interface impedance may vary greatly, the current magnitude in the latter case cannot be known a priori. Undesired effects such as pain or burns to the skin may occur when excessive current is applied, especially at low frequencies. We therefore recommend the injection of a controlled current and measurement of the resulting voltage for the study of the electrode-skin interface. In electrical impedance spectroscopy, very small current amplitudes of less than 10 μA should be used to avoid nonlinearity of the skin impedance.[18] The major source of nonlinear behavior is the skin's parallel resistance, which affects the overall skin impedance, especially at low frequency.[19]

In the past, nearly all impedance measurements carried out in the field of transdermal drug delivery were based on a four-electrode or two-electrode configuration (FIGURE 3). Unfortunately, both of these configurations are unsuitable for measurement of the impedance of the electrode-skin interface at a single skin site. In the two-electrode setup, both the sum of the two electrode-skin impedances and the tissue impedance between the electrodes are measured.[20–22] The general assumption that the tissue impedance is negligibly small compared to the skin impedances is not always valid, especially in the case of iontophoresis since the applied current drastically decreases the skin impedances below the electrodes, making them comparable to that of the tissue. Additionally, the impedance at each skin site may have different values due to intrahuman variations, such as the varying presence and activity of sweat glands, or due to differences in the measuring electrodes. Summing together the impedances of both skin sites can mask subtle changes occurring at one or the other site.

When the measurement of deep body tissue alone is required, the electrode-skin interface impedances can be eliminated, at least in theory, using a "four-electrode" technique.[20,22] Two independent pairs of electrodes are necessary for the current injection and the voltage measurements. Such a technique is obviously not appropriate for the accurate monitoring of the effects of transdermal drug delivery at a single skin site.

We have suggested that the study of the effects of transdermal drug delivery on the electrical properties of the skin treatment site is best carried out by only investigating the properties of the electrode-skin interface in question, without the contributions of the

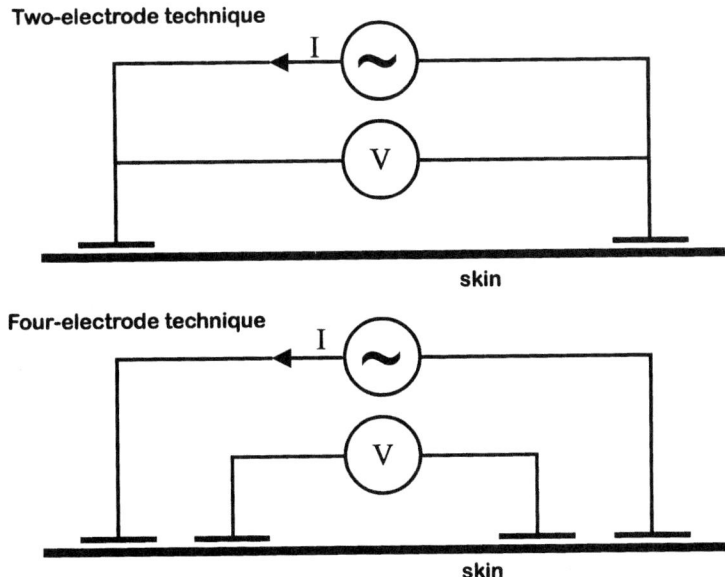

FIGURE 3. Two- and four-electrode configurations.

internal tissues and any other electrode-skin interface. A "three-electrode" technique[23] as shown in FIGURE 4 is therefore used. An alternating current is injected through the "test" electrode site and an "indifferent" electrode is used to complete the current loop. The potential V_A immediately beneath the electrode-skin interface under test is sensed by a third electrode, termed the "sensing" electrode, located on the skin surface directly next to the test electrode. The input potential ΔV to the voltmeter can be calculated by

$$\Delta V = V_A + V_B \tag{15}$$

$$\Delta V = I_A Z_A + I_B Z_B \tag{16}$$

$$I = I_A + I_B \text{ with } I_B \text{ negligibly small.} \tag{17}$$

If the voltmeter consists of an electronic instrumentation amplifier with an extremely high input impedance, then the current I_B flowing through the instrumentation amplifier and the skin site below the sensing electrode is negligibly small. Therefore, only a negligibly small voltage V_B develops below the sensing electrode, and the voltage difference ΔV is thus equal to the voltage drop V_A generated across the electrode-skin interface under test. The electrode-skin interface impedance is obtained by dividing the measured voltage drop ΔV by the applied current I.

TIME DEPENDENCE AND ASSOCIATED PROBLEMS

The application of gels and electrode solutions generally causes the skin's parallel resistance to decrease with time in a pseudoexponential manner as the ions in the gel grad-

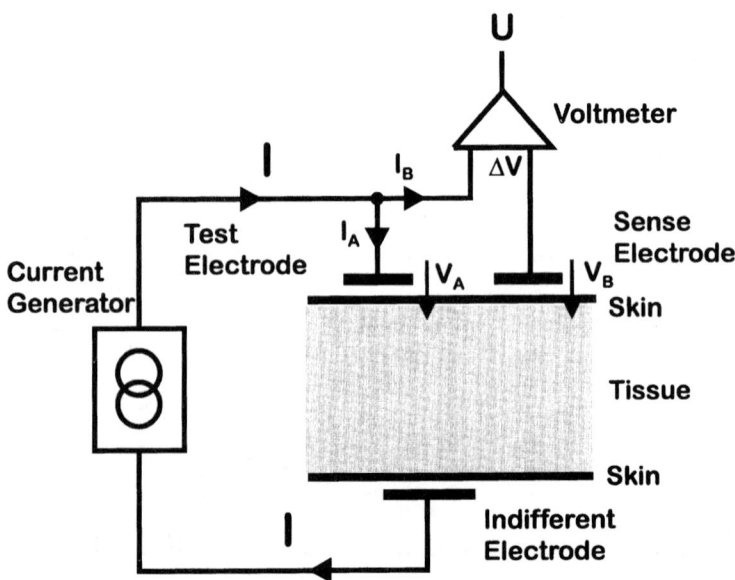

FIGURE 4. Three-electrode configuration.

ually diffuse through the skin and make it more conductive. The time constant for this decay is inversely proportional to the concentration and ionic strength of the gel.[4,8]

On occasions, when cold gel is first applied to a skin site, the measured value of the parallel resistance is observed to initially increase.[24] This is thought to be due to the cold gel causing the sweat pores to contract or at least reduce their activity. Once the gel has warmed up, the value of R_p is observed to decrease pseudoexponentially as the electrolyte ions diffuse through the epidermal layer. It is therefore important to note that the temperature of the applied gel/medication can have a significant effect on one's experimental results and should be monitored or controlled. It should also be noted that, when comparing several skin sites, the timing and ordering of experiments after disrobing of the treatment area may be of great importance due to the gradual cooling down of the skin sites and the resultant increase in their impedances.

Although the parallel capacitance varies with gel concentration and composition, it does not exhibit as strong a time dependence.[10] Psychophysiological studies in which a subject was instructed to induce a stressful state for 10 minutes by reliving a previous free-fall experience and to relax afterwards have shown that stress can cause the skin's parallel resistance to decrease rapidly and was attributed to an increased sweat gland activity.[25]

A frequency range between 1 Hz and 2 kHz is often used by us as it has been found to be sufficient for skin impedance measurements while avoiding the low-frequency problems that can occur. This range encompasses a major portion of the impedance arc since the "characteristic frequency" f_0, at which the reactive component is maximal, tends to be around 10 Hz to 100 Hz for human skin.[10] For the determination of the impedance spectrum, only a small number of frequencies, equally distributed across the frequency range, need to be used to enable the rapid monitoring of the electrical properties of the skin in situations where the impedance is changing rapidly with time. For example, over the first minute of data acquisition, the skin impedance will normally be expected to decrease rapidly with time. It is therefore desirable to measure fewer frequency points per spectrum and to decrease the time interval between spectra in order to follow the variation in the skin during this initial period. Later, the impedance tends to decrease less with time, and hence spectra involving more frequency points are feasible and longer intermeasurement intervals are appropriate.

Under certain conditions, especially at low frequencies, the epidermal ac impedance locus has been observed to deviate from the expected depressed semicircular impedance arc. Given that R_p dominates the impedance at low frequencies and that the measurement of each low-frequency point can take several minutes, we[26] have pointed out that the observed distortions are due to time-dependent changes in the skin's parallel resistance. The system under investigation is thus in a dynamic state and can change too rapidly for the recording device. FIGURE 5 shows a complex impedance plot of a subject's skin impedance (subject is relaxing) measured using a PALS T.E.N.S. hydrogel electrode[11] and illustrates how the measured impedance is often found to be elongated (in this case) at the low-frequency end. As the measurement frequency is decreased, the value of R_p, which is increasing with time, causes the observed distortion. The arc would have been truncated if the skin's parallel resistance had been decreasing with time. Kalia and Guy[4] have also observed this behavior. It is important to recognize that such distorted arcs are a result of artifacts and efforts similar to those outlined above should be made to minimize the effects of time-dependent variations in skin impedance.

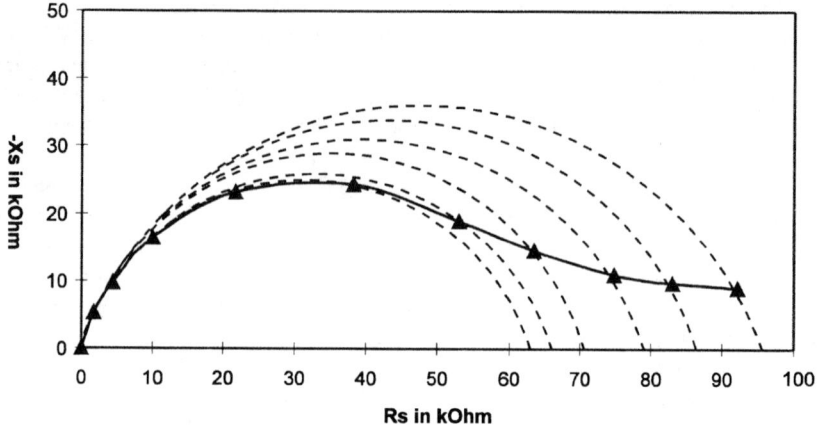

FIGURE 5. Complex impedance plot using a PALS T.E.N.S. hydrogel electrode illustrating the time-dependency changes in the skin's parallel resistance.

The dependence of skin impedance on a large number of time-dependent factors often makes it difficult to compare a set of measurements carried out sequentially and draw meaningful conclusions. *In vivo* measurements are greatly affected by time-dependent factors such as the degree of hydration, sweat gland activity, and emotional state and alertness of the subject. Contact problems or differing contact pressures may also affect the measurements. Unfortunately, all these factors have a major impact on the measured data. If a set of experiments are required to investigate the effect of a certain parameter of interest (e.g., drug concentration) on a measured skin impedance, then the ordering of the experiments and the experimental protocol are very important as time-dependent factors will distort the results.

In order to minimize the adverse effects of at least some of these extraneous time-dependent variables, it would be most advantageous to carry out comparisons in parallel under identical conditions.

THE NIBEC RESEARCH SYSTEM

The above requirements can be met, in part at least, by the use of a multichannel impedance analyzer, enabling the simultaneous *in vivo* comparison of several skin sites under a range of conditions. Such a device was developed at the Northern Ireland Bio-Engineering Center (NIBEC) and was successfully employed for the *in vivo* assessment of biosignal monitoring electrodes[27] and for the *in vivo* ac impedance monitoring of percutaneous drug delivery.[6] It consists of four impedance meters, used on up to four skin sites, which calculate the complex ratio of the voltage developed across each treated skin site (three-electrode technique) and the current flowing through it (FIGURE 6). The system is fully programmable and allows the easy setting of acquisition parameters according to the

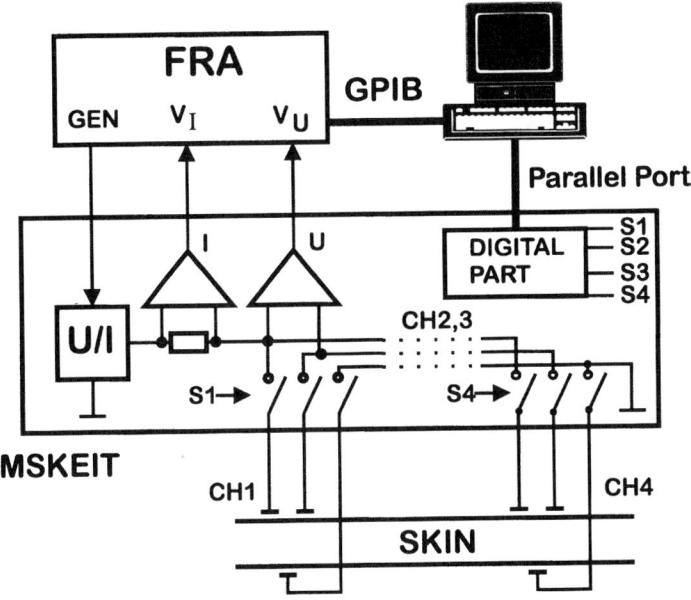

FIGURE 6. Multiskin electrical impedance analyzer (MSKEIT).

requirements of the particular experiment. The principal parameters involved are the number and values of frequencies used for a given spectrum, the measurement interval between the acquisition of spectra, the current amplitudes, and the number of parallel channels used. With the developed software, it is possible to program a series of time segments with combinations of the above-mentioned parameters. For example, over the first minute of data acquisition, the skin impedance will normally be expected to decrease rapidly with time. It is therefore desirable to measure fewer frequency points per spectrum and to decrease the time interval between spectra in order to follow the rate of variation in the skin in this initial period.

The impedance of the skin is known to vary greatly from subject to subject and from body site to body site. These variations are largely due to differences in the skin's parallel resistance.[10] The skin's resistance is dependent on the presence and activity of sweat glands and on the presence of other appendageal pathways. The density of sweat glands varies over the body surface, with estimated values of 370 per cm^2 on the palms and soles and approximately 160 per cm^2 on the forearm.[28] The stratum corneum thickness can vary greatly for different body sites. Chien[29] reported that the stratum corneum can be as thick as 400 to 600 μm in the palm and plantar areas and as little as 10 to 20 μm on the back, legs, and abdomen. Therefore, when comparing different gels, etc., experiments should be carried out simultaneously with the treated skin sites in close vicinity of each other to minimize as far as possible variations in impedance due to differences in the skin site. This would enable the researcher to better isolate parameters of interest and thus enable more meaningful assessment and comparisons.

NOVEL ELECTRODE DESIGN

When applying a drug to the skin, it is important to provide a reservoir for the formulation that incorporates an electrode system enabling the monitoring of the underlying skin-electrode impedance while ensuring unhindered passage of the drug. As pointed out above, it is also important to test differing formulations, etc., on adjacent skin sites to minimize effects due to variations in the thickness and structure of the skin.

At the NIBEC, these problems have been addressed by the use of a novel electrode template (FIGURE 7). For reported passive drug delivery experiments,[6] a placebo and three active gels were applied to adjacent skin sites and tested by means of a template with four wells. The wells were formed by cutting 2×2-cm-square apertures out of a 1.6-mm-thick sheet of adhesive foam (3M 9751). A nylon mesh coated with silver was attached to the adhesive side of the template across each aperture to assure direct electrical contact with the skin. Before the template was applied to the subject's skin, the mesh was fed through to the top of the foam template and aluminum foil was folded around the exposed mesh to provide a "tab" contact for connection to the impedance monitor system. The use of the mesh electrodes allowed the drug to flow through each electrode while enabling the direct monitoring of the resultant change in the electrical properties of the underlying epidermis.

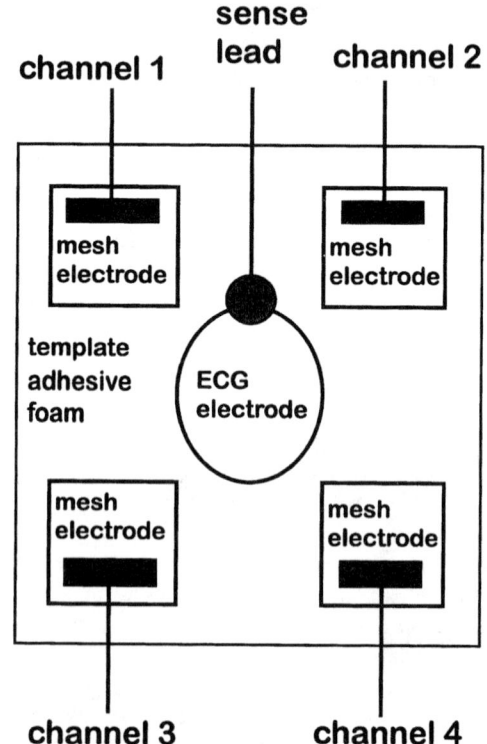

FIGURE 7. Multichannel electrode template.

The four-electrode template was attached to the front, right upper leg of the subject. A standard ECG electrode (Medicotest T-00-S) centered between the four mesh electrodes and applied through a fifth aperture, cut centrally in the foam template, served as a reference electrode to the four skin sites under test. A second standard ECG electrode, connected to the back of the thigh, acted as the indifferent electrode in the "three-electrode technique" employed.

BODY-WORN DEVICE

The above system is well suited as a laboratory or clinical research tool. The use of a novel electrode system design, a three-electrode technique, multifrequency measurement, and multichannel recording all help to remove or minimize many of the problems encountered in EIS studies of the skin. However, problems still do remain and experiments need to be carefully controlled and must be repeated on a range of subjects to clearly establish the relative performances of differing electrodes, formulations, etc.

The situation is therefore even more difficult when one endeavors to incorporate impedance measurements into a body-worn device with the aim of monitoring such things as drug delivery rate, presence of skin irritation, etc.

It would be ideal if one could simply measure the magnitude or phase angle of the skin site impedance at a certain frequency and have value ranges clearly and unequivocally linked to, for example, acceptable and unacceptable performances. Such a system could then be used to activate an alarm, when necessary, or used as part of a feedback mechanism to ensure acceptable long-term performance. However, the impedance of the skin at one frequency reflects the combined effects of several underlying processes and generally cannot be related to the process that one wishes to study. If one uses the equivalent circuit model of FIGURE 2A or the Cole equation (1), four parameters are needed to fully characterize the electrode-skin impedance and hence a minimum of three frequency points must be measured. If one carries out extensive testing, one may be able to show that a monofrequency point, suitably chosen, can act as a "rule of thumb". However, the extensive range in intra- and intersubject impedances would tend to make such an approach unreliable and, when used to control a body-worn device such as a transdermal drug delivery unit, even dangerous. There is a distinct possibility that an extraneous factor, such as a rare or ignored skin condition, or the effect of an uncommon combination of factors could lead to the drawing of erroneous conclusions.

The measurement of two frequency points, if properly chosen, can lead to more meaningful monitoring. For example, if both impedance measurements are made at high frequencies, relatively sound conclusions can be drawn on the variations of R_∞, K, and α (using the equivalent circuit in FIGURE 2A) and on the underlying processes they are thought to represent. Hence, for example, skin integrity and moisturization can be relatively well studied in this way. On the other hand, if impedance measurements are made at both the high- and low-frequency end of the impedance arc shown in FIGURE 1 (assuming of course that one knows the values of frequency required), the diameter of the arc and hence R_p can be derived and the underlying process it is thought to represent can be monitored.

An approach related to the above has been used by Ollmar and colleagues,[30] who have used ratios of the magnitudes and phase angles as well as ratios of the real and imaginary parts of the impedance at two different frequencies. The studies of the magnitudes and relative changes in these indices have enabled Ollmar and his colleagues to successfully quantify and classify a range of different skin conditions.

Occasionally, the presence within a given measurement frequency range of an additional "dispersion" or impedance arc, due to some extraneous process, has been observed and this can adversely affect the validity of models or ratios used. It is therefore suggested that more than two frequencies should be used to monitor the skin's impedance and that some feedback is obtained on the quality of fit between the measured data and the equivalent circuit/mathematical model used. This will also help to detect unforeseen changes in the system due, for example, to low-frequency time-dependent distortion of the impedance locus (see FIGURE 5).

As previously mentioned, the wide range of intra- and intersubject skin impedance generally rules out the use of absolute measurements in skin monitoring, even when a multifrequency approach is employed. Monitoring relative changes in a parameter appears to hold some promise of success. The value of a monitored parameter or a given impedance value at a given skin site can be compared either to its value at a given moment in time, say at the beginning of the experiment, or to the value measured at another adjacent reference skin site. To illustrate some of the possibilities, we carried out the experiments detailed in the following section.

METHODS

The impedance properties of healthy skin in a human volunteer were investigated during percutaneous local anesthesia in order to establish the feasibility of using ac impedance techniques to study *in vivo* the effects of transdermal delivery of medication. Percutaneous local anesthesia occurs when a local anesthetic agent penetrates the stratum corneum and desensitizes the underlying nociceptors.

A placebo and three active amethocaine gels were applied to adjacent skin sites on the front of the left thigh of a 32-year-old male by means of a four-well (each well 2 cm × 2 cm) adhesive foam template (3M 9751), as previously described. The subject remained seated and relaxed during the experiment. An *in vivo* four-channel impedance analyzer developed at the NIBEC was used in conjunction with a Solartron 1260 frequency response analyzer and a custom-designed data-acquisition software to monitor the impedances of the four sites simultaneously. A current of 1 μA_{rms} was used. Only a relatively small number of frequencies (f = 2000 Hz, 300 Hz, 44 Hz, 6 Hz, 1 Hz) were used to enable rapid monitoring of the electrical properties of the skin in a situation where the impedance was likely to initially change rapidly with time, thus distorting the lower frequency data. The experiment was run for 50 minutes. The channels of the device were allocated as follows—channel 1: placebo; channel 2: 1% amethocaine; channel 3: 2% amethocaine; channel 4: 4% amethocaine.

RESULTS AND DISCUSSION

There were distinct differences between the electrical properties of the skin sites treated with amethocaine (especially for the higher concentrations) and the site treated with placebo. The values of R_p, K, and α were generally lowest for the skin site with the highest drug concentration, especially for application times longer than around 10 minutes, indicating a higher rate of drug diffusion through the stratum corneum. FIGURE 8 displays a typical set of results. Only the R_p results are reproduced in this paper.

Somewhat surprisingly, in the experimental results presented, the skin sites treated with 2% and 4% gels had very much higher initial R_p values (around 600 kOhm) compared to those measured at the other sites (around 300 kOhm). This was probably due, however, to a range of "background" factors, including concentration-related variations in the gel consistency, variations in the skin site, order of gelling, etc. After approximately 10 minutes, R_p decreased pseudoexponentially for the drug-treated sites over the observation period, indicating that the drug amethocaine was gradually diffusing into the skin. The skin site with the highest amethocaine concentration experienced a faster decrease in R_p values, reaching lower values than the other sites.

Similar distortions due to "background" factors were also observed for plots of K and α in this series of experiments and also in other unreported experimental data. Obviously, these background variations make meaningful comparisons of drug-treated site impedances something of an art based on the researcher's intuition and previous experience of similar experiments. Thus, it is not an approach particularly well suited to the automated monitoring of drug-treated sites.

In an effort to correct for these distortions, it was decided to normalize the calculated data. Several options are possible. In FIGURE 9, the R_p values presented in FIGURE 8 have been normalized by dividing the data points on each curve by the maximum value of R_p reached by that curve. The results now show the relative order of R_p value magnitudes that the researchers have learned from prior experience. The placebo-treated site changes the least with time, while R_p values decrease progressively more for higher amethocaine concentrations.

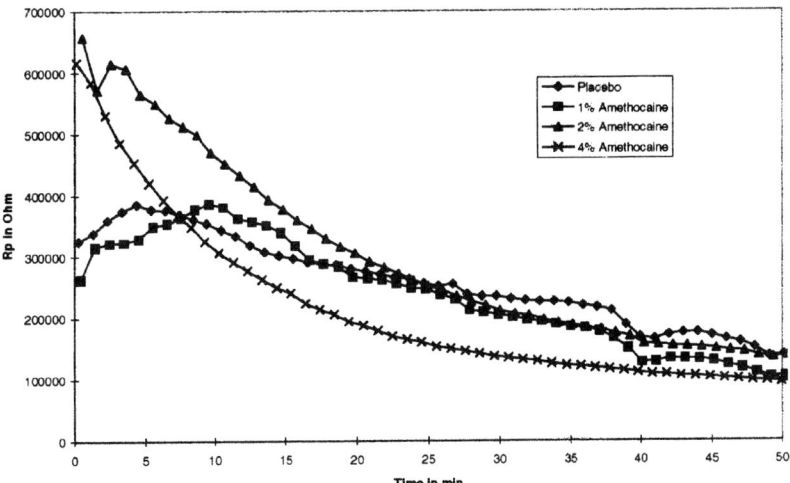

FIGURE 8. Calculated values of the skin's parallel resistance, R_p, plotted against time following application of amethocaine (1%, 2%, and 4%) and placebo.

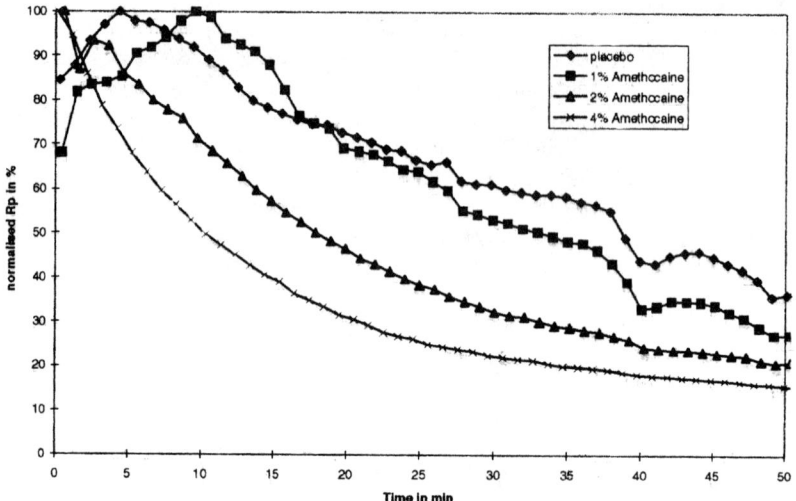

FIGURE 9. Normalized values of the skin's parallel resistance, R_p, plotted against time following application of amethocaine (1%, 2%, and 4%) and placebo.

CONCLUSIONS

Results indicate that ac impedance techniques are potentially useful in the *in vivo* investigation of percutaneous drug delivery. However, as the electrical properties of skin are dependent on a wide range of parameters, the task is difficult. In an effort to minimize several potential problem sources,[31] we have already developed a multichannel analyzer, an electrode template, a mesh electrode, and a rigorous experimental protocol. Notwithstanding these improvements, intersite differences, for example, still make meaningful comparison of treatment site impedances difficult, certainly not suitable for use in an automated skin monitoring system.

The normalization of calculated data has been shown to be a further step in the right direction. The problem is by no means solved, though, and further work is required before EIS can be used reliably in such applications. It is hoped that it will be eventually possible to identify one or several impedance-related parameters that, when suitably calculated from readily detectable data, will enable the monitoring of important processes, such as drug delivery or tissue injury, with sufficient accuracy to prove clinically useful.

REFERENCES

1. BURNETTE, R. R. & T. M. BAGNIEFSKI. 1988. Influence of constant current iontophoresis on the impedance and passive Na^+ permeability of excised nude mouse skin. J. Pharm. Sci. **77**(no. 6): 492–497.
2. BURNETTE, R. R. & B. ONGPIPATTANAKUL. 1987. Characterization of pore transport properties and tissue alteration of excised human skin during iontophoresis. J. Pharm. Sci. **76**: 765–773.
3. FOLEY, D., J. CORISH & O. I. CORRIGAN. 1992. Iontophoretic delivery of drugs through membranes including human stratum corneum. Solid State Ionics **53**: 184–196.

4. KALIA, Y. N. & R. H. GUY. 1995. Interaction between penetration enhancers and iontophoresis: effect on human skin impedance *in vivo*. J. Controlled Release **44**: 33–42.
5. KONTTURI, K. *et al*. 1993. Electrochemical characterization of human skin by impedance spectroscopy: the effect of penetration enhancers. Pharm. Res. **10**(no. 3): 381–385.
6. MCADAMS, E. T. *et al*. 1995. *In vivo* impedance monitoring of percutaneous drug delivery. *In* Proceedings of the Ninth International Conference on Electrical Bio-Impedance, Heidelberg, p. 344–347.
7. NOLAN, L. M. A., J. CORISH & O. I. CORRIGAN. 1993. Electrical properties of human stratum corneum and transdermal drug transport. J. Chem. Soc. Faraday Trans. **15**: 2839–2845.
8. OH, S. Y. *et al*. 1993. Effect of current, ionic strength, and temperature on the electrical properties of skin. J. Controlled Release **27**: 115–125.
9. EDELBERG, R. 1971. Electrical properties of the skin. *In* A Treatise of the Skin. Wiley. New York.
10. MCADAMS, E. T. & J. JOSSINET. 1991. The importance of electrode-skin impedance in high resolution electrocardiography. Automedica **13**: 187–208.
11. COLE, K. S. 1940. Permeability and impermeability of cell membranes for ions. Cold Spring Harbor Symp. Quant. Biol. **8**: 110–112.
12. MCADAMS, E. T., J. JOSSINET & A. LACKERMEIER. 1995. Modelling the "constant phase angle" behavior of biological tissues: potential pitfalls. Innov. Technol. Biol. Med. **16**(6): 662–669.
13. SALTER, D. C. 1981. A study of some electrical properties of normal and pathological skin *in vivo*. Ph.D. thesis, University of Oxford, United Kingdom.
14. COLE, K. S. & R. H. COLE. 1941. Dispersion and absorption in dielectrics. I. Alternating characteristics. J. Chem. Phys. **9**: 341–351.
15. MACDONALD, J. R. & W. B. JOHNSON. 1987. Impedance Spectroscopy: Emphasizing Solid Materials and Systems. Wiley. New York.
16. MCADAMS, E. T. & J. JOSSINET. 1995. Tissue impedance: a historical overview. Physiol. Meas. **16**: A1–A13.
17. MCADAMS, E. T., J. JOSSINET & A. LACKERMEIER. 1996. Factors affecting the electrode-gel-skin interface impedance in electrical impedance tomography. Med. Biol. Eng. Comput. **34**: 397–408.
18. LACKERMEIER, A. *et al*. 1996. Non-linearity in the skin's a.c. impedance. *In* Eighteenth Annual Conf. on IEEE Eng. in Med. and Biol. Soc., Amsterdam (paper no. 6.7.1–7).
19. MCADAMS, E. T. *et al*. 1995. The linear and nonlinear electrical properties of the electrode-electrolyte interface. Biosens. Bioelectronics **10**: 67–74.
20. SALTER, D. C. 1979. Quantifying skin disease and healing *in vivo* using electrical impedance measurements. *In* Non-invasive Physiological Measurements. Volume 1, p. 21–64. Academic Press. New York/London.
21. TRAEGER, R. T. 1966. Physical Functions of the Skin. Academic Press. New York/London.
22. YAMAMOTO, Y. 1994. Measurement and analysis of skin electrical impedance. Acta Dermato-Venereol. **S185**(SI5): 34–38.
23. BARNETT, A. 1938. The phase angle of normal human skin. J. Physiol. **93**: 349–366.
24. ROSELL, J. *et al*. 1988. Skin impedance from 1 Hz to 1 MHz. IEEE Trans. Biomed. Eng. **35**: 649–651.
25. MCADAMS, E. T., A. LACKERMEIER & J. JOSSINET. 1994. A.C. impedance of the hydrogel-skin interface. *In* Sixteenth Annual Conf. on IEEE Eng. in Med. and Biol. Soc., Baltimore, p. 870–871.
26. MCADAMS, E.T. *et al*. 1993. Epidermal ac impedance: low frequency distortion. *In* Fifteenth Annual Conf. on IEEE Eng. in Med. and Biol. Soc., San Diego, p. 1497–1498.
27. MCADAMS, E. T. *et al*. 1993. *In vivo* assessment of ECG electrodes. *In* Second European Conference on Engineering and Medicine, Stuttgart, p. 391–392.
28. REILLY, J. P. 1992. Electrical Stimulation and Electropathology. Cambridge University Press. London/New York.
29. CHIEN, Y. W. 1982. Transdermal controlled-release drug administration. *In* Novel Drug Delivery Systems, p. 149. Dekker. New York.
30. OLLMAR, S. & L. EMTESTAM. 1992. Electrical impedance applied to non-invasive detection of irritation in skin. Contact Dermatitis **27**: 37–42.
31. MCADAMS, E. T. & J. JOSSINET. 1996. Problems in equivalent circuit modelling of the electrical properties of biological tissues. Bioelectrochem. Bioenerg. **40**: 147–152.

On Assessment of Skin Reactivity Using Electrical Impedance[a]

MIRUNA NYRÉN, LENA HAGSTRÖMER, AND LENNART EMTESTAM[b]

Department of Dermatology and Venereology, Karolinska Institute, Huddinge University Hospital, S-141 86 Huddinge, Sweden

ABSTRACT: Pathophysiological events in biological tissue are characterized by a shift in electrical impedance spectra of the tissue under study. In this paper, techniques based on electrical impedance are reviewed with emphasis on their possible role in evaluating the skin reactivity of an individual, including results from impedance measurement studies on patients with allergic contact reactions, wheals, tuberculin tests, and irritant contact reactions and on an appropriate number of controls. The results show that, compared to relevant controls, at different types of experimental cutaneous reactions, both of allergic and irritant type, statistically significant changes of the impedance parameters have been detected. Each reaction type had a specific impedance index pattern. Data up to now indicate that the improved impedance technique offers not only a noninvasive alternative for characterization and perhaps differentiation between the skin responses induced by either an allergen or an irritant, but also a capability to distinguish responses induced by chemically different irritants.

INTRODUCTION

Pathophysiological events in biological tissue are related to changes of the electrical impedance of the tissue.[1] Technology based on electrical impedance for medical purposes has existed since the early 1920s, but it is not until recently, through technical development, that research groups have developed more or less successful instruments for a variety of clinical applications other than skin, such as cardiopulmonary tomography[2,3] and the detection of dental decay.[4] Several techniques for the skin have been proposed.[5–12] Methods for investigating allergies and the immune status of an individual exist. For the skin, the T-cell specific mediated response of delayed type IV in contact allergic reactions, that is, against nickel salts, is the most widely used model both *in vivo* and *in vitro*. The tuberculin skin reaction is also of the delayed type. Finally, the immediate wheal type I reaction may often be used in diagnosing allergy. In experimental work, different chemicals induce irritant contact reactions. The aim of this report is to review the use of electrical impedance as a noninvasive tool for evaluating skin reactivity, both of immunologic and nonimmunologic types. References to other noninvasive techniques in relation to skin impedance measurements are found elsewhere.[13]

---

[a]This study was supported by grants from the Swedish Council for Work Life Research, the Swedish Society of Medicine, the Karolinska Institute, the Edvard Welander Foundation, the Finsen Foundation, and the Tore Nilson Foundation for Medical Research.
[b]To whom all correspondence should be addressed.

ELECTRICAL IMPEDANCE TECHNIQUES

Biologic tissue has both resistive and reactive electrical properties. The impedance will be frequency-dependent, and an impedance spectrum, that is, the magnitude and phase for a number of frequencies, will be represented by a characteristic graph in the complex number space.[1]

The first studies on skin electrical impedance were published around 1920. Already by then, it was known that the skin constituted the major barrier to the passage of electrical current through the body. After that, many attempts to use impedance for assessment of skin have been published, but the studies undertaken have shown a wide variation in the sophistication of the equipment and techniques employed, in the objectives of the studies, and in the complexity of the models used to aid in the interpretation of data. The pioneering works of Salter,[5] Yamamoto,[6] and others[7–12] have added important insights in the field of skin bioimpedance, although limitation to one dispersion or one single frequency restricted the obtained information from the outermost part of the skin, the stratum corneum. A most promising instrument has recently been marketed, developed by Martinsen and Grimnes, using 88 Hz, which seems ideal for studies of the important hydration status of the stratum corneum, the outermost part of the skin (Sensoderm™ 970, Skinstrument AS, Sellebakk, Norway).

Over the last couple of years, we have been working with a multifrequency, depth-controlled impedance technique, originally invented by Stig Ollmar.[14] In our first trials, a provisional experimental setup was used, consisting of a number of standard laboratory instruments plus a dedicated driver box for the special probe. This first probe had a fixed geometry that determined the depth penetration.[12,15] This system was operated in a Faraday cage in order to avoid electromagnetic interference from sources in the surroundings. For analysis, a simple impedance index was used, defined as the quotient between the absolute values of the impedance at the frequencies of 20 kHz and 1 MHz. Results from studies with this simple early technique indicated that the initial and recovery phases of the irritant contact reaction induced by sodium lauryl sulfate were readily monitored.[16] The impedance technique was at least as sensitive as measurement of transepidermal water loss and the naked eye, perhaps even more sensitive since data also indicated that concentrations of the compound inducing subclinical reactions could be detected.[16] Daily measurements of the impedance index from the same skin site showed little day-to-day variations of the index. Significant differences in normalized skin impedance levels between six different anatomical regions were found.[15]

The initial promising results prompted the development of a computer-controlled prototype instrument followed by an updated and simplified version. Also, the simple impedance index was further developed since we were looking for practical ways to use more of the information inherent in the impedance spectra and to avoid the limits of electrical models widely used by other investigators.[5,6] In short, a set of four indices, representing changes with frequency along the four major aspects of electrical impedance in complex number space, were used:[17]

(1) magnitude index, MIX = $\mathrm{abs}(Z_{20\mathrm{kHz}})/\mathrm{abs}(Z_{500\mathrm{kHz}})$

(2) phase index, PIX = $\mathrm{arg}(Z_{20\mathrm{kHz}}) - \mathrm{arg}(Z_{500\mathrm{kHz}})$

(3) real part index, RIX = $\mathrm{Re}(Z_{20\mathrm{kHz}})/\mathrm{abs}(Z_{500\mathrm{kHz}})$

(4) imaginary part index, IMIX = $\text{Im}(Z_{20\text{kHz}})/\text{abs}(Z_{500\text{kHz}})$,

where $\text{abs}(Z_i)$ is the magnitude (modulus) of the complex electrical impedance at the frequency i, $\arg(Z_i)$ is the argument (phase angle) in degrees, $\text{Re}(Z_i)$ is the real part, and $\text{Im}(Z_i)$ is the imaginary part of the complex electrical impedance. The processing of the data and calculations of the indices were performed with a special software. The technical design allowed measurements from five different, stepwise inclusive skin depths, the deepest being approximately 2 mm. The instrument in its updated version now definitely seems suitable for noninvasive assessment of skin. Results on allergic and irritant contact reactions, wheals, and tuberculin tests, as well as some preliminary data on a large baseline impedance study, are discussed below.

IRRITANT CONTACT DERMATITIS

Irritant contact dermatitis accounts for the majority of industrial cases of hand eczema. The dermatitis is initiated as a direct chemical injury on the main skin barrier, the stratum corneum. Strong irritants elicit an acute reaction and weak irritants need prolonged exposure over weeks or years to cause eczema. There is a wide range of susceptibility between individuals, and those with dry skin or atopic dermatitis are especially vulnerable. In 40 healthy volunteers, we explored the use of measurements of impedance to discriminate between the effects of different irritant substances on the volar forearm skin as well as the relationship between impedance and histopathological change.[14,17] Three compounds with different chemical profiles were tested: sodium lauryl sulfate, benzalkonium chloride, and nonanoic acid. The concentrations were chosen to produce a response of a similar order as judged by visual scoring. Impedance measurements were performed and the above-mentioned four indices were calculated and statistically analyzed. The three irritants produced different skin effects, giving distinct impedance patterns (summarized in TABLE 1), which were also reflected in three different types of histopathological skin responses. The results suggested that the indices can be used to classify irritant contact reactions. In another study where 21 healthy subjects were patch-tested with mild and subthreshold doses (0.004%, 0.02%, 0.1%, and 0.5% for 24 h) of sodium lauryl sulfate, the impedance index patterns of our previous studies were confirmed in a larger material (Nicander and Ollmar,

TABLE 1. Summary of Electrical Impedance Measurements in Some Experimental Skin Reactions[a]

	MIX	PIX	RIX	IMIX
Nickel sulfate 0.1%	+		−	+
Sodium lauryl sulfate 0.5%	−	+		−
Nonanoic acid 40%	−			−
Benzalkonium chloride 0.5%		−	+	
Tuberculin (PPD) 2TU ic	+			+
Wheals		−		

[a]The table represents a summary of results from several uniquely designed studies. + and − represent skin responses (increase or decrease) as reflected in the four indices.

submitted). In addition, the previous assumption that the electrical impedance method is a sensitive technique for detection of macroscopically negative skin responses induced by sodium lauryl sulfate was confirmed. To see if the instrument could be used to discriminate individuals with different susceptibility to irritants, work is currently in progress comparing irritant reactivity in eczema patients with healthy controls.

ALLERGIC CONTACT DERMATITIS

The mechanism of allergic contact dermatitis is that of delayed (type IV) hypersensitivity. Previous contact is needed to induce allergy. All areas of the skin react to the allergen, and this reactivity is specific. Upon renewed contact with the sensitizer, specific migratory CD4+ T cells will proliferate in the skin and produce a cascade of inflammatory events in the exposed area. Interaction between T cells and an allergen–HLA class II antigen complex on Langerhans' cells initiates the response. Also, skin endothelial cells, keratinocytes, and cytokines participate in the regulation of the immune response. Only 2% of the infiltrating cells in allergic contact dermatitis seem antigen-specific. Since the end results of both allergic and irritant contact reactions are clinically and microscopically similar, it is important to select appropriate time intervals for making measurements. The most common cause for contact allergy is nickel, especially in women. In a pilot study on 8 nickel-allergic individuals, skin reactions were induced on the forearm by exposure to nickel sulfate in petrolatum in various concentrations.[18] The changes in impedance indices of the nickel reactions were found to follow a particular pattern (summarized in TABLE 1) that significantly diverged not only from controls, but also from the patterns obtained from irritant contact reactions as shown in our previous studies. The results support the notion that the impedance method might be used to characterize the allergic contact reaction and to differentiate between skin responses induced by allergens and irritants. However, this has to be confirmed in a larger study, which is in progress.

WHEAL FLARE REACTIONS

The immediate hypersensitivity reactions (type I) are characterized by vasodilatation and an outpouring of fluid from blood vessels. Such reactions can be induced directly by toxins and chemicals, but they are most commonly mediated by immunologic mechanisms: IgE antibodies attached to mast cells combine with antigens, leading to a liberation of mediators into the surrounding tissue. Histamine and leukotrienes induce the typical redness and swelling. In 10 allergic patients, on which prick tests of relevant antigens were performed on the volar forearm and compared to the controls, there were significant changes in the impedance parameters of the wheals, especially in the index related to the phase angle (TABLE 1).[19] The patterns of the statistically significant changes of the impedance indices differed from those obtained in contact skin reactions of both allergic and irritant types. Also, the results indicated that the allergic skin reactions of the immediate type could be characterized by the impedance technique, and the instrument is a candidate tool for evaluation of the efficacy of antihistamines. On the other hand, in a recent study by Magnusson and Koskinen[20] on topical application of capsaicin, which induced wheal-like lesions, the electrical impedance measurements did not correlate to clinical findings nor to laser Doppler flowmetry measurements.

TUBERCULIN TESTS

The tuberculin skin test (Mantoux test) is the traditional method to determine past or present infection with *M. tuberculosis*. Besides being a classic model for the cell-mediated immune system in humans, it is a guide for prognosis and a measure of delayed sensitivity in an individual. Tuberculin is a mixture of proteins (PPD) prepared from cultural extract of the tubercle bacilli.

In 16 tuberculin-positive individuals, PPD (2TU) was injected intracutaneously (ic), and the reactions were compared with irritant contact reactions induced by 2% sodium lauryl sulfate (SLS). PPD-negative medium ic and normal skin served as controls (Nyrén *et al.*, under preparation). The preliminary data show that the skin reactions induced by PPD created a pattern of the impedance indices in contrast to the pattern of the SLS reactions. Interestingly, the impedance pattern of the PPD reactions was similar to the one found in nickel allergic contact reactions (TABLE 1), another delayed cell-mediated immune response.

BASELINE ELECTRICAL IMPEDANCE

In a total of 131 healthy subjects divided into 4 groups according to sex and age, the impedance baseline values were measured in 10 different skin locations.[21] The result of the variance analysis from that study clearly demonstrates that, as for other noninvasive methods, it is necessary to carefully select the sites for controls as well as the actual test sites since, due to structural differences, the electrical impedance of skin varies significantly between different skin regions. Also, there are significant alterations in the impedance parameters related to age, but to a lesser extent between men and women.

CONCLUSIONS

The immune system defends the host against infectious and other agents that threaten it, and many skin reactions are good examples of immune mechanisms at work. At least in theory, by the use of sound noninvasive techniques, experimental skin studies would benefit from being performed in a relatively small material number of patients or study subjects in contrast to the ordinary techniques based on ocular inspection. However, before the technique based on electrical impedance could become more than just another potential candidate for noninvasive assessments, the solutions of some problems are necessary. At the moment, the typical experimental dermatologist may not even consider electrical impedance when selecting appropriate tools for his/her work. The interpretation of the large amount of data is complicated and perhaps difficult to comprehend by investigators with a limited knowledge in electrophysics, and pedagogic improvements of the software for processing the data are needed. Also, the use of artificial neural networks seems to increase the rational handling of data.[22] Our own recent results indicate that the data analysis could be automated and, at the same time, the diagnostic power of the impedance technique could be increased by the use of neural network methodology.[23] However, the main point remains: although pathophysiological events of the tissue under study lead to significant changes of the impedance parameters, little is known about their structural and chemical correlates and further collaborative work including chemical, other physical, and histopathological techniques are needed.

In conclusion, changes in the four indices derived from data obtained by the improved electrical impedance instrumentation create patterns that discriminate between skin responses of different origin. Our data up to this point indicate that electrical impedance seems suitable for dynamic and precise analysis of skin reactions.

ACKNOWLEDGMENTS

All persons involved in the skin impedance work at the Huddinge Hospital are gratefully acknowledged, especially Stig Ollmar, Barbro Lundh Rozell, Ingrid Nicander, and Gun-Britt Karlberg.

REFERENCES

1. FOSTER, K. R. & H. P. SCHWAN. 1989. Dielectric properties of tissues and biological material: a critical review. Crit. Rev. Biomed. Eng. **17:** 25–104.
2. METHERALL, P., D. C. BARBER, R. H. SMALLWOOD & B. H. BROWN. 1996. Three-dimensional electrical impedance tomography. Nature **380:** 509–512.
3. DIJKSTRA, A. M., B. H. BROWN, A. D. LEATHARD, N. D. HARRIS, D. C. BARBER & D. L. EDBROOKE. 1993. Clinical applications of electrical impedance tomography. J. Med. Eng. Technol. **17:** 89–98.
4. LONGBOTTOM, C., M-C. D. N. J. HUYSMAN, N. B. PITTS, P. LOS & P. G. BRUCE. 1996. Detection of dental decay and its extent using a.c. impedance spectroscopy. Nat. Med. **2:** 235–237.
5. SALTER, D. C. 1979. Quantifying skin disease and healing *in vivo* using electrical impedance measurements. *In* Non-invasive Physiological Measurements. Volume 1, p. 21–64. Academic Press. New York/London.
6. YAMAMOTO, T. & Y. YAMAMOTO. 1977. Analysis for the change of skin impedance. Med. Biol. Eng. Comput. **15:** 219–227.
7. BERARDESCA, E., G. BORRONI, P. GABBA, V. BRAZZELLI, R. PERICOLI & P. T. PUGLIESE. 1986. Dermal changes in progressive systemic sclerosis assessed by skin impedance measurements. Bioeng. Skin **2:** 181–189.
8. BORRONI, G., E. BERARDESCA, P. GABBA & G. RABBIOSI. 1988. Skin impedance in psoriatic epidermis. Bioeng. Skin **4:** 15–22.
9. MORKRID, L. & Z-G. QIAO. 1988. Continuous estimation of parameters in skin electrical admittance from simultaneous measurements at two different frequencies. Med. Biol. Eng. Comput. **26:** 633–640.
10. GRIMNES, S. 1983. Impedance measurements of individual skin surface electrodes. Med. Biol. Eng. Comput. **21:** 750–755.
11. MARTINSEN, O. G., S. GRIMNES & J. KARLSEN. 1993. An instrument for the evaluation of skin hydration by electrical admittance measurements. Innov. Technol. Biol. Med. **14:** 588–596.
12. OLLMAR, S. & L. EMTESTAM. 1992. Electrical impedance applied to non-invasive detection of irritation in skin. Contact Dermatitis **27:** 37–42.
13. EMTESTAM, L. & M. NYRÉN. 1997. Electrical impedance for quantification and classification of experimental skin reactions. Am. J. Contact Dermatitis **8:** 202–206.
14. NICANDER, I., S. OLLMAR, B. LUNDH ROZELL, A. EEK & L. EMTESTAM. 1995. Electrical impedance measured to five skin depths in mild irritant dermatitis induced by sodium lauryl sulphate. Br. J. Dermatol. **132:** 718–724.

15. EMTESTAM, L. & S. OLLMAR. 1993. Electrical impedance index in human skin: measurements after occlusion, in 5 anatomical regions and in mild irritant dermatitis. Contact Dermatitis **28:** 104–108.
16. OLLMAR, S., M. NYRÉN, I. NICANDER & L. EMTESTAM. 1994. Electrical impedance compared with other non-invasive bioengineering techniques and visual scoring for detection of irritation in human skin. Br. J. Dermatol. **130:** 29–36.
17. NICANDER, I., S. OLLMAR, A. EEK, B. LUNDH ROZELL & L. EMTESTAM. 1996. Correlation of impedance response patterns to histological findings in irritant skin reactions induced by various surfactants. Br. J. Dermatol. **134:** 221–228.
18. NICANDER, I., S. OLLMAR, B. LUNDH ROZELL & L. EMTESTAM. 1997. Allergic contact reactions in the skin assessed by electrical impedance—a pilot study. Skin Res. Technol. **3:** 121–125.
19. NYRÉN, M., S. OLLMAR, I. NICANDER & L. EMTESTAM. 1996. An electrical impedance technique for assessment of wheals. Allergy **51:** 923–926.
20. MAGNUSSON, B. M. & L. O. KOSKINEN. 1996. Effects of topical application of capsaicin to human skin: a comparison of effects evaluated by visual assessment, sensation registration, skin blood flow, and cutaneous impedance measurements. Acta Dermato-Venereol. **76:** 129–132.
21. NICANDER, I., M. NYRÉN, L. EMTESTAM & S. OLLMAR. 1997. Baseline electrical impedance measurements at various skin sites—related to age and sex. Skin Res. Technol. **2:** 126–132.
22. BAXT, W. G. 1995. Application of artificial neural networks to clinical medicine. Lancet **346:** 1135–1138.
23. OLLMAR, S., I. NICANDER, J. OLLMAR & L. EMTESTAM. 1997. Information in full and reduced data sets of electrical impedance spectra from various skin conditions compared by using a holographic neural network. Med. Biol. Eng. Comput. **35:** 415–419.

Electrical Bioimpedance Related to Structural Differences and Reactions in Skin and Oral Mucosa

INGRID NICANDER[a] AND STIG OLLMAR[a,b]

[a]*Center for Oral Biology*
[b]*Division of Medical Engineering, Karolinska Institute at NOVUM, SE-14104 Huddinge, Sweden*

ABSTRACT: Electrical bioimpedance can reflect structural and chemical changes of the skin and the oral mucosa in the β-dispersion frequency range. From our measured multifrequency data set, four physically distinct indices have been formulated to distinguish the electrical properties for different anatomical locations and to detect different reactions and conditions of the skin and the oral mucosa. In comparison with the skin, the differences for various anatomical regions were greater in the oral cavity, which showed as well a different impedance pattern after irritant responses. We conclude that the impedance technique is able to classify and quantify different responses and conditions, preferably by using contralateral reference sites, or following a site in time; however, mapping of baseline properties facilitates the use of the method even if a large part of the skin or the oral mucosa is involved. The method has the potential of becoming a diagnostic decision support tool.

INTRODUCTION

Living tissues have different electrical properties, and both structural and chemical alterations are reflected in impedance changes. With increasing frequencies, a decrease of the impedance magnitude is seen. This decrease is characterized by plateaus separating steeper changes, dispersions (α, β, and λ), which were first defined by Schwan in 1957.[1] For interpretation of impedance changes, it is important to understand what dispersions are involved and what they might reflect. For structural changes, such as edema and necrosis, the β-dispersion is the most informative. A general review of the electrical properties of living tissues has been compiled by Foster and Schwan.[2] It should be noted that the α- and β-dispersions are partially overlapping for both skin and oral mucosa.

Yamamoto and Yamamoto[3] have made significant contributions to the understanding of the electrical properties of the skin, but limited to the α-dispersion (Hz to some kHz). A noninvasive multifrequency impedance spectrometer covering the upper part of the α-dispersion and the essential part of the β-dispersion range has been developed to measure reactions in the skin and in the oral mucosa. The device is also facilitated with variable depth penetration by electronically varying the effective size of the electrode system.[4,5] The instrument is equipped with either a skin probe or an intraoral probe depending on the measurement situation.[6,7] Four impedance indices have been used to extract information from the impedance spectra. These indices have been shown to be useful for characterization of changes in the invisible or barely visible range of alterations in both the skin and the oral mucosa.[8–10] For the skin, responses to other irritants have also been studied, that is, benzalkonium chloride and nonanoic acid.[8] Allergic responses to nickel[9] and alterations induced by removing lipids from the stratum corneum[11] have also been studied. Knowledge about normal variation between and within different anatomical locations of both the skin and the oral mucosa is important when assessing the usefulness of methods or evaluating skin reactions, especially if reference sites (contra- or ipsilateral) cannot be made available, for example, in situations where large parts of the skin or the oral mucosa are involved.[6,7]

MATERIALS AND METHODS

The baseline studies were performed on a total number of 94 healthy volunteers: nonsmokers without known skin diseases or allergy, men and women, 20 to 40 years of age. For evaluation of the electrical impedance technique's ability to detect mild irritant responses, men and women without a history of skin diseases or allergy were recruited, 33 for the skin studies and 26 for studies of the oral mucosa. Before the intraoral measurements, the test subjects had refrained from eating and drinking for at least 1 h.

For mapping of the normal electrical impedance, measurements at 10 different anatomical skin locations (forehead, cheek, postauricular, chest, forearm, dorsum of the hand, neck, back, thigh, and ankle) and at 6 different locations of the oral cavity (hard palate, floor of the mouth, anterior and posterior part of the buccal mucosa, dorsal surface of tongue, and vermilion border of lower lip) were done.

Irritant reactions of the skin and the oral mucosa were produced using sodium lauryl sulfate (SLS). The irritant was applied in 12-mm Finn chambers in the concentration of 0.5% for 24 h on the skin of the volar forearm. For the buccal musosa, 2% SLS was used for 15 min in 18-mm Finn chambers. An unoccluded contralateral reference site was used for both the skin and the oral mucosa. Electrical impedance measurements were done before application of the irritant and at 24 h after the removal of the chamber for the skin and after 5 min for the oral mucosa. Before the skin measurements, the surface of the skin was soaked with physiological saline solution to obtain good electrical contact. In the oral cavity, the wet milieu provides easy contact.

The instrument records magnitude and phase at 31 logarithmically distributed frequencies between 1 kHz and 1 MHz. From the magnitude and phase at 20 kHz and 500 kHz, the following four indices were calculated, representing changes with frequency along the four major aspects of the electrical impedance space:[12]

$$\text{Magnitude index, MIX} = \text{abs}(Z_{20kHz})/\text{abs}(Z_{500kHz}),$$

$$\text{Phase index, PIX} = \text{arg}(Z_{20kHz}) - \text{arg}(Z_{500kHz}),$$

$$\text{Real part index, RIX} = \text{Re}(Z_{20kHz})/\text{abs}(Z_{500kHz}),$$

$$\text{Imaginary part index, IMIX} = \text{Im}(Z_{20kHz})/\text{abs}(Z_{500kHz}),$$

where abs is the magnitude, arg is the phase angle in degrees, and Re and Im are the real and imaginary parts of the impedance Z at the frequencies indicated.

RESULTS AND DISCUSSION

Even before the present impedance spectrometer had been developed, it was found that electrical impedance had the potential of a highly sensitive method for detection of irritation in both skin and oral mucosa.[13–16] A simple manual impedance bridge was used in these early studies, and a simple index reflecting mainly edema was used, inspired by studies from the field of body composition analysis.[17] Pioneers in the field of skin impedance such as Yamamoto[3] and Salter[18] limited the investigated frequency range to relatively low frequencies, where the hydration of the outermost layer of the skin, the stratum corneum, provides the dominating contribution to the signal, as demonstrated by Rosendal.[19] For historical reasons, many users still seem to consider electrical impedance as a method only to measure skin moisturization, and indeed several instruments based on the measurement of electrical capacitance, drawing on the relatively high dielectric constant of water, are available. However, it must be emphasized that electrical impedance is more general and offers the potential to both quantify and classify a number of reactions and conditions of the skin (and the oral mucosa), provided that more than one frequency is used and that the frequencies are wisely chosen. A short review has been compiled in reference 20.

Baseline values of the impedance indices varied at different anatomical locations for both the skin and the oral mucosa. In FIGURE 1, the results of the indices MIX and PIX are presented as box plots for both the skin and the oral mucosa. The chest showed the highest electrical impedance values for the skin and the face showed the lowest; the corresponding values for the oral mucosa were the hard palate and the tongue. The impedance indices showed greater differences between the oral sites than those encountered in the skin. The

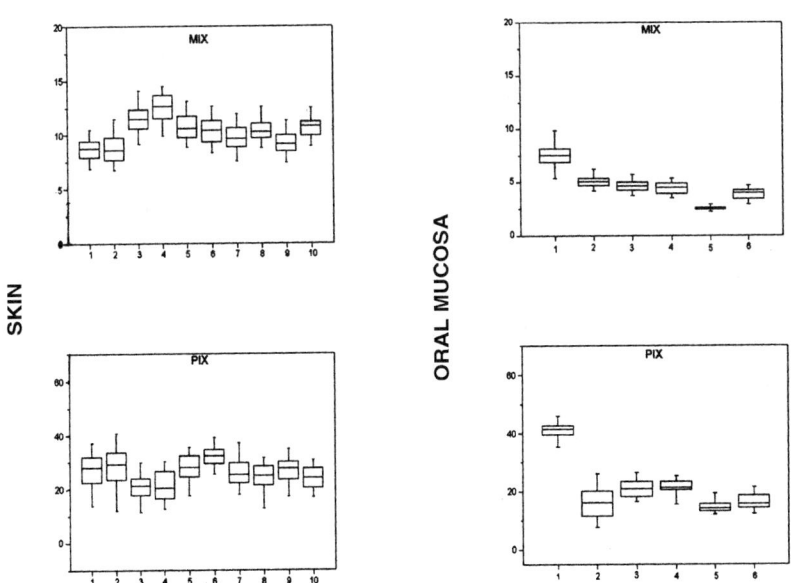

FIGURE 1. Box charts for the MIX and PIX indices. Each box marks the twenty-fifth to seventy-fifth percentile. A horizontal line indicates the median value. A vertical line marks the fifth to ninety-fifth percentile. Left boxes: 1 = forehead, 2 = cheek, 3 = postauricular, 4 = chest, 5 = forearm, 6 = dorsum of the hand, 7 = neck, 8 = back, 9 = thigh, 10 = ankle. Right boxes: 1 = hard palate, 2 = floor of the mouth, 3 = bucca ant., 4 = bucca post., 5 = dorsal surface of tongue, 6 = vermilion border of lower lip.

four indices in general showed lower values for the oral mucosa than for the skin, and the main reasons seem to be the degree of keratinization and the water content of the tissues. The electrical impedance properties of the most keratinized part of the oral mucosa, the hard palate, showed the most similarity to the skin sites. Notably, the variations for the skin at each anatomical site were larger than those for the oral mucosa.

The results after exposure to SLS of the skin and the oral mucosa are presented in TABLE 1. The skin showed statistically significant decreases for the indices MIX and IMIX and an increase for PIX, while the buccal mucosa showed significant decreases for all four impedance indices.

When contralateral (or ipsilateral) reference sites are not available, for example, because of extensive involvement by a skin or mucosal condition, the baseline values will be useful.[6,7] In TABLE 2, some preliminary results from the electrical impedance measurements show that different conditions of the skin and the oral mucosa seem to manifest in different impedance patterns when the tolerance range of the baseline values for a particular anatomical location has been used as a reference.

The indices have been shown to extract and condense most of the information in the measured spectrum and entail a normalization that reduces interindividual and intersite variation. This has also been demonstrated using a holographic neural network.[21] The measured values of the magnitude and the phase for the two used frequencies showed lower values for the mucosa, and the differences were more obvious at 20 kHz. After exposure to SLS, the changes of the measured values were largely due to alteration at the lower frequency. This is consistent with the fact that the measured values at low frequencies are dominated by contributions from the most superficial layer of the oral mucosa or the skin, whereas the higher frequencies are more readily transmitted by capacitive coupling through this layer and include more information about tissue properties below the superficial layer.

In order to simplify interpretation, and possibly establish the impedance technique as a differential diagnostic decision support tool, a catalogue with typical examples of spectra from various reactions, conditions, and diseases of the skin and oral mucosa should be compiled. To facilitate information exchange, some standard will have to be used and we recommend the four indices as a minimum set of parameters. Also, validated training sets intended for use with artificial neural networks would be helpful. The high sensitivity of the electrical impedance technique should make it particularly useful to assess lesions below or barely above the visual threshold.

TABLE 1. Results after Exposure to SLS[a]

	MIX	PIX	RIX	IMIX
Skin:				
SLS 0.5%, 24 h	↓	↑		↓
Buccal mucosa:				
SLS 2.0%, 15 min	↓	↓	↓	↓

[a]The arrows indicate the direction of statistically significant changes ($P \leq 0.001$) in the four impedance indices after the exposure to SLS for the skin and the buccal mucosa.

TABLE 2. Preliminary Results[a]

	MIX	PIX	RIX	IMIX
Skin:				
atopic dermatitis	↓	↑	↓	↓
Buccal mucosa:				
lingua geographica		↑	↓	

[a]The arrows indicate values outside the tolerance range of the baseline values in the direction of the arrow.

CONCLUSIONS

Electrical impedance is a powerful tool for quantification and classification of different reactions and conditions of the skin and the oral mucosa.

As controls, we recommend the use of contralateral (or ipsilateral) sites, or following a site in time, if possible; however, mapping of baseline electrical properties at different anatomical locations of the skin and the oral cavity facilitates the impedance method as a noninvasive diagnostic support tool even when large parts of the skin or the oral mucosa are involved.

REFERENCES

1. SCHWAN, H. P. 1957. Electrical properties of tissue and cell suspensions. Adv. Biol. Med. Phys. **5:** 147–224.
2. FOSTER, K. R. & H. P. SCHWAN. 1989. Dielectric properties of tissues and biological materials: a critical review. Crit. Rev. Biomed. Eng. **17:** 25–104.
3. YAMAMOTO, T. & Y. YAMAMOTO. 1977. Analysis for the change of skin impedance. Med. Biol. Eng. Comput. **15:** 219–227.
4. OLLMAR, S., A. EEK, F. SUNDSTRÖM & L. EMTESTAM. 1995. Electrical impedance for estimation of irritation in oral mucosa and skin. Med. Prog. Technol. **21:** 29–37.
5. NICANDER, I., S. OLLMAR, B. LUNDH ROZELL, A. EEK & L. EMTESTAM. 1995. Electrical impedance measured to five skin depths in mild irritant dermatitis induced by sodium lauryl sulphate. Br. J. Dermatol. **132:** 718–724.
6. NICANDER, I., L. RUNDQUIST & S. OLLMAR. 1997. Electric impedance measurements at six different anatomic locations of macroscopically normal human oral mucosa. Acta Odontol. Scand. **55:** 88–93.
7. NICANDER, I., M. NYRÉN, L. EMTESTAM & S. OLLMAR. 1997. Baseline electrical impedance measurements at various skin sites—related to age and sex. Skin Res. Technol. **3:** 252–258.
8. NICANDER, I., S. OLLMAR, A. EEK, B. LUNDH ROZELL & L. EMTESTAM. 1996. Correlation of impedance response patterns to histological findings in irritant skin reactions induced by various surfactants. Br. J. Dermatol. **134:** 221–228.
9. NICANDER, I., S. OLLMAR, B. LUNDH ROZELL & L. EMTESTAM. 1997. Allergic contact reactions in the skin assessed by electrical impedance—a pilot study. Skin Res. Technol. **3:** 121–125.
10. NICANDER, I., B. LUNDH ROZELL, L. RUNDQUIST & S. OLLMAR. 1997. Electrical impedance: a method to evaluate subtle changes of the human oral mucosa. Eur. J. Oral Sci. **105:** 576–582.
11. NICANDER, I., L. NORLÉN, U. BROCKSTEDT, B. LUNDH ROZELL, B. FORSLIND & S. OLLMAR. 1998. Electrical impedance and other physical parameters as related to lipid content of human stratum corneum. Skin Res. Technol. **4:** 213–221.

12. OLLMAR, S. & I. NICANDER. 1995. Information in multi-frequency measurement on intact skin. Innov. Technol. Biol. Med. **16:** 745–751.
13. NILSSON, R., J. O. FALLAN, K. S. LARSSON, S. OLLMAR & F. SUNDSTRÖM. 1992. Electrical impedance—a new parameter for oral mucosal irritation tests. J. Mater. Sci.: Mater. Med. **3:** 278–282.
14. OLLMAR, S. & L. EMTESTAM. 1992. Electrical impedance applied to non-invasive detection of irritation in skin. Contact Dermatitis **27:** 37–42.
15. EMTESTAM, L. & S. OLLMAR. 1993. Electrical impedance index in human skin: measurements after occlusion, in 5 anatomical regions and in mild irritant contact dermatitis. Contact Dermatitis **28:** 104–108.
16. OLLMAR, S., M. NYRÉN, I. NICANDER & L. EMTESTAM. 1994. Electrical impedance compared with other non-invasive bioengineering techniques and visual scoring for detection of irritation in human skin. Br. J. Dermatol. **130:** 29–36.
17. LUKASKI, H. C. 1987. Methods for the assessment of human body composition: traditional and new. Am. J. Clin. Nutr. **46:** 537–556.
18. SALTER, D. C. 1979. Quantifying skin disease and healing *in vivo* using electrical impedance. *In* Non-invasive Physiological Measurements. Volume 1, p. 21–64. Academic Press. New York/London.
19. ROSENDAL, T. 1945. Concluding studies on the conducting properties of human skin to alternating current. Acta Physiol. Scand. **9:** 39–45.
20. OLLMAR, S. 1998. Methods of information extraction from impedance spectra of biological tissue, in particular skin and oral mucosa—a critical review and suggestions for the future. Bioelectrochem. Bioenerg. **45:** 157–160.
21. OLLMAR, S., I. NICANDER, J. OLLMAR & L. EMTESTAM. 1997. Information in full and reduced data sets of electrical impedance spectra from various skin conditions, compared using a holographic neural network. Med. Biol. Eng. Comput. **35:** 415–419.

Stress Action on Biological Tissue and Tissue Models Detected by the *Py* Value

FRITZ PLIQUETT[a] AND UWE PLIQUETT[b]

[a]*Institute of Medical Physics and Biophysics, University of Leipzig, D-04103 Leipzig, Germany*

[b]*Department of Physical and Biophysical Chemistry, University of Bielefeld, D-33615 Bielefeld, Germany*

> ABSTRACT: The *Py* value, a fast measurable combination of the conductivity at the corner frequencies of the β-dispersion, is a measure of the relative cell volume concentration in tissue. In many cases, if the biological object is stressed, for instance, by mechanical deformation, shortage of oxygen, electric field strength, temperature rise, or ischemia, *Py* increases. Depending on the object and the kind of stress, *Py* plateaus for minutes up to hours and then it decreases continuously. Values of passive electrical parameters of biological tissues are often given without information about the time following a stimulation or stress situation, for example, death, surgery, field application, etc. However, since the passive electrical properties change with time, information about their history, for example, time after death, should be given.

INTRODUCTION

The most interesting frequencies for impedance measurements of tissues range from about 1 kHz to some MHz. This dispersion (β-dispersion) is mostly influenced by the polarization of membrane structures. Thus, one can gain information about the behavior of membrane structures by measuring the passive electrical behavior in this frequency range.

In the case of linear, time-invariant objects, the passive electrical parameter of interest is the electrical impedance or its reciprocal, the admittance (complex conductivity). After Ohm's law, the admittance is the quotient of the current through an object and the voltage dropping across. Linear and time-invariant indicate here that the admittance does not change with voltage and is stable at least for the time of the measurement. A nearly linear behavior for biological objects was found below several hundred millivolts, strongly depending on the object itself.

The admittance is often measured over the whole frequency range of the β-dispersion. This is today a very convenient approach since a great number of devices for this purpose (gain-phase analyzers, network analyzers) are commercially available.

Often, the locus diagram of the biological tissue is presented (FIGURE 1). It can be characterized by four parameters: the conductance at high and low frequencies, G_∞ and G_0, respectively; the characteristic frequency, f_{0y}; and the distribution and interaction parameter, α. The relation of these parameters to morphologic structures is not always clear. The normalized extent of the β-dispersion is termed the *Py* value:

$$Py = \frac{G_\infty - G_0}{G_\infty}.$$

Introduction of the conductivity $\kappa = cG$ shows that *Py* is independent of the geometry of the probe:

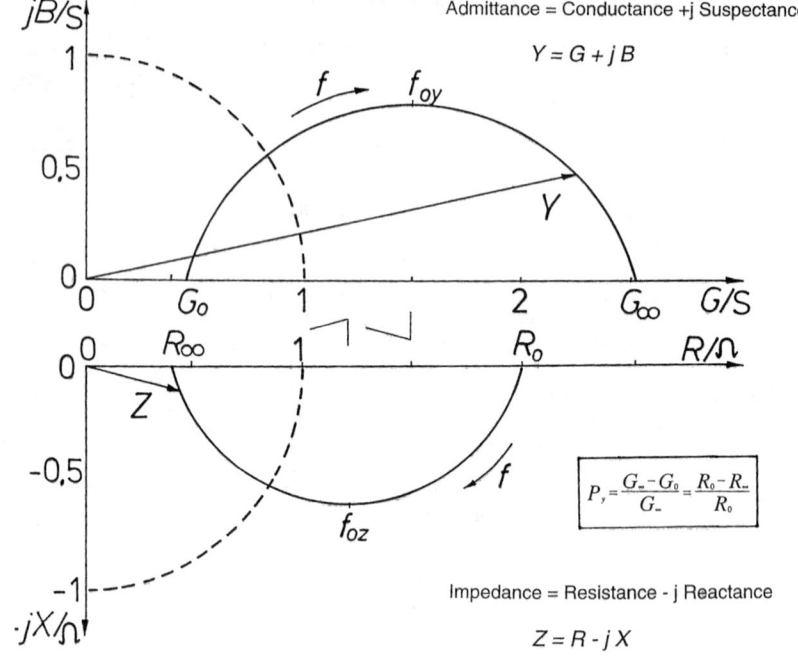

FIGURE 1. Definition of Py from the loci circuit in the admittance and impedance representation.

$$Py = \frac{\kappa_\infty - \kappa_0}{\kappa_\infty}$$

where $c = \kappa/G$ is the probe constant.

Py was found at high volume concentrations (p) of the cells as a logarithmic function of p (FIGURE 2). Therefore, it is a useful parameter for practical purposes, where often only one value significantly describing one object parameter is required.

This Py value is determined by the resistance R or the conductance G at the corner frequencies of the β-dispersion as shown in FIGURE 1. It expresses the passive electrical properties only partially and does not take into account the shape of the locus diagram and the characteristic frequencies f_{0z} or f_{0y}.

A number of commercially available devices reduce the passive electrical properties to one parameter; some devices, for instance, measure the magnitude of the conductivity at only one empirical frequency. Thus, in comparison, several advantages of Py should be pointed out:[1]

- Py as a ratio of conductances (or resistances) is independent of the probe constant c;

- Py depends only negligibly on the temperature if the object is stable over the temperature range considered;

- Py is a well-defined relation to the volume fraction of cells surrounded by an isolating membrane;

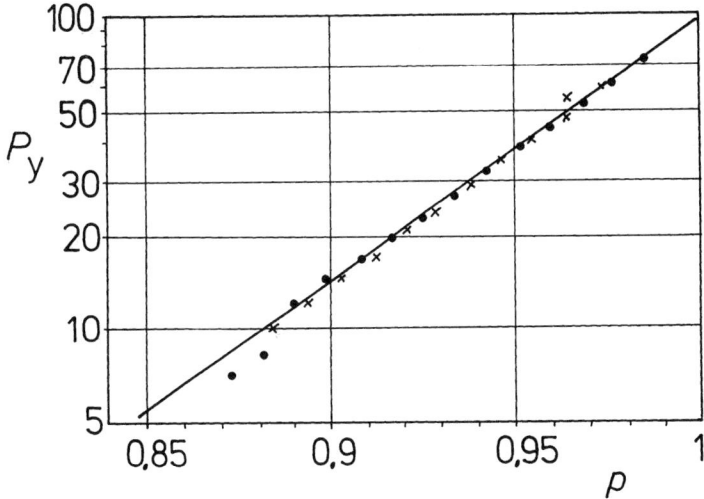

FIGURE 2. P_Y versus p of a concentrated RBC suspension. $p = V_{cell}/V_{tissue}$ is the fraction of V_{cell} of the cell volume in the tissue or suspension volume V_{tissue}.

- P_Y is an adequate parameter for many practical aims, for example, meat quality,[2,3] tumor diagnostics,[4,5] changes during storage of fruits or vegetables,[6] and detection of cryo-effects.[7]

A stress situation can alter the passive electrical behavior of tissues. For instance, the influence of ischemia and postmortal alterations can be sensitively detected by passive electrical properties.[8,9]

For practical purposes, a fast measurable and easy to interpret parameter such as the P_Y value is required.

MATERIALS AND METHODS

Materials and Preparation Procedures

The tissues under investigation were muscle, liver, and human skin *in vitro* or *ex vivo*. Furthermore, model tissues like erythrocytes and spheroids were used.

Human skin was harvested from donors by surgery or was taken from the body. Both the fresh skin and the cadaver skin were carried over in physiological solution. The fatty layer of the skin was carefully removed so that the integrity of the stratum corneum was not compromised. A round-shaped slide with a thickness of about 3 mm and a diameter of 8 mm was cut out and clamped into a Ussing-type chamber. Both compartments were filled with 150 mM PBS (phosphate buffered saline, pH 7.4) and held two electrodes (Ag/AgCl, In Vivo Metric, Healdsburg, California) for contacting a gain-phase analyzer (Solar-

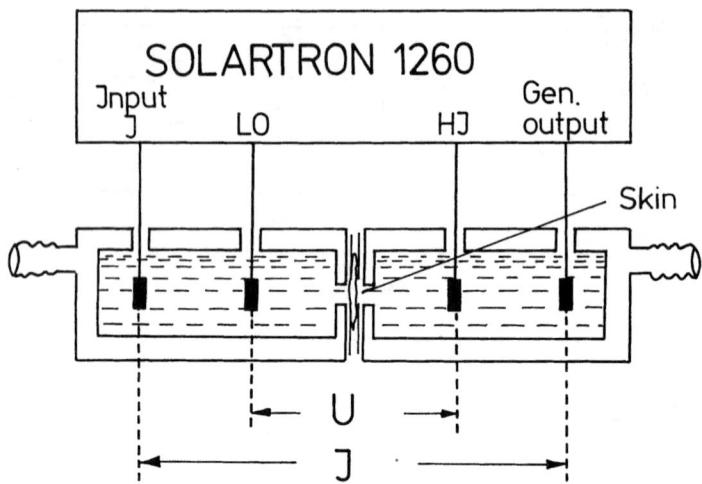

FIGURE 3. Experimental setup for impedance measurements of the skin *in vitro* or *ex vivo*. The skin is clamped in a Ussing chamber, which was thermostated by using a water jacket: I = current electrodes, U = voltage electrodes.

tron 1260, Schlumberger, GB) as shown in FIGURE 3. The chamber was thermostated at different temperatures using a water jacket.

The muscle and liver tissues obtained from animals (canine or pig) were contacted with needle or plate stainless-steel electrodes at room temperature. For some experiments, AgCl or gold electrodes were used.

Red blood cells (RBC) taken from a human donor were washed in phosphate buffer, centrifuged, and concentrated ($p = 0.95$) as described in reference 10.

Spheroids are clusters of cells with an extracellular matrix and behavior close to tissues. They are more homogeneous than real tissues and they can be easily observed under physiological conditions. Therefore, we employed spheroids as a model for biological tissue.

HeLa–Cx 43 spheroids were prepared according to reference 11. These spheroids consist of an aggregation of equal cells transfected with connexin-43 in their membrane and interconnected by gap junctions. The diameter of each spheroid was about 200 μm. For measurement purposes, a single spheroid was soaked in a micropipette tip and placed like a bridge between two compartments, filled with physiological solution (FIGURE 4). Each compartment facilitated two electrodes (stimulus and sensing electrodes), connected to the measuring device (Solartron 1260).

Measurements in the Frequency Domain

The β-dispersion (from about 1 kHz to 10 MHz) is caused by the cellular or membrane structures of biological tissue. The measurement of the impedance or admittance in this region is a sensitive method for investigation of the membrane behavior of these structures. Special devices are commercially available.

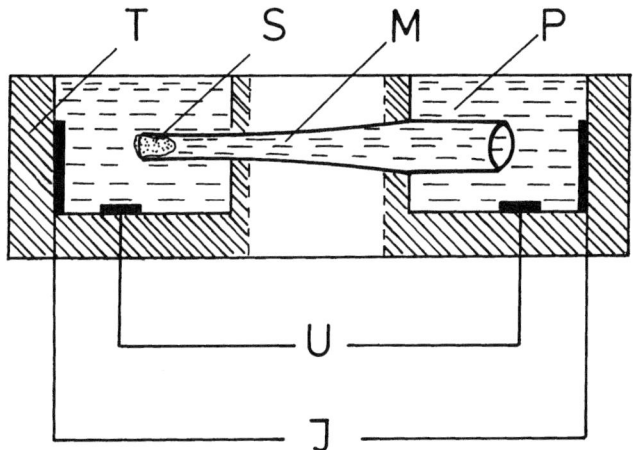

FIGURE 4. Measuring probe for spheroids: T = Teflon vessel, S = spheroid, M = micropipette, P = physiological solution, U = sensing electrodes, I = stimulus electrodes.

We used a computer-controlled setup based on a gain-phase analyzer (Solartron 1260 or HP 4194A) for impedance measurements (four-electrode interface). Simultaneously, the temperature was recorded. The impedance values as a function of the frequency are stored in a PC for subsequent processing. For more convenient data presentation, the parameters of the equivalent circuit were calculated.

Measurements in the Time Domain

Often, the available time for measurements is short: for example, in the case of investigation of fast events, such as recovery after electroporation; in medical diagnostics; and for quality checking in the food industry. In these cases, the values of the passive electrical properties are calculated from the deformation of an applied high bandwidth signal, such as a square wave.

The principle of the pulse deformation is shown in FIGURE 5. A voltage pulse $U(t)$ results in a current pulse $I(t)$ through the object. The time course of the current differs from that of the applied voltage and carries information about the passive electrical properties of the object.

An example for a current response $I(t)$ to a square wave voltage excitation is given in FIGURE 5.

The Py can be determined straightforward by

$$Py = \frac{I(0) - I(\infty)}{I(0)}.$$

The frequency range assessable in this way is determined by the voltage pulse form—in this case, the highest frequency by the pulse rise time and the lowest frequency by the pulse length.

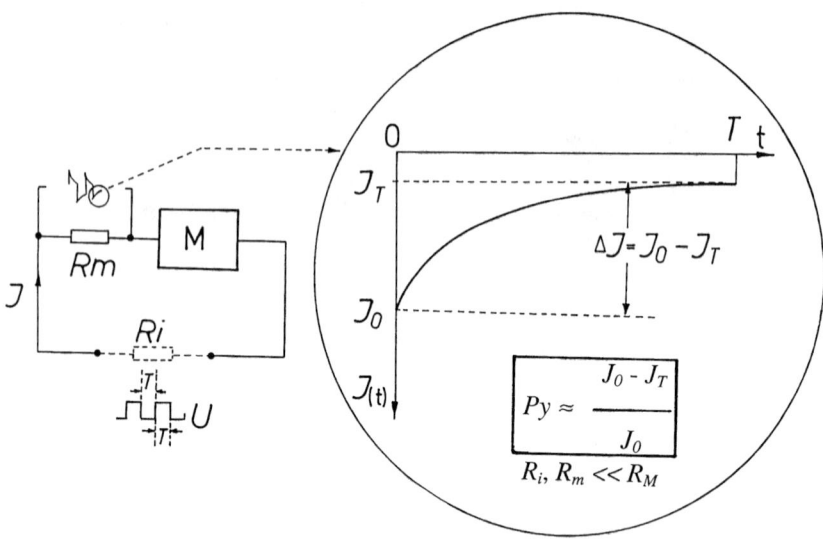

FIGURE 5. Principle of the measurement in the time domain. A square wave voltage $U(t)$ with a periodicity T yields a current response $I(t)$ depending on the passive electrical behavior of the object. If both the intrinsic resistance R_i and the measuring resistance R_m are low as compared to the impedance of M, the Py value is determinable from the current at the pulse beginning and at its end.

Meatcheck—A Device for Direct Measurement of the Py

A device for direct check of the Py value on the basis of the pulse deformation analyses is the "Meatcheck", manufactured by Sigma Electronic Erfurt.[2] This instrument is designed for use in a slaughterhouse, but is also a suitable tool for research work on any biological tissues.

RESULTS

Several biological tissues *in vitro* were under investigation and similar characteristic behaviors of Py versus time after various stress action were observed. In most cases, Py first increases, then reaches a plateau, and finally decreases irreversibly (FIGURE 6).

Muscle Tissue and Meat Quality

The Py value of meat was measured in some thousand pigs (m. long. dorsi) and cattle in several slaughterhouses.[2,3] In all cases, the Py value of living muscle tissue is around 70. After a short time, Py increases between points A and B in FIGURE 6 and reaches a maximum. After about 1 hour postmortem, it starts to decrease. The time of points A, B, C, and D depends on the meat quality, especially the behavior of the cell membranes. The meat

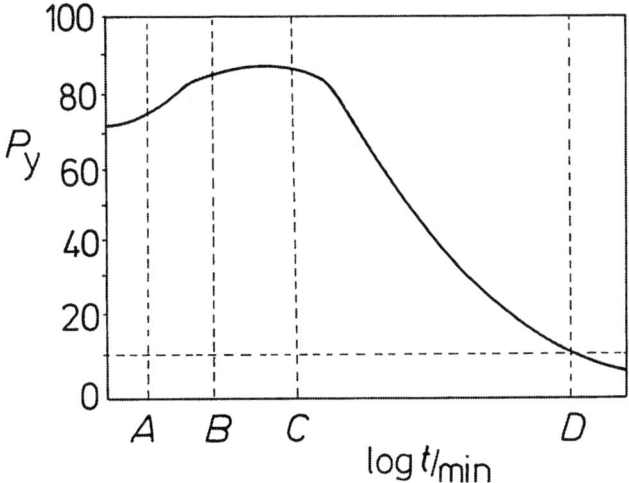

FIGURE 6. P_y of muscle tissue (m. long. dorsi) stored at 6 °C and measured at 20 °C versus time after sacrifice (schematically). The time points A, B, C, and D depend on the meat quality.

quality feature used as a reference is the so-called drip loss, the independently determined liquid efflux during a standardized time (24 h).

The distance between C and D takes a time from some hours up to 2 weeks depending on the meat quality in different muscles (m. long. dorsi, m. semitendinosus, m. semimembranosus, etc.). Here, the influence of the storage temperature should be taken into account. As standardized in meat processing, the temperature is 6 °C. The C-D distance is short for bad meat quality (high liquid loss between 24 and 48 hours ≈ 5–10%) and rises with increasing quality (2–3% liquid loss).

The "meatcheck" device is suitable for measuring the actual quality of the meat. If the procedure, especially the time postmortem, is standardized, a clear distinction between different meat qualities is possible.

Skin after Excision

It is tricky to check the passive electrical properties of living skin because they depend in a complicated manner on different factors. Most of the skin's resistance resides in its outer layer, the 10- to 20-μm-thick stratum corneum. The behavior of the stratum corneum can vary over almost an order of magnitude, depending on the body location, the extent of hydration, the open state of sweat ducts, the density of hair follicles, and many other things. Thus, the influence of the electrode location and ambient conditions are important. To minimize these influences, *in vitro* measurements are useful; however, in this case, the excision and the measuring procedure induce a stress causing a reaction on skin that is still vital.

FIGURE 7 shows the time course of P_y for skin obtained from a cadaver at 3.5 days postmortem (curve I) and for freshly excised skin from a living donor at 90 min after surgery

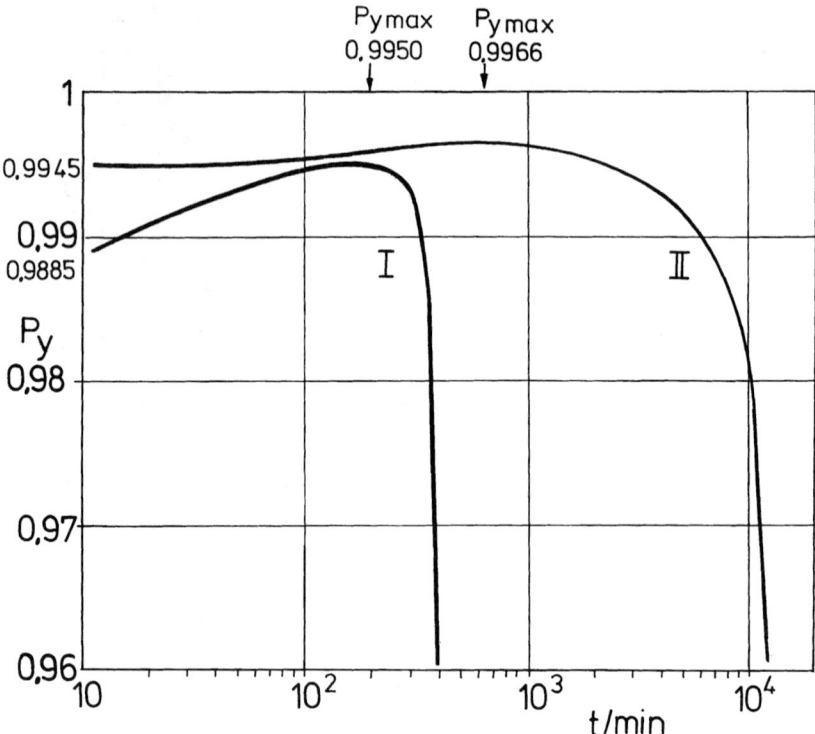

FIGURE 7. Py of human skin as a function of time after clamping into the chamber, which induces a stress: (I) cadaver skin, 3.5 days after death; (II) fresh skin after excision (*ex vivo*), 90 min after surgery.

(curve II). The temperature during the measurement was held constant at 35 °C. The Py of the dead skin plateaued after 2–3 hours, while the plateau for the freshly excised skin was reached after 10 hours. An exponential function fits well the decrease in Py after the plateau was reached; however, the mechanism still needs more investigation.

Liver Perfused with Different Solutions

A typical time course for the Py value of liver tissue is shown in FIGURE 8. Immediately after killing the animal and excision of the liver, Py increases and reaches a plateau with a flat maximum. The time for achieving the plateau can be influenced by the perfusion liquid.[8] Vitamin A enhances this time and formaldehyde (a fixation substance) diminishes it drastically. It is interesting that the time up to the rapid decrease of Py does not change significantly with different perfusion solutions.

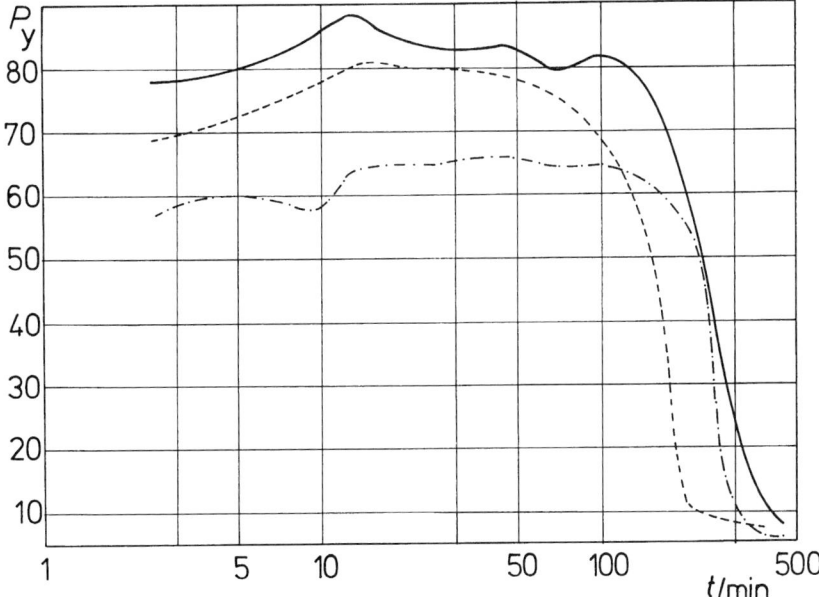

FIGURE 8. Py of rat liver tissue, perfused with different solutions, measured at 37 °C: --- physiological NaCl solution; — vitamin A, high dose; -·-·- 0.5% formaldehyde solution (fixation).

RBC and Electric Fields

The action of an electrical field jump below the breakdown condition ($E < 1$ kV/cm; $t < 20$ ms) yields a maximum of Py at about a half second after the pulse application.[9,12] However, if a breakdown is induced, a drastic decrease of Py is observed at 0.1 s after the pulse (FIGURE 9). This is interpreted as the compromising of the cell's barrier function, reducing the volume fraction of cells surrounded by isolating membranes, which correlates to the Py value.

Spheroids and Oxygen

During the measurement procedure, the spheroids are situated in a narrow (about 200 μm diameter) capillary (see FIGURE 4). The volume of the surrounding culture medium is comparable to the spheroid volume. Since the metabolism of the cells will change the medium and exchange processes in the capillary will take up considerable time (negligible convection), the stress action is here assumed to be the change of the culture solution and the oxygen shortage experienced by the spheroid.

During the first 20 minutes, the Py increases. This coincides with a volume increase of the spheroid as determined under a microscope (Leica MS 5 Leitz, Wetzlar), which is attributed to cell swelling (FIGURE 10). Then, the Py decreases because of membrane

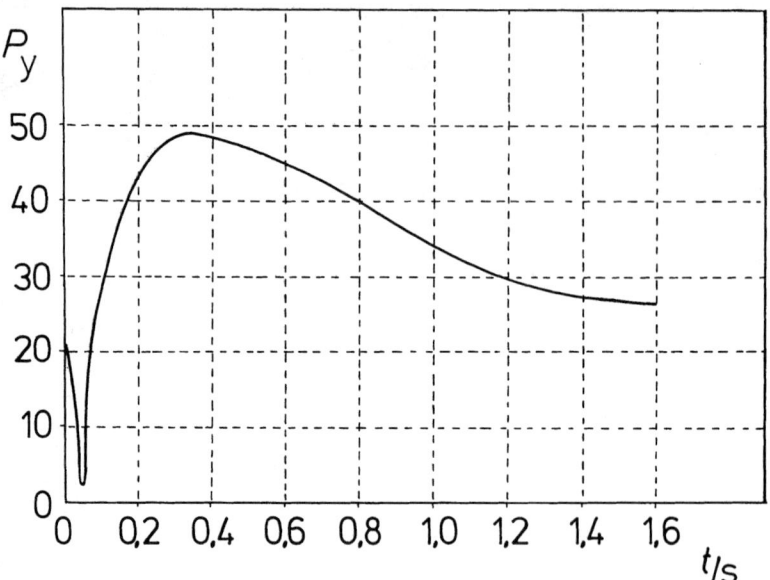

FIGURE 9. P_y of an RBC suspension versus time after action of an electric field jump (schematically).

destruction (breakdown of the barrier function). The cells remain swollen until further destruction by membrane leakage.

DISCUSSION

The P_y value is a measure of the relative cell volume in tissue. This was proven experimentally by comparison of P_y and cell concentration (see FIGURE 2) in RBC suspensions. Furthermore, it was observed that the volume change of the spheroid is closely connected to changes in its P_y value (FIGURE 10).

It seems to be a general fact that different stresses lead to a similar effect, that is, the cell swelling (= P_y increase).

The time dependence of the passive electrical properties postmortem has already been investigated earlier.[8,13] From the findings, presented in these publications, the time course of P_y was calculated. During an initial phase, P_y increases, plateaus for a shorter or longer time depending on the specific tissue, and decreases subsequently. With respect to Gersing,[13] we suggest that the P_y value is good for assessment of the vitality of the tissue; for example, the tissue is vital until the maximum is achieved. Later processes involve an increasing leakage of the cell membranes, resulting in tissue destruction and therefore decreased P_y.

A qualitatively similar time course of P_y was found for the skin.[14] Here, P_y is mostly influenced by the behavior of the 10- to 20-μm-thick stratum corneum, the dead outer

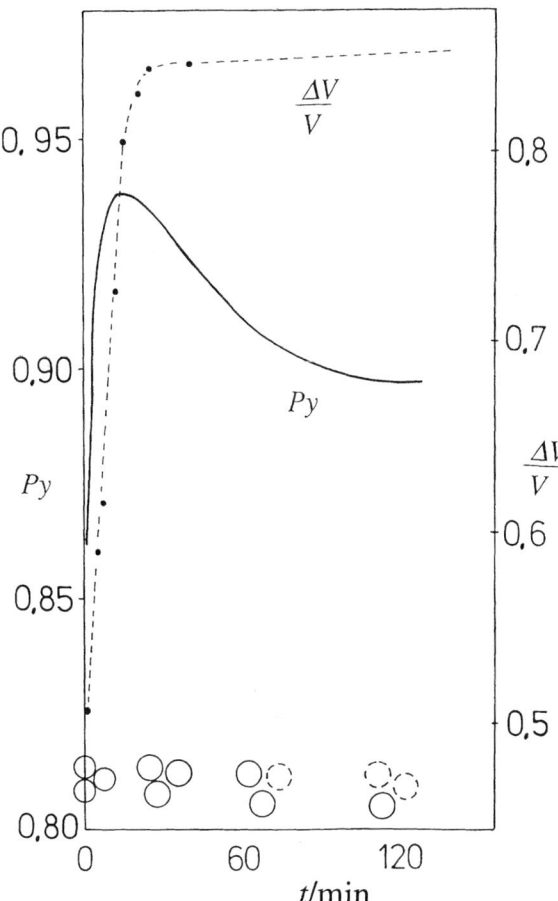

FIGURE 10. Py of HeLa–Cx 43 spheroids and the relative volume change versus measuring time. At $t = 0$, the spheroid was introduced into the measuring capillary. Spheroid swelling and membrane destruction are shown on the bottom.

layer of the skin with a resistance of orders of magnitude higher than that of the underlying tissue.

As shown in FIGURE 7, the Py value of fresh skin (90 min after surgery) is, at the beginning of the measurement, higher than the Py of the cadaver skin (after the influence of 3.5 days postmortem). In both cases, the Py then rises for hours.

The time of the Py increase is specific for different tissues. While the maximum of Py for muscle and liver tissue was achieved after about 30 min, the maximum of Py is reached after 10 hours for fresh skin and after about 3 hours for skin from a cadaver at 3.5 days after death.

Spheroids are a simple model of biological tissue with the important property of the cell-cell interaction and an extracellular matrix. This model shows the same behavior after a stress action as biological tissues in general.

It seems that cell swelling (indicated by Py increase) is an unspecified answer to a general stimulus—for instance, ischemia after death or excision from the living organism. The postmortal changes in tissue lead to changes in the passive electrical behavior and can be easily assessed for research purposes and practical applications as well.

In many papers,[15,16] impedance values for several biological tissues are given, but without the measuring conditions. What does a skin conductivity of 0.25 Sm^{-1} at 13.56 MHz mean without a remark as to the history? For suitable interpretation of impedance measurements *in vitro*, the measuring conditions are necessary, especially the time after death and the storage conditions.

REFERENCES

1. PLIQUETT, U. & F. PLIQUETT. 1998. Kritische Bemerkungen zur Leitfähigkeit als Qualitätsmerkmal für Fleisch. Fleischwirtschaft **78**(9): 1010–1012.
2. PLIQUETT, F., U. PLIQUETT, L. SCHÖBERLEIN & K. H. FREYWALD. 1995. Impedanzmessungen zur Charakterisierung der Fleischbeschaffenheit. Fleischwirtschaft **75**(4): 496–498.
3. PLIQUETT, F., U. PLIQUETT & W. RÖBEKAMP. 1990. Beurteilung der Reifung des M. long. dorsi und M. semitendinosus durch Impulsimpedanzmessungen. Fleischwirtschaft **70**(12): 1468–1470.
4. PLIQUETT, F. & J. HEINITZ. 1989. Veränderung passiv elektrischer Gewebeeigenschaften eines experimentellen Tumors während der Kanzerogenese. Z. Exp. Chir. Transplant. Künstliche Organe **22**: 38–44.
5. PLIQUETT, F., S. STAFRI & K. KÜHNDEL. 1988. Passiv elektrische Gewebeparameter des normalen und pathologisch veränderten Portioepithels. Arch. Geschwulstforsch. **58**: 105–111.
6. PLIQUETT, F. & R. VOLKMANN. 1991. Beurteilung der Lagerfähigkeit von Speisemöhren durch Impulsimpedanzmessung. Arch. Züchtungsforsch. Berlin **21**: 65–71.
7. PLIQUETT, F. 1989. Passiv elektrische Verfahren zur Untersuchung von Kryoeffekten. *In* Kryotherapie in Ophthalmologie und Dermatologie, p. 107–116. Barth. Leipzig.
8. TAUBERT, G., F. PLIQUETT, Y. A. VLADIMIROV & Y. M. PETRUSEVIC. 1979. Untersuchungen physikochemischer Veränderungen von Lebergewebe mit passiv elektrischen, redoxometrischen, und Lumineszenzmethoden in Abhängigkeit von der Zeit nach der Isolierung. Wiss. Z. Karl-Marx-Univ. Leipzig Math. Naturwiss. Reihe **28**: 141–147.
9. PLIQUETT, F. & U. PLIQUETT. 1995. Electrical field effects on biological cells, detected by pulse deformation. Phys. Chem. Biol. Med. **2**: 11–19.
10. FOMEKONG, R. D., U. PLIQUETT & F. PLIQUETT. 1998. Passive electrical properties of RBC suspensions: changes due to distribution of relaxation times in dependence on the cell volume fraction and medium conductivity. Bioelectrochem. Bioenerg. In press.
11. HÜLSER, D. F. 1992. Intercellular communication in three-dimensional culture. *In* Spheroid Culture in Cancer Research, p. 172–193. CRC Press. Boca Raton, Florida.
12. PLIQUETT, F. & S. WUNDERLICH. 1983. Relationship between cell parameters and pulse deformation due to these cells as well as its change after electrically induced membrane breakdown. Bioelectrochem. Bioenerg. **10**: 467–475.
13. GERSING, E. 1991. Measurement of electrical impedance in organs. Biomed. Tech. **36**: 6–11 and 70–77.
14. PLIQUETT, F. & U. PLIQUETT. 1996. Passive electrical properties of human stratum corneum *in vivo* depending on time after separation. Biophys. Chem. **58**: 205–210.
15. FOSTER, K. R. & H. P. SCHWAN. 1989. Dielectric properties of tissues and biological materials: a critical review. Crit. Rev. Biomed. Eng. **17**: 25–104.
16. PETHIG, R. & D. B. KELL. 1987. The passive electrical properties of biological systems: their significance in physiology, biophysics, and biotechnology. Phys. Med. Biol. **32**: 933–970.

From Concept to Market in Industrial Impedance Applications

CHRISTOPHER DAVEY,[a] ROBERT TODD,[b] AND JOHN BARRETT[a]

[a]*Institute of Biological Sciences, University of Wales, Aberystwyth, Ceredigion, Wales SY23 3DA, United Kingdom*

[b]*Aber Instruments Limited, Science Park, Aberystwyth, Ceredigion, Wales SY23 3AH, United Kingdom*

ABSTRACT: This paper discusses some of the technical aspects of converting a laboratory idea into a commercial product. The example used is the development of the Aber Instruments Biomass Monitor, which is now used worldwide in industry for the pitching of yeast in breweries and for biomass measurements in the pharmaceutical industry. Although the issues raised will relate to instrumentation in a production environment, many of the themes will be equally applicable to medical instruments.

INTRODUCTION

This paper aims to bring to the attention of academics some of the issues that they will face if they try to commercialize an impedance instrument. In a text of this size, it is not possible to discuss all facets of such a project and so the emphasis here will be on the technical aspects of product development and support. The problems encountered during the development of the Aber Instruments Biomass Monitor (BM) will be used as a case study as this is a project that we were actively involved in. The evolution of the BM over the past 12 years and its establishment in the marketplace provide very important lessons that one should consider before embarking on such a course.

This paper will consist of a brief history of the origins of the BM, including the theory behind the machine. After this, there is a discussion of the market that the BM is aimed at and why it sells successfully into it. The rest of the paper consists of six subsections that outline areas of importance that we found to be crucial during the development and commercialization of the BM.

THE BIOMASS MONITOR (BM)

The origins of the BM came from purely academic studies on the structure of biological materials carried out in Aberystwyth by Douglas Kell. He was using an HP4192A impedance analyzer to look at the dielectric properties of cells and the β-dispersion in particular.[1–3] The dielectric properties of a cell suspension are characterized by the frequency dependence of its relative permittivity (ε') and conductivity (σ').[4] In the radio-frequency range, the dielectric properties of cells are dominated by this β-dispersion, which causes permittivity to fall and conductivity to rise as frequency increases, due to a falling off of the charging of the plasma membrane capacitance. The permittivity falls from a high low-frequency plateau to a low high-frequency plateau (see FIGURE 1). The height of this plateau above the residual high-frequency permittivity (ε_∞') is called $\Delta\varepsilon'$ and for the β-dispersion is given by equation 1:[5,6]

$$\Delta\varepsilon' = 9PrC_m/4\varepsilon_0 \tag{1}$$

where P is the volume fraction of cells, r is the cell radius, C_m is the plasma membrane capacitance, and ε_0 is the permittivity of free space.

It was realized that P provides a measure of the biomass (concentration of viable cells) in the suspension. For most fermentations, rC_m remains approximately constant. This means that measuring the $\Delta\varepsilon'$ of the β-dispersion allows the on-line and real-time measurement of biomass, which has been at the top of the fermentation industries' "wish list" for many years.

It rapidly became apparent that the HP4192A was not suitable for industrial applications of this measurement (see later sections for reasons). Hence, Aber Instruments was formed to build and exploit the Biomass Monitor (formerly called the βugmeter),[7,8] a machine purposely built for this application.

The main market for the BM has been in the inoculation of the fermentors in breweries ("yeast pitching"), where it is used by major companies worldwide.[9] Its main selling point is that the BM can save very considerable sums of money because the better control of inoculation gives increased brewing capacity, consistent fermentation performance, reduced labor costs, quicker fermentation start-up, and reduced product losses. The machine has also found application in the pharmaceutical industry to quantify the biomass of filamentous organisms, which are otherwise difficult to measure.[10] Lab-based research has shown its application to bacteria,[11,12] yeast,[13,14] animal[15,16] and plant cells,[17] immobilized cells,[18] and solid substrate fermentations of filamentous fungi,[19] and in assessing cytotoxicity.[20,21]

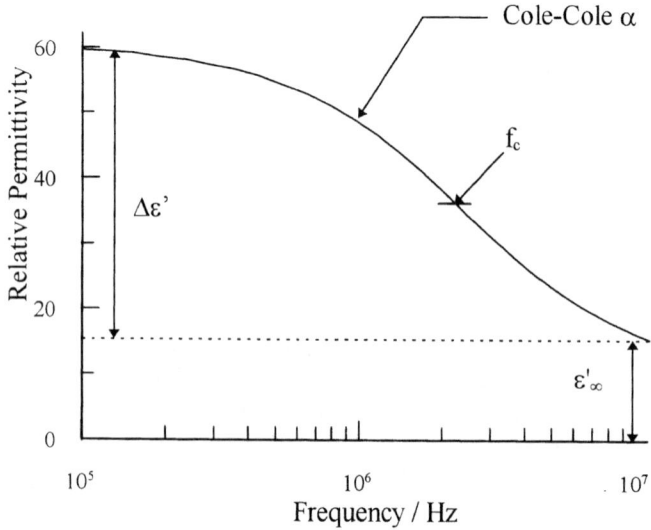

FIGURE 1. The dielectric β-dispersion of a suspension of cells. See text for details.

FACTORS FOUND TO BE IMPORTANT DURING THE DEVELOPMENT OF THE BM

Identifying the Physical Properties of the Target Markets' Cell Suspensions

To develop an instrument that will sell, you must know the physical properties of the material that you want to measure. In the case of the BM, this was cell slurries inside yeast-pitching mains or cells in suspension in fermentors. Thus, when designing the machine, one has to consider the many factors that influence the electrical properties measured. The conductivity of the cell growth medium is critical. The BM operates from 0.2 to 10 MHz. Hence, highly conducting suspensions would cause serious electrode polarization[22–26] at the lower frequencies, thereby swamping the $\Delta\varepsilon'$ that one wishes to measure, and at higher frequencies cross talk could severely distort the permittivity (or equivalently, the capacitance) measured. Yeast slurries have very low conductivity media, while some commercial *Escherichia coli* and animal cell applications have very high conductivities.

Other physical factors inside fermentors that were found to be important were high, fluctuating gas holdups; large temperature changes; and high concentrations of nonbiomass solids. The biomass concentration range that needed to be measured was also found to be very wide. During a fermentation run, the initial concentration is very low and thus the BM needs to be very sensitive; in contrast, in pitching slurries, the biomass concentration is so high that linearizers are needed.[13] This need for sensitive registration of permittivity (capacitance) in the presence of a high conductivity meant that the phase detector design was critical.[7]

Identifying the Locations where the BM Would Be Used

Industrial fermentation halls can be extremely hostile environments. Thus, the measuring electronics and the housing box must be designed to cope with such a situation. Likely conditions that will be encountered and that need to be designed against include water and steam, personnel climbing on the equipment, very large and sudden ambient temperature fluctuations, and the presence in the hall of potential sources of electrical interference (the BM itself fulfills the EMC regulations). In addition, the machine must be capable of operating for many days *in situ* without drift. The system must be physically robust and this includes the electronics being able to survive transportation.

It is likely that the measuring electronics will be some distance from the electrode probe. Hence, signal conditioning, cable design, and connectors need consideration.

Identifying the Users' Expectations

The industrial users of a BM want to treat it like any other fermentor monitoring probe (e.g., a pH electrode); they just want to put it into the fermentor and get biomass readings out. This fact affects the whole design philosophy of the BM. Its probes fit standard fermentor ports; the calibrations required are simple and are needed very infrequently; the machine is simple to use; and the electrical output of the data is compatible with commercial fermentor control systems. The cost of the machine is well within the range that users can afford and a multiplexer is available to reduce the cost per measurement even further.

A vital area is documentation. Time and money must be spent on getting this right. Those who wish to get straight on and use the machine must be catered for, as well as those requiring in-depth knowledge of the physics behind it.[27,28]

Electrode Design

The electrode design for the BM took a lot of work. To reduce electrode polarization, a four-terminal electrode arrangement was developed[7,23] and *in situ* electrolytic cleaning was implemented to prevent growth of cells on the electrodes during fermentations. The materials used must be inert; they must not leach toxins into the fermentation; the electrode metal pins must be strong and stable over time; the probes should be robust to physical shocks and designed to allow repeated *in situ* chemical/heat sterilization; they must survive the high pressures encountered; they must not present a risk of loss of sterility; they must be relatively inexpensive; they must not introduce excessive strays; and they need to be designed to minimize ensnarement of bubbles and solids.[29] The BM electrodes fulfill all these criteria.

Product Developments and Developing a Market

Vital to the success of the BM were those people in industry who championed its use.[9,10] These people not only established links into a market and the product's credibility, but also provided feedback on areas of weakness that could be rectified in later designs. However, it is vital that a stable product range is achieved as soon as possible and one must not develop the habit of building custom machines for each customer's requirements. It is far better to build a generic product line optimized to a specific market.

Once a sales base has been established, one can then develop related business areas. These include establishing an international distributors network, training workshops, and (in the case of the BM) forming links to companies that sell complete brewery yeast-pitching systems so that a BM is an integral part of their product lines.

Dealing with Customers

The BM is an expensive machine and thus customers need to be able to have their samples tested at Aber Instruments or on-site before purchasing. Customer applications are carefully screened to ensure that sales are only made in areas where they will work. Advice is given on interfacing and software development and on any operating difficulties encountered when the BM is in use. Aber Instruments also provides advice on interpreting the data produced by the BM.

CONCLUSIONS

This paper has outlined some of the areas that were found to be important in bringing dielectric biomass measurements to the market. For industrial applications, it will be clear that this process can take many years, requires a large investment in research and development and in customer support personnel, and needs strong customer interest and feedback.

ACKNOWLEDGMENTS

C. Davey wishes to thank the Wellcome Trust for financial support and Aber Instruments Limited for allowing him to discuss his and their past experiences in product development.

REFERENCES

1. KELL, D. B. 1985. Dielectric properties of bacterial chromatophores. Bioelectrochem. Bioenerg. **15:** 405–415.
2. HARRIS, C. M. & D. B. KELL. 1983. The radio-frequency dielectric properties of yeast cells measured with a rapid, automated, frequency-domain dielectric spectrometer. Bioelectrochem. Bioenerg. **11:** 15–28.
3. DAVEY, C. L., D. B. KELL, R. B. KEMP & R. W. J. MEREDITH. 1988. On the audio- and radio-frequency dielectric behaviour of anchorage-independent, mouse L929-derived LS fibroblasts. Bioelectrochem. Bioenerg. **20:** 83–98.
4. PETHIG, R. 1979. Dielectric and Electronic Properties of Biological Materials. Wiley. New York.
5. FOSTER, K. R. & H. P. SCHWAN. 1986. Dielectric properties of tissues. In CRC Handbook of Biological Effects of Electromagnetic Fields, p. 27–96. CRC Press. Boca Raton, Florida.
6. DAVEY, C. L. & D. B. KELL. 1995. The low-frequency dielectric properties of biological cells. In Bioelectrochemistry of Cells and Tissues, p. 159–207. Birkäuser. Basel.
7. HARRIS, C. M., R. W. TODD, S. J. BUNGARD, R. W. LOVITT, J. G. MORRIS & D. B. KELL. 1987. The dielectric permittivity of microbial suspensions at radio-frequencies: a novel method for the estimation of microbial biomass. Enzyme Microb. Technol. **9:** 181–186.
8. KELL, D. B. & R. W. TODD. 1998. Dielectric estimation of microbial biomass using the Aber Instruments Biomass Monitor. Trends Biotechnol. **16:** 149–150.
9. BOULTON, C. A., P. S. MARYAN & D. LOVERIDGE. 1989. The application of a novel biomass sensor to the control of yeast pitching rate. In Proceedings of the European Brewing Convention Congress, p. 653–661. Zurich.
10. FEHRENBACH, R., M. COMBERBACH & J. O. PÊTRE. 1992. On-line biomass monitoring by capacitance measurement. J. Biotechnol. **23:** 303–314.
11. FERRIS, L. E., C. D. DAVEY & D. B. KELL. 1990. Evidence from its temperature dependence that the β-dielectric dispersion of cell suspensions is not due solely to the charging of a static membrane capacitance. Eur. Biophys. J. **18:** 267–276.
12. MARKX, G. H. & D. B. KELL. 1990. Dielectric spectroscopy as a tool for the measurement of the formation of biofilms and of their removal by electrolytic cleaning pulses and biocides. Biofouling **2:** 211–227.
13. DAVEY, C. L., H. M. DAVEY & D. B. KELL. 1992. On the dielectric properties of cell suspensions at high volume fractions. Bioelectrochem. Bioenerg. **28:** 319–330.
14. MARKX, G. H., C. L. DAVEY & D. B. KELL. 1991. The permittistat: a novel type of turbidostat. J. Gen. Microbiol. **137:** 735–743.
15. CERCKEL, I., A. GARCIA, V. DEGOUYS, D. DUBOIS, L. FABRY & A. O. A. MILLER. 1993. Dielectric-spectroscopy of mammalian cells. 1. Evaluation of the biomass of Hela-cell and CHO-cell in suspension by low-frequency dielectric-spectroscopy. Cytotechnology **13:** 185–193.

16. DAVEY, C. L., Y. GUAN, R. B. KEMP & D. B. KELL. 1997. Real-time monitoring of the biomass content of animal cell cultures using dielectric spectroscopy. *In* Animal Cell Technology: Basic and Applied Aspects, p. 61–65. Kluwer. Dordrecht.
17. MARKX, G. H., C. L. DAVEY, D. B. KELL & P. MORRIS. 1991. The dielectric permittivity at radio frequencies and the Bruggeman probe: novel techniques for the on-line determination of biomass concentrations in plant cell cultures. J. Biotechnol. **20:** 279–290.
18. SALTER, G. J., D. B. KELL, L. A. ASH, J. M. ADAMS, A. J. BROWN & R. JAMES. 1990. Hydrodynamic deposition: a novel method of cell immobilization. Enzyme Microb. Technol. **12:** 419–430.
19. DAVEY, C. L., W. PENALOZA, D. B. KELL & J. N. HEDGER. 1991. Real-time monitoring of the accretion of *Rhizopus oligosporus* biomass during the solid-substrate fermentation. World J. Microbiol. Biotechnol. **7:** 248–259.
20. STOICHEVA, N. G., C. L. DAVEY, G. H. MARKX & D. B. KELL. 1989. Dielectric spectroscopy: a rapid method for the determination of solvent biocompatibility during biotransformations. Biocatalysis **2:** 245–255.
21. DAVEY, C. L., G. H. MARKX & D. B. KELL. 1993. On the dielectric method of monitoring cellular viability. Pure Appl. Chem. **65:** 1921–1926.
22. SCHWAN, H. P. 1968. Electrode polarization impedance and measurements in biological materials. Ann. N.Y. Acad. Sci. **148:** 191–209.
23. SCHWAN, H. P. & C. D. FERRIS. 1968. Four-terminal null techniques for impedance measurement with high resolution. Rev. Sci. Instrum. **39:** 481–485.
24. DAVEY, C. L., G. H. MARKX & D. B. KELL. 1990. Substitution and spreadsheet methods for fitting dielectric spectra of biological systems. Eur. Biophys. J. **18:** 255–265.
25. DAVEY, C. L. & D. B. KELL. 1998. The influence of electrode polarisation on dielectric spectra, with special reference to capacitive biomass measurements: (I) Quantifying the effects on electrode polarisation of factors likely to occur during fermentations. Bioelectrochem. Bioenerg. **46:** 91–103.
26. DAVEY, C. L. & D. B. KELL. 1998. The influence of electrode polarisation on dielectric spectra, with special reference to capacitive biomass measurements: (II) Reduction in the contribution of electrode polarisation to dielectric spectra using a two-frequency method. Bioelectrochem. Bioenerg. **46:** 105–114.
27. DAVEY, C. L. 1993. The Biomass Monitor Source Book. Aber Instruments Limited. Aberystwyth.
28. DAVEY, C. L. 1993. The Theory of the β-Dielectric Dispersion and Its Use in the Estimation of Cellular Biomass. Aber Instruments Limited. Aberystwyth.
29. HARRIS, C. M. & D. B. KELL. 1985. The estimation of microbial biomass. Biosensors **1:** 17–84.

Orientation and Deformation of Erythrocytes in Flowing Blood

MAMIKO FUJII,[a] KENGO NAKAJIMA,[a] KATSUYUKI SAKAMOTO,[b] AND HIROSHI KANAI[a]

[a]*Department of Electrical and Electronics Engineering, Sophia University, Tokyo 102-0094, Japan*

[b]*Department of Biomedical Engineering, Kitasato University, Kanagawa, Japan*

ABSTRACT: The effects of flow on the changes of electrical resistivity and light-scattering characteristics of blood are experimentally and theoretically discussed. Studies indicate that most erythrocytes deform and orient themselves in the flow direction when blood flows in a conduit. Such oriented blood shows anisotropic properties. Anisotropic electrical resistivity of flowing blood is measured in three rectangular directions with a measurement cell of coaxial cylindrical type. From these experimental results, the orientation and deformation of erythrocytes are discussed. The orientation ratio and the deformation are calculated using a simplified spheroidal model of an erythrocyte. Calculated results show that the fractions of erythrocytes with their short axis parallel to each direction and the equivalent axis ratio for a simplified spheroidal model change with the shear rate of flow.

INTRODUCTION

The physical properties of blood are of practical interest in medical engineering and various fields of medicine because the electrical impedance of blood is much less and the absorption coefficient of blood for visible and infrared light is much larger than those of all other living tissues. These characteristics can be utilized for various purposes in biomedical engineering, such as in impedance and optical plethysmographies, in impedance and optical CT, and in the study of the rheological behavior of blood.

When blood flows, its physical properties—such as viscosity, optical reflection, and electrical resistivity—are different from those of quiescent blood and change with the shear rate. It is assumed that the main cause of these changes is the same and is attributed to the orientation and deformation of red blood cells. From an electrical point of view, it can be assumed that blood is a suspension of small insulated particles (erythrocytes) in a conductive fluid (plasma) when the frequency of supplied voltage is lower than several hundred kHz because the β-dispersion frequency of blood is about 3 MHz.[1] When blood flows, the erythrocytes deform and rotate. The rotation velocity of an erythrocyte depends on the angle between the long axis of the erythrocyte and its flow direction.[2] Therefore, it seems that the erythrocytes orient themselves in the flow direction,[2–7] and flowing blood shows anisotropic electrical and optical properties.[3,4] For example, the electrical resistivity of flowing blood depends on the direction of the applied electrical field and the rate of flow. The resistivity longitudinal to laminar flow decreases with the flow rate, and the transverse resistivity increases. We have already reported the effects of steady flow on the electrical properties of flowing blood.[4] The results of measuring the longitudinal and the transverse resistivity changes, the optical reflection change, and the viscosity change of sinusoidally flowing blood in a rectangular conduit have also been discussed.[5]

In this paper, the effects of Couette blood flow on electrical resistivity in the three rectangular directions are experimentally and theoretically discussed. The effects of flow on light scattered from flowing blood are also discussed. Couette flow is produced in a concentric cylindrical cell. This cell is used to measure the resistivity of flowing blood in the circumferential, axial, and radial directions. The angular distribution of light scattered from flowing blood can also be measured simultaneously. From experimental results, the apparent orientation ratio in each direction is calculated. To estimate the deformation, the equivalent axis ratio for the spheroidal model is also calculated.

THEORY AND METHODS

The principal factors affecting the resistivity of flowing blood are the deformation and orientation of erythrocytes. Many researchers have thoroughly studied this effect.[3–7] From an electrical point of view, it can be assumed that blood is a suspension of small insulated particles in a conductive fluid when the frequency of supplied current is much lower than the β-dispersion frequency of blood, about 3 MHz. In order to simplify our theoretical analysis, it is assumed that erythrocytes have a spheroidal shape. The left diagram in FIGURE 1 shows the schematic cross-sectional view of an erythrocyte and the right one shows the simplified spheroidal model used for the calculation in this paper.

Although each erythrocyte in flowing blood rotates itself along its own constant orbit, the probability of the erythrocytes being oriented in various directions can be calculated.[2] In this paper, it is assumed that all of the erythrocytes orient themselves so that their short axes are parallel to one of the Cartesian axes.[3]

The conductivity (inverse of resistivity) of a suspension of ellipsoidal particles is given by equation 1:[3]

$$\sigma_i = \sigma_s + \frac{\rho}{1-\rho} \sum_{j=x,y,z} \frac{2k_j(\sigma_p - \sigma_i)}{2 + abcL_{ij}(\sigma_p/\sigma_s - 1)} \tag{1}$$

where i indicates the direction of the conductivity measurement along one of the three x, y, z rectangular axes; j is the orientation direction of those erythrocytes whose short axis is parallel to one of the three x, y, z rectangular axes; σ_i is the blood conductivity value in the i direction; σ_s is the conductivity of plasma; σ_p is that of an erythrocyte; ρ is the hematocrit value; L_{ij} is the fraction of erythrocytes oriented to the j direction, $k_x + k_y + k_z = 1$; L_{ij} is the shape factor when the applied current flows in the i direction and the short axis of the erythrocyte is parallel to the j direction; and a, b, and c are the respective half-lengths of

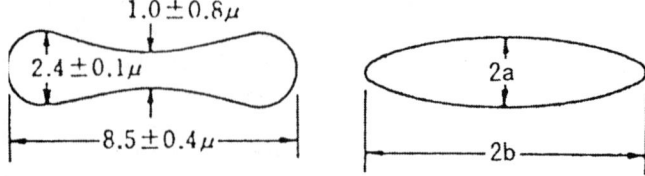

FIGURE 1. Schematic cross-sectional view of an erythrocyte and its spheroidal model.

the three axes of the ellipsoid shown in FIGURE 2. For a spheroid, $b = c$. The axis ratio, $a{:}b{:}c$, of the erythrocyte in quiescent blood is assumed to be 1:4:4 as shown in FIGURE 2.

In flowing blood, each erythrocyte rotates itself along its own constant orbit. The rotation velocity of the erythrocyte depends on the angle between the long axis of the erythrocyte and the flow direction.[2] When this angle is 90°, the velocity is fastest; when it is zero, the velocity is slowest. Although all of the erythrocytes do not effectively orient themselves in the same direction simultaneously, it seems that each erythrocyte statistically orients itself in one of the three rectangular axes, and most of them orient themselves in the flow direction.[2,3,7]

From equation 1, the conductivity of flowing blood is obtained as

$$\sigma_i = \sigma_p + \frac{\sigma_s - \sigma_p}{1 + \frac{2k_x}{m_{ix}} + \frac{2k_y}{m_{iy}} + \frac{2k_z}{m_{iz}}}. \quad (2)$$

Here,

$$m_{ij} = [(1-\rho)/\rho][2 + (2-M)(\sigma_p - \sigma_s)/\sigma_s] \quad \text{when } i = j \quad (3)$$

$$= [(1-\rho)/\rho][2 + M(\sigma_p - \sigma_s)/\sigma_s] \quad \text{when } i \neq j \quad (4)$$

$$M = [\Phi - 0.5\sin(2\Phi)]\cos\Phi/\sin^3\Phi \quad (5)$$

where $\Phi = \cos^{-1}(a/b)$ and a/b is the axis ratio of a spheroid.

When blood is quiescent, erythrocytes orient themselves at random. Because $k_x = k_y = k_z = 1/3$ and $\sigma_x = \sigma_y = \sigma_z = \sigma_r$, the conductivity σ_r is given by

$$\sigma_r = \sigma_p + \frac{\sigma_s - \sigma_p}{1 + \frac{2}{2m_{xx}} + \frac{4}{3m_{xy}}}. \quad (6)$$

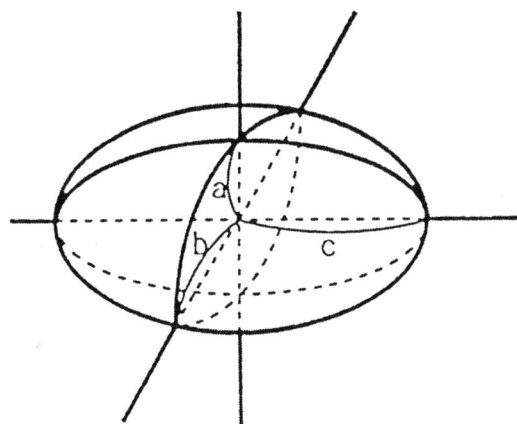

FIGURE 2. Spheroidal model of an erythrocyte—$a{:}b{:}c$ = 1:4:4.

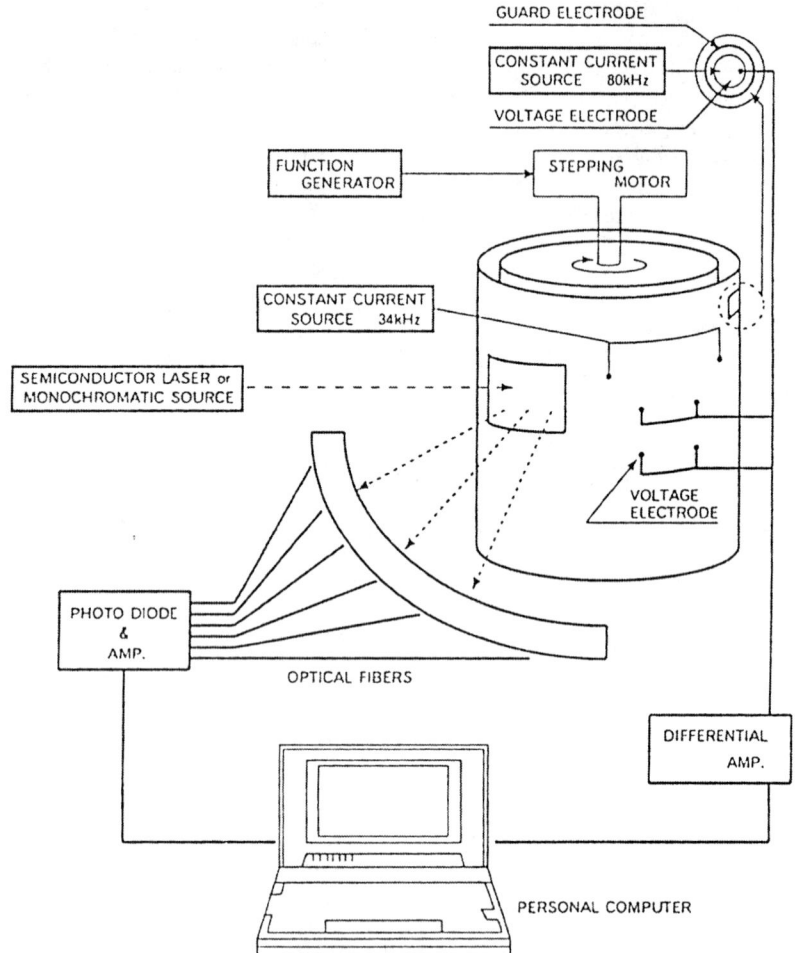

FIGURE 3. Schematic diagram of the experimental system.

At our measurement frequencies of 30 kHz and 80 kHz, $\sigma_p \ll \sigma_s$ and σ_p can be neglected. From the measurement results of σ_r, σ_x, σ_y, σ_z, the apparent orientation ratio (k_x, k_y, k_z) and the equivalent axis ratio (a/b) are calculated.

The physical properties of living tissues are quite complicated because of the inhomogeneity due to hierarchical structures of cells, tissues, and organs. The optical properties of living tissues are not yet understood well because of their complicated structure and their large scattering coefficient compared with their absorption coefficient. However, optical methods have often been used in the wide field of biomedical engineering because the absorption coefficient of visible light is very small for living tissues, except for blood. The optical properties of blood are very important not only for the development of optical methods for biomedical measurement and therapy, but also for the study of flowing blood itself. We have theoretically and experimentally discussed the optical properties of flowing blood, such as scattering, absorption, reflection, and transmission.

The scattering and absorption coefficients of blood change with the change of flow rate, just as the electrical properties of blood do. We have already reported that the intensity and the angular distribution of light scattered from flowing blood are remarkably affected by the orientation and deformation of erythrocytes due to shear flow. The cause of this phenomenon is the orientation and deformation of erythrocytes.

In this paper, in order to discuss the optical properties of flowing blood, the angular distribution of light scattered from flowing blood is measured. FIGURE 3 shows a schematic diagram of our experimental system. The flow cell is a coaxial cylindrical device in which fluid flows in the 1.4-mm space between the inner and outer cylinders. To obtain a uniform shear rate, the inner cylinder rotates to create various patterns of Couette flow, such as steady, sinusoidal, and step shape, with a stepping motor.

The directions of the three rectangular axes are shown in FIGURE 4. It is assumed that the erythrocytes orient themselves in one of the three directions, namely, the circumferential, axial, and radial directions shown in FIGURE 4.

On the inner surface of the outer cylinder, current electrodes and detecting electrodes are arranged to measure the electrical resistivities in the circumferential, axial, and radial directions. The measurement method of anisotropic resistivity will be shown elsewhere.

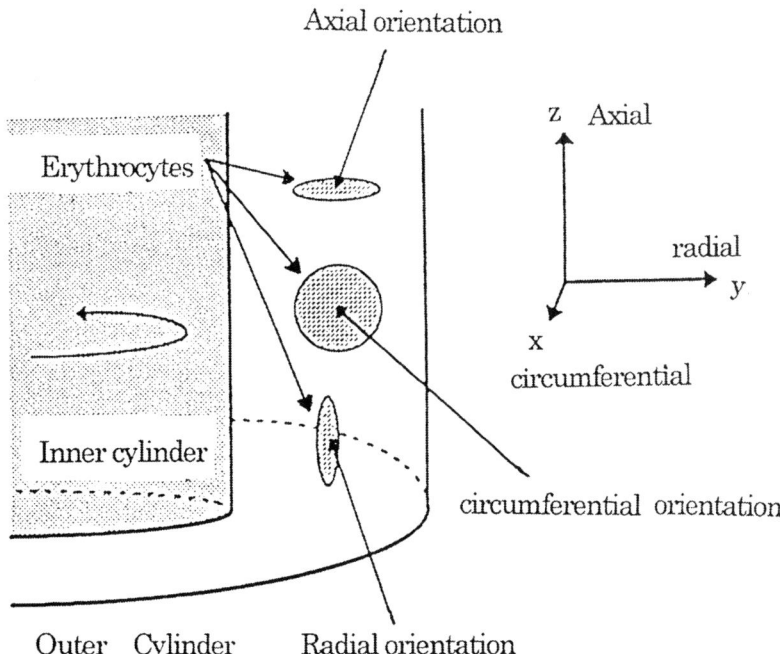

FIGURE 4. Rectangular system and orientation direction.

The frequencies of the applied electrical current are 35 kHz for the circumferential and axial measurements, and 80 kHz for the radial measurement.

For optical measurement, monochromatic light is irradiated onto blood in the cell through the transparent outer cell, and the light scattered from the blood is measured with six optical fibers arranged at scattering angles of 10, 15, 20, 25, 35, and 45 degrees to detect the angular distribution of scattering light.[8] Using this system, the electrical resistivities in the three rectangular directions and the angular distribution of the scattering light intensity are measured for various types of flow at various shear rates and for human blood of various hematocrit. From these measurement results, the orientation ratios of the three rectangular directions and the effective axis ratio of the spheroidal model are calculated.

RESULTS AND DISCUSSION

The shear rate of flow and the typical resistivity are shown in FIGURE 5 when blood flows stepwise repeatedly. The shear rates are 0 and 10 s^{-1}, and the sample is human whole blood of 45% in hematocrit.

After the blood flow stops, the resistivities in the three directions change rapidly at first, and then approach the same value obtained when the blood is at rest. After the blood flow is increased stepwise, the resistivity in the radial direction increases remarkably and then approaches a certain steady value, about a 20% increase. The change of the circum-

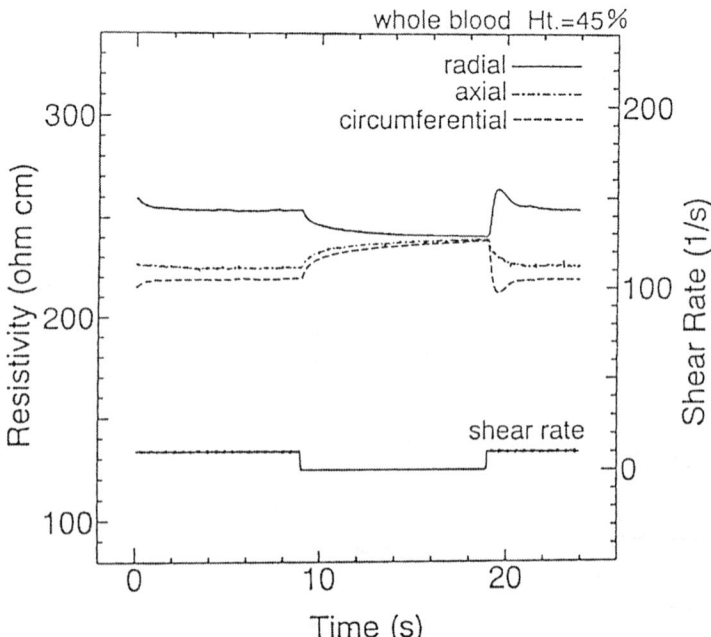

FIGURE 5. Repeated stepwise flow and measurement resistivities of three rectangular directions. Sample: whole blood of 45% hematocrit. Shear rate: 10 s^{-1}.

ferential resistivity decreases inversely to the radial one and reaches a steady value about 15% lower than the initial value. The resistivity in the axial direction decreases slowly and approaches a steady value, about 10% less. From these results, it can be seen that when blood flows, the number of radial-oriented erythrocytes will increase and circumferential ones will decrease rapidly. This means that, at first, the circumferential-oriented erythrocytes change their direction to a radial direction. Then, the axial-oriented erythrocytes increase and the proportions oriented in each direction approach steady values. After the blood stops flowing, the resistivities in the three directions approach the same initial value within a few seconds.

Some of the measurements are shown in FIGURE 6. This graph shows the relation between the shear rate and the resistivity change measured at steady states. From these measurements, it seems that the fraction of radial-oriented erythrocytes increases with the increase in shear rate. At a high shear rate, the directional resistivities approach each saturation value. The resistivity in the radial direction increases about 20% from the initial value, whereas the resistivities in the circumferential and axial directions decrease about 15% to the same saturation value.

The main causes of this resistivity change are erythrocyte orientation and deformation. Using our simplified spheroidal model for an erythrocyte, the orientation ratio and the equivalent axis ratio of the spheroid are calculated with equations 2, 5, and 6 from the measurement resistivities in the three rectangular directions and the resistivity of quiescent blood.

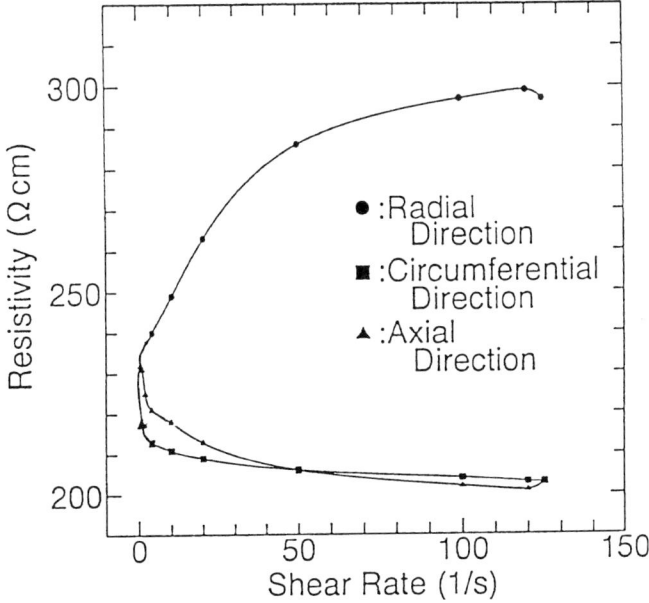

FIGURE 6. Measurement resistivity vs. shear rate of flow. Sample: whole blood of 45% hematocrit.

Some of the calculated results are shown in FIGURES 7 and 8. FIGURE 7 shows the relation between the shear rate and the calculated orientation ratio in each direction when blood flows intermittently stepwise. For blood at rest, the orientation ratio is 1/3 in all three directions.

These results show that the fractions of erythrocytes oriented in each direction change with the shear rate of flow and approach a saturation value at a rather low shear rate of about 50 s^{-1}. At the shear rate of 100 s^{-1}, the fraction of radial-oriented erythrocytes is about 74%, and those in both the circumferential and axial directions are each about 13%. These values of the orientation ratio agree well with the theoretical results.[4]

From Jeffery's equation, it would be expected that the orientation ratio is not dependent on the shear rate of flow[2,4,6] if the shape of the erythrocyte does not change due to flow. Our results suggest that the erythrocytes in flowing blood not only change their orientation, but also deform their shape.

FIGURE 8 shows some calculated results for an equivalent axis ratio of our spheroidal model of an erythrocyte. The change in the equivalent axis ratio reflects the erythrocyte deformation. The axis ratio of low hematocrit blood abruptly increases at a very low shear rate of less than 10 s^{-1}; then, it slowly increases and approaches a saturation value. The saturation axis ratio is about 0.27 for the blood of 32% in hematocrit, 0.29 for that of 45%, and 0.35 for that of 61%. The axis ratio of the spheroidal model in quiescent blood is assumed to be 0.25. The change in the axis ratio is rather small; however, this small

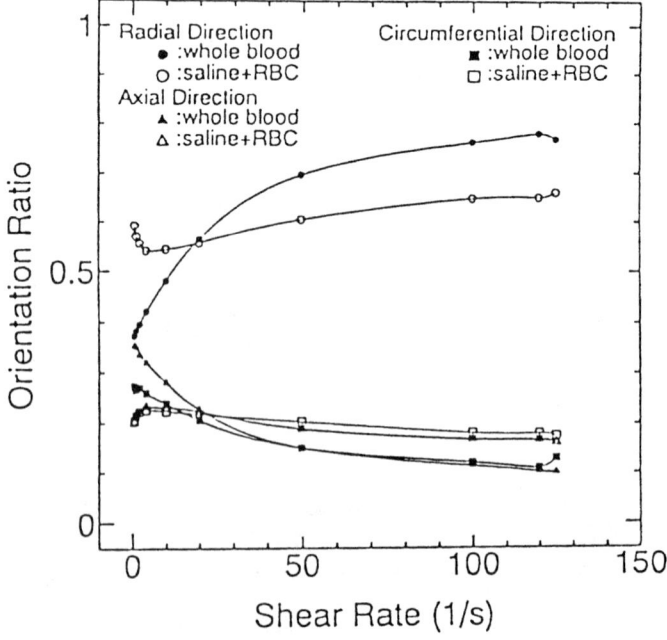

FIGURE 7. Orientation ratio vs. shear rate of flow calculated from measurement results shown in FIGURES 6 and 12.

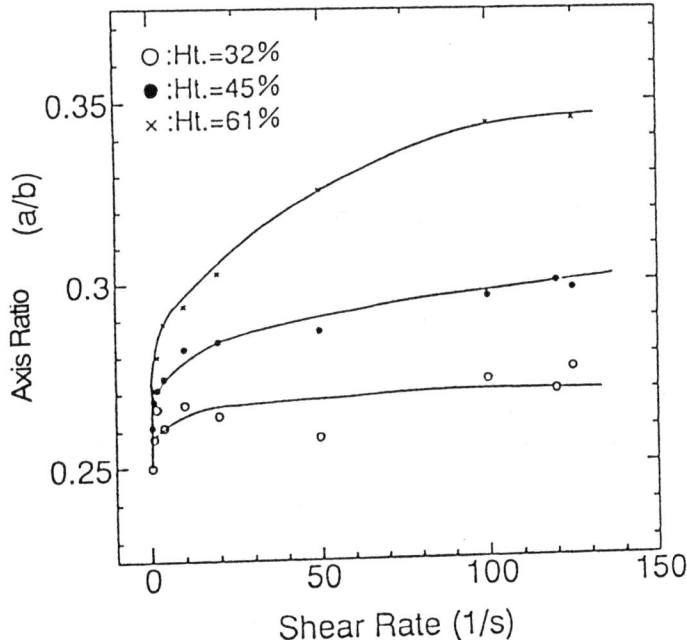

FIGURE 8. Axis ratio vs. shear rate of flow calculated from the results shown in FIGURE 6.

change causes a large change of the resistivity. FIGURE 9 shows the calculated relative change of the resistivity of quiescent blood due to the change in the axis ratio.

The light scattered from flowing blood depends on the shear rate of flow as shown in FIGURE 10. This figure shows the measurement intensity change of light scattered from flowing blood measured simultaneously with electrical resistivity.

When erythrocytes orient themselves parallel to the surface of the outer cylinder, that is, in the radial direction, the light-scattering intensity increases because of the increase of the scattering cross section.[8] Therefore, from these results, it can be concluded that the number of radial-oriented erythrocytes will increase with the increase of shear rate. These results agree well with those for electrical resistivity.

The saturation value of the scattering light intensity is about three times larger than that of quiescent blood. This remarkable increase of light-scattering intensity will be discussed elsewhere.

FIGURE 11 shows the angular distribution of light scattered from flowing blood of various hematocrit values measured simultaneously with the electrical resistivity shown in FIGURE 6. When blood is at rest, erythrocytes orient themselves at random; therefore, resting blood can be considered to be a perfect scatterer. The angular distribution of scattering light from quiescent blood gives a cosine curve, the so-called Lambertian distribution, shown by the broken line in this figure.

FIGURE 11 shows very interesting results. When blood flows, the angular distribution of light scattered from flowing blood becomes asymmetrical. The angular distribution of the light scattering depends on the angle between the measurement direction and the direction

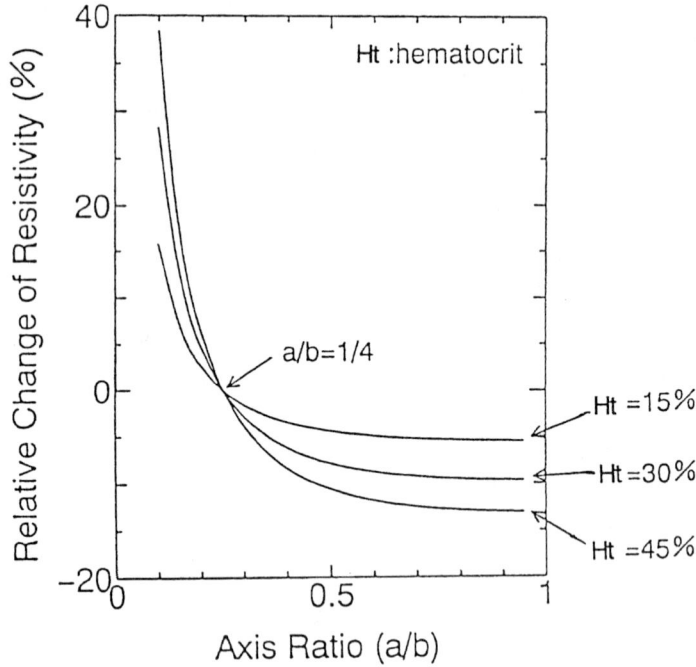

FIGURE 9. Relative resistivity change vs. axis ratio normalized by the resistivity of a spheroid of 1:4 in axis ratio.

of flow. The light scattering in the flow direction is much larger than that in the reverse direction. If the shape of the erythrocytes in flowing blood is spheroidal, the light-scattering intensities in both the flow and reverse directions should be the same. Therefore, the measurement of angular distribution shows that the shape of the erythrocytes in flowing blood is asymmetric and not spheroidal.[8]

The equivalent axis ratio calculated above is obtained under the assumption that the erythrocytes in flowing blood are spheroidal. However, the equivalent axis ratio reflects the degree of deformation and is useful in analyzing the behavior of erythrocytes in flowing blood. From the asymmetry of the angular distribution, we conclude that the erythrocytes in flowing blood not only reorient themselves, but also are deformed into some asymmetrical form shaped like a parachute. A more detailed discussion is still needed.

When the sample is a suspension of erythrocytes in saline solution, the measurements are quite different from those in a whole blood experiment. Some of the measurements are shown in FIGURE 12. This sample shows anisotropic resistivity even when the liquid is at rest. It seems that some of the erythrocytes in resting saline solution orient themselves in a radial direction because the 1.4-mm gap of the measurement cell is very narrow and the mutual force between erythrocytes in saline solution is very small. The resistivities in the axial direction are similar to those in the circumferential direction. The shear rate does not greatly affect the resistivity of the fluid.

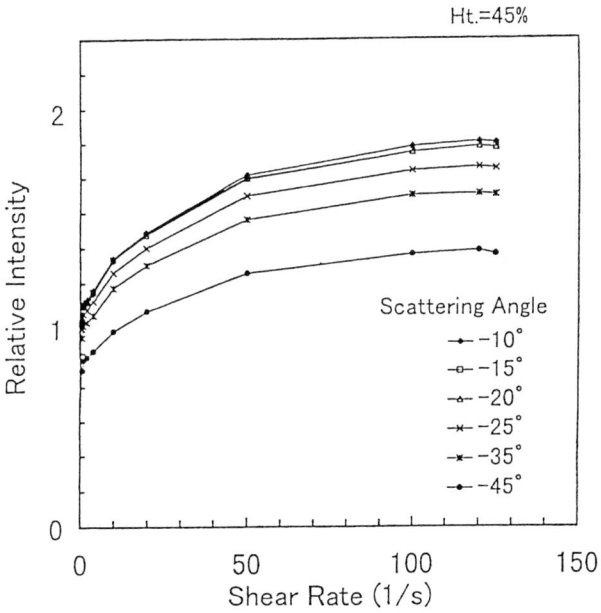

FIGURE 10. Relative intensity of scattering light vs. shear rate of flow for various scattering angles measured simultaneously with the resistivity shown in FIGURE 6.

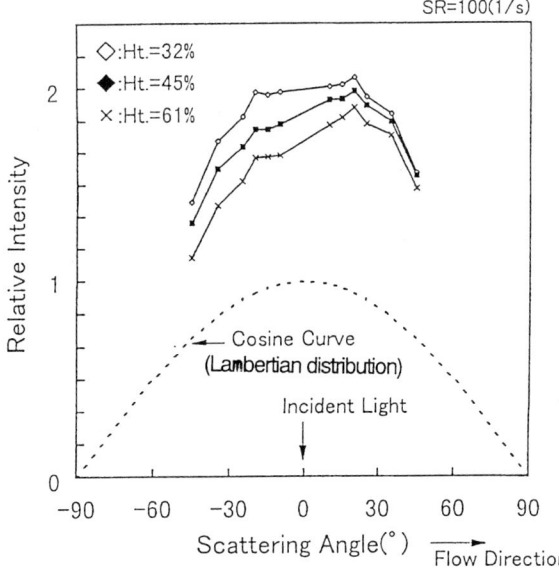

FIGURE 11. Angular distributions of scattering light from flowing blood and the Lambertian distribution.

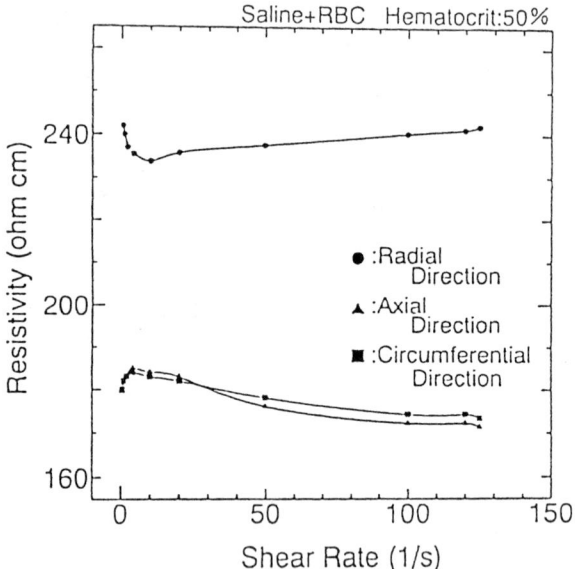

FIGURE 12. Electrical resistivity vs. shear rate. Sample: suspension of erythrocytes in saline solution. Hematocrit (Ht): 50%.

These results agree well with those obtained from optical measurements, as shown in FIGURE 13. The light-scattering intensity is very large, even when the fluid is at rest, and does not change much with the increase in the shear rate of flow. The angular distribution is almost symmetrical and is not affected much by the shear rate, as shown in FIGURE 14.

The calculated results of the orientation ratio in the three rectangular directions are shown in FIGURE 7 for comparison with whole blood. The changes of the orientation ratio for whole blood depend greatly on the shear rate; however, those erythrocyte suspensions in saline do not depend on the shear rate of flow and, even at a very low shear rate, the orientation ratio in the radial direction is very large. A detailed discussion will be given elsewhere.

When the membrane of the erythrocytes is hardened by glutaraldehyde, the measurements are quite different from those of other suspensions. The resistivities of the suspension of hardened erythrocytes in plasma, the so-called hardened blood, are shown in FIGURE 15. The resistivities of hardened blood in the three rectangular directions are almost all the same when blood is at rest, but when blood flows, even at the very small shear rate of $1\ s^{-1}$, the resistivities change abruptly to a certain value. These results agree quite well with Jeffery's theorem.[2,4,7] These results certify that the resistivity of blood is not dependent at all on the shear rate of flow if the erythrocytes in the flowing blood do not deform.

FIGURE 16 shows the angular distributions of hardened blood measured from various scattered angles. The light scattered from flowing hardened blood is independent of the shear rate. The shape of the angular distribution is symmetrical. From these results, it is assumed that the hardened erythrocytes are not deformed due to flow.

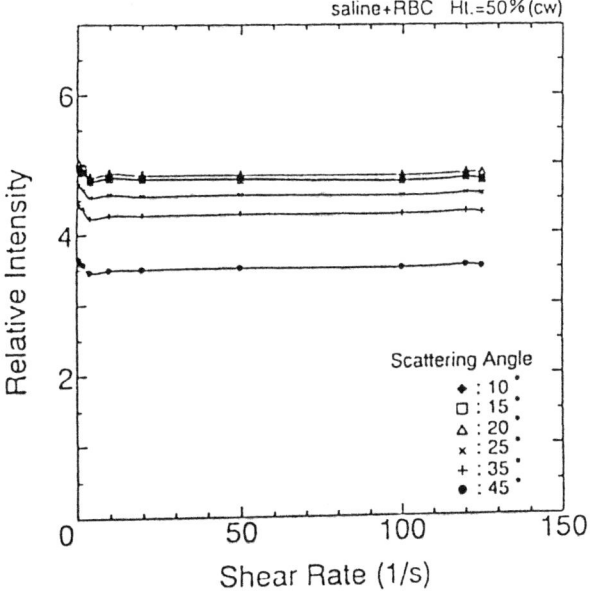

FIGURE 13. Relative intensity of scattering light vs. shear rate measured simultaneously with the resistivity shown in FIGURE 12.

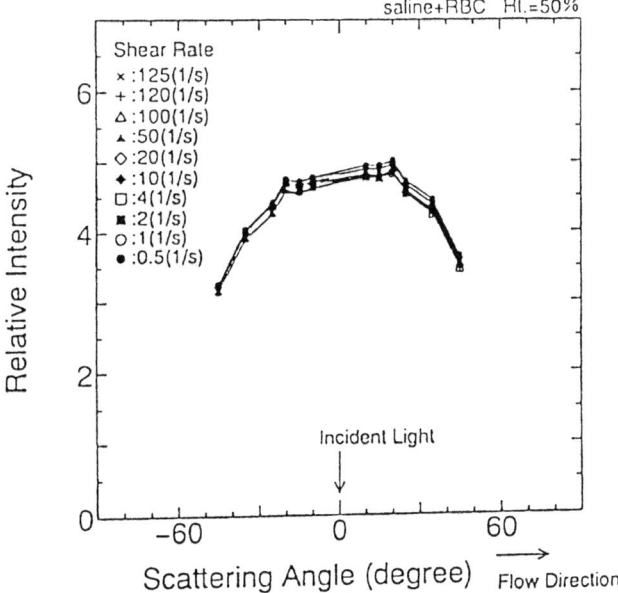

FIGURE 14. Angular distributions of scattering light calculated from FIGURE 13.

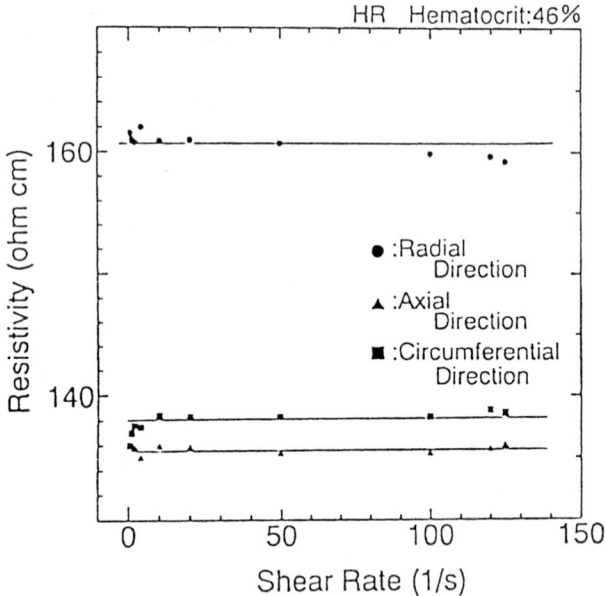

FIGURE 15. Resistivity vs. shear rate. Sample: hardened erythrocytes in plasma. Hematocrit: 46%.

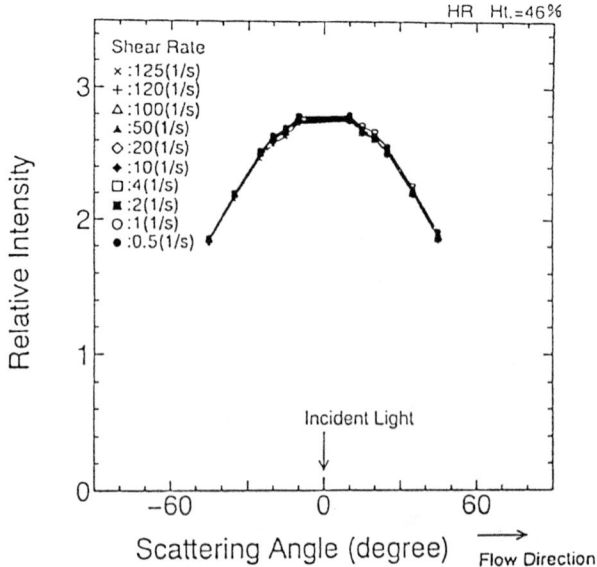

FIGURE 16. Angular distributions of hardened blood measured simultaneously with the resistivity shown in FIGURE 15.

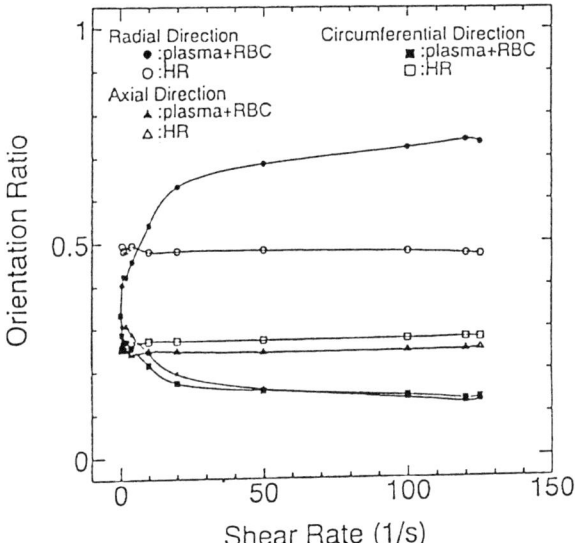

FIGURE 17. Orientation ratio of erythrocytes in whole blood and hardened blood.

The calculated results of the orientation ratio are shown in FIGURE 17 with the results obtained for a suspension of erythrocytes in plasma for comparison. The calculated results from these measurements show that the orientation ratio of hardened blood in the radial direction is about 0.48, that in the circumferential direction is about 0.28, and that in the axial direction is about 0.24. The calculated axis ratio of hardened erythrocytes is about 0.24. This value agrees quite well with the model of erythrocyte having an axis ratio of 0.25. The results calculated based on Jeffery's theorem for the orientation ratio of 0.50 in the radial direction show that the orientation ratio in the circumferential direction is 0.30 and that in the axial direction is 0.20, and the axis ratio of the spheroid is 0.35.[2,4,7] The orientation ratio and axis ratio do not change at all with the shear rate.

CONCLUSIONS

In this paper, a coaxial cylindrical-type flow cell is used to produce various patterns of uniform Couette flow such as steady, sinusoidal, and repeated stepwise flow. The electrical resistivities of flowing blood are affected by the shear rate of flow. In flowing blood, each erythrocyte rotates itself along its own constant orbit. The rotation velocity of the erythrocyte depends on the angle between the long axis of the erythrocyte and the flow direction.[2] When this angle is 90°, the velocity is fastest; when it is zero, the velocity is slowest. Although all of the erythrocytes do not effectively orient themselves in the same direction simultaneously, it seems that most of them orient themselves in the flow direction.[2,4,7]

From Jeffery's equation, it would be expected that the orientation ratio is not dependent on the shear rate of flow[2,4,6] if the shape of the erythrocyte does not change due to flow.

Our results suggest that the erythrocytes in flowing whole blood not only change their orientation, but also deform their shapes.

The resistivity in the radial direction increases with the increase of shear rate and approaches its saturation value. The resistivities in the circumferential and axial directions decrease with the increase of shear rate and approach their saturation values. The resistivity in the radial direction increases about 20% from its initial value for whole blood of 45% in hematocrit; in the circumferential and axial directions, it approaches the same saturation value, about 15% less than the initial value.

From the measurements of resistivities, the orientation ratio of erythrocytes is calculated for the three rectangular directions. At high shear rate, for whole blood of 45% in hematocrit, the fraction of radial-oriented erythrocytes is about 75% and that of both circumferential- and axial-oriented erythrocytes is 13%. The equivalent axis ratio for the spheroidal model of an erythrocyte is also calculated from the measurements.

The light scattered from flowing blood also increases with the increase of shear rate and approaches a saturation value. It seems that the ratio of the erythrocytes parallel to the surface of the measurement cell increases with the increase in shear rate and increases the scattering cross section of blood.

The angular distribution of light scattered from flowing whole blood depends on the angle between the measurement direction and the flow direction, and shows an asymmetrical shape. These results suggest to us that the erythrocytes in flowing whole blood are deformed asymmetrically. In this paper, the erythrocyte is simulated as a spheroid. Since a spheroid is symmetrical, this model is inconsistent with the results obtained by optical measurements. Although this model is not suitable for an erythrocyte in flowing blood, the orientation ratio and axis ratio are easily calculated from the measurements of resistivity and reflect the orientation and deformation of erythrocytes in flowing blood. These parameters are useful in understanding the behavior of erythrocytes in flowing blood because these phenomena can be attributed to the orientation and deformation of erythrocytes due to flow.

When the sample is the suspension of erythrocytes in saline solution, quite different results are obtained. It seems that some of the erythrocytes in a quiescent saline solution orient themselves in the radial direction, when the gap of the measurement cell is very narrow, because the mutual force between erythrocytes in saline solution is very small.

To confirm Jeffery's theorem, the resistivity of hardened blood and the light scattered from hardened blood are measured at various shear rates. The measurements show that both the resistivity and the light intensity do not depend on the shear rate for hardened blood. This means that the resistivity and the light scattered from hardened blood change at a very low shear rate, less than 1 s^{-1}, and keep a constant value up to a high shear rate.

From the above results, it is concluded that Jeffery's theorem is valid for the analysis of flowing blood if the erythrocytes are not deformed due to flow. A more detailed discussion will be given elsewhere.

REFERENCES

1. SCHWAN, H.P. 1959. Alternating current spectroscopy of biological substances. Proc. IRE **47:** 1841–1855.
2. JEFFERY, G.B. 1922. The motion of ellipsoidal particles immersed in a viscous fluid. Proc. R. Soc. Lond. **A102:** 161–179.

3. FRICKE, H. 1924. A mathematical treatment of the electric conductivity and capacity of disperse systems. Phys. Rev. **24:** 575–587.
4. SAKAMOTO, K. & H. KANAI. 1979. Electrical characteristics of flowing blood. IEEE Trans. Biomed. Eng. **BME-26:** 686–695.
5. NINOMIYA, N. et al. 1988. Physical properties of flowing blood. Biorheology **25:** 319–328.
6. DELLIMORE, J.W. & R.G. GOSLING. 1973. Use of electrical conductance measurements in studies of the orientation of microscopic particles in stationary and flowing suspensions. J. Appl. Phys. **44:** 5599–5606.
7. EDGERTON, R.H. 1974. Conductivity of sheared suspension of ellipsoidal particles with application to blood flow. IEEE Trans. Biomed. Eng. **BME-21:** 33–43.
8. KANAI, H., M. FUJII, M. YOSHIDA, F. MASUJIMA & K. SAKAMOTO. 1996. Optical properties of steadily and sinusoidally flowing blood. In Proceedings of the Tenth Nordic-Baltic Conference on BME, p. 167–168.

On the Limits of Ellipsoidal Models when Analyzing Dielectric Behavior of Living Cells

Emphasis on Red Blood Cells

EUGEN GHEORGHIU

NIB-UNESCO Center for Biodynamics, Calea Plevnei 46-48, 77102 Bucharest 1, Romania

ABSTRACT: The dielectric behavior of red blood cells is simulated by taking into account the real shape (consistent with microscopic observations) and the ellipsoids (prolate and oblate spheroids) having the same surface and volume. We have pointed out that the spectra of the imaginary versus the real part of polarizability, which can be directly derived from the measured data, provide quantitative insight to cell morphology. We emphasize that ellipsoidal approximation is fairly good for random oriented cells, but rather poor whenever oriented cells are measured. This fact is assumed to be the reason for the differences between the reported parameters derived from measurements on single cells and those from observations on (random oriented) cells in suspension.

INTRODUCTION

In view of the virtues of dielectric spectroscopy to reveal cell morphology, as well as the challenging applications to hematology, we endeavored to investigate the extent to which information on cell shape is able to be provided by this technique.

Theoretical and computational difficulties restricted the treatment of dielectric behavior of nonspherical cells mainly to ellipsoidal models (described by analytical expressions; e.g., see reference 1). Recently, we have developed a new procedure able to describe the dielectric properties of a wider class of shapes (not necessarily spheroids) (see reference 2).

This study emphasizes the results of applying this procedure on red blood cells, with shapes consistent with microscopic observations.

THEORY

To compute the dielectric spectra, we have used the theory described in reference 2.

We consider a regular distribution of particles; that is, the suspension is equivalent to a rectangular lattice containing one cell (of volume V_c) in the center of each element.

A uniform electrical field, $\vec{E}_0 = E_0\vec{N}$, is applied to the entire ensemble. Suspension permittivity (ε_{sus}) relates the volume averages of the displacement (D) and electrical field:

$$\langle \vec{D} \rangle = \varepsilon_{sus} \langle \vec{E} \rangle. \qquad (1)$$

Suspension permittivity is derived using the mean field method, taking into account the mutual dipole-dipole interaction between suspended particles.

The electrical field is assumed to exhibit the same distribution regardless of the lattice unit emplacement. The total electrical field is given by means of two sources:

$$E = E_e + E_1 \Rightarrow \langle E_e \rangle = \langle E \rangle - \langle E_1 \rangle \tag{2}$$

where E_e denotes the effective field due to the external sources (including the dipoles of the particles outside the respective lattice unit), while E_1 represents the electrical field of the dipole induced by cell polarization in the effective field. Thus,

$$\varepsilon^*_{sus} \cdot \langle \vec{E} \rangle =$$

$$\frac{1}{V}\int_V \varepsilon^* \vec{E} dV \Rightarrow (\varepsilon^*_{sus} - \varepsilon^*_0) \cdot \langle \vec{E} \rangle = E_e \cdot p \cdot \varepsilon^*_0 \cdot \underbrace{\frac{1}{V_p}\frac{1}{4\pi}\int_{V_p}\int_\Omega \frac{\varepsilon^* - \varepsilon^*_0}{\varepsilon^*_0} \cdot \frac{\vec{E}\cdot\vec{N}}{E_e} dV \cdot d\Omega}_{\alpha} \tag{3}$$

where α denotes the particle's polarizability.

Considering the field-induced polarization, we have

$$\varepsilon_{sus} = \frac{\langle P \rangle}{\langle E \rangle} + \varepsilon_0. \tag{4}$$

Here, P stands for the polarization due to the effective field in the center of the lattice element:

$$\langle P \rangle = \varepsilon_0 \cdot \alpha \cdot E_e \big|_c \cdot \frac{V_c}{V}; \quad \langle E_1 \rangle = -\frac{C}{\varepsilon_0} \cdot \langle P \rangle \tag{5}$$

where C is the interaction constant; in dipole approximation, $C = 1/3$ for spheres in a periodic lattice. For a low concentration of suspended particles, we assumed that C has the same value regardless of the particle shape. Consequently, one obtains

$$\frac{1}{V_p}\int_{V_p} \vec{E}_1 \, dV = -(1/3)p\alpha\vec{E}_e \Rightarrow \langle \vec{E} \rangle = [1 - (1/3)p\alpha] \cdot E_e. \tag{6}$$

Subsequently, the suspension permittivity is given by

$$\varepsilon^*_{sus} = \varepsilon^*_0 \cdot \left[1 + p \cdot \frac{\alpha}{1 - p \cdot \left(\frac{\alpha}{3}\right)}\right]; \quad \varepsilon^* = \varepsilon + \frac{\kappa}{j\omega \cdot \varepsilon_v} \tag{7}$$

where p represents the volume fraction, ε^*_0 stands for the complex permittivity of the medium, ε_v is the dielectric constant of the vacuum, and α is the polarizability specific to the respective shape and electrical properties.

The problem is to find a proper way to compute the polarizability of an arbitrarily shaped particle. To do this, we have derived the field distribution in relation to the effective electrical field. Single-layer potential has been considered. By assuming the usual boundary conditions, we have obtained an integral equation for the surface charge distributions. The key idea for solving the integral equation is to transform it into an algebraic one using decomposition on the eigenvectors of the integral operator. Based on these ideas, we have developed a homemade algorithm able to provide cell polarizability for shelled particles with a shape exhibiting axial symmetry.

Aiming to describe the dielectric (β_1) dispersion of red blood cells, we have considered the shapes given by the following expression (consistent with reference 3):

$$R[x] = \sqrt{-A \cdot \cos[2x] + \sqrt{C^2 - (A \cdot \sin[2x])^2}}; \quad A = \frac{(d^2 - t^2)}{8}; \quad C = \frac{(d^2 + t^2)}{8} \tag{8}$$

TABLE 1. Red Blood Cell Parameters

No.	d (μm)	t (μm)
1	7	0.8
2	7.5	0.9
3	8	1

where d is the diameter and t is the least thickness of the actual red blood cell.

Three shapes (corresponding to the values given in TABLE 1) and the sphere with a radius $R_s = 3.356$ μm have been considered (FIGURE 1).

In our present application, we have considered shelled particles (membrane thickness = 10^{-2} μm) with the following values for the electrical parameters: $\varepsilon_{in}^* = 70.1 - 0.2/(\varepsilon_v w)$, $\varepsilon_{shell}^* = 12$, $\varepsilon_0^* = 78 - 0.377/(\varepsilon_v w)$, and $p = 0.5 V_{shape}/(4\pi/3 R_s^3)$; that is, for all shapes, the

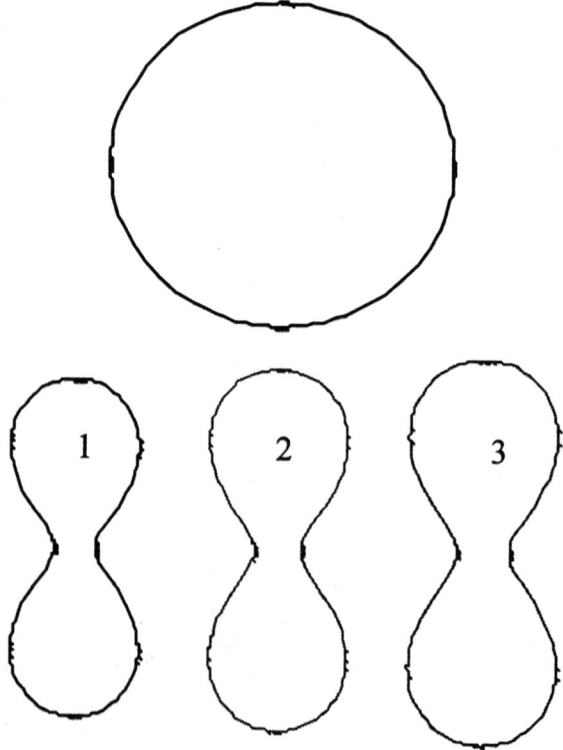

FIGURE 1. The shapes (1–3) considered for the red blood cells and the sphere with a similar surface.

same number of cells have been considered. The dielectric behaviors of the prolate and oblate spheroids, having the same volume and surface as the actual red blood cell, have been computed and compared with the spectra of the real shapes.

RESULTS

FIGURE 2 shows the permittivity spectra for suspensions of random oriented cells with shapes given by the parameters in TABLE 1. It is worth noting that the dielectric spectra are distinct for each shape. However, the dielectric behavior for oblate spheroids is similar to that derived from the "real" shape consistent with equation 8.

It is worth emphasizing that the imaginary versus the real part of the polarizability, α in equation 7, does not depend on the cell volume fraction and might be straightforwardly derived from experimental data.[4] This representation has the advantage of being more sensitive to shape than the permittivity spectra. FIGURE 3 shows the $Im[\alpha]/Re[\alpha]$ spectra of shape 2 and the corresponding spheroids for random oriented cells.

Aiming to find out if impedance spectroscopy is able to provide more detailed information, that is, to "see" the difference between the real red blood cells and the related oblate spheroids, we have considered suspension of oriented (not random) cells.

The permittivity spectra for shape 1 and the corresponding oblate spheroid when the electric field is perpendicular to the cell rotation axes are plotted in FIGURE 4.

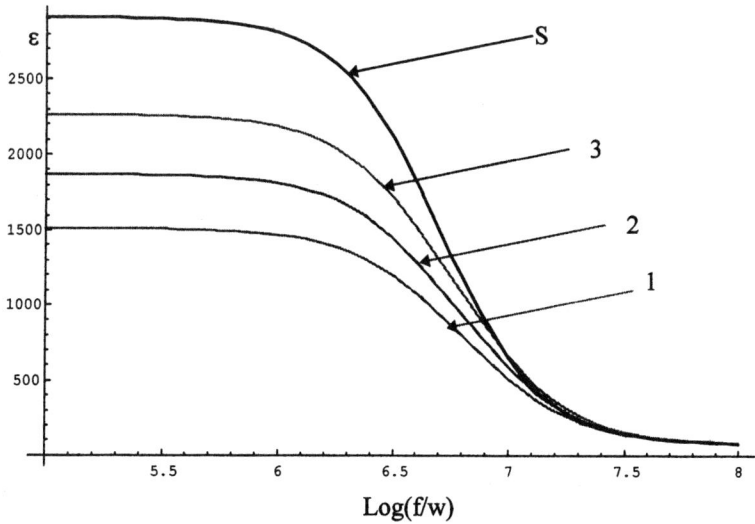

FIGURE 2. The permittivity spectra of three red blood cells (1–3) and the sphere (S).

266   **ANNALS NEW YORK ACADEMY OF SCIENCES**

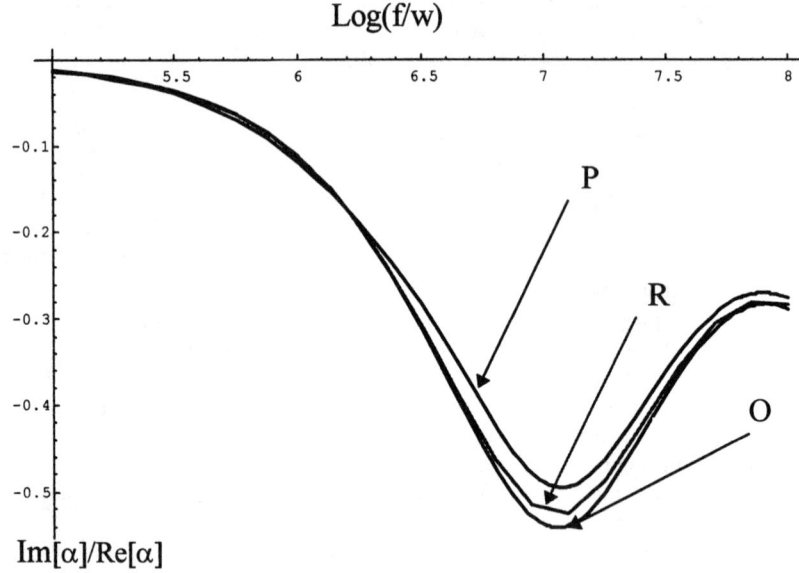

FIGURE 3. Spectra of $Im[\alpha]/Re[\alpha]$: R, suspensions of red blood cells with shape 2; P and O, suspensions of the corresponding prolate and oblate spheroids, respectively.

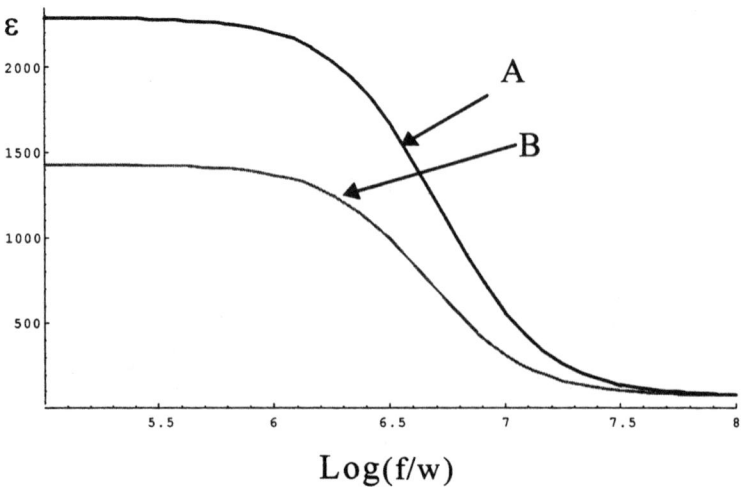

FIGURE 4. The permittivity spectra for (A) shape 1 and (B) the corresponding oblate spheroid.

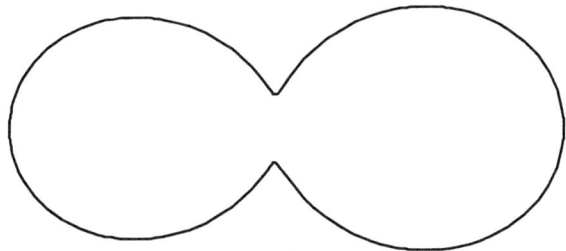

FIGURE 5. Budding yeast slightly before cell splitting.

DISCUSSION

Dielectric spectroscopy is able to reveal subtle information on living cell shape, especially when measurements on oriented cells are available. In the case of red blood cells, ellipsoidal models should be considered only for random oriented cells, with the challenging exception of spectra of $\text{Im}[\alpha]/\text{Re}[\alpha]$.

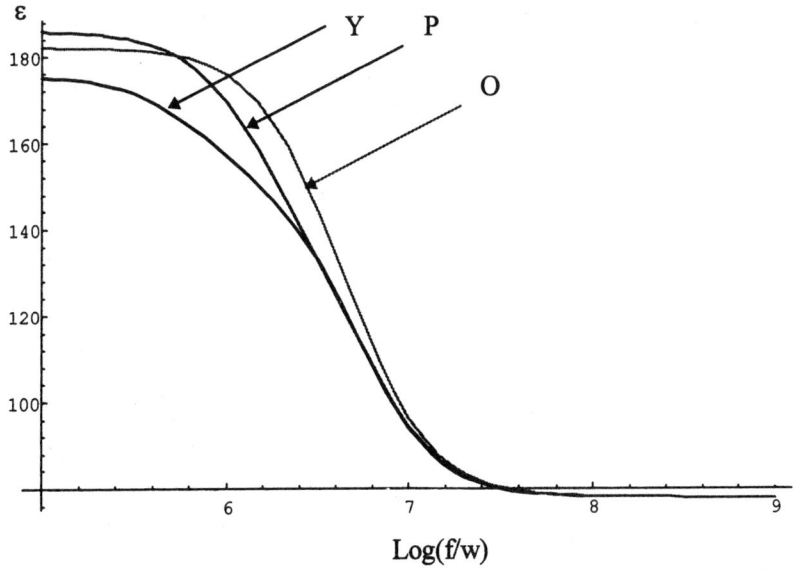

FIGURE 6. Permittivity spectra: suspensions of budding yeasts, Y (prototype shown in FIGURE 5), and of the related oblate, O, and prolate, P, spheroids.

We emphasize that ellipsoidal approximation is fairly good for random oriented cells, but rather poor whenever oriented cells are measured. This fact is assumed to be the reason for the differences between the reported parameters derived from measurements on single cells and those from observations on (random oriented) cells in suspension. It is worth emphasizing that the fitted plots (using spheroid models) could nicely match the experimental data on nonspherical cells, but the relevance of the derived parameters should be carefully considered.

However, for other types of nonspheroidal cells, even for suspensions of arbitrarily oriented cells, ellipsoidal approaches should be carefully considered. The differences between the permittivity spectra computed for the budding yeast (FIGURE 5) and the related prolate and oblate spheroids are revealed in FIGURE 6.

REFERENCES

1. ASAMI, K., T. HANAI & N. KOIZUMI. 1980. Dielectric approach to suspensions of ellipsoidal particles covered with a shell in particular reference to biological cells. Jpn. J. Appl. Phys. **19:** 359–365.
2. VRINCEANU, D. & E. GHEORGHIU. 1996. Shape effects on the dielectric behaviour of arbitrarily shaped particles with particular reference to biological cells. Bioelectrochem. Bioenerg. **40:** 167–170.
3. VAYO, W.H. & M.K. SHIBATA. 1982. Numerical results on red blood cell geometry. Jpn. J. Physiol. **32:** 891–894.
4. GHEORGHIU, E. & K. ASAMI. 1998. Monitoring cell cycle by impedance spectroscopy: experimental and theoretical aspects. Bioelectrochem. Bioenerg. **45:** 139–143.

Electrical Impedance Tomography Study of Biological Processes in a Single Cell

TERRY C. CHILCOTT AND HANS G. L. COSTER[a]

UNESCO Center for Membrane Science and Technology and Department of Biophysics, School of Physics, University of New South Wales, Sydney 2052, Australia

ABSTRACT: An *in vivo* electrical impedance tomography (EIT) study of single plant cells of *Chara corallina* is reported. When these aquatic cells grow in alkaline conditions, proton-translocating ATP synthases in the plasma membrane operate in reverse, utilizing ATP to translocate protons against an electrochemical gradient to the periplasm and creating localized acidic regions along the cell's cylindrical surface. These acidic regions, which appear as radial bands, ~5 mm long, between narrower alkaline bands, facilitate the uptake of bicarbonate, the plant's source of inorganic carbon for photosynthesis in the carbon dioxide–depleted alkaline conditions. Our EIT study of cell ultrastructure in the acidic and alkaline regions provides evidence that the plasma membrane is folded in localized regions (e.g., charasomes) in the acidic bands. The very low frequency capacitance dispersions were very similar to those of double fixed-charge structures. Such charge distributions are known to be present in the membrane-bound F_0 portion of the ATP synthase. The theoretical dependence of the fixed-charge concentrations on pH in the proteins is shown to broadly account for the observed correlations between pH, membrane potential, conductance, and capacitance in these regions. In synthetically formed double fixed-charge membranes, electric field–induced dissociation of water into H^+ and OH^- occurs. This leads to the speculation that H^+/OH^- fluxes in ATP synthases located in the alkaline regions of *Chara* cells might also involve the electric field–induced dissociation of water.

INTRODUCTION

Electrochemical Physiology of the Characeae Family

Since the diffusion coefficient for carbon dioxide (CO_2) in water is some five orders of magnitude slower than that in the gas phase and since aquatic plants are surrounded by unstirred layers, only turbulent and slightly acidic streams can supply carbon dioxide fast enough to support photosynthesis in some aquatic plants. In eutrophic waters, especially when stagnant, bicarbonate (HCO_3^-) is usually abundant; however, unlike carbon dioxide, it is not available directly for photosynthesis as it has a low permeability in the plasma membrane.[1] Nonetheless, many aquatic plants can utilize bicarbonate via an active uptake mechanism.

In highly alkaline eutrophic waters, the *Characeae* family of water plants supplies metabolic energy to drive the proton-translocating ATP synthases in reverse for establishing localized acidic regions along the cylindrical cellular surfaces and thereby increasing rates of bicarbonate uptake. The interconversion reaction between bicarbonate and carbon dioxide in water is

---

[a]To whom all correspondence should be addressed.

$$H_2CO_3 \Leftrightarrow H^+ + HCO_3^- \Leftrightarrow CO_2 + OH^- \quad (1)$$

and shows how local acidic conditions and an abundance of bicarbonate favor the conversion of bicarbonate into carbon dioxide, which is permeable in the plasma membrane. In some cells, the presence of the enzyme carbonic anhydrase catalyzes the reaction

$$H_2CO_3 \Leftrightarrow CO_2 + H_2O \quad (2)$$

and has been shown to play a role in bicarbonate uptake in some unicellular algae. An active mechanism has also been proposed for bicarbonate uptake[2] and is similarly dependent on the establishment of a pH gradient across the plasma membrane.

Single cells of the *Chara* genus are cylindrical with diameters of 1–2 mm and lengths reaching 150–200 mm. For survival in alkaline conditions (~pH 9.5), these cells develop unique, intricate, membranous globular organelles called charasomes that are 0.5–1 μm in diameter and that consist internally of three-dimensional branched tubular invaginations of the plasma membrane (see first inset of FIGURE 1). Electron micrograph studies have revealed that these charasomes are found at higher densities in acidic regions[3] and, significantly, high densities have been correlated with high rates of bicarbonate uptake,[4] presumably because plasma membrane folding in charasomes further concentrates ATP synthase activity in the acidic regions to offset the extreme alkaline conditions elsewhere in the bathing media.

Associated with the pH gradients along the cylindrical surfaces of *Chara* cells are large electrical currents that generally emanate from acidic regions and terminate in alkaline regions. The cell generate electrical potential differences along the surface between these regions that drive these currents. The electrical potential differences can be measured most effectively with a movable water-film electrode[5] that makes contact with the surface of a vertically mounted cell exposed to moist air (FIGURE 1). Although exposure to air removes the main electrical connection between the acid and alkaline regions and significantly reduces the current magnitudes that can flow along the surface of the cell through the cell

FIGURE 1. Longitudinal cross section of the cylindrical *Chara* cell and schematic of the water-film apparatus. Shown are the circulating H^+/OH^- electric currents that emerge from the cell in acidic regions and reenter in alkaline regions. The main difference between the ultrastructure in the acidic and alkaline regions is the predominant presence of charasomes in the acidic regions. Charasomes are intricate, highly ordered globular structures (0.5–1 mm in diameter) in which there is a network of branched tubular (~50 nm long by ~30 nm in diameter) invaginations of the plasma membrane[3] (see first inset). The second inset depicts the plasma membrane-bound (F_0) portion of an ATP synthase and a proposed distribution of charged acidic amino acids.[17] The water film was supported by the cell and an agar-coated Ag/AgCl circular electrode attached to a movable rod, which in turn was attached to a computer-controlled linear stepping motor (not shown) capable of positioning the film at any longitudinal position along the cell to within a 0.1-mm accuracy. The top of the cell was submerged in artificial pond water (APW) in a chamber with a flexible silicone rubber disk bottom. The cell protruded through a small hole (~0.5 mm in diameter) in the disk which formed a watertight seal around the cell and supported it in a vertical position. The lower portion of the cell was confined in a chamber that was flooded for 30–45 minutes with APW in between electrical measurements. During measurements, the chamber was drained, leaving the lower tip of the cell emersed in APW. Alternating current, $i_0 \sin(\omega t)$, used for impedance measurements, was injected into the cell via the water film (arrows) and a reference electrode located in the lower solution. The ac electrical potential was measured with a separate Ag/AgCl electrode located in the water film and a reference electrode located in the upper solution. The electrodes were connected to a computer-controlled digital impedance spectrometer[11] (not shown).

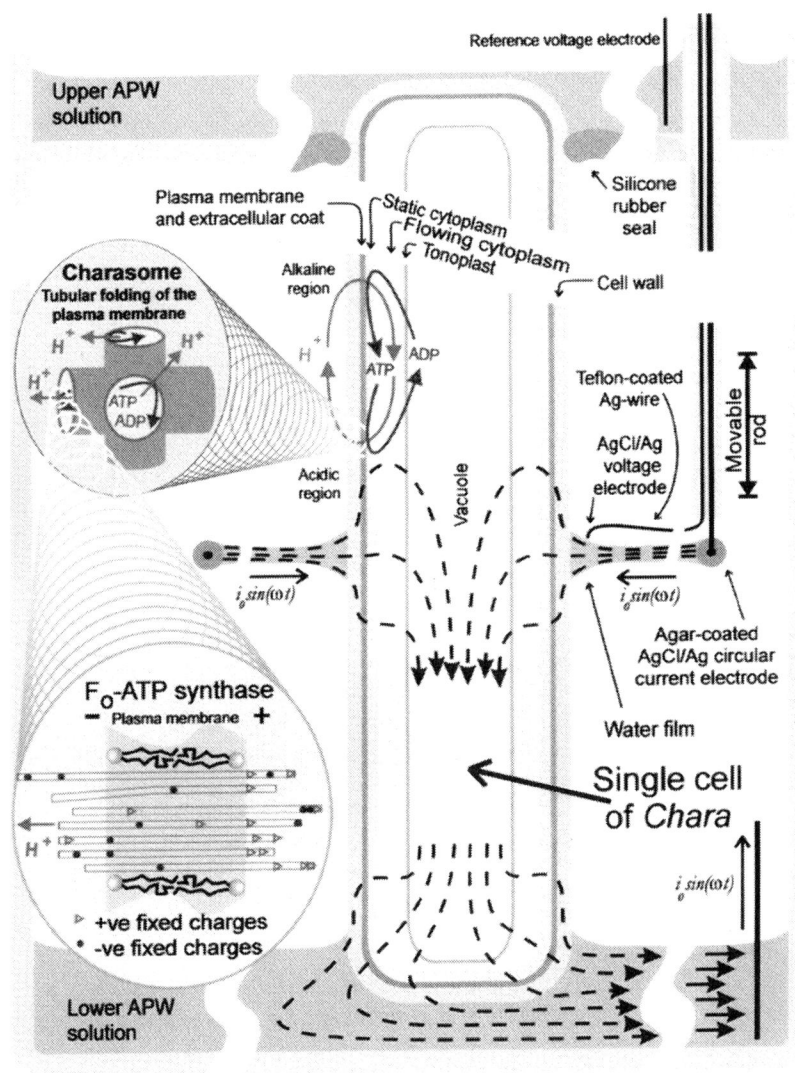

wall, it facilitates the measurement of the "open circuit" potential differences that drive the currents in aquatic conditions. The electric potential of the acid region is positive with respect to adjacent alkaline regions. In these experiments, the "open circuit" potential difference was on some occasions as large as 50 mV (e.g., see FIGURE 4).

Electrical Impedance Tomography

Early biophysics studies[6] utilized impedance techniques to establish the ubiquitous presence of the membrane surrounding biological cells and to provide the first estimate of membrane thickness. Our impedance spectroscopy studies have focused on noninvasive, high-resolution studies of reconstituted bimolecular lipid membranes[7] and the determination of cell ultrastructure, such as that of the giant *Chara* cell.[8] In order to observe spatial differences in the ultrastructure, we obtained impedance spectra at various longitudinal positions along this cell's cylindrical surface using our version of the "Ogata water-film electrode apparatus"[5] (FIGURE 1). The spectra revealed differences in radial ultrastructure (first inset of FIGURE 1) as well as differences in the electrical properties of the plasma membrane that correlated with a proposed fixed-charge structure for the membrane-bound F_0 portion of the ATP synthase (second inset of FIGURE 1). This structure is analogous to that of polymer bipolar membranes. Under appropriate nonequilibrium conditions, bipolar membranes also exhibit proton-translocating properties that have their origin[9] in the electric field–induced dissociation of water into H^+ and OH^-.

MATERIALS AND METHODS

Electrophysiology and Apparatus

A detailed description of the water-film apparatus and physiological protocols has been published[10] and we only describe the principles of operation such as are illustrated in FIGURE 1.

The cell was held vertically by a silicone rubber disk clamped in a cylindrical Perspex chamber that contained moist air during impedance measurements, but was at other times kept flooded with artificial pond water (APW: 1 mM NaCl, 0.1 mM KCl, 0.5 mM $CaCl_2$, 2 mM Hepes, pH 7). The water film was formed by dipping an agar-coated Ag/AgCl circular electrode into the APW solution, into which the bottom of the cell was immersed throughout the experiment.

FIGURE 1 shows that the film and the lower solution provided the necessary electrical connections to the cell for injecting ac current used for the impedance measurements. Since the ac current was injected into the lower portion of the cell below the film, the measured ac electrical potential could only arise from ac current injected radially into the cell via the film. Hence, the measured impedance was that for the region of the cell directly in contact with the film and for regions in very close proximity where the injected current could leak along the cell-wall surface before flowing radially into the cell.

The electrical leakage along the cell wall is analogous to that which occurs during electrical transmission along coaxial cables. The consequence of the cell's cable properties was that the effective surface area of the cell involved in the impedance measurements was always larger than the actual area in contact with the film. We adapted the cable property theory to determine the effective area of the measurement for cells whose electrical properties were not spatially uniform. The theory, thus so modified, was tested using numerical simulations of measurements on model cells with highly nonuniform properties.[11] The tests confirmed that it was possible to determine the effective area of the measurement and that the experimental apparatus had ample spatial resolution to identify acidic and alkaline regions.

Impedance Spectroscopy

Impedance measurements were made by injecting a very small alternating current (ac) of known amplitude i_0 and frequency ω radially into the cell at a particular longitudinal position. The amplitude[b] v_0 and the phase ϕ of the concomitant ac electrical potential that develops across the cell were monitored with a separate electrode immersed in the water film. The impedance magnitude and phase are given by v_0/i_0 and ϕ, respectively. Here, we choose to express impedance in terms of conductance [$G(\omega) = i_0 \cos \phi / v_0$] and susceptance [$S(\omega) = -i_0 \sin \phi / v_0$], which are, respectively, the real and imaginary parts of the admittance or the reciprocal of the impedance. The capacitance [$C(\omega) = S(\omega)/\omega$] can be readily calculated from the susceptance.

Impedance Model for a Folded Layer

For a homogeneous layer of thickness t, the conductance and capacitance per unit area are

$$g = \alpha \frac{\sigma}{t} \quad \text{and} \quad c = \alpha \frac{\varepsilon}{t}, \tag{3}$$

respectively, where σ and ε are constants in ω and characterize the electric conduction and charge-storing capacitive properties of the material comprising the layer, and α is an area factor that is either unity, if the layer is flat, or greater than unity, if the layer is folded. The impedance of the layer of material is

$$z = \frac{1}{g + j\omega c}. \tag{4}$$

At sufficiently high frequencies, a heterogeneous system can be modeled as several layers of material in series, in which case the total impedance is the sum of the impedances of the individual layers. An approach for analyzing impedance spectra that applies generally for all frequencies is to determine the transfer function of the system. This has the form

$$TF_N(s) = \sum_{n=1}^{N} \frac{r_n}{\omega_n + s} \tag{5}$$

where r_n are the residues of the function, ω_n are the frequency constants (reciprocal time constants) of the system, and s is the Laplace variable, which for impedance measurements equals the complex angular frequency $j\omega$ (cf. equations 4 and 5 for $N = 1$).

It should be pointed out that contributions to the transfer function are not restricted to the elements arising purely from the presence of layers of materials.

---

[b]This was always less than 10 mV, too small to induce an action potential or to interfere with electrophysiological processes occurring in the cell.

Impedance Model for a Double Fixed-Charge Module

Consider a module of total width w consisting of two juxtaposed regions with fixed charge of opposite sign, but with the same dielectric permittivity ε_l. If the diffusion constant D for anions and cations is the same throughout the module and the concentration for the fixed charges C_{fix} is also the same, then Nernst-Planck theory gives the conductivity for either the positive or negative fixed-charge region as

$$\sigma_l \approx \frac{q^2 D C_{fix}}{kT}. \qquad (6)$$

However, when these regions are in tight opposition to each other, ions preferentially permeate those regions with a fixed charge that is opposite in sign to their own charge. Thus, the concentration of a particular ionic species will be enhanced in one region, but depressed in the other, and vice versa for species of opposite charge. At the junction of these juxtaposed regions, a localized layer is then established that is depleted of ions of either charge (see FIGURE 2). Since there are very few ions in this layer to neutralize the fixed charges, there is a net charge distribution that gives rise to an electrical potential difference V_d across the depletion layer. If we assume that the boundary of the depletion layer is sharp, then Gauss' law yields the width of the layer, which is given by

$$\lambda = \sqrt{\frac{\varepsilon V_d}{4 q C_{fix}}}. \qquad (7)$$

The theoretical conductivity for this layer[12] is approximately

$$\sigma_d \approx 2\sigma_l \sqrt{\frac{kT}{qV_d}} e^{\frac{-qV_d}{kT}} \qquad (8)$$

and is orders of magnitude less than σ_l and, at low frequencies, largely determines the total conductance of the system, which is approximately σ_d/λ. This layer has a capacitance ε_l/λ that is very large since λ is very small ($< w$). Thus, its impedance will diminish as the

FIGURE 2. Howitt and Cox's proposed arrangement of transmembrane segments for the F_0-ATP synthase depicting a double fixed-charge structure.[17] Transmembrane helices of F_0 form a core of a and b subunits surrounded by a ring of c subunits (a, b, and c are present in a stoichiometry of 1:2:6–12). Only one c subunit is shown. The b subunit helices (not shown) do not possess charged residues, but are required for the binding of F_1 to F_0. Structures for F_0 have been formulated by considering hydrophobicity plots and functional studies involving site-directed substitution experiments. Proposed structures for b and c, which identify helices that form the proton pore, are well accepted.[16] Replacement of lysine for R210 completely prevents proton translocation, suggesting a functional role for the double fixed-charge structure. Positive ions (cations) preferentially permeate the region, which has a net negative charge, and vice versa for negative ions (anions). The ionic concentration profiles show that a region develops toward the center of the membrane where ions with a charge of either sign are depleted. V_d is the electric potential that develops across the depletion layer. This contributes to the membrane potential, which is[13]

$$V_m \approx V_d - \frac{kT}{q} \ln\left\{\frac{C_{fix}^2}{\gamma_+ \gamma_- C_{out} C_{in}}\right\}.$$

The second term defines the contribution from Donnan potentials, where the γ's are partition coefficients for the cations and anions, and C_{out} and C_{in} are the respective solution concentrations outside and inside the cell. Our analysis predicts that V_d will be 35 mV larger in the acidic regions.

frequency increases, as will its contribution to the total impedance. At these higher frequencies, the total conductance will therefore derive from regions external to the depletion layer, which have a conductivity of σ_l. Thus, the total conductance will disperse from approximately

$$\frac{\sigma_d}{\lambda} \text{ at low frequencies to } \frac{\sigma_l}{w} \text{ at high frequencies.} \qquad (9)$$

Similarly, the total capacitance will disperse from approximately

$$\frac{\varepsilon_l}{\lambda} \text{ at low frequencies to } \frac{\varepsilon_l}{w} \text{ at high frequencies.} \qquad (10)$$

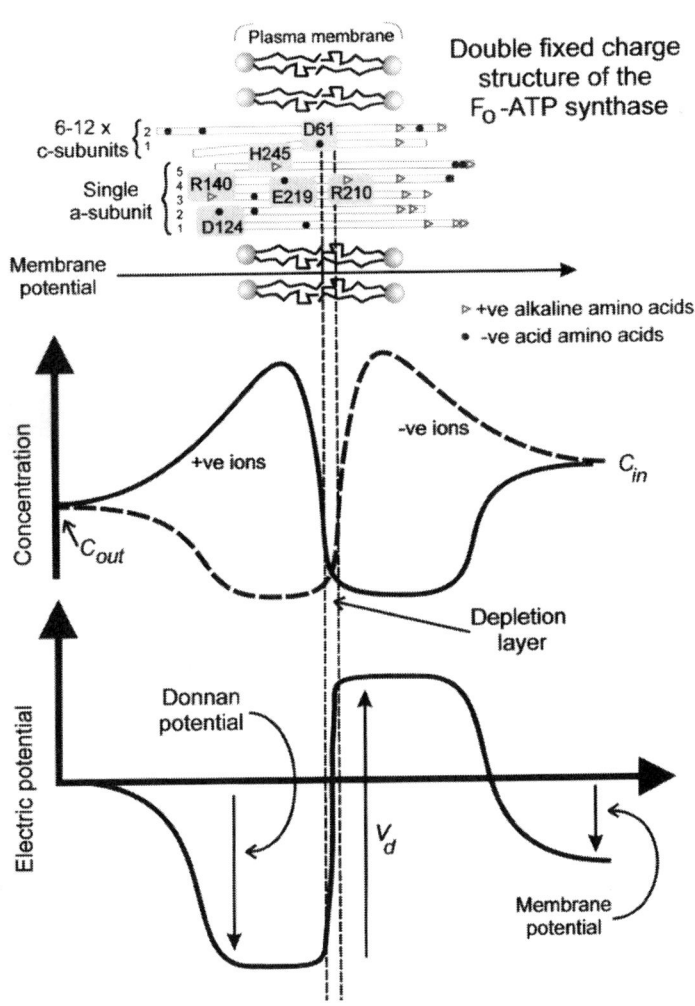

The expression[12] describing these dispersions, although very complicated when derived from the Nernst-Planck equations (see APPENDIX), can be described more simply[13] by the transfer function, that is,

$$TF_l(s) = \frac{r_1}{\omega_1 + s} + \frac{r_2}{\omega_2 + s}. \tag{11}$$

In a biological membrane, fixed charges derive from the NH_3^+ and COO^- groups on alkaline and acidic amino acids that form proteins. As shown in FIGURE 2, these amino acids can be distributed so that fixed charges of positive sign predominate on one side and those of opposite sign predominate on the other.

Impedance Model for the Membrane Mosaic

The plasma membrane consists of protein modules embedded in a lipid bilayer membrane matrix.[14] Impedance measurements on artificially reconstituted lipid bilayers[7] show that the conductivity of the lipid matrix is much less than that of a cell membrane and that protein modules provide the main pathway for ionic movement across the membrane. Some proteins form pores lined with amino acids with charge of one sign and facilitate the movement of ions of opposite charge. These proteins are called ion channels. There will be many such modules operating in parallel in a membrane, each module with pore properties selective for one or more of the many ionic species that permeate a membrane. Although the conductance properties of these modules will be diverse, the total impedance of the parallel combination will be indistinguishable from that for a single layer. If the effective conductivity of this network of modules is σ_0, then the conductance of this membrane mosaic will be σ_0/w, where w denotes the width of the membrane. The capacitance will be ε_l/w, where we have assumed that the bulk dielectric permittivity of the modules is the same throughout the mosaic. Note that the transfer function remains that for a single layer (i.e., $N = 1$ in equation 5).

Impedance of a Mosaic Membrane Containing Double Fixed-Charge Modules

Membrane proteins also form modules that transport ions against their respective electrochemical gradients, expending free energy in the process. The ATP synthase is one such protein for which there is a proposed structure involving a bipolar distribution of charged amino acids (FIGURE 2). However, the transfer function for this type of module is second order (see equation 11), that is, distinctly different from that for the other "ion channel" proteins in the membrane mosaic.

We assume that the double fixed-charge modules have the same width w and dielectric permittivity ε_l as the membrane and, collectively, they occupy a fraction p of the membrane. The system now acquires a conductance and capacitance that disperse with frequency. The dispersions will be modulated from that for the double fixed-charge module alone (equations 9 and 10) by the parallel contributions from the membrane mosaic with conductance σ_0/w and capacitance ε_l/w. The total conductance will disperse with increasing frequency from approximately

$$\frac{\sigma_d}{\lambda}p + \frac{\sigma_0}{w}(1-p) \quad \text{to} \quad \frac{\sigma_l}{w}p + \frac{\sigma_0}{w}(1-p). \tag{12}$$

Similarly, the capacitance of the system will disperse with increasing frequency from approximately

$$\frac{\varepsilon_l}{\lambda}p + \frac{\varepsilon_l}{w}(1-p) \approx \frac{\varepsilon_l}{\lambda}p \quad \text{to} \quad \frac{\varepsilon_l}{w}. \tag{13}$$

Note that the capacitance dispersion remains strongly dependent on the depletion layer capacitance at low frequencies (since $\lambda < w$) and is unchanged at high frequencies (cf. equations 10 and 13).

Although the transfer function for these modules is second order and that for modules that form channels is first order, it can be readily shown that the transfer function for the parallel combination of these different modules remains second order and, hence, as defined by equation 11.

Most significantly, the physical properties in a system containing fixed charges can be obtained by equating the limiting values of equations 11 at low and high frequencies to the corresponding limits for the capacitance and conductance of the system. Equations 12 and 13 then yield

$$\frac{\omega_1 \omega_2}{\omega_1 r_2 + \omega_2 r_1} = \alpha\left[\frac{\sigma_d}{\lambda}p + \frac{\sigma_0}{w}(1-p)\right], \quad \frac{r_1^3 \omega_2 + r_2^3 \omega_1}{r_1 r_2(r_1 + r_2)^2} = \alpha\left[\frac{\sigma_l}{w}p + \frac{\sigma_0}{w}(1-p)\right],$$

$$\frac{\omega_1^2 r_2^3 + \omega_2^2 r_1^3}{(\omega_1 r_2 + \omega_2 r_1)^2} \approx \alpha p\frac{\varepsilon_l}{\lambda}, \quad \text{and} \quad \frac{1}{r_1 + r_2} = \alpha\frac{\varepsilon_l}{w}, \tag{14}$$

where we have also introduced an area factor α to take into account the folding of the membrane.

EXPERIMENTAL RESULTS

FIGURE 3 shows the conductance tomograph of two *Chara* cells joined by a node. The upper cell had good turgor and its cytoplasm was flowing. In contrast, the lower cell was limp (poor turgor) and its cytoplasm was stationary. It can be seen that the conductance for the upper cell was strongly dependent on frequency, indicating the presence of membranes and internal substructures that had vastly differing electrical properties. In contrast, the conductance for the lower cell was independent of frequency, indicating homogeneity and the absence of a membrane structure (which is necessary for maintaining cell mobility and turgor). Further tomographs from another cell are shown in FIGURE 4. These reveal that both the susceptance (imaginary part of the admittance) as well as the conductance (real part of the admittance) are strong functions of frequency in a healthy cell.

The other distinguishing feature of the tomographs is the spatial constancy of the conductance dispersion with frequency for the healthy cell shown in FIGURE 3. This contrasts with tomographs in FIGURE 4 that reveal marked spatial variations in both the conductance and susceptance dispersions.

The spatial variations in the conductance and susceptance at certain frequencies generally correlate with spatial variations in the surface electrical potential (FIGURE 4A). A strong correlation exists between electrical potential minima and (low-frequency) conductance peaks (FIGURE 4B). These correlations identify the alkaline regions (shown shaded) that separate the acidic regions. The susceptance exhibited a less general correlation with

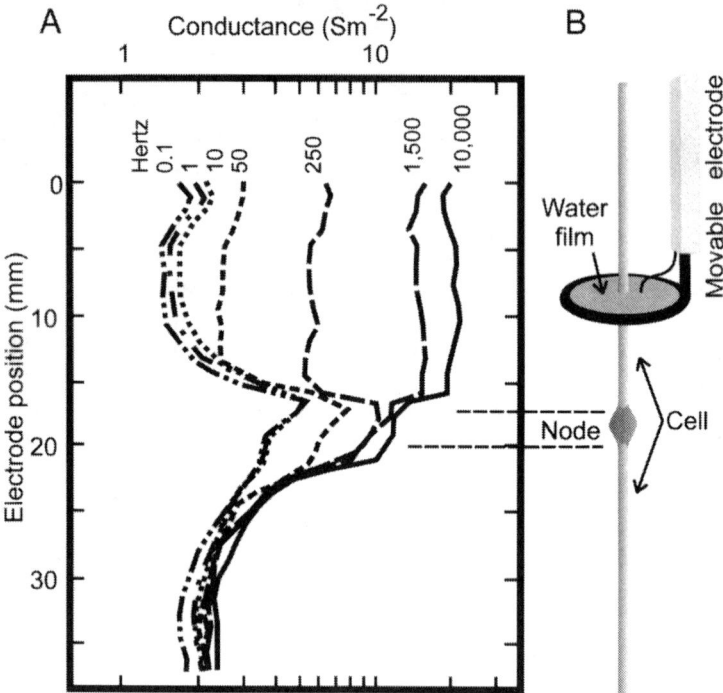

FIGURE 3. A conductance tomograph from two *Chara* cells separated by a node (shown in geometrically accurate proportions in B). Three characteristic dispersions of conductance with frequency (A) can be seen to correlate spatially with the upper cell, node, and lower cell: that for the upper cell disperses significantly, indicating the presence of structure such as a plasma membrane; this contrasts with that for the lower cell, which is independent of frequency, indicating homogeneity and the absence of structure; that for the node disperses to a lesser extent than that for the upper cell and reflects the fact that nodes contain an array of smaller cells with intact plasma membranes.

the conductance. For instance, FIGURE 4C shows that minima in the susceptance at the highest frequency correlate with alkaline regions. The opposite trend is seen for the susceptance at low frequencies (FIGURE 4D), where susceptance peaks generally correlate with alkaline regions. The impedance tomographs for even higher frequencies (>244 Hz) were poorly correlated with the acidic-alkaline bands and are not shown. Measurements at these frequencies have been shown to derive substantially from the plasma membrane coat[8] and the static cytoplasm.[10]

Impedance spectra over a broader range of frequencies were obtained in adjacent acid and alkaline regions that exhibited the largest differences in electrical properties (not shown). The transfer functions (equation 5) fitted to these spectra identified contributions from the static cytoplasm, plasma membrane, charasomes, and extracellular coat.[8] These yielded a conductance of 10^6 S m^{-2} for the static cytoplasm[c] and a conductance and capac-

---

[c]The capacitance of the static cytoplasm was modeled as a single conductance element.

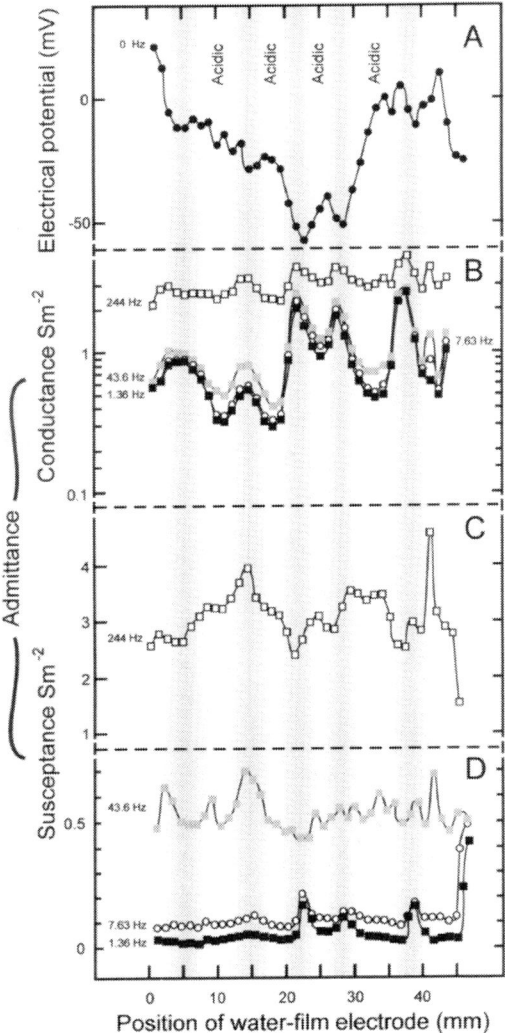

FIGURE 4. Electrical impedance tomographs of a *Chara* cell revealing correlations between the electric potential and the admittance. The shaded areas identify alkaline regions, which are at a more negative potential than adjacent acidic regions (A). Further, the conductance (at low frequencies) is higher than in the adjacent acidic regions (B). The imaginary part of the admittance, the susceptance, also exhibits differences that correlate with acidic and alkaline regions. The susceptance at high frequencies (C) derives substantially from the dielectric geometrical capacitance of the plasma membrane. Generally, this is larger in the acidic regions than in adjacent alkaline regions, indicating that plasma membrane folding (charasomes) predominates in acidic regions. (Note that the second alkaline region is the exception to this trend, although consistent with another electron micrograph study suggesting that charasomes are not essential for the establishment of the acidic regions.[21]) The opposite relationship is observed for the susceptance at lower frequencies (D) and suggests that the plasma membrane capacitance is more enhanced in the alkaline regions. Measurements are expressed in terms of the contact area of the water film.

itance of 20 S m^{-2} and 15 mF m^{-2}, respectively, for the plasma membrane coat. These values were the same for both regions.

The dielectric geometrical capacitance for the biological membrane, including the plasma membrane and tonoplast, has been shown in numerous experiments to be ~8 mF m^{-2}. Further, it has been shown that the tonoplast has the same two natural frequencies (i.e., ω_1 and ω_2) as those for the plasma membrane.[15] Based on these assumptions and using the smallest reported area factor (= 3) describing folding of the tonoplast, it was possible to identify the following transfer-function parameters for the plasma membrane:

$r_1 \sim 17.85$ m^{2}F^{-1}, $\omega_1 \sim 2.73$ Hz, $r_2 \sim 107$ m^{2}F^{-1}, and $\omega_2 \sim 29.6$ Hz **(15)**

for the acidic region and

$r_1 \sim 1.38$ m^{2}F^{-1}, $\omega_1 \sim 2.75$ Hz, $r_2 \sim 123.6$ m^{2}F^{-1}, and $\omega_2 \sim 122$ Hz **(16)**

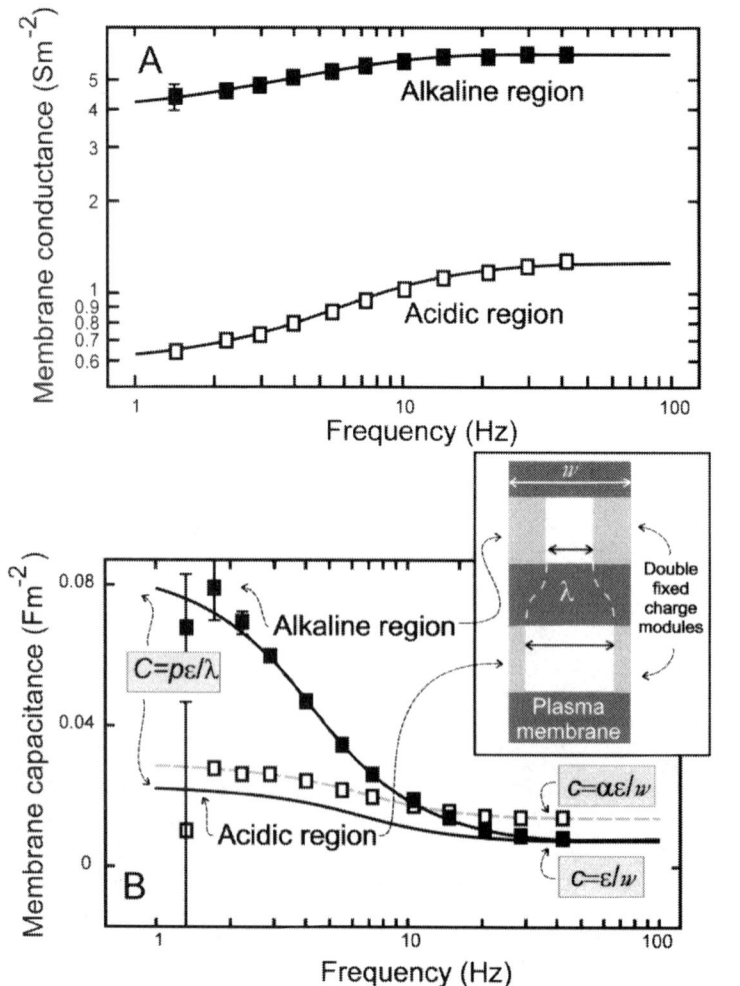

for the alkaline region. This second-order transfer function was used to generate the theoretical curves shown in FIGURE 5 and can be seen to fit the conductance and capacitance data after contributions from other ultrastructures were extracted.

DISCUSSION

In this study, we have specifically identified the contribution of the plasma membrane and have shown that it has the form of a second-order transfer-function in both the acidic and alkaline regions of the cell. We have also shown that the transfer-function parameter values are different for acidic and alkaline regions (e.g., compare values in equations 15 and 16). In these two regions, the local electrochemical environment (pH and membrane potential) is very different. If we assume that the terms derive from substructural layers in the plasma membrane, then equations 3 and 5 yield dielectric geometrical capacitances that are not related to pH or electric potential. However, in some instances, these capacitances are too large to be attributed to the possible presence of substructural layers. Since intrinsic dielectric properties of materials are generally only weakly dependent on pH and electric potential, the numerical differences in the parameter values in equations 15 and 16 cannot originate from differences in such substructural layers in either the acidic or alkaline regions.

Origin of the Conductance and Capacitance Dispersions for the Plasma Membrane

If we assume that the transfer-function terms derive from double fixed-charge modules embedded in a membrane mosaic, such as described by equations 6–9, then equation 13 yields a dielectric geometrical capacitance of ~8 mF m^{-2} for the plasma membrane in the alkaline region and a value ~1.44 times this in the acidic region. This corresponds to values for the area factor α of ~1 and ~1.44, respectively. These values are consistent with electron microscopy evidence of plasma membrane folding, such as that found in organelles called charasomes (see first inset of FIGURE 1), predominating in acid regions.[3]

Additionally, equations 7, 8, 12, and 13 indicate that all the transfer-function parameters for the fixed-charge system may be dependent on the electrical potential term V_d. Changes in V_d along the cell were observed from the electrical potential measurements (FIGURE 4), which indicate that V_d was larger in acidic regions than in adjacent alkaline

---

FIGURE 5. Conductance (A) and capacitance (B) dispersions from the plasma membrane of *Chara*. The impedance dispersions differ significantly in acidic (□) and alkaline (■) regions (bands) that form along the cell's cylindrical surface. Values in the acidic region for the capacitance at high frequencies are 1.44 times greater than those in the alkaline region and represent the geometrical factor α in equation 14 arising from folding. The curves are theoretical plots of the impedance of a membrane containing double fixed-charge modules after membrane folding has been accounted for. The fixed charges in the modules establish a "depletion" layer of low conductance (width λ) sandwiched by layers of high conductance (see inset). The theory predicts that the capacitance of the membrane decreases from approximately $p\varepsilon_l/\lambda$ to ε_l/w as the frequency increases over the indicated range ($p \sim 0.5$). The different dispersions can be explained if the acidic and alkaline conditions in the different regions induce the indicated changes in λ through the dependency of this parameter on the fixed-charge concentration. Data have been corrected for "cable property" effects.[11]

regions. The model predicts that the conductance of the double fixed-charge modules, which at low frequencies is substantially determined by the conductivity of their depletion layers (equation 8), will be lower in acidic regions than in adjacent alkaline regions as a consequence of these spatial variations in V_d. In addition, the capacitance at low frequencies will be lower in the acidic region than in the alkaline region because of the dependence of the depletion layer width λ on V_d (see equation 7). These general trends were all observed (e.g., see FIGURES 4 and 5).

Equation 14 determines that the conductance of the protein modules in the membrane mosaic, that is, σ_0/w, was 1.18 S m^{-2} in the acidic region and 7.8 S m^{-2} in the alkaline region. This indicates that these modules are also modulated by the local electrochemical environment in these regions. To reconcile this, we would need to conclude that these spatial variations could arise from direct effects of local pH on the degree to which ionizable moieties in these modules are ionized and/or from the influence of the electric potential on channels that are voltage-gated. For instance, alkaline conditions would be expected to increase the ionization of those negatively charged amino acids that form cation-selective pores, thus making these channels more permeable to cations. Since cation channels predominate in the plasma membrane of *Chara*, one would generally expect that the conductance of the membrane mosaic would be smaller in acidic regions than in adjacent alkaline regions.

Equation 14 further yields values for the diffusion constant D, the electrical potential across the depletion layer V_d, and the concentration of fixed charges C_{fix}. These were

$$D = 2.2 \times 10^{-17} \text{ m}^2 \text{ s}^{-1}, \quad V_d = 100 \text{ mV}, \quad \text{and} \quad C_{fix} = 200 \text{ mM} \quad \text{for the acidic region} \quad \textbf{(17)}$$

and

$$D = 2.2 \times 10^{-17} \text{ m}^2 \text{ s}^{-1}, \quad V_d = 65 \text{ mV}, \quad \text{and} \quad C_{fix} = 840 \text{ mM for the alkaline region} \quad \textbf{(18)}$$

and are physiologically realistic.

Origin of the Double Fixed-Charge Modules in Chara

Given the sequence homology for the ATP synthases in a variety of biological systems,[16] it seems probable that the ATP synthase from *Chara* will also exhibit high homology to these others. Further, detailed site-directed substitution experiments have identified functionally important amino acids in the ATP synthase from these systems and have led to the proposal of a double fixed-charge structure (FIGURE 2) for its membrane-bound (F_0) segments.[17] Additionally, our electrical impedance tomography study of macroscopic spatial electrochemical structures established by the ATP synthase in *Chara* suggests the presence of double fixed-charge structures in the plasma membrane of *Chara*. We therefore suggest that the double fixed-charge structure, which provides a basis to account for our electrical impedance measurements in *Chara*, might be the F_0 segments of its ATP synthase.

Putative Role for the F_0–ATP Synthase in Dehydration and Water-Splitting

The fact that synthetically formed double fixed-charge membranes, called bipolar membranes, exhibit proton-translocating properties suggests a role for the double fixed-charge structure of the ATP synthesis. It is now widely accepted[9] that the proton currents in bipolar membranes originate in the electric field–induced dissociation of water into H$^+$

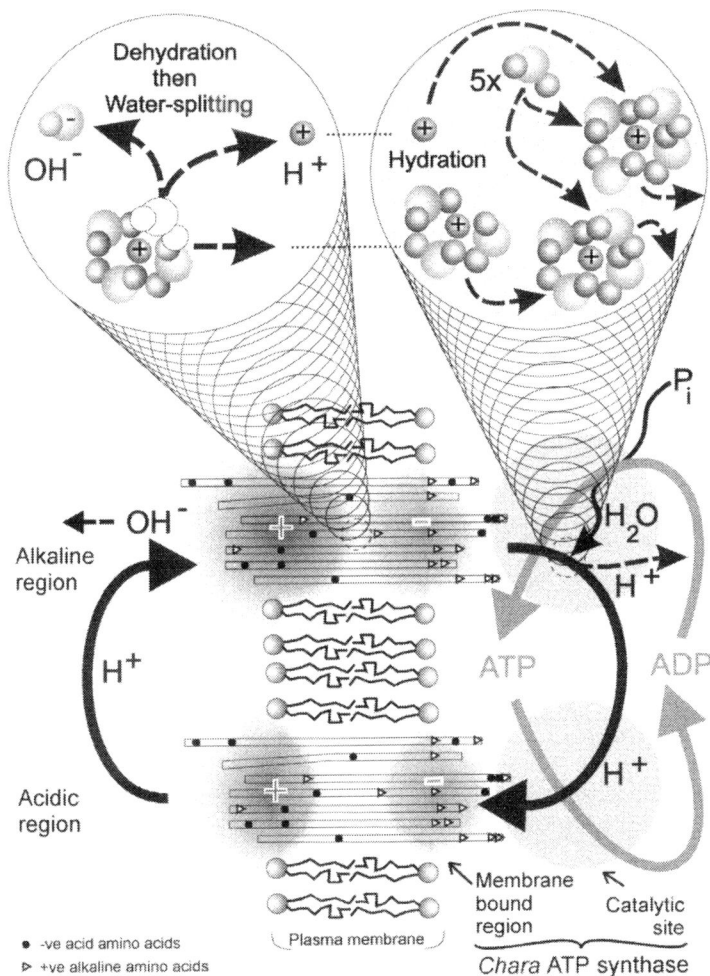

FIGURE 6. Proposed bioelectrochemical role for the F_0-ATPase. We propose that hydration assisted by "water-splitting" occurs in the F_0-ATPase located in the alkaline region. "Water-splitting" would induce an outward OH^- flux, inducing further ionization of negative fixed charges. We further propose that the inward flux of protons will be rehydrated in the catalytic reaction center of the ATP synthase (F_1-ATPase), where H_2O is the by-product of ATP synthesis. The ATP thus synthesized is shown to be recycled in the acidic region, where it provides energy for pumping H^+.

and OH^- at this junction. The depletion layer width in both systems is of similar magnitude, and fields are of sufficient strength (V_d/λ; ~8.6×10^7 V/m for the acidic region and ~1.4×10^8 V/m for the alkaline region) to induce "water-splitting".

Thermodynamic calculations reveal that a proton will most likely permeate a membrane if it is hydrated with four water molecules.[18] We propose that such a hydrated proton enters the membrane-bound portion of the *Chara* ATP synthase, whereupon the strong electric field across the depletion layer induces partial dehydration as the result of the dissociation of one water molecule into H^+ and OH^-. When the partially dehydrated proton enters the catalytic site of the ATP synthase (F_1-ATPase), it can rehydrate with water produced as a by-product of ATP synthesis (see FIGURE 6). The fully dehydrated proton could similarly remove additional water (up to four molecules) from the catalytic site, further favoring the synthesis of ATP.

Note that the water-splitting process involves the disposal of OH^- externally, thereby creating a region external to the cell that will be alkaline. The alkaline conditions externally and the acidic conditions internally would be expected to further increase the degree to which the ionizable sites in the F_0-ATPase would be ionized, thereby further strengthening the electric field and hence the likelihood of inducing dehydration by "water-splitting" and ATP synthesis. Indeed, our data and the analysis in terms of double fixed-charge modules indicate that the fixed-charge concentration was largest in the alkaline region, as was the electric field (cf. values in equations 17 and 18).

Our study further indicates that the membrane potential is more positive in the acidic regions. This is consistent with notions widely accepted in the literature that the ATP synthase, in this instance, is utilizing ATP for pumping protons into the external solution. The external acidic conditions, thus maintained, would reduce the degree of ionization of the negative fixed charges in the outer regions of the F_0-ATPase, resulting in a wider depletion layer and hence a lower membrane conductance for this region, as was observed. The low conductance would help to sustain the high H^+ concentration externally by minimizing the back-diffusion of protons into the cell.

CONCLUSIONS

The electrical impedance tomography study of the acidic and alkaline regions of a single *Chara* cell has revealed structural and electrical differences that can be interpreted in terms of a model of the plasma membrane in which there are proteins that form double fixed-charge regions. The origin of the double fixed-charge modules may be the proton-translocating ATP synthases involved in establishing the acidic regions. We propose that electric field–induced dissociation of water into H^+ and OH^- is relevant to the modus operandi of the F_0 portion of the ATP synthases in alkaline regions. Our theoretical studies of the double fixed-charge structure in conjunction with chemiosmotic theory[19] and kinetic studies[20] generally support this hypothesis. However, more detailed structural-functional studies will shed further light on this proposed role for the fixed charges in the ATP synthase.

REFERENCES

1. WALKER, N.A. 1983. The uptake of inorganic carbon by freshwater plants. Plant Cell Environ. **6:** 323–328.
2. LUCAS, W.J. 1983. Photosynthetic assimilation of exogenous bicarbonate by aquatic plants. Annu. Rev. Plant Physiol. **34:** 71–104.
3. FRANCESCHI, V.R. & W.J. LUCAS. 1980. Structure and possible function(s) of charasomes, complex plasmalemma–cell wall elaborations present in some *Characean* species. Protoplasma **104:** 253–271.

4. PRICE, G.D., M.R. BADGER, M.E. BASSETT & M.I. WHITECROSS. 1985. Involvement of plasmalemma and carbonic anhydrase in photosynthetic utilisation of bicarbonate in *Chara corallina*. Aust. J. Plant Physiol. **12**: 241–256.
5. OGATA, K. 1983. The water-film electrode, a new device for measuring the *Characean* electropotential and conductance distributions along the length of the internode. Plant Cell Physiol. **24**: 695–703.
6. COLE, K.S. 1972. Membranes, Ions, and Impulses. University of California Press. Berkeley.
7. ASHCROFT, R.G., H.G.L. COSTER & J.R. SMITH. 1977. Local anaesthetic benzyl alcohol increases membrane thickness. Nature **269**: 819–820.
8. CHILCOTT, T.C. & H.G.L. COSTER. 1994. AC impedance measurements on *Chara corallina*: III. Characterisation of the plasma membrane using a new presentation of impedance spectra. Aust. J. Plant Physiol. **21**: 147–168.
9. SIMONS, R. 1985. Water splitting in ion exchange membranes. Electrochim. Acta **30**(3): 275–282.
10. CHILCOTT, T.C. & H.G.L. COSTER. 1991. AC impedance measurements on *Chara corallina*: I. Characterisation of the static cytoplasm. Aust. J. Plant Physiol. **18**: 191–199.
11. CHILCOTT, T.C. 1988. Admittance tomography of cells of *Chara corallina*: a study of the electrical spatial structures associated with photosynthesis. Ph.D. thesis, University of New South Wales, Sydney.
12. CHILCOTT, T.C., H.G.L. COSTER & E.P. GEORGE. 1995. AC impedance of the bipolar membrane at low and high frequencies. J. Membr. Sci. **100**: 77–87.
13. CHILCOTT, T.C., H.G.L. COSTER & E.P. GEORGE. 1995. Novel method for the characterisation of the bipolar membrane using impedance spectroscopy. J. Membr. Sci. **108**: 185–198.
14. SINGER, S.J. & G.L. NICOLSON. 1972. The fluid mosaic model of the structure of cell membranes. Science **175**: 720.
15. COSTER, H.G.L. & J.R. SMITH. 1977. Low-frequency impedance of *Chara corallina*: simultaneous measurements of the separate plasmalemma and tonoplast capacitance and conductance. Aust. J. Plant Physiol. **4**: 667–674.
16. SENIOR, A.E. 1990. The proton-translocating ATPase of *Escherichia coli*. Annu. Rev. Biophys. Chem. **19**: 7–41.
17. HOWITT, S.M. & G.B. COX. 1992. Second-site revertants of an arginine-210 to lysine mutation in the *a* subunit of the F_0-F_1-ATPase from *Escherichia coli*: implications for structure. Proc. Natl. Acad. Sci. U.S.A. **89**: 9799–9803.
18. ASHCROFT, R.G. & H.G.L. COSTER. 1978. The hydration number of protons in membranes: thermodynamic implications. Bioelectrochem. Bioenerg. **5**: 37–42.
19. MITCHEL, P. 1979. Keilin's respiratory chain concept and its chemiosmotic consequences. Science **206**: 1148–1159.
20. FISAHN, J., U. HANSEN & W.J. LUCAS. 1992. Reaction kinetic model of a proposed plasma membrane two-cycle proton-transport system of *Chara corallina*. Proc. Natl. Acad. Sci. U.S.A. **89**: 3261–3265.
21. BISSON, M.J., A. SIEGEL, R. CHAU, S.A. GELSOMINO & S.L. HERDIC. 1991. Distribution of charasomes in *Chara*: banding pattern and effect of photosynthetic inhibitors. Aust. J. Plant Physiol. **18**: 81–93.

APPENDIX

The expression[12] for the admittance of a double fixed-charge membrane (DFCM) system exhibits a complicated dependence on the diffusion constant D for ions (assumed to be the same for anions and cations), the electric potential V_d that develops between the fixed-charge regions of concentration C_{fix}, the thickness λ of the region (called the depletion layer) over which V_d develops, and the thickness of the DFCM system w. Specifically,[d]

---

[d]Equations quoted in this appendix correct a typographical error in references 12 and 13.

$$y_{\text{DFCM}} = \frac{1}{z_{\text{DFCM}}} = \frac{2\dfrac{\vartheta\varepsilon\omega_P}{\lambda} + j\omega\dfrac{\beta\varepsilon}{\lambda}}{1 + \dfrac{w-\lambda}{\lambda}\left[1 + \beta\dfrac{j\omega - \omega_P}{j\omega + \omega_P}\left(1 - \dfrac{2x_1}{w-\lambda}\tanh\left\{\dfrac{w-\lambda}{2x_1}\right\}\right)\right]} \quad \text{(A1)}$$

where

$$\vartheta = \frac{\zeta e^{-qV_d/kT}}{1 + (2\zeta - 1)e^{-qV_d/kT}}, \quad \beta = \frac{1 - e^{-qV_d/kT}}{1 + (2\zeta - 1)e^{-qV_d/kT}}, \quad \text{(A2)}$$

$$x_0 = \sqrt{\frac{D}{j\omega}}, \quad x_1 = \sqrt{\frac{D}{j\omega + \omega_P}}, \quad \omega_P = \frac{q^2 D C_{\text{fix}}}{kT\varepsilon}, \quad \text{and} \quad \zeta = \frac{x_1 \tanh\left\{\dfrac{w-\lambda}{2x_1}\right\}}{x_0 \tanh\left\{\dfrac{w-\lambda}{2x_0}\right\}}. \quad \text{(A3)}$$

New Light-Scattering and Field-Trapping Methods Access the Internal Electric Structure of Submicron Particles, like Influenza Viruses[a]

JAN GIMSA

Institut für Biologie, Humboldt-Universität zu Berlin, D-10115 Berlin, Germany

ABSTRACT: A variety of AC-electrokinetic field effects can be exploited for handling or electric characterization of microscopic and submicroscopic particles, like cells, organelles, supramolecular structures, and artificial colloids. Despite the fact that dielectric spectroscopy methods by AC-electrokinetics, like common impedance methods, are based on the impedance properties of the different constituents of the particles, the first methods yield higher parameter resolutions. A drawback of the electrokinetic methods was that they required microscopic observability of field-induced particle movements. New AC-electrokinetic methods like electrorotational light scattering (ERLS), dielectrophoretic phase-analysis light scattering (DPALS), and dielectrophoretic field trapping (DFT) solve this problem and access the submicroscopic particle range. This paper gives an introduction to the new methods and presents measurements on influenza viruses. To develop a dielectric virus model, experiments of ERLS were combined with DFT of viruses in microstructured electric-field cages. The model assumes a spherical virus with a radius of 50 nm and a single-shell dielectric structure. The shell thickness of 18 nm summarizes the dimensions of the lipid and viral surface protein layers. For this model, the conductivities of core and shell of 0.1 mS/m and 0.1 µS/m, respectively, and the relative permittivities of 30 and 80, respectively, were obtained.

INTRODUCTION

Currently, the number of applications of AC-electrokinetic effects for characterization, sorting, collection, orientation, fusion, poration, particle forming, or segregation of colloids, DNA, proteins, and other biological particles is rapidly growing.[1–5] All exploited effects exhibit a frequency dependence that is mediated by dispersion processes of different physical nature. For cells, α-dispersions at the low-frequency end below 1 kHz are based on hydrodynamic relaxations of electroosmotically induced convections around the particles, as well as on particle electrophoresis.[6,7] Similar processes, electrochemical electrode polarizations, and electroosmosis may occur within the field chambers.[8] Dispersions at higher frequencies are based on the structuration of the material (Maxwell-Wagner)[9–12] or are caused by the frequency dependence of the orientation of molecular dipoles (Debye).[2,10] A classification according to frequencies originally yielded a scaling where the dispersions with increasing frequencies were assigned to the α-, β-, and γ-range.[13] Generally, the characteristic frequency of a dispersion decreases with increasing size of the structure responsible for dispersing the hydrodynamic, charge transport, redox, or field-orientation process. Thus, "α-dispersions" of virus-sized particles or "γ-dispersions" of large proteins can be found in the β-range from kHz to MHz.

---

[a]This study was supported by Grant No. Gi 232/1-2 from Deutsche Forschungsgemeinschaft.

In principle, impedance and the AC-electrokinetic single-particle methods yield the same information on dielectric particle properties.[9,12] The frequency range of the methods, reaching from AC-electrophoresis techniques in the Hz range up to impedance measurements in the GHz range, covers more than twice as many orders of magnitude than optical spectroscopy techniques, ranging from IR to UV light. For particle characterization, two complementary AC-electrokinetic effects—dielectrophoresis (DP) and electrorotation (ER)—are of special importance. DP and ER analyze the translation and rotation of single particles in an inhomogeneous and rotating external field, respectively. Registration of the frequency dependence yields DP and ER spectra. The different motions in DP and ER depend on the different spatial properties of the field determining the interaction with the induced dipole moment of the particles. In DP, in the regions of high field, particles or suspension media are displaced, depending on their frequency-dependent relative polarizabilities. Dispersion processes lead to the frequency dependence of the DP force. In ER, the rotating field induces a particle dipole moment that rotates at the angular frequency of the field. Any dispersion process causes a spatial phase shift of the field vector and the induced dipole moment, giving rise to a torque. The torque, and therefore particle rotation, is at a maximum if the relaxation time of the dispersion process and field frequency match. The different principles of DP and ER result in the complementary nature of the methods. While DP is proportional to the real part of the induced dipole moment, ER depends solely on the imaginary or "out of phase" part. To verify a certain dielectric model and to determine its dielectric parameters for particles of unknown structure, advantage can be taken of this strict interrelation of DP and ER.[12,14,15] Models for multishell spherical, cylindrical, and ellipsoidal geometries are available.[16–18]

DP and ER avoid several problems of commonly used impedance methods. Electrode polarizations do not influence the measurement. In contrast to impedance, DP and ER are based on the difference of particle and medium polarizability, and particle movement is measured relative to the suspension medium. Electric and hydrodynamic particle-particle interactions can be avoided since the measuring effect is independent of the solution volume and, in principle, one particle is sufficient for measurements. Ultramicroelectrode chambers widen the accessible frequency and conductivity range, a previous limitation of the methods.[1,2,19]

Microscopic measurements of particle kinetics are tedious and restricted to the microscopic-size range. Movement of submicroscopic particles like viruses can be investigated by dynamic light-scattering (DLS) techniques, which are widely used to characterize the size and surface charge of colloidal particles. Recently developed light-scattering methods—ER light scattering (ERLS) and dielectrophoretic phase-analysis light scattering (DPALS)—overcome these drawbacks.[20–22] Both methods allow the simultaneous, computerized registration of the individual movement of many particles within a population, yielding statistical significance at short measuring times. ERLS is a homodyne dynamic light-scattering method with a single beam and a single detector (FIGURE 1A).[21,23] The field-frequency-dependent ER of the particles generates field-frequency-dependent autocorrelation functions (ACF) of the scattered light intensity (FIGURE 1C). For this, a deviation of the particles from perfect optical rotational symmetry is essential. As a measure of the induced rotation speed, the inverse of the decay time of the ACF to 75% of its initial value ($1/\tau_{75}$) was used. The $1/\tau_{75}$ spectra allow the determination of the frequency dependence of the particle rotation speed from the ACF.[21] Unfortunately, the criteria depend not only on the rotation speed, but also on particle shape and translational DP motion. As a

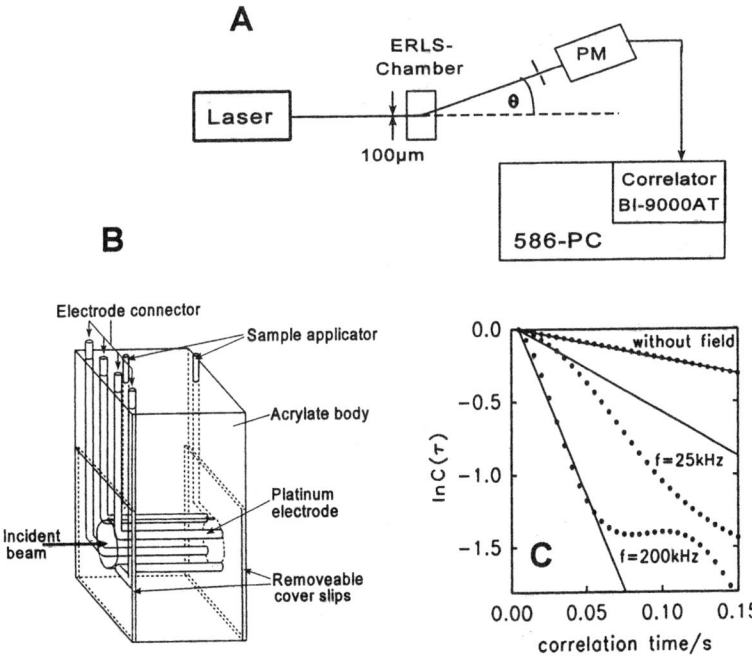

FIGURE 1. Schemes of the ERLS setup (A) and ERLS chamber (B). The dots in graph C are an example for baseline-subtracted ACFs of red blood cells undergoing ER. The lines designate the initial slopes of the ACFs without field and for two different external field frequencies inducing different rates of rotation.

result, a lower limit for clear detection of particle rotation exists.[20] However, above a certain speed, ER clearly dominates the ERLS spectra, allowing determination of the characteristic frequencies of ER. A notorious problem of the homodyne method was the inability to detect the rotation sense of the particles. This problem could be partly solved by a compensation method according to FIGURE 2. The compensation method alternatingly applies a reference and measuring field.[23] The inertia of the particles results in a smooth rotation detectable by ERLS. The mode allows detection of the rotation sense for the measuring field relative to that of the reference field frequency.

To take advantage of the Kramers-Kronig relation between DP and ER (see above), field-induced translational motions also need to be registered. In light scattering, particle translations are commonly analyzed by heterodyne single- or dual-beam laser Doppler setups.[24] The advantage of the dual-beam setup is that heterodyne mixing occurs by the particle itself and no problems due to different light intensities of the two mixed beams arise. Another advantage is that the measuring volume, which is restricted to the crossing region of the two beams, can be adjusted to an area of known field distribution. In contrast to ERLS, no optical anisotropy of the particles is required for detection. The major disadvantage of the classical laser Doppler method is that the detectable particle displacement is limited. This restriction can be overcome by phase-analysis light scattering (PALS). In

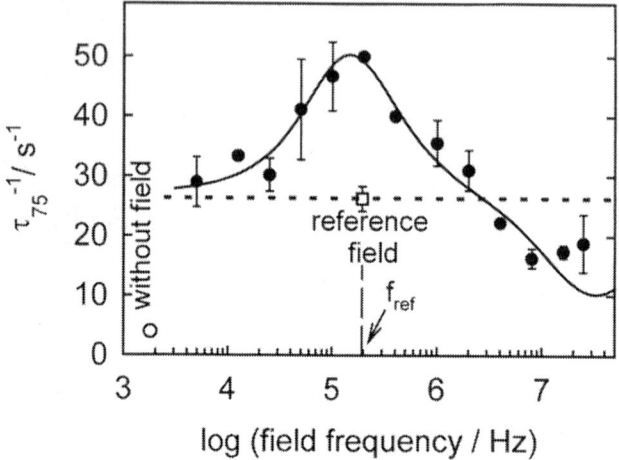

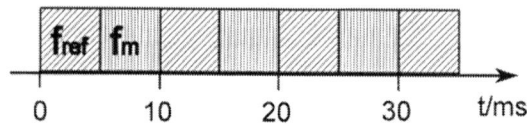

FIGURE 2. ERLS compensation measurements for detection of the relative rotation sense. The solid circles are the means of the $1/\tau_{75}$ spectra of three red blood cell suspensions at 10 mS/m. The solid line is a linear transformation of a theoretical ER spectrum.[2,21] For measurements, a compensation field mode with a constant reference (f_{ref}) of 194 kHz and with a variable measuring frequency (f_m) was used. Open square: Reference field only. The fields were applied according to the bottom scheme. Note that the original peak directions of the lower and higher frequency peaks are negative (antifield) and positive (cofield), respectively.

PALS, a small optical frequency difference between the two laser beams is used to create an interference region with a moving fringe pattern (FIGURE 3).[22,24,25] Thus, the intensity of the scattered light of a fixed particle within the crossing region varies with the frequency difference of the two laser beams. When the optical frequency difference is used as a reference, phase demodulation of the Doppler signal yields the particle velocity. Lock-in detection makes the registration of very slow field translations possible. This method was successfully applied to characterize traveling-wave micropumps.[22] Special optical chambers were developed for DPALS.[25]

Besides DPALS, field caging is another way to register the real part of the induced dipole moment. Three-dimensional field cages for trapping or caging of microparticles were first introduced by Fuhr et al.[26] Also, collection of viruses in the central field minimum of a cage was demonstrated by this group.[1] Cages consist of a system of ultramicroelectrodes fabricated by semiconductor technology, preferably on glass substrates. Such electrodes, with typical dimensions between 100 nm and several tens of micrometers, also

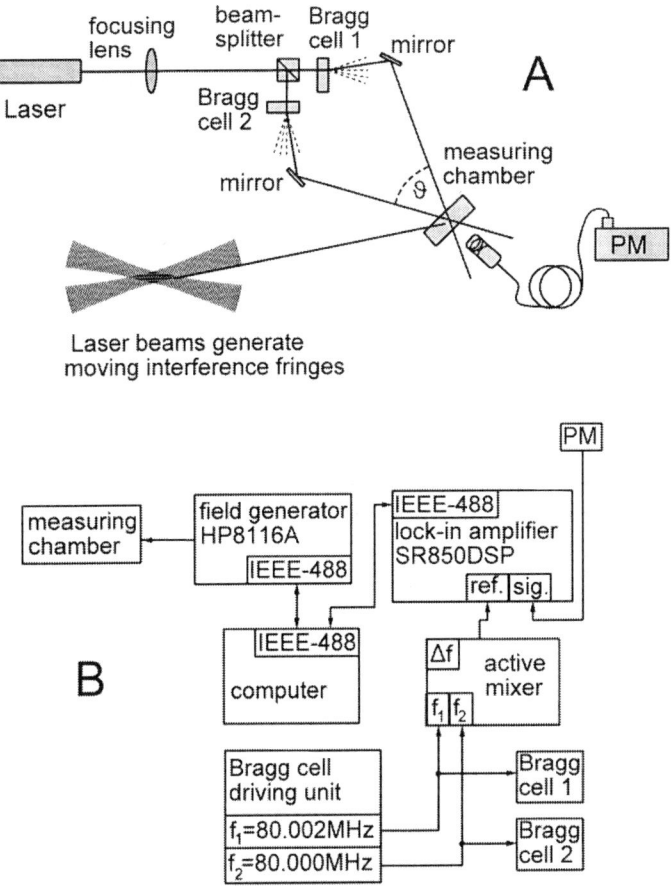

FIGURE 3. DPALS setup. The measuring chamber is illuminated by two laser beams with a frequency difference of 2 kHz (A). The scattered light intensity of the interference region is detected by a photomultiplier (PM). For DPALS, the interference region is located in an inhomogeneous field region. (B) Electronic setup.

allow the application of strong electric fields in highly conductive aqueous media. A cage repels particles from the electrodes by negative DP, a behavior analogous to a dielectric with higher permittivity (medium) tending to replace a dielectric of lower permittivity (particle).[11] For biological membrane-covered particles like cells, negative DP is achieved for electric-field frequencies below the capacitive membrane bridging at around 100 kHz and in the upper MHz range. The latter range is based on the volume properties of the cell causing a polarizability that is lower than that of the medium. The reasons for this are restricted ion mobility and a disturbed water structure. In highly conductive solutions, the two ranges may merge to a purely negative DP spectrum. The low-frequency range is disadvantageous for caging of biological particles because of a large transmembrane potential being induced. When a sufficient number of submicroscopic particles are trapped, microscopic observation of the collection efficiency of submicroscopic particles by DFT becomes possible and can be exploited for characterization of the frequency-dependent polarizability of the particles.

By conventional techniques, the internal dielectric structure of small particles like viruses is hardly accessible. One reason is that their electric properties are dominated by surface properties even above 10 kHz due to their small size. Common impedance methods require large probe volumes at high particle concentrations and are not as sensitive for the dielectric particle properties as single-particle spectroscopy. This paper gives an introduction to DPALS, ERLS, and DFT and presents results of combined ERLS and DFT experiments on influenza viruses. It proposes dielectric parameters for a single-shell viral model.

MATERIALS AND METHODS

ERLS Setup

For ERLS, an optically transparent ER chamber was used (FIGURE 1B; for details, see reference 21). The distance between two opposing electrodes was 1.4 mm. The chamber electrodes were driven by four 90° phase-shifted symmetrical square-wave signals of 20 V_{pp} amplitude and variable frequency. In the chamber, the ER field rotated in a plane perpendicular to the optical axis. The scattered light intensity was detected by a photon multiplier through a pinhole at a fixed detection angle θ of 6.5° and processed by a BI-9000AT-correlator (Brookhaven Instruments). Field frequencies and amplitudes of a measuring protocol could be programmed to a personal computer, which contained the correlator card and also drove the field generator.

Field Cage

The field cage was kindly provided by G. Fuhr (Humboldt-Universität zu Berlin). Details are given elsewhere.[1,27] In short, semiconductor technology was used to fabricate arrays of three planar four-electrode cages (FIGURE 5A). Gold electrodes, 950 nm thick, were processed on a 40-nm chrome base on a glass substrate. The chip was inserted and bonded in a ceramic carrier and driven with high-frequency electric signals of up to 10 V amplitude. The field cage was closed by a coverslip at a distance of half the electrode distance (FIGURE 5B). The device could be cleaned in an ultrasonic bath, cold or hot sterilized, or rinsed with alcohol.

Virus Measurements

For ERLS measurements, influenza viruses [A/PR/8/34 (H1N1)] from a 13-mg protein/mL suspension in phosphate buffer solution (pH 7.4) were resuspended in a 300-mOsm sucrose solution to a final concentration of 65 μg protein/mL (approximately 1.6 × 10^{11} viruses/mL). At the start of each experiment, irregularly shaped aggregates of up to

10 μm diameter were microscopically observed. To determine the rotation sense of ER peaks, virus aggregates were also microscopically observed in a microstructured four-electrode chamber at about 25 kV/m (see reference 2). In virus trapping experiments, a concentration of 1 mg protein/mL was used. Viruses were fluorescence-labeled with 10 μM octadecylrhodamine B chloride (R18; Molecular Probes) (for details, see reference 1).

RESULTS

For biological cells, the inverse of the characteristic decorrelation time of the normalized ACF to 0.75, $1/\tau_{75}$, is an approximately linear measure for the induced rotation speed.[21] Thus, registration of the frequency dependence of $1/\tau_{75}$ yields ERLS spectra that can be interpreted by common ER theory (see FIGURE 1C and FIGURE 2). At an external conductivity of 6.5 mS/m, the ERLS spectrum exhibited peaks at 29 kHz and 1.5 MHz (FIGURE 4A). Microscopic observation of the ER of virus aggregates at the two peak frequencies revealed a co- and antifield rotation sense, respectively. It also indicated that the rotation speed for the antifield peak is about twice as high as that for the cofield peak. Nevertheless, even at the higher antifield peak, the observable rotation of sedimented virus aggregates was too poor for microscopic registration of a smooth ER spectrum. This was only possible by ERLS.

In DFT experiments, the cage was filled with an influenza virus suspension with a conductivity of 74 mS/m. After field-on, formation of a central aggregate occurred within a few seconds if a frequency and an external conductivity were used where the viruses showed negative DP. Field-induced liquid streaming transported viruses over a longer distance to the trap, producing large virus aggregates. The growth rate and final size of the aggregate for a given viral concentration depended on the voltage and frequency of the field. Qualitative results are given in FIGURE 4B. After field-off, the aggregate disappeared within a few seconds. In the frequency range of positive DP, a shiny edge at the electrode surfaces could be observed. Measurements were possible down to a concentration of 1 μg protein/mL. At the bottom of FIGURE 4B, the frequency dependence of the trapping efficiency is given. Note the correspondence of the decrease of trapping efficiency above 10 MHz to the absolute value of the Clausius Mossotti factor. Obviously, the efficiency decrease below 1 MHz corresponds to another dispersion. Although this is not predicted by the structural model, it is in qualitative agreement with the cofield α-peak of the ERLS spectrum (see below).

DISCUSSION

ERLS detection of the field-induced particle rotation requires an optical inhomogeneity of the particles. In principle, the induced rotation does not change the location of the individual particles. Since field-induced medium convections only cause particle number fluctuations within the measuring volume, they have minor impact on the light-scattering results.[21] Further, the deterministic, field-induced rotation component is independent of particle size because electrically induced and frictional torques are both proportional to the cube of the particle radius. Nevertheless, lower limits for ERLS detection are imposed by

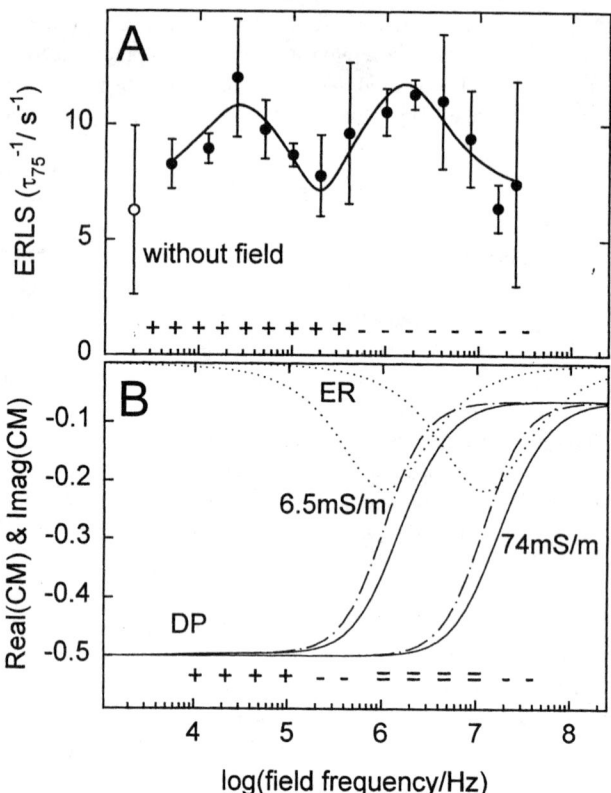

FIGURE 4. (A) ERLS spectrum of suspended influenza viruses at a conductivity of 6.5 mS/m. Each point represents three ACF measurements on the same sample. The double-Lorentzian fit reveals two ER maxima. The signs at the bottom denote the microscopically observed rotation sense of the aggregates. (+) and (−) stand for co- and antifield sense, respectively. (B) Model calculations of the real and imaginary part of the Clausius Mossotti factor (CM) of the virus model for external conductivities of 6.5 and 74 mS/m. Dotted, broken, and solid lines are the imaginary, real, and absolute values of the CM, respectively. Note the correspondence of the imaginary part at 6.5 mS/m to the high-frequency peak of panel (A). At the bottom, the frequency dependence of the DP trapping efficiency at 74 mS/m is indicated. (−), (=), and (+) stand for moderate trapping, very efficient trapping, and no trapping, respectively.

translational and rotational diffusion, which are proportional to r^{-1} and r^{-3} of the particle radius r.[20]

DPALS does not require an optical anisotropy of the particles. Since the method is based on detection of particle translations, field-induced convections influence the results. Up to now, it was not possible to develop a DPALS chamber design allowing a clear separation of particle DP from convections of the suspension medium.[25] The reason is that the inhomogeneous field required for DP also gives rise to induced temperature gradients, which in turn generate gradients in the dielectric constant and conductivity of the medium.

In consequence, not only thermal, but also electrically driven convections disturb DPALS detection. Translational diffusion imposes a lower limit for DPALS detection for a given field strength.

Of advantage is the proportionality of the induced ER torque and DP force to the square of the field strength. There is hope that the current field-strength limits can be overcome by miniaturization of the electrode system.

In a cage, the rate of heat production per unit volume depends on the field strength and medium conductivity. Extreme miniaturization may solve the problem of severe temperature rises by increasing the surface-volume ratio of the cage. Size, driving mode, and arrangement of electrodes determine the field distribution. The cage forces increase with the gradient of the electric field. Although electrode spacing can be more than 100 times larger than the particle diameter, smaller cages operate more efficiently.[1] Closed field cages require a three-dimensional, for example, octopole, arrangement of electrodes or, as in this paper, a planar arrangement generating a funnel-like field structure (FIGURES 5A and 5B). A funnel can be achieved by geometrically restricting the field cage or by gravitational forces.[1,27] Fast and strong trapping occurs if the electrode spacing is of the same order of magnitude as the particles. Suppositions for trapping are sufficient polarizability differences between the particle and the surrounding solution. Of course, trapping is frequency-dependent. For interpretation, one has to consider single-particle trapping as well as particle-particle and particle-aggregate interactions. Since the frequency dependence of the polarizability of individual virus particles is identical, they tend to attract each other, forming small aggregates. Commonly, the frequency dependence of aggregate polarization is very similar to that of the individual particles. Thus, small particle aggregates will grow and the central particle aggregate formed in the field minimum of the cage will facilitate

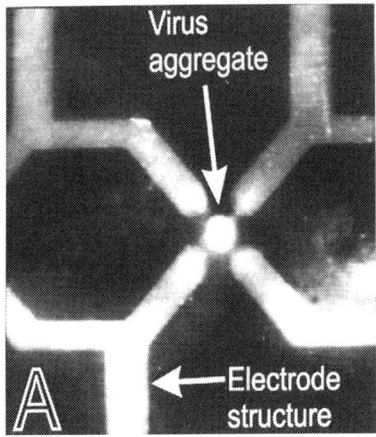
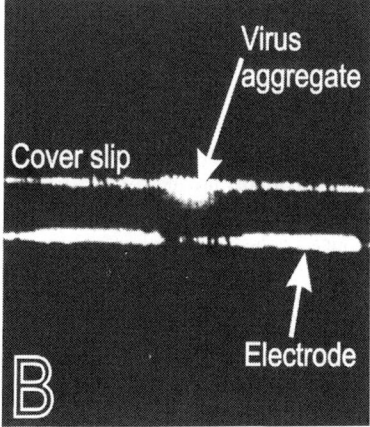

FIGURE 5. (A) Trapped virus particles in a planar DFT chamber covered with a microscope slide. The electrode distance was 25 μm. Electrodes were driven at 7 MHz and an amplitude of 3 V_{rms}. (B) Cross-sectional view of the chamber. The image is a 90° perspective obtained by a confocal laser-scan microscope. Videoframes were reprocessed using Leica Confocal Microscopy image-processing software (Leica, Göttingen, Germany).

collection of further particles or smaller aggregates by its attractive force. The attraction force of two particles is proportional to the absolute value of their induced dipole moments. Nevertheless, the frequency dependence of the attraction force is very similar to the real part of the induced dipole moment since the imaginary part contributes only in the case of dispersions (FIGURE 4B).

Schnelle et al.[27] derived a virus model from trapping experiments at 5 MHz and described the virus as a homogeneous sphere (conductivity of 0.8 mS/m, permittivity of 3). In this paper, the internal dielectric parameters were deduced from modeling the whole antifield peak in the range from 200 kHz to 25 MHz. As a rough description of the actual structural composition of influenza viruses, a spherical geometry with an external radius of 50 nm and a single shell of 18 nm thickness was assumed.[28] The shell summarizes the dimensions of the lipid and surface protein (hemagglutinin and neuraminidase) layers. Model calculations were conducted to optimize the dielectric parameters for the model. An optimal fit for the high-frequency peak was achieved for core and shell conductivities of 0.1 mS/m and 0.1 μS/m, respectively, and relative permittivities of 30 and 80, respectively. A problem is that rotation sense and trapping efficiencies were deduced from the behavior of aggregates. Nonetheless, from experiments on biological cells, it is known that, for structural dispersions, aggregates have no qualitatively changed ER behavior, but only exhibit slight peak shifts.

Although the low-frequency cofield peak below 100 kHz is consistent with the observed transition in the DFT behavior (FIGURES 4A and 4B), it cannot be described in the framework of a structural dispersions model. This peak is caused by the dispersions of electrophoretic particle movement and the electroosmotic streaming within its electric double layer.[6,29]

A very rough explanation for the effect is to consider the disturbance of the ζ-potential by the external field. For negatively charged particles in a DC field, the electric double layer would be deformed, resulting in a weaker screening at the side of the positive electrode. Now, according to the Einstein-Smoluchovski model, a perpendicular field component would induce asymmetric particle electrophoresis, generating a torque on the particle. Disturbance of the double layer requires a characteristic time, T_α, which is related to the characteristic particle size and the diffusion coefficients of the ions involved in double-layer polarization. In a rotating field for an external field frequency much lower than $1/T_\alpha$, a maximum disturbance of the double layer would occur. Nevertheless, since the process can follow field rotation, no field component perpendicular to the orientation of the induced polarization exists and no torque is induced. At very high frequencies, double-layer polarization is too slow to build up. The optimum of the polarization and the perpendicular field component, inducing a maximum α-torque, will occur at the frequency $f_\alpha = 1/(2\pi T_\alpha)$. Assuming a diffusion coefficient of ions ($D = 1.5 \times 10^{-5}$ cm^2/s) and a characteristic length r, T_α can be estimated to be $T_\alpha = r^2/D$. For the frequency of 29 kHz measured for the α-peak, a characteristic length r of 91 nm can be estimated. It must be taken into account that a very low ionic strength of about 1 mM was used. Therefore, the Debye length is about 10 nm and cannot be neglected. This leaves a characteristic particle radius of about 81 nm. These rough estimations suggest that most of the ERLS signal was probably generated by small aggregates of a few viruses. Further considerations should include the amplitude of the peak, which is related to the amount of viral surface charges.[6,7,29] Alas, data on the surface charge were not available from the literature.

Combination of DPALS, ERLS, and DFT offers a promising method to explore the dielectric structure of submicroscopic particles. The transparency of field cages suggests direct combination not only with ERLS or DPALS, but also with laser tweezers. For viruses, supramolecular particles, or macromolecules, electric characterization is the prerequisite for possible field-enhanced crystallization or the improvement of particle sorting techniques, etc.

ACKNOWLEDGMENTS

I thank G. Fuhr and A. Herrmann for providing the field cage and the viruses, respectively. T. Müller is acknowledged for many fruitful discussions and help with the experiments. B. Prüger, Ch. Mrosek, and D. Wachner are acknowledged for help with the experiments and figures.

REFERENCES

1. FUHR, G., T. SCHNELLE, S.G. SHIRLEY & R. HAGEDORN. 1995. Dielectrophoretic field-cages—a new technique for cell, virus, and macromolecule handling. Cell. Eng. **1:** 47–57.
2. GIMSA, J., T. MÜLLER, T. SCHNELLE & G. FUHR. 1996. Dielectric spectroscopy of single human erythrocytes at physiological ionic strength: dispersion of the cytoplasm. Biophys. J. **71:** 495–506.
3. ASBURY, C.L. & G. VAN DEN ENGH. 1998. Trapping of DNA in nonuniform oscillating electric fields. Biophys. J. **74:** 1024–1030.
4. HUANG, Y., X-B. WANG, F.F. BECKER & P.R.C. GASCOYNE. 1997. Introducing dielectrophoresis as a new force field for field-flow fractionation. Biophys. J. **73:** 1118–1129.
5. BECKER, F.F., X-B. WANG, Y. HUANG, R. PETHIG, J. VYKOUKAL & P.R.C. GASCOYNE. 1995. Separation of human breast cancer cells from blood by differential dielectric affinity. Proc. Natl. Acad. Sci. U.S.A. **92:** 860–864.
6. GEORGIEWA, R., B. NEU, V. SHILOV, E. KNIPPEL, A. BUDDE, R. LATZA, E. DONATH, H. KIESEWETTER & H. BÄUMLER. 1998. Low frequency electrorotation of fixed red blood cells. Biophys. J. **74:** 2114–2120.
7. MAIER, H. 1997. Electrorotation of colloidal particles and cells depends on surface charge. Biophys. J. **73:** 1617–1626.
8. MOUSSAVI, M., H.P. SCHWAN & H.H. SUN. 1994. Harmonic distortions caused by electrode polarisation. Med. Biol. Eng. Comput. **32:** 121–125.
9. GIMSA, J. & D. WACHNER. 1998. A unified RC-model for impedance, dielectrophoresis, electrorotation, and induced transmembrane potential. Biophys. J. **75:** 1107–1116.
10. PETHIG, R. & D.B. KELL. 1987. The passive electrical properties of biological systems: their significance in physiology, biophysics, and biotechnology. Phys. Med. Biol. **32:** 933–977.
11. POHL, H.A. 1978. Dielectrophoresis: The Behavior of Neutral Matter in Nonuniform Electric Fields. Cambridge University Press. London/New York.
12. WANG, X-B., Y. HUANG, R. HÖLZEL, J.P.H. BURT & R. PETHIG. 1993. Theoretical and experimental investigations of the interdependence of the dielectric, dielectrophoretic, and electrorotational behaviour of colloidal particles. J. Phys. D Appl. Phys. **26:** 312–322.
13. SCHWAN, H.P. 1957. Electrical properties of tissue and cell suspensions. *In* Advances in Biological and Medical Physics, p. 147–209. Academic Press. New York.
14. PASTUSHENKO, V. PH., P.I. KUZMIN & YU. A. CHIZMADSHEV. 1985. Dielectrophoresis and electrorotation: a unified theory of spherically symmetrical cells. Stud. Biophys. **110:** 51–57.
15. GIMSA, J., P. MARSZALEK, U. LOWE & T.Y. TSONG. 1991. Dielectrophoresis and electrorotation of neurospora slime and murine myeloma cells. Biophys. J. **60:** 749–760.
16. PAULY, H. & H.P. SCHWAN. 1959. Über die Impedanz einer Suspension von kugelförmigen Teilchen mit einer Schale. Z. Naturforsch. **14b:** 125–131.

17. FUHR, G., J. GIMSA & R. GLASER. 1985. Interpretation of electrorotation of protoplasts. I. Theoretical considerations. Stud. Biophys. **108:** 149–164.
18. PAUL, R. & M. OTWINOWSKI. 1991. The theory of the frequency response of ellipsoidal biological cells in rotating electrical fields. J. Theor. Biol. **148:** 495–519.
19. FUHR, G., T. MÜLLER, T. SCHNELLE, R. HAGEDORN, A. VOIGT, S. FIEDLER, M. ARNOLD, U. ZIMMERMANN, B. WAGNER & A. HEUBERGER. 1994. Radio-frequency microtools for particle and live cell manipulation. Naturwissenschaften **81:** 528–535.
20. EPPMANN, P., J. GIMSA, B. PRÜGER & E. DONATH. 1996. Dynamic light scattering from oriented, rotating particles: a theoretical study and comparison to electrorotation data. J. Phys. III (France) **6:** 421–432.
21. PRÜGER, B., P. EPPMANN, E. DONATH & J. GIMSA. 1997. Measurement of inherent particle properties by dynamic light scattering—introducing electrorotational light scattering (ERLS). Biophys. J. **72:** 1414–1424.
22. GIMSA, J., P. EPPMANN & B. PRÜGER. 1997. Introducing phase analysis light scattering for dielectric characterization: measurement of traveling-wave pumping. Biophys. J. **73:** 3309–3316.
23. PRÜGER, B., P. EPPMANN & J. GIMSA. 1998. Particle characterization by AC-electrokinetic phenomena: 3. New developments in electrorotational light scattering (ERLS). Colloids Surf. **A136:** 199–207.
24. SCHÄTZEL, K. 1987. Correlation techniques in dynamic light scattering. Appl. Phys. **B42:** 193–213.
25. EPPMANN, P., B. PRÜGER & J. GIMSA. 1999. Particle characterization by AC-electrokinetic phenomena: 2. Dielectrophoresis of latex particles measured by dielectrophoretic phase analysis light scattering (DPALS). Colloids Surf. A. **149:** in press.
26. FUHR, G., W.M. ARNOLD, R. HAGEDORN, T. MÜLLER, W. BENECKE, B. WAGNER & U. ZIMMERMANN. 1992. Levitation, holding, and rotation of cells within traps made by high-frequency fields. Biochim. Biophys. Acta **1108:** 215–223.
27. SCHNELLE, T., T. MÜLLER, S. FIEDLER, S.G. SHIRLEY, K. LUDWIG, A. HERRMANN, G. FUHR, B. WAGNER & U. ZIMMERMANN. 1996. Trapping of viruses in high-frequency electric field cages. Naturwissenschaften **83:** 172–176.
28. MURPHY, B.R. & R.G. WEBSTER. 1990. Orthomyxoviruses. *In* Virology, p. 1091–1152. Raven Press. New York.
29. GROSSE, C. & V. SHILOV. 1996. Theory of the low-frequency electrorotation of polystyrene particles in electrolyte solution. J. Phys. Chem. **100:** 1771–1778.

Biomass Monitoring Using Impedance Spectroscopy[a]

R. BRAGÓS,[b] X. GÁMEZ,[c] J. CAIRÓ,[c] P. J. RIU,[b] AND F. GÒDIA[c]

[b]*Departament d'Enginyeria Electrònica, Universitat Politècnica de Catalunya, 08034 Barcelona, Spain*

[c]*Departament d'Enginyeria Química, Facultat de Ciències, Universitat Autònoma de Barcelona, 08193 Bellaterra, Barcelona, Spain*

ABSTRACT: The biomass density in biotechnological processes is often determined by indirect and manual methods. Electrical impedance spectroscopy can provide on-line viable biomass density estimators. In this work, we present two linear estimators obtained with this technique. Four different microorganisms were measured. The detection threshold was approximately 1 g/L (dry weight) for bacteria and 0.5 g/L for yeast. Liposome suspensions were also used to validate the methods. The monitoring of the continuous growth of a yeast culture is also presented.

INTRODUCTION

One of the most important variables in biotechnological processes is the density of viable biomass in a bioreactor. Most of the methods used to obtain an estimation of this value are indirect and off-line, and they often require the manipulation of the sample in order to adjust it to the dynamic range of the measurement system.[1] Some on-line methods are based on electrical measurements and use the dependence of electrical parameters (σ,ε) on the cell volume fraction (p) at one or two frequencies. Some published results have been obtained using a two-electrode system.[2–4] This method has a high sensitivity, but mainly measures the variation of the electrode impedances due to the biomass changes on the surface, and is more suited to the study of response to antibiotics, for example. Other groups have measured the properties of the cell suspension by using the four-electrode method to obtain estimations of viable biomass density based on the variation of the conductivity[5] or the capacitance.[6] There is at least a commercial system (Aber Instruments Biomass Monitor) based on this last technique.

Since 1994, our group has been working on the development of biomass density estimators directly derived from electrical impedance measurements. In reference 7, we presented an estimator obtained from the measurement of the impedance magnitude at two frequencies. This estimator was derived from a numerical model of a double time-constant relaxation in the β region. In this paper, the results obtained with two other estimators are shown: the first estimator (E_2, equation 1) also uses measurements at two frequencies and is derived from the RC model of a generic cell suspension and the dependence of its parameters on the cell volume fraction p. This model is described in reference 8. Using this model as a starting point, we make the approximation that the capacitance ε_∞ can be canceled by the calibration process due to its slight dependence on the cell volume fraction p; that is, it can be considered constant. The impedance of this reduced RC model shows a single relaxation in the β region and varies not only with p, but also with the intra- and

---

[a]This work was supported by Spanish CICYT Project No. SAF98-0121.

extracellular conductivities, the membrane capacitance, and the cell radius. Making the assumption that the intra- and extracellular conductivities are similar, the impedance of the model has a simpler expression. The estimator E_2 (equation 1) defined over this impedance has an exact linear dependence with p and does not depend on the other parameters. In practice, the intracellular conductivity can be considered constant, but the extracellular medium displays conductivity changes. This means that a correction should be made for high conductivity changes. HF and LF in the estimator formula mean two frequencies higher and lower enough with respect to the central relaxation frequency. The reduction of the frequency range leads to a sensitivity loss. This problem has practical implications, due to the fact that the smallest cells have relaxation frequencies above 10 MHz:

$$E_2\ (\%) = 100 \cdot \left(1 - \frac{|Z(\mathrm{HF})|}{|Z(\mathrm{LF})|}\right). \quad (1)$$

The second estimator (E_{2m}, equation 2) can be considered as an extension of the first and uses the parameters R_0 and R_∞ of the Cole-Cole impedance model (equation 3), which most closely fitted the measured spectrum. A least-squares noniterative method was employed to fit the measured data to the model:

$$E_{2m}\ (\%) = 100 \cdot \left(1 - \frac{R_\infty}{R_0}\right), \quad (2)$$

$$Z(f) = R_\infty + \frac{R_0 - R_\infty}{1 + \left(j\frac{f}{f_c}\right)^{1-\alpha}}. \quad (3)$$

MATERIALS AND METHODS

Measurement System

The impedance spectrum measurements in the 10 kHz–10 MHz range were performed using an HP4192A impedance analyzer. To reduce the errors caused by the combined effect of the electrodes and coaxial cables, the analyzer was connected to the electrodes through a remote front end.[9] This front end consisted of a wide-bandwidth current-mode differential amplifier with a common mode rejection ratio (CMRR) of 56 dB at 10 MHz. A triple reference calibration method, adapted from reference 10, was used to reduce the effect of residual errors.

The measurements were made in two modes:

(a) Off-line: Highly concentrated static suspensions of each microorganism were measured in a prism-shaped cell with four stainless steel rod electrodes. Each suspension was then successively diluted to one-half of its density until the detection threshold was reached. The aim of this experiment was to determine the linearity and sensitivity of both biomass estimators using cells of different size.

(b) On-line: Monitoring the growth of a cell culture in a B. Braun Biostat bioreactor (2000 mL) using an on-line, *ex situ* probe based on a thermostatized cell continuously filled with a sample of the bioreactor contents, using a closed circuit that maintained the sterile barrier.

Samples of the cell and bioreactor contents were also measured by determining their dry weight (DW) and their optical densitometry (OD) as reference methods.

Microorganisms

Two yeast species (*Saccharomyces cerevisiae* and *Candida rugosa*) and two bacteria (*Escherichia coli* and *Rhodobacter capsulata*) were measured using the off-line method. The on-line method was employed with *E. coli* and *S. cerevisiae*. Suspensions of liposomes were also measured to validate the method and to determine the relation between the particle size and the estimator sensitivity.[11]

RESULTS AND DISCUSSION

Off-line Measurements

As an example, FIGURE 1 shows the magnitude and phase angle of the impedance of a suspension of *C. rugosa* and the first four dilutions. It clearly shows how the frequency range of the instrument does not completely cover the β relaxation. As expected, successive dilutions have a lower impedance as well as a lower relaxation ratio. FIGURE 2 shows the complex plane plot of the impedance spectrum of the initial suspension and the result of the fitting to a Cole-Cole model for the impedance. It can be seen how more than half of the arc is extrapolated. FIGURE 3 shows the behavior of the estimators versus the dry weight of the samples. The E_2 estimator (circles) has a linear range that reaches a threshold below 0.3 g/L dry weight. However, the E_{2m} estimator (squares) obtained from the parameters of the whole spectrum has a smaller linear range than E_2. This is because the process of model fitting has large errors for low relaxations in the presence of noise. We can also see

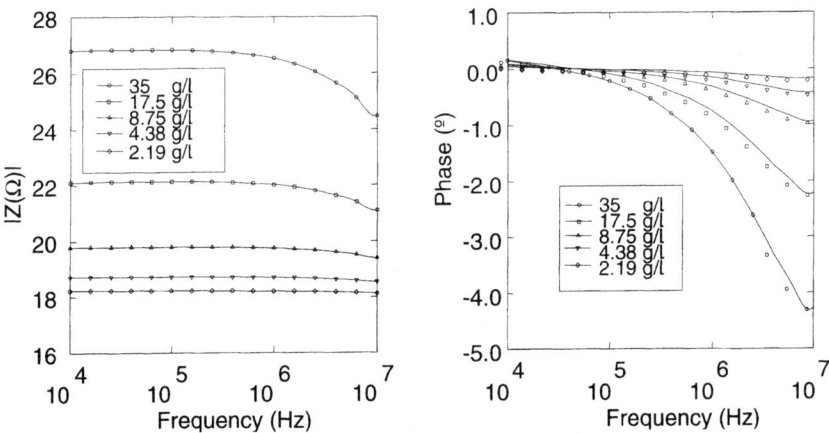

FIGURE 1. Magnitude and phase angle of the electrical impedance of successive dilutions of *C. rugosa*.

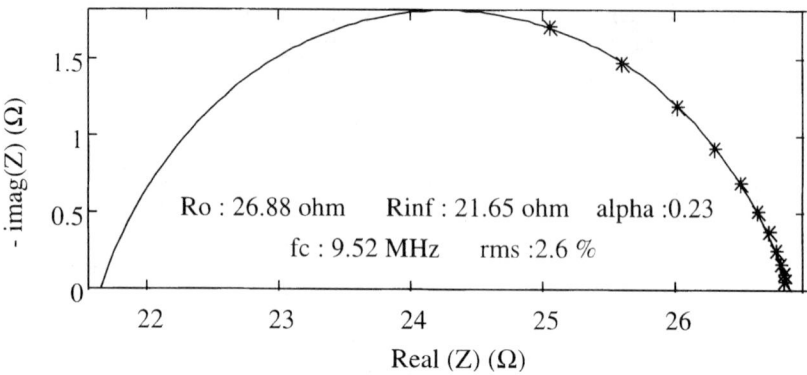

FIGURE 2. Complex plane plot and model fitting of the initial suspension of *C. rugosa*.

how E_{2m} has a larger sensitivity. This is because it uses the full relaxation instead of the reduced range employed by E_2. TABLE 1 summarizes the results obtained with the four microorganisms. As expected, the larger microorganisms have lower central relaxation frequencies and show a higher sensitivity and a lower detection threshold. The estimation for the *E. coli* threshold (*) is pessimistic. The correlation coefficient for the linear regressions is also included.

To overcome the limitations of the instrumentation in the high-frequency range, with the aim of validating the theoretical performance of both estimators, we also measured

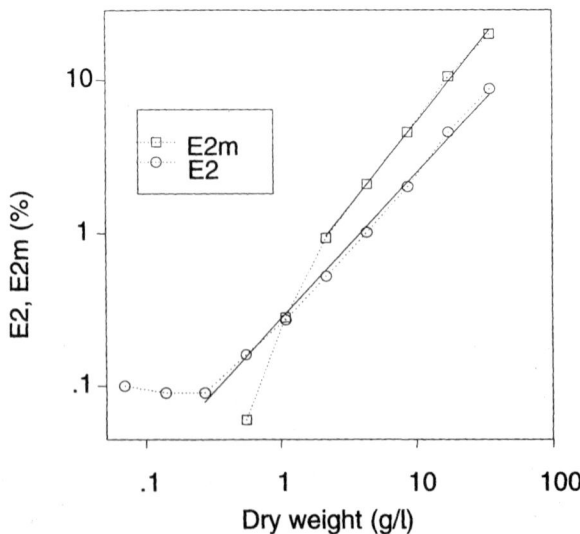

FIGURE 3. E_2 and E_{2m} estimators for *C. rugosa*.

TABLE 1. Summary Results of the Off-line Measurements with Yeast and Bacteria[a]

Microorganism	Diameter (μm)	Threshold (g/L)	Sensitivity [%/(g/L)]	Correlation Coefficient r
R. capsulata	0.5–1.2	0.9	0.06	0.995
E. coli	1.5–2.7	1.5*	0.07	0.998
S. cerevisiae	3.5–4.5	0.6	0.13	0.997
C. rugosa	5.0–6.0	0.3	0.25	0.999

[a]An asterisk indicates that the estimation for the *E. coli* threshold is pessimistic.

suspensions of liposomes. These particles allow the use of low-conductivity intra- and extracellular medium, resulting in high relaxations with low central frequencies that could be easily measured by the system. This means that the high-frequency measurement is closer to the R_∞ obtained from the model fitting and, therefore, both estimators should have the same sensitivity. FIGURE 4 shows the complex plane plot of the impedance spectrum for a liposome suspension of 1.1 μm ϕ and 60 g/L dw. We can see how the data set is now centered around the central frequency and almost covers the whole arc. FIGURE 5 displays the behavior of both estimators for the successive dilutions of this suspension. We can observe the predictable coincidence of the sensitivities and detection thresholds.

On-line Measurements

FIGURE 6 shows the continuous growth monitoring of an *S. cerevisiae* culture over a period of 7 hours. The curve is plotted from 140 readings taken every 3 minutes and has been filtered using a moving average filter (5 points). The result can be compared with the dry weight and optical density of the samples extracted every hour. As can be seen, the E_2 estimator begins to show a response at the end of the second hour, when the dry weight is about 0.2 g/L, and has a slight overshoot at the end of the exponential growth. The model fitting of each spectrum gives the time course of the Cole-Cole model parameters (not

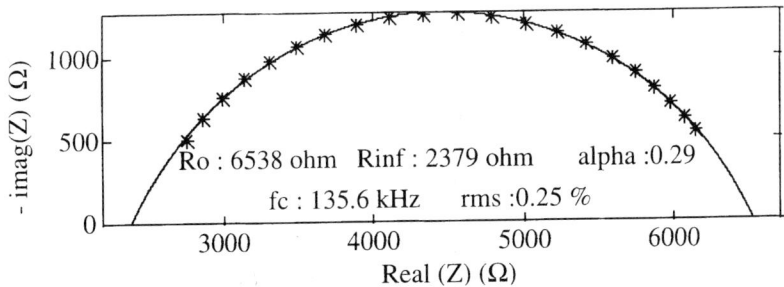

FIGURE 4. Complex plane plot and model fitting of the initial suspension of liposomes.

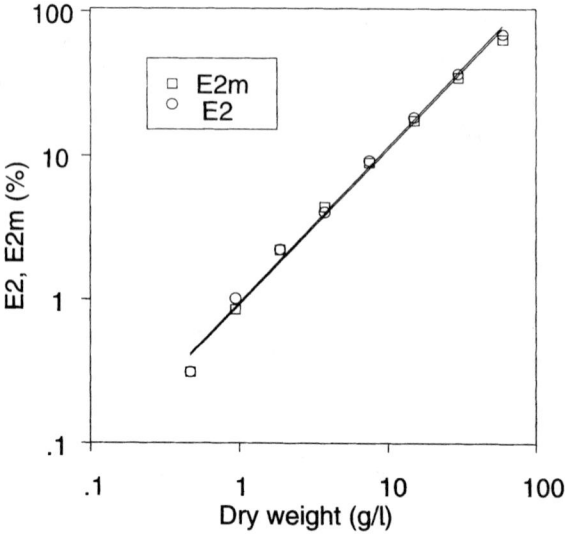

FIGURE 5. E_2 and E_{2m} estimators for the successive dilutions of liposomes.

shown). The fitting error falls below 5% at 3 hours and below 2% at 4 hours. R_0 and R_∞ show a continuous increase and allow the E_{2m} estimator to be obtained. The central frequency and the α parameter show a decrease (16 MHz to 5 MHz and 0.18 to 0.1, respectively). This could be interpreted as an increase and homogenization of the average dimensions of the cells.

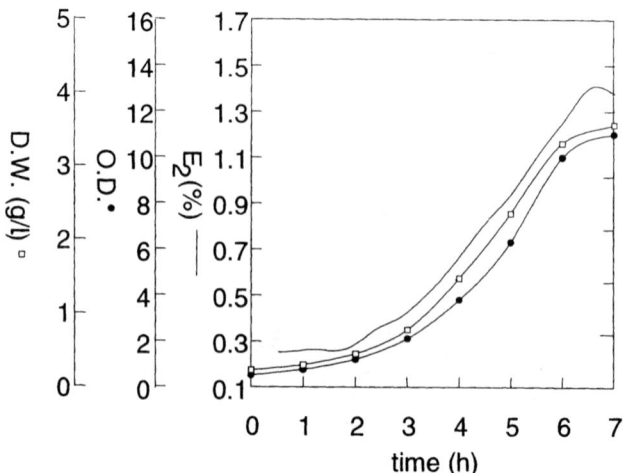

FIGURE 6. Continuous growth monitoring of *S. cerevisiae*.

CONCLUSIONS

This communication presents two estimators for the viable biomass density in a cell culture based on impedance spectrum measurements. The off-line results show their linearity, sensitivity, and detection threshold. Paradoxically, the estimator based on model fitting for the whole spectrum has a higher threshold than the estimator based on two frequencies. This is due to errors in the model adjustment of low relaxations. The presented method allows the continuous monitoring of yeast growth. The biomass density estimator based on two frequency measurements can be obtained after 2 hours from the inoculation of the bioreactor. The estimator based on the parameters of the Cole-Cole model can be obtained after 3 hours. The time course of these parameters can provide additional information about the evolution of the cell morphology.

REFERENCES

1. LOCHER, G., B. SONNLEITNER & A. FIECHTER. 1992. On-line measurement in biotechnology: techniques. J. Biotechnol. **25:** 235–253.
2. KEESE, C.R. & I. GIAEVER. 1994. A biosensor that monitors cell morphology with electrical fields. IEEE Eng. Med. Biol. **13:** 402–408.
3. MADRID, R.E., M.I. VERCELLONE, C.J. FELICE & M.E. VALENTINUZZI. 1994. Multichannel bacterial growth analyzer by impedance and turbidity. Med. Biol. Eng. Comput. **32:** 670–672.
4. MISHIMA, K., A. MIMURA & Y. TAKAHARA. 1991. On-line monitoring of cell concentrations during yeast cultivation by dielectric measurements. J. Ferment. Bioeng. **72:** 296–299.
5. LOVITT, R.W., R.P. WALTER, J.G. MORRIS & D.B. KELL. 1986. Conductimetric assessment of the biomass content in suspensions of immobilised (gel-entrapped) microorganisms. Appl. Microbiol. Biotechnol. **23:** 168–173.
6. DAVEY, C.L., H.M. DAVEY & D.B. KELL. 1992. On the dielectric properties of cell suspensions at high volume fractions. Bioelectrochem. Bioenerg. **28:** 319–340.
7. BRAGÓS, R., P. RIU, J. CAIRÓ, J.L. MONTESINOS & A. TINTÓ. 1995. On-line estimation of biomass in free and immobilized cell cultures using two-frequency measurements. Presented at the Ninth ICEBI Conference, Heidelberg, Germany.
8. FOSTER, K.R. & H.P. SCHWAN. 1989. Dielectric properties of tissues and biological materials: a critical review. Crit. Rev. Biomed. Eng. **17:** 25–104.
9. GERSING, E. 1991. Measurement of electrical impedance in organs—measuring equipment for research and clinical applications. Biomed. Tech. **36:** 6–11.
10. BOLK, W.T. 1985. A general digital linearizing method for transducers. J. Phys. E Sci. Instrum. **18:** 61–64.
11. GÁMEZ, X., M. SABÈS, R. BRAGÓS, P.J. RIU, J. CAIRÓ & F. GÒDIA. 1996. Biomass monitoring using multifrequency impedance measurements: relationship between particle size and electrical impedance. Presented at the First European Symposium on Biochemical Engineering Science, Dublin, Ireland.

Improvement of a Front End for Bioimpedance Spectroscopy[a]

DAVID YÉLAMOS, ÓSCAR CASAS, RAMON BRAGÓS, AND JAVIER ROSELL[b]

Department of Electronic Engineering, Universitat Politècnica de Catalunya, 08034 Barcelona, Spain

ABSTRACT: This paper describes the main changes that have been introduced into the design of a new front end to be used with commercial impedance analyzers for the measurement of biological samples. This bioimpedance adapter has been specially designed to improve the accuracy at low frequencies and to increase the frequency range. The use of very accurate current conveyor circuits, together with the use of common-mode negative feedback, leads to an improvement in the impedance measurements at low frequencies, reducing the effect of electrode impedance.

INTRODUCTION

Front end nonidealities determine the accuracy of impedance measurement systems and, consequently, the quality of the parameters estimated in impedance spectroscopy. This is particularly true for wide-band multifrequency systems. Bioimpedance measurements at low frequencies (below 100 Hz) are not only of interest in particular situations such as ischemia processes monitored throughout the time evolution of the α-relaxation, but also have general-purpose applications such as broadening the frequency range of electrical impedance spectroscopy or imaging systems.

In a four-electrode measurement method, the impedance of current-injecting electrodes introduces a common-mode voltage that hides the measures (the differential voltage). This effect is especially noticeable at low frequencies when the electrode impedance is higher. In addition, electrode impedance on the voltage detection side degrades the differential amplifier effective CMRR.[1]

There are two ways of reducing the influence of electrode impedance. The first one is to reduce the electrode impedance, for example, by increasing the electrode effective area by sputtering or electrolysis of a stable, good conductor metal like platinum or iridium. The second one is to use a specific front end[2] to improve the critical input specifications of commercial equipment when used in bioimpedance measurements.

Previous published front ends[2-5] are based on a high input impedance instrumentation amplifier (IA) that detects the differential voltage across the impedance under measurement (rejecting the common-mode voltage). This differential voltage is then transformed into a unipolar voltage that is measured by the impedance analyzer.

We designed two front ends following this philosophy: front end 1 and front end 2. They were designed to improve the performance of bioimpedance measurements at high frequencies (up to 1 MHz) using small needle electrodes and a commercial impedance analyzer. The first front end has been implemented with a differential amplifier working in current mode (MAX436). This circuit operates in open loop, so it has lower accuracy and

---

[a]This work was supported by Spanish CICYT Project No. SAF 98-0121.
[b]To whom all correspondence should be addressed.

more drifts in gain. However, this is necessary at high frequencies because negative feedback leads to closed-loop phase shifts (the primary cause of circuit oscillation in conventional high-speed amplifiers). Between the inputs of this IA and the two voltage detection electrodes, we used two buffers in order to increase the input impedance and to supply a signal with low output impedance to drive the shield of the cable between the electrode and the front end circuit.[1] The buffers are of bipolar technology (EL2244). For this reason, the input resistance is poor (2 MΩ), but the input capacitance is very low (1 pF). They also have a good bandwidth (60 MHz) and are stable at unity gain. This front end has a high CMRR at high frequencies: 56 dB at 10 MHz, 76 dB at 1 MHz, and 85 dB at lower frequencies.

The second front end was built with a difference differential amplifier (DDA) (AD830) as the IA. The DDA circuit is based on two OTAs followed by a buffer. Altogether, within a loop, this achieves higher accuracy (0.6%) and stability in the gain. In this case, the buffers were CBFET (AD843). Also, active guarding has been used to avoid cross talk and to maintain high input impedance. With this front end, we get an effective CMRR greater than 110 dB until 200 Hz and greater than 90 dB at 1 MHz.[4]

This paper presents a new design that uses an IA to detect the differential voltage, but also uses common-mode feedback to reduce the common-mode voltage at the IA input.[6] This front end could be used in conjunction with equipment such as HP and Solartron impedance analyzers. Another difference is to inject a constant current instead of a constant voltage supplied by the impedance analyzer. The new front end is compared with previous IA-based front ends and with a commercial front end developed by Solartron.

FRONT END DESIGN

The newly developed front end (FIGURE 1) introduces three main changes compared to previous front end designs:

(1) injects a constant current instead of a constant voltage across the impedance under measurement using current conveyors (CCII);[7]

(2) a common-mode negative feedback was connected between the IA inputs and the current sink electrode to reduce the common-mode voltage;

(3) gives an estimate of the electrode impedance during the measurement.

The voltage supplied by the analyzer (H_{CUR}) is copied to node X through the voltage buffer of a CCII. This voltage, divided by the resistor connected to L_{CUR} and L_{POT}, determines the reference current i, which will be measured by the impedance analyzer. A copy of this current (i') is injected into the bioimpedance through the high impedance output Z. A composite[8] CCII configuration was used to improve the accuracy of the copied current.

The differential voltage of the bioimpedance is measured using an IA based on the AD830 commercial high bandwidth differential amplifier and an FET input stage based on the AD843. The output of this IA goes directly to the analyzer measurement input (H_{POT}). The common-mode voltage is detected at the differential amplifier input and is fed back to the current sink electrode through a gain stage based on a single operational amplifier (OP42).

Electrode impedance is estimated by measuring the magnitude of the voltage at the output of the feedback amplifier divided by the magnitude of the injected current (i'). This gives an approximation to the modulus of the current sink electrode. This approximation is

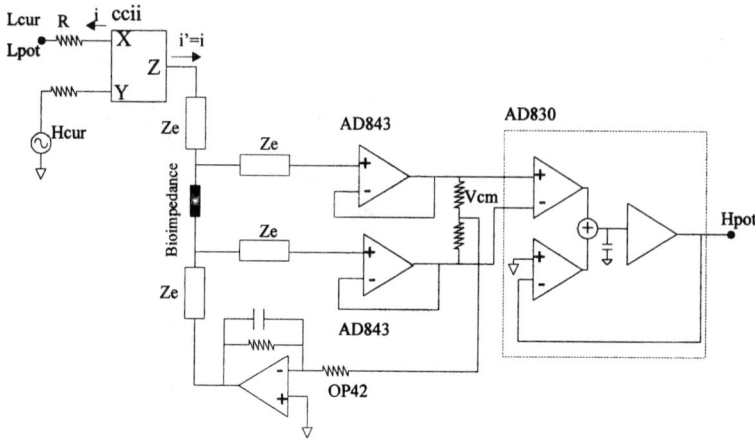

FIGURE 1. Electronic diagram of the new front end design.

valid when the impedance under measurement is much smaller compared to the electrode impedance and when the feedback closed-loop gain is much bigger than unity.

The whole circuit has been simulated to include high-order effects in the analysis and to guarantee its stability. The feedback lead compensation technique was used to prevent oscillations. This resulted in a phase margin of more than 45° with a feedback loop gain of about 40 dB. The dominant pole is placed around 1 kHz; this frequency is above the corner frequency of the electrode impedance and assures that the feedback gain is maximum at the frequencies when the electrode impedance is larger.

To simulate the front end, we developed a CCII model based on the characteristic parameters given by the manufacturer. This is a hierarchical block that can be reused in any schematic and can even be repeated within the same one, as is the case of the composite CCII. Extreme care should be taken when designing the printed circuit board, especially for the ground plane and for the power supply distribution in order to prevent the occurrence of a resonant circuit in the operating range.

RESULTS AND DISCUSSION

The front end was built and measurements of low-value pure resistive impedance (10–40 Ω) were made using discrete components. Each electrode impedance was simulated with 100 Ω in series with a 1-μF capacitor and in parallel with 100 kΩ. These values are used to simulate the electrode impedance of black platinum needles of 4 mm in length and 0.5 mm in diameter.

FIGURE 2 compares the two previous front ends with the new one, and also with the nominal value of the pure resistive impedance measured (36.5 Ω). Front end 1 is based on an open-loop differential amplifier with high bandwidth, but with comparatively low input impedance due to its bipolar input. It does not have enough CMRR at low frequency (85 dB). Front end 2 is based on a closed-loop IA with higher gain accuracy and input impedance (the buffers have

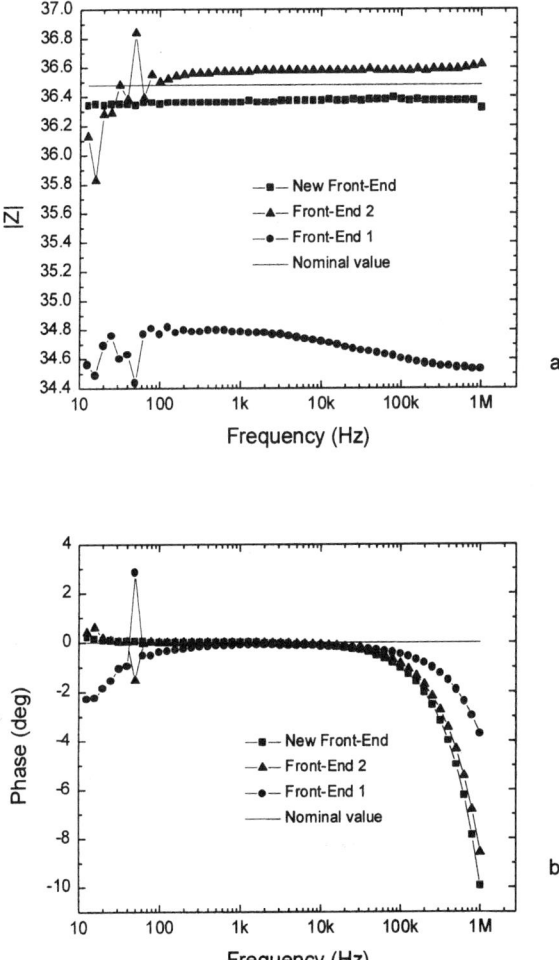

FIGURE 2. Comparison between different front ends over the whole frequency range: (a) module of impedance vs. frequency and (b) phase vs. frequency.

FET inputs), but it has a lower bandwidth than front end 1. The module and phase versus frequency curves have better behavior with the new front end at low frequencies.

Although front ends 1 and 2 have less accuracy, the high-frequency behavior can be corrected using a single reference calibration method and any residual load-dependent errors can be compensated for by using a three-reference method.[4] The performance of these calibration methods requires exactly the same conditions during the acquisitions of references and measurements. Due to the thermal and temporal variability of the electrode impedance, calibration does not work at low frequencies. In FIGURE 2, we can see how the new front end improves the accuracy throughout the frequency range and more especially at low frequencies as it is more resistant to the effects inherent to the electrodes as well as those caused by noise. The limit of resolution is determined only by the quantification step in the impedance analyzer used (HP4192A).

To complete the performance measurements of the new front end, we used very high impedance electrodes, equivalent to ECG electrodes over the skin. Each electrode impedance was simulated with 220 Ω in series with a 15-nF capacitor and in parallel with 220 kΩ. These values give an impedance modulus of 150 kΩ at 10 Hz and 200 kΩ at 1 Hz. We analyzed the results of measuring the previous pure resistive impedance with three different designs. The squares in FIGURE 3 correspond to the points obtained with the new front

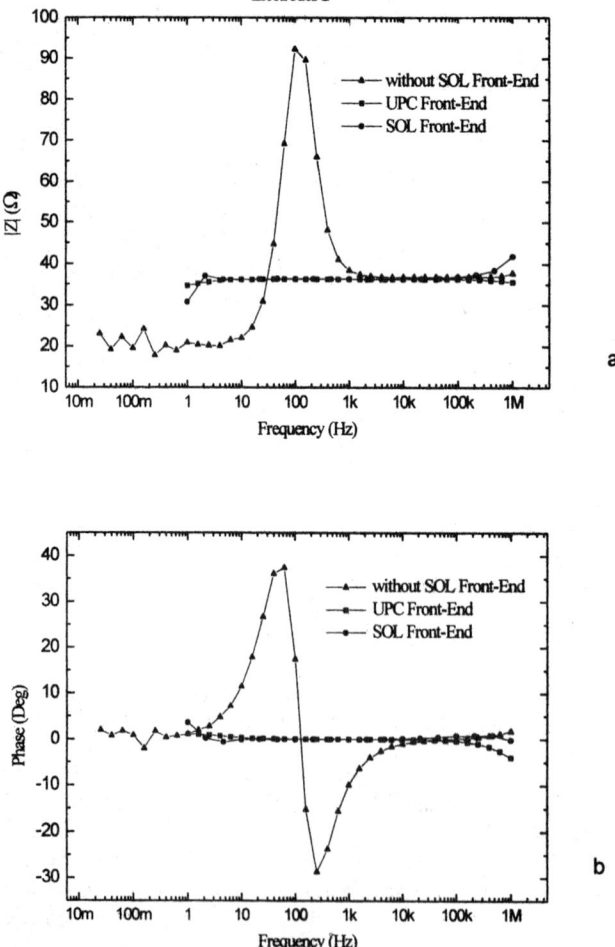

FIGURE 3. Comparison between the impedance measures done with balanced electrodes and obtained without a front end (triangles), with the Solartron front end (circles), and with the new front end (squares): measures of the module of impedance (a) and the corresponding phase (b).

end (NFE); the circles correspond to the impedance measured by a Solartron front end (SFE); and triangles correspond to the behavior of the latter equipment, but without front end, that is, only the Solartron impedance analyzer. We can appreciate at low frequencies that the SFE seems to pick up some induced common-mode noise; then, at high frequencies (at 100 kHz), it begins to move away from the expected behavior. Also, without a front end, it can be seen that the measured impedance has an error greater than 50%; for this reason, we are forced to use a different scale axis. Only at high frequencies, when the

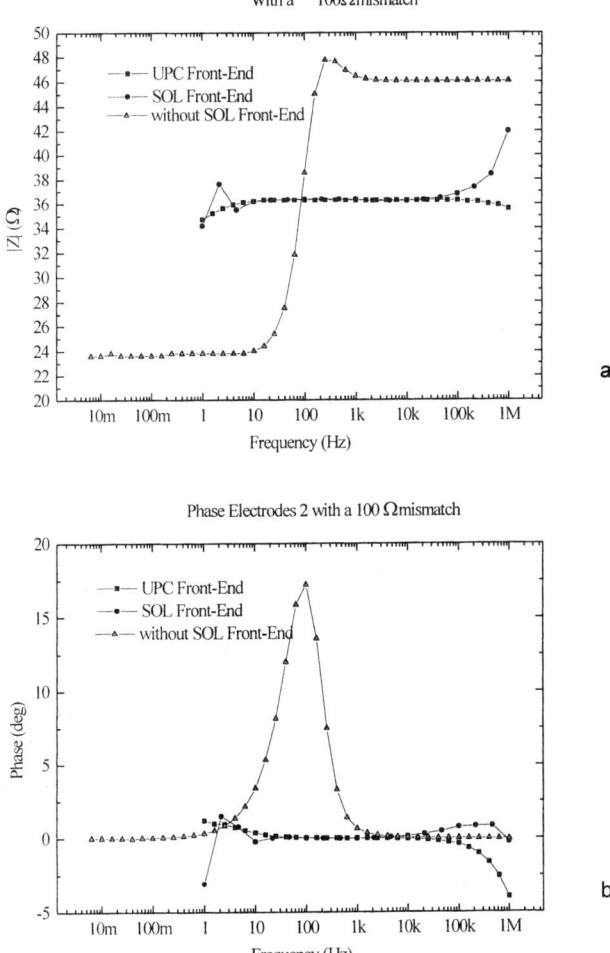

FIGURE 4. Comparison between the impedance measures done with unbalanced electrodes and obtained without a front end (triangles), with the Solartron front end (circles), and with the new front end (squares): measures of the module of impedance (a) and the corresponding phase (b).

electrode effect has disappeared, will the measurement of an impedance analyzer alone be similar to the nominal value.

From the previous test, the difference between the SFE and the NFE is negligible, but this is because the electrodes are balanced. If we now unbalance the electrodes placed in the detection side (see FIGURE 4), we will find more pronounced differences. To take into account the mismatch, we simulate the impedance of one of the electrodes at the differential voltage channel with a low-value resistor (100 Ω) and we keep the other with the same impedance used previously (200 kΩ at 1 Hz). Besides the differences described, we can see in contrast with the previous test that the measures of the impedance analyzer without a front end have more than 20% error over the frequency range.

CONCLUSIONS

The new front end improves the accuracy of impedance measurement at low frequencies and this allows an increase of the frequency range of measurements. This was basically achieved by the use of common-mode feedback. This technique cancels the systematic error that appears at low frequency due to the high electrode impedance, as well as the random error induced as common mode by interference. At high frequencies, common-mode voltage is not as crucial because the electrode impedance is lower, and the feedback is not effective because the feedback gain at these frequencies is low.

From the last test, we also emphasize that this new design is very robust against electrode mismatches.

REFERENCES

1. ROSELL, J., D. MURPHY, R. PALLÁS ARENY & P. ROLFE. 1988. Analysis and assessment of errors in parallel data acquisition system for electrical impedance tomography. Clin. Phys. Physiol. Meas. **9**(A): 93–100.
2. GERSING, E. 1991. Measurement of electrical impedance in organs—measuring equipment for research and clinical applications. Biomed. Tech. **36**(1–2): 6–11.
3. CASAS, Ó., J. ROSELL, R. BRAGÓS, A. LOZANO & P.J. RIU. 1996. A parallel broadband real-time system for electrical impedance tomography. Physiol. Meas. **15**(4): 1–6.
4. BRAGÓS, R. 1997. Contribution to the tissue characterization and biological systems through electrical impedance spectroscopy techniques. Ph.D. thesis, Universitat Politècnica de Catalunya, Barcelona, Spain.
5. BRAGÓS, R., P. RIU, J. CAIRÓ, J.L. MONTESINOS & A. TINTÓ. 1996. On-line estimation of biomass in free and immobilized cell cultures using two-frequency measurements. In Proceedings of the Ninth International Conference on Electrical Bio-Impedance, Heidelberg, p. 59–62.
6. ROSELL, J. & P.J. RIU. 1992. Common-mode feedback in electrical impedance tomography. Clin. Phys. Physiol. Meas. **13**(A): 11–14.
7. TOUMAZOU, C. et al. 1990. Analogue IC Design: The Current-Mode Approach. Peter Peregrinus. London.
8. LTP ELECTRONICS. 1993. CCII01 current conveyor amplifier (data sheet).

Virtual Biopsies in Barrett's Esophagus Using an Impedance Probe

C. A. GONZÁLEZ-CORREA,[a,b,c] B. H. BROWN,[a] R. H. SMALLWOOD,[a] N. KALIA,[d]
C. J. STODDARD,[d] T. J. STEPHENSON,[d] S. J. HAGGIE,[e] D. N. SLATER,[e]
AND K. D. BARDHAN[e]

[a]*Department of Medical Physics and Clinical Engineering, University of Sheffield, Sheffield, United Kingdom*

[b]*Departamento de Física, Universidad de Caldas, Manizales, Colombia*

[d]*The Sheffield Central University Hospitals, Royal Hallamshire Hospital, Sheffield, United Kingdom*

[e]*Rotherham District General Hospital, Rotherham, United Kingdom*

ABSTRACT: Preliminary results of electrical impedance measurements in squamous and columnar epithelia in rat and human tissues are presented. The aim of this work is to show the possibility of differentiating these two types of epithelia in terms of their electrical characteristics. For the measurements, we employed a 1.95-m-long, 3.2-mm-diameter, four-electrode probe designed to be used transendoscopically in the diagnosis of Barrett's esophagus (BE). BE is a condition in which the normal squamous epithelium of the esophagus is replaced by columnar epithelium of the intestinal type. This metaplasia is considered as a premalignant condition that puts patients at a 30–125-fold risk of developing adenocarcinoma of the esophagus. The diagnosis and surveillance of BE involve taking multiple biopsies, an expensive and time-consuming procedure. This study constitutes the first stage in the replacement of tissue biopsy by "virtual biopsies".

INTRODUCTION

Biological tissue characterization in terms of the electrical impedance spectrum has been studied by different authors.[1] One way of doing this is to fit the Cole model with the impedance data.[2] The three main parameters of this model are an extracellular resistance (R), an intracellular resistance (S), and a membrane capacitance (C). R is in parallel to a series combination of S and C. Knowing R, S, and C, it is then possible to calculate f_c, a characteristic frequency for the tissue. The use of this approach to differentiate between normal and pathological tissues has been called virtual biopsy[1] and is based on the well-known facts that each biological tissue has a specific electrical impedance (Z) and that this specific Z decreases with frequency. Impedance characteristics are basically determined by the tissue structure.[3]

Barrett's esophagus (BE) is widely accepted as a premalignant condition that puts patients bearing it at a 30- to 125-fold risk of developing adenocarcinoma of the esophagus (ACE) when compared to the normal population.[4] The incidence of ACE has been growing since the 1970s "at a rate exceeding that for any other cancer".[5] The diagnosis and life-long surveillance of patients with BE involves the transendoscopic taking of several

---

[c]Address for correspondence: Royal Hallamshire Hospital, Glossop Road, Sheffield, South Yorkshire S10 2JF, United Kingdom.

biopsies. This is an invasive (each biopsy is an excised sample of tissue, which implies some bleeding), time-consuming (2–3 days to know the results), expensive, and relatively complicated procedure that involves qualified staff (at least a gastroenterologist and a pathologist). BE is defined as "intestinal metaplasia in the lower esophagus".[6] This means that the normal squamous (multilaminar) epithelium of the esophagus is replaced by intestinal epithelium (columnar and, therefore, unilaminar). BE affects almost exclusively white patients and is considered as a complication of chronic gastroesophageal reflux disease (GERD).[7] The incidence of BE among the general population of Western countries has been estimated by different authors to be between 1.0% and 4.3%.[5]

For the electrical measurements, we have designed and built a 1.95-m-long, 3.2-mm-diameter, four-electrode probe that fits into the large instrument channel (3.8 mm diameter) of some endoscopes.

Preliminary measurements on rat squamous and columnar epithelia show that it is possible to distinguish clearly between these two types of tissue. We also present data from *in vitro* studies on specimens taken from patients with ACE that confirm these measurements. The results reported in this paper are part of the first step in the development of a full *in vivo* measurement system and aim to answer the following question: is it possible to separate squamous from columnar epithelium in terms of their electrical characteristics? The second step will be to differentiate columnar metaplastic from dysplastic and carcinomatous tissue.

METHODS

The four electrodes of the probe are made of 0.8-mm-diameter gold wire and the distance between the centers of adjacent electrodes is 1.27 mm. The interelectrode separation is therefore 0.47 mm. Each electrode is connected to an individually screened coaxial cable with an outer diameter of 1.02 mm (Habia Cable, Bristol, United Kingdom). The cables are held together by means of a polytetrafluoroethylene (PTFE) tube with an internal diameter of 2.71 mm and an outer diameter of 3.33 mm (Jencons Scientific Limited, Beds, United Kingdom). FIGURE 1 shows the dimensions of the tip of the probe. To minimize the relatively large cable capacitance due to the length of the probe, the "bootstrapping" technique is used. An electrical current of 20 μA_{p-p} is applied through two of the electrodes (A and B), while the voltage drop is measured between the other two (C and D). The probe is attached to a multifrequency tissue impedance meter designed and built in Sheffield, using the same electronics architecture as has been used for electrical impedance tomography.[8,9] For the measurements reported in this paper, the following frequencies were used: 9.6, 19.2, 38.4, 76.8, 153.6, 307.2, and 614.4 kHz. The real part or the impedance is measured, and the data are digitized and stored in a microcomputer using a PCM-DAS16S/12 board (Computer Boards, Incorporated, U.S.A.). The probe has been calibrated against saline solutions of known conductivities and its sensitivity at different depths was calculated using Geselowitz's theory.[10] According to this author, the change in the mutual impedance can be considered as a means for determining the sensitivity distribution under a planar array. The mutual impedance is defined as the ratio of the voltage measured between two sense terminals to the current passed between two drive terminals and should be "proportional to the dot product of the transfer impedances associated, respectively, with the current terminals and voltage terminals." Each transfer impedance is

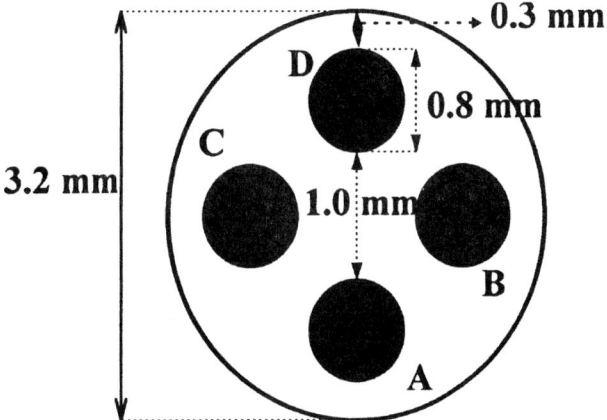

FIGURE 1. Dimensions of the tip of the probe. A and B are current electrodes, while C and D are sense electrodes. The probe is to be fitted into a large instrument channel (3.8 mm diameter) of an endoscope.

associated with a lead field and this, in turn, is considered to be "identical at each point to the electrical field that would exist at that point if unit current were injected into the lead."[10] A normalized sensitivity results from dividing the sensitivity of different points or regions by that of a common point or region used as a reference. For these calculations, a subroutine using a vectorial approach to this theory was written in MatLab®.

Measurements were made at room temperature on 9 rats immediately after death. The stomach was exteriorized under anesthesia (hypharm and diazepam in a 1:1 ratio). The epithelium of the glandular (posterior) stomach is columnar in nature, whereas that of the forestomach is squamous and similar to the esophageal epithelium. Differentiation between the two areas of the rat stomach is easy visually. In most of the rats, measurements were made at 3–4 different randomly selected positions on each tissue for a total of 61 measurements (30 on glandular stomach, 31 on forestomach).

We also used resected human specimens from 6 patients with ACE, after partial gastroesophagectomy, and from 1 patient with gastric carcinoma, after gastrectomy. Measurements were made at room temperature immediately after the surgical resection. In most of the cases, a pin was inserted in the vicinity of the place where each electrical measurement was taken and the pathologist took a sample later. In other cases, we cut the samples of the mucosa immediately after taking the electrical measurement, put them in separated boxes filled with formalin, and sent them for histopathological analysis. In all cases where epithelium was identified, it was of one of the following types: squamous, glandular (gastric) body type, glandular (gastric) fundic type, or glandular intestinal type. When intestinal type is found either in the esophagus or in the stomach, pathologists talk of intestinal metaplasia, and of gastric metaplasia when gastric type mucosa is found in the esophagus. The condition of any of the epithelia can be normal, inflamed, hyperplastic, dysplastic, or malignant (adenocarcinoma). Any sample analyzed under the microscope can show a single or a mixed pattern. In the present study, we have classified as squamous those samples displaying the single pattern (16 cases). Those either with cancer alone (without epithelium) or with a mixture of squamous and columnar epithelia were excluded. All others were considered as glandular (32 samples). The classification of the human samples was done independently by a histopathologist who was unaware of the impedance results.

The equation for the Cole model is

$$Z = R_\infty + (R_0 - R_\infty)/[1 + (if/f_c)^{(1-\alpha)}]$$

where R_∞ is the impedance at very high frequency, R_0 is the impedance at low frequency, f is the frequency, f_c is the relaxation or characteristic frequency for the tissue, and α is a constant that characterizes the Cole-Cole distribution function.[8] Based upon R, S, C, and f_c described in the INTRODUCTION, we assume $R_0 = R$ (the value read at the lowest frequency of our system) and the constant α is given a value of 0.2. S and C are calculated with a least-sum-of-squares fit, $R_\infty = RS/(R + S)$, and the relaxation frequency is obtained with $f_c = 1/2\pi C(R + S)$.

RESULTS

FIGURE 2 shows the decrease of the sensitivity with depth. FIGURES 3a, 3b, and 3c show the calculated distribution of the sensitivity of the electrode arrangement at the surface and at depths of 0.55 and 0.8 mm, respectively. All values are normalized against the value of the middle point on the surface. The normal squamous epithelium has a thickness between 0.3 and 0.8 mm (see reference 11, p. 1752). Therefore, a depth of 0.55 mm represents the average of these two values.

FIGURES 4a, 4b, and 4c show the electrical impedance spectra of squamous and columnar epithelia of rats in terms of R, S, and f_c, and FIGURES 5a, 5b, and 5c show the same using human tissue. For the measurements on rats, the maximum error of the estimates in

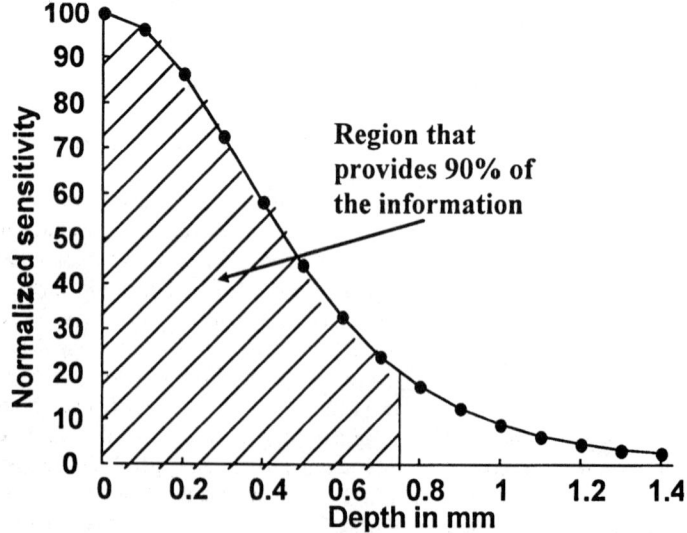

FIGURE 2. Decrease of the sensitivity of the array with depth.

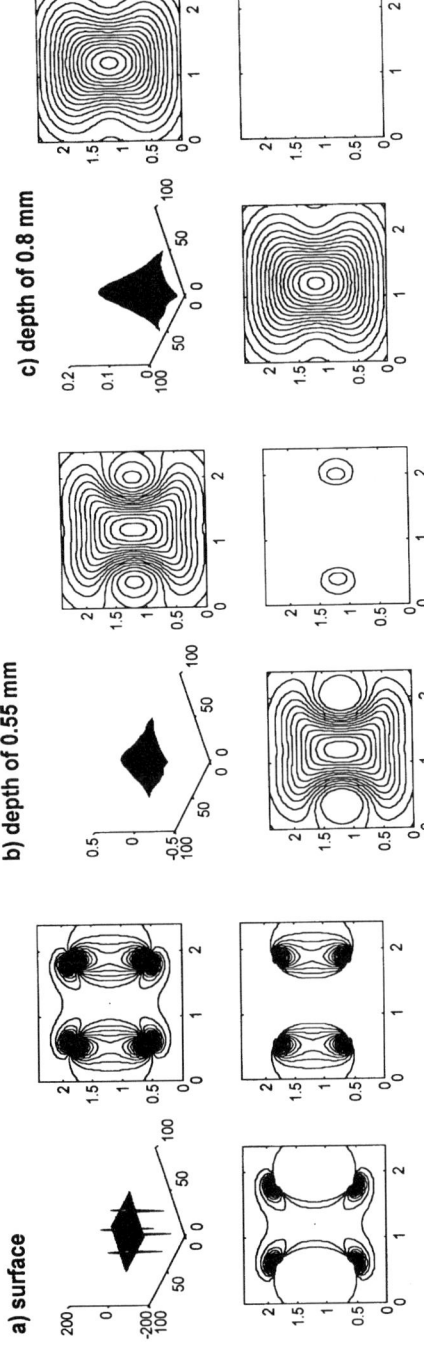

FIGURE 3. Sensitivity distribution of the electrical array at three different depths (a,b,c). In each figure, the upper left graph is a 3-D representation of the values, whereas the upper right graph shows the contour lines of those values in the *X-Y* plane. In the lower two graphs, contours of positive (left) and negative (right) values are separated. In part c, we only find positive sensitivity. See text for more details.

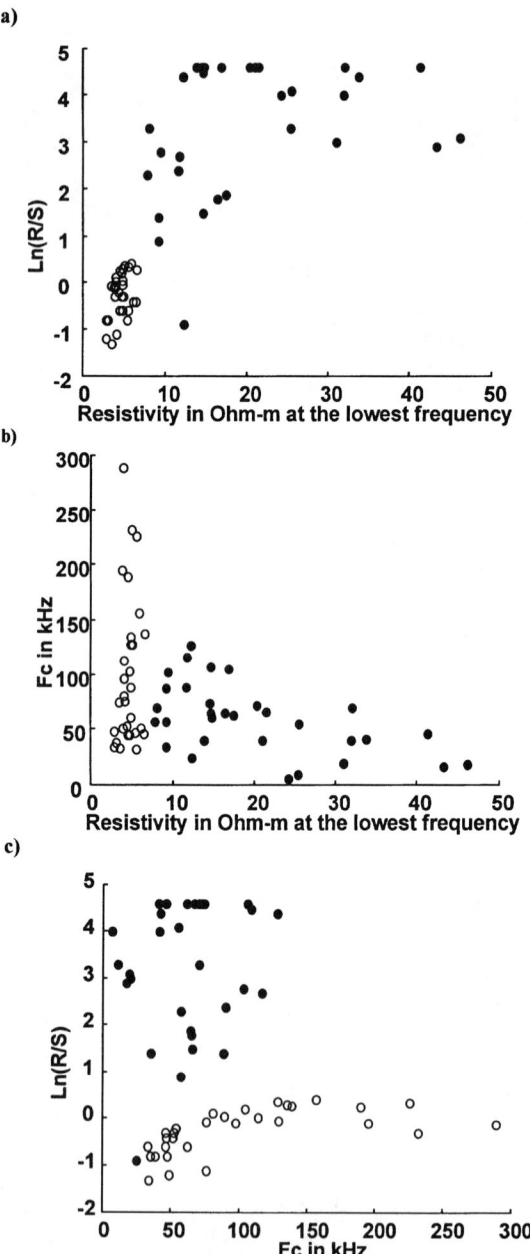

FIGURE 4. Electrical parameters for rat tissue. Open circles ($n = 30$) show measurements made from columnar epithelium, while filled circles ($n = 31$) are from squamous epithelium.

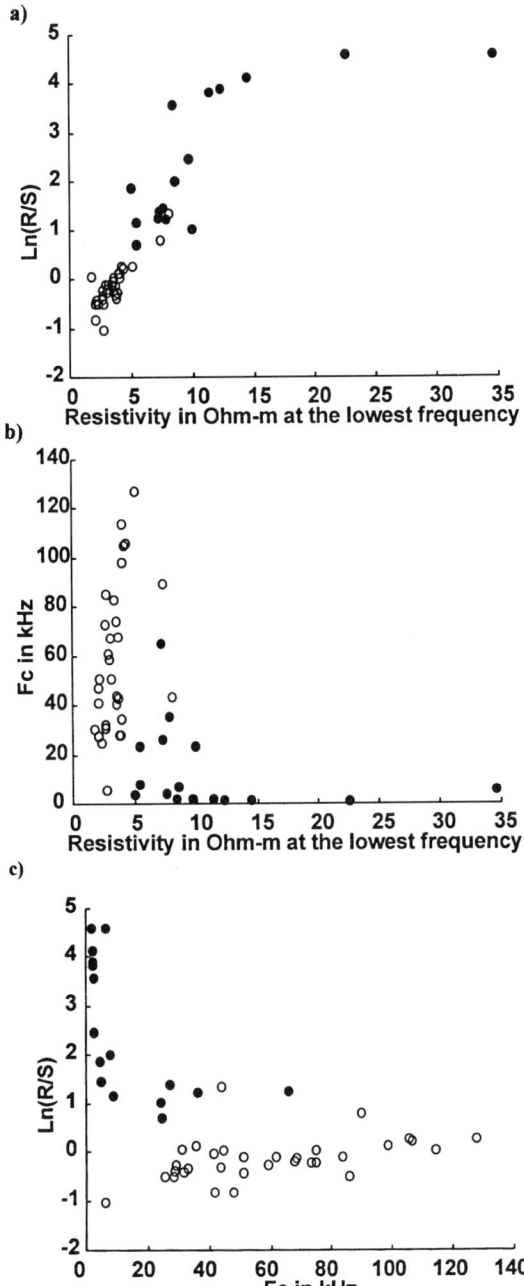

FIGURE 5. Electrical parameters for human tissue. Open circles ($n = 32$) represent columnar epithelium, while filled circles ($n = 16$) represent squamous epithelium.

the fitting was 0.093 with an average of 0.019. In the measurements on human tissue, these two values were 0.084 and 0.022, respectively.

For rat tissue as well as for human tissue, the Mann-Whitney test shows a significant difference ($p \ll 0.001$) between the means of the values of R and the index R/S. In terms of f_c the values for both tissues overlap, but it is interesting to notice that they are widely spread out, a fact that we will explore in the second step of our project. The overlap of f_c for the two tissue types seems to be less in human tissues. The p value of the Mann-Whitney test for f_c is 0.0218 for rat tissue and $\ll 0.001$ for human tissue. On the basis of R/S alone, with a division made at ln $R/S = 0.6$, from all the 61 measurements made on rat tissue, only 1 (1.6%) is not correctly assigned. On the same basis (R/S), with a division made at ln $R/S = 0.5$, from the 48 measurements on human tissue, 2 (4.2%) are not correctly assigned.

DISCUSSION

The sensitivity of any array of electrodes placed on a surface decreases with depth. The values for the middle of our array are shown as a graph in FIGURE 2. For our configuration, we see that the sensitivity at a depth of 0.8 mm is still about 17% of that on the surface. Another way to use these results is to integrate the curve to find the region from which 90% of the information comes. In this case, it is formed by the region above a depth of 0.77 mm. We consider this as appropriate for our purposes.

According to Geselowitz's theory, the sensitivity of the array shows very high values in the regions close to the electrodes, as seen in FIGURE 3a. We also see here two regions with negative sensitivity between electrodes A and C, on the left, and B and D, on the right. With depth, these two regions reduce in size and we do not see them at 0.8 mm (FIGURE 3c). All of this suggests that the readings made with the probe can be affected by its placement, and this is an issue to be considered in the future.

It is known that at low frequencies the current flows mainly through the extracellular space, whereas at higher frequencies the current flows both through the extracellular space as well as through the intracellular space. Therefore, in the squamous epithelium, where many cells are very tightly packed, the impedance at low frequency is expected to be high and to decrease quite rapidly with increasing frequency. In the columnar epithelium, as we only find a single row of cells, the difference between low and high frequencies is not expected to be very large since most of the current flows through the extracellular space (lamina propria) all the time. At the same time, the impedance at low frequencies in the columnar tissue should be much lower than that of squamous epithelium.

The results obtained with both rat and human tissues agree with the theoretical assumptions and show a very good separation between squamous and columnar tissue. Of the three parameters shown here, the index R/S and R seem to be good indicators of the tissue structure. The small degree of overlap in terms of R and R/S in human tissues could be possibly explained either by the fact that, in some cases, biopsies may not have been taken from the precise points from which the electrical readings were obtained or by the presence of more than one type of tissue in the same area. The electric characteristics of tissue with mixed patterns will be explored in detail in the future.

CONCLUSIONS

The results presented in this paper show that it is possible to differentiate between squamous and columnar epithelium in terms of their electrical characteristics. This constitutes the first step in our attempt to develop an *in vivo* measurement system to perform what we have called virtual biopsies of the esophagus. This procedure is aimed to reduce the number of real biopsies needed for the diagnosis and long-term surveillance of patients with Barrett's esophagus and, with refinement, should eventually replace them.

We are about to begin measurements transendoscopically and thus to collect *in vivo* data from patients with BE. At the same time, we will begin to deal with the second question and try to differentiate between simple metaplastic change and tissues with dysplastic changes that have already begun a cancerous pathway.

ACKNOWLEDGMENTS

C. A. González-Correa is sponsored by the Universidad de Caldas (Colombia) and the University of Sheffield (United Kingdom) and wishes to thank Liliana Robledo, Tulio Marulanda, and Guido Echeverry for their support.

REFERENCES

1. RIGAUD, B. *et al.* 1995. *In vitro* characterization and modelling using electrical impedance measurements in the 100 Hz–10 MHz frequency range. Physiol. Meas. **16:** A15–A28.
2. GRIFFITHS, H. 1995. A Cole phantom for EIT. Physiol. Meas. **16:** A29–A38.
3. LU, L. *et al.* 1995. A fast parametric modelling algorithm with the Powell method. Physiol. Meas. **16:** A39–A47.
4. CLARK, G.W.B. & T.R. DEMEESTER. 1995. Biopsy of upper gastrointestinal tract lesions. Surg. Oncol. Clin. North Am. **4**(1): 81–102.
5. SPECHLER, S.J. 1994. Barrett's esophagus. Gastroenterologist **2:** 273–284.
6. RIDDELL, R.H. 1996. The biopsy diagnosis of gastro-esophageal reflux disease, "carditis", and Barrett's esophagus, and sequelae of therapy. Am. J. Surg. Pathol. **20**(suppl. 1): S31–S50.
7. FALK, G.W. 1994. Barrett's esophagus. Gastrointest. Endosc. Clin. North Am. **4**(4): 773–789.
8. BROWN, B.H. *et al.* 1994. High frequency EIT data collection and parametric imaging. Innov. Technol. Biol. Med. **15:** 1–8.
9. LU, L. & B.H. BROWN. 1994. The electrode and electronic interface in an EIT spectroscopy system. Innov. Technol. Biol. Med. **15:** 97–103.
10. GESELOWITZ, D. 1971. An application of electrocardiographic lead theory to impedance plethysmography. IEEE Trans. Biomed. Eng. **BME-18**(1): 38–41.
11. WILLIAMS, P.L., Ed. 1995. Gray's Anatomy: The Anatomical Basis of Medicine and Surgery. Chapter 12: Alimentary System, p. 1683–1812. Thirty-eighth edition. Churchill Livingstone. New York.

Inductively Coupled Wideband Transceiver for Bioimpedance Spectroscopy (IBIS)[a]

HERMANN SCHARFETTER,[b] WOLFGANG NINAUS,[b] BERNHARD PUSWALD,[b]
GALIDIA I. PETROVA,[c] DIMITER KOVACHEV,[d] AND HELMUT HUTTEN[b]

[b]*Institute for Biomedical Engineering, Technical University Graz, A-8010 Graz, Austria*
[c]*Technical University of Plovdiv, Plovdiv 4000, Bulgaria*
[d]*Technical University of Varna, Varna 9010, Bulgaria*

ABSTRACT: Most measurement devices for bioimpedance spectroscopy are coupled to the measured object (tissue) via electrodes. At frequencies > 500 kHz, they suffer from artifacts due to stray capacitances between electrode leads as well as between the ground and object. The noninvasive measurement of the brain conductivity is hardly possible with surface electrodes. These disadvantages can be obviated by inductive coupling. The aim of this work was the development of a wideband transceiver for inductive impedance spectroscopy. In order to define its specifications, a feasibility study has been carried out with a simulation model for three different coil systems above a homogeneous conducting plate. According to simulation results, all systems render it possible to resolve conductivity changes down to 10^{-3} $(\Omega m)^{-1}$ at frequencies > 50 kHz. The transceiver electronics must then provide a resolution of ≥ 1 μV and an excitation current of up to 1 A. The realized receiver matches these specifications with an S/N ratio of 22 dB at 1 μV in the frequency range of 50 kHz to 5 MHz.

INTRODUCTION

Bioimpedance spectroscopy (BIS) has been recognized as a valuable tool for the noninvasive assessment of biological tissue via measurement of the electrical conductivity. Among others, methods for the monitoring of the hydration state[1–3] and episodes of ischemia[4] have been developed. A very challenging possible application of BIS is the monitoring of brain edema. As reviewed in reference 5, ischemic states or lesions can be detected from changes in the impedance within minutes, whereas in CT or MRI the first changes appear with a marked delay. Moreover, the imaging methods do not allow a bedside monitoring of patients.

During the past decade, fairly advanced instrumentation has been developed for BIS. However, most published systems are coupled to the tissue via electrodes. Such devices are difficult to apply above 500 kHz because of leakage currents via stray capacitances. The major stray capacitances appear between the object under measurement and the ground as well as between the electrode leads.[6,7] Moreover, the measurement of the brain conductivity poses a major methodological problem with surface electrodes attached on the scalp because the electrical current cannot penetrate through the skull. Inductively coupled transducers have been suggested for different single-frequency applications.[8–12] In principle, they are also applicable at multiple frequencies in the β-dispersion range of the conductivity of most tissues (some few kHz to some MHz).

---

[a]The appendix at the end of this paper lists the variables and abbreviations used.

The device proposed in reference 5 enables the measurement of brain impedance changes, but it operates at a single frequency. Hence, it is not possible to distinguish between intra- and extracellular edema. A multifrequency approach can reveal more information on the hydration state of tissue as it allows the application of structural fluid distribution models. Such models have been developed in the past based on the theory of disperse dielectrics.[2] An inductive multifrequency probe for the frequency range of 100 kHz to 30 MHz has become commercially available recently.[13] However, since this sensor is only applicable for fluids into which it can be immersed, it is not suitable for *in vivo* measurements.

The aim of this work was the development of the necessary measurement electronics for *in vivo* inductive bioimpedance spectroscopy (IBIS). In order to define the specifications, a theoretical feasibility study has been carried out with a simple model of eddy current flow in a homogeneous object. Based on the theoretical results, a wideband transceiver has been realized for the frequency range of 50 kHz to 5 MHz.

METHODS

Measurement Principle

Exposure of a conducting medium to an alternating magnetic field induces an eddy current field, the strength of which depends on the conductivity of the medium. The eddy currents cause a field disturbance that manifests itself as a change ΔV of the induced voltage in a pickup coil. Moreover, the power dissipation in the medium causes an impedance change ΔZ in the excitation coil (EXC). The conductivity of most biological tissues is about 0.1–1.5 $(\Omega m)^{-1}$;[14] hence, a resolution of 10^{-3} $(\Omega m)^{-1}$ is required in order to keep the relative measurement error $\leq 1\%$. As the Colpitts oscillator method suggested in reference 11 is very insensitive at frequencies below 1 MHz, three alternative sensors have been considered, which shall be abbreviated as S-1, S-2, and S-3. In all cases, it is reasonable to integrate the EXC into a tunable series resonance circuit in order to keep the load impedance for the driving circuitry as low as possible.

S-1 represents a circuitry for the measurement of the impedance change ΔZ of the EXC. This ΔZ manifests itself as a change ΔV of the voltage V_0 along the resonant circuit as depicted in FIGURE 1. V_0 is the voltage drop along the ohmic loss resistance of the undisturbed circuit. As ΔV is much lower than V_0, a compensation technique must be employed in order to suppress V_0. This is achieved by adding a compensation voltage V_C that drops along a compensation resistor R_C. As a consequence, only a small residual offset voltage V_{OR} remains, which is due to inevitable inaccuracies in the balancing process. The sum $\Delta V + V_{OR}$ can then be amplified with high gain.

The excitation current I is provided by two wideband power amplifiers, PA1 and PA2, one of which must be adjustable in both magnitude and phase. Phase adjustments are necessary because capacitive leakage currents across stray capacitances cause deviations of the circuit impedance from the ideal ohmic behavior even at the resonant frequency. If $\Delta V \ll V_0$, the impedance change ΔZ produces a ΔV according to equation 1:

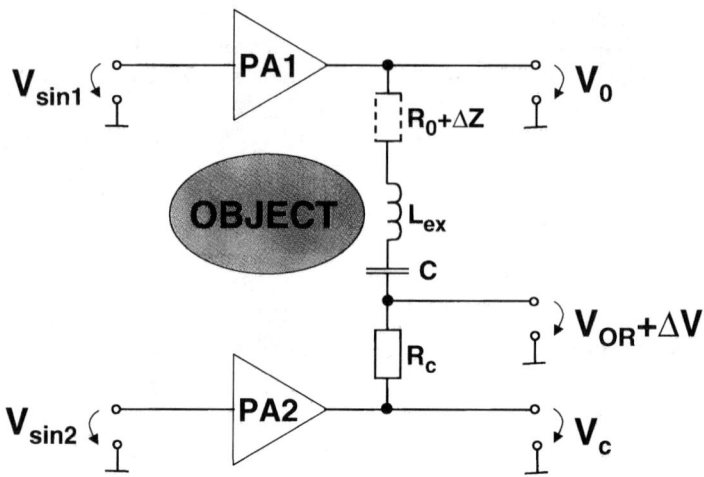

FIGURE 1. Sensor S-1 with compensation circuit. The PAs are fed by the adjustable sinusoidal voltages V_{sin1} and V_{sin2}. The voltage V_C is adjusted such that it opposes exactly V_0. Hence, the signal at the middle node vanishes in the undisturbed system.

$$\Delta V = V_0 \Delta Z \frac{R_0}{(R_0 + R_C)^2}. \tag{1}$$

The maximum ΔV is $0.25 V_0 \Delta Z/R_0$ if $R_0 = R_C$.

In contrast to S-1, the sensors S-2 (FIG. 2) and S-3 (FIG. 3) measure the change ΔV of the voltage when the object is brought into the magnetic field. ΔV is due to an alteration of

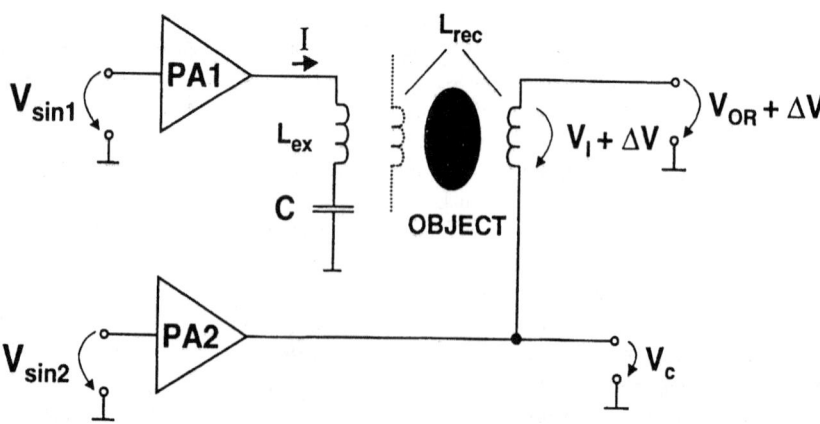

FIGURE 2. Sensor S-2 (transformer): The receiving coil L_{rec} can be placed either between the EXC and the object or on the opposite side of the object. The voltage V_C is adjusted such that it opposes exactly V_I. The PAs are fed by the adjustable sinusoidal voltages V_{sin1} and V_{sin2}.

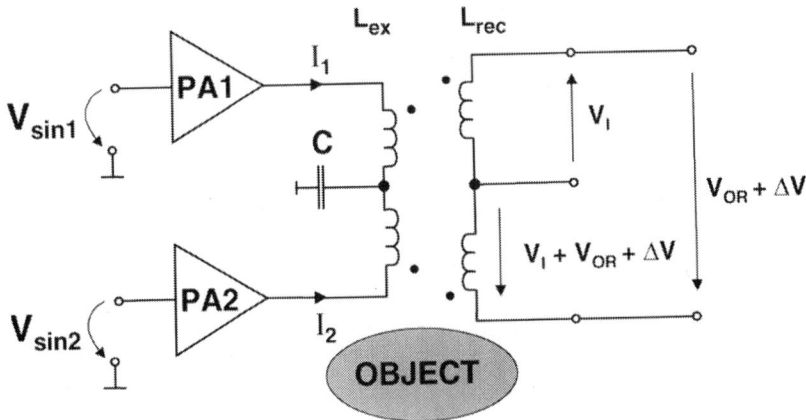

FIGURE 3. Sensor S-3 (magnetometer): Two receiving coils are connected such that the induced voltages V_I cancel out mutually. Electronic balancing can be achieved by adjusting I_1 and I_2 properly. This is possible by feeding the PAs with adjustable sinusoidal voltages V_{sin1} and V_{sin2}.

the mutual inductance between the primary and secondary coil of a transformer. V_I denotes the voltage that is induced in the undisturbed pickup coil. This configuration is suitable for measuring the conductivity distribution along a magnetic flux tube through the object as suggested in references 10 and 12. It is also possible to place the receiver coil between the EXC and the object, which allows the combination of the EXC and the receiver coil into a compact and easily applicable sensor. In our calculations, however, the receiving coil was assumed to be placed always on the opposite (distal) side of the object.

Sensor S-3 works on the same basis, but the compensation of V_I is achieved via a gradiometer arrangement on the secondary side (differential transformer or magnetometer).[5,8] The gradiometer is arranged symmetrically around the EXC and coaxially with it. A mismatch of the two receiver coils due to mechanical tolerances can be canceled out in principle by feeding both halves of the EXC with currents I_1 and I_2, respectively, which differ by an appropriate ΔI ("field compensation").

Model for Sensitivity Estimation of Sensors

We define the sensitivity $s = \Delta V/\Delta \kappa$ as the voltage change ΔV in the sensor due to a conductivity change $\Delta \kappa$ in a homogeneous infinite plate with thickness h_Z at a distance d_G apart from the receiving coil. For the estimation of s, the model in FIGURE 4 is employed.[15] The EXC is modeled by an infinitely thin monolayered solenoid with height h_{EX} and n_{EX} turns. It is placed at a distance d_{EX} above a conducting plate with thickness h_Z and infinite radial extension. The receiving configuration consists of a cylindrical gradiometer with

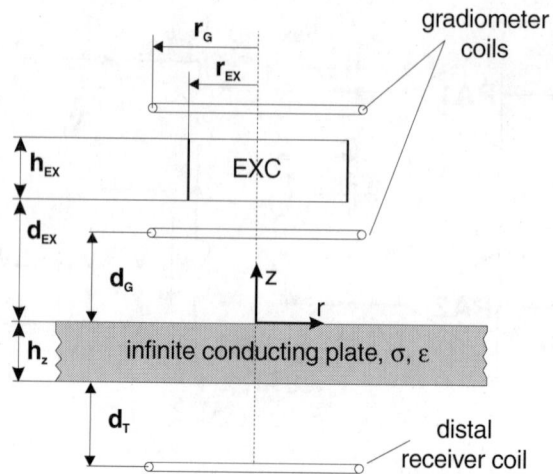

FIGURE 4. Model for the sensitivity estimation as published in reference 15.

infinitely thin coils (n_G turns) and an additional receiver coil on the opposite side of the conducting plate (n_T turns). For sensor S-1, the ΔZ in the EXC is calculated from the apparent power of the eddy current field in the object. We calculated s at 50–200 kHz as the sensitivity is lowest at low frequencies. As a consequence, this range is critical for the design of the receiver electronics. The geometrical data were $r_{EX} = r_G = r_T = 40$ mm, $h_Z = 20$ mm, $d_T = d_G = 20$ mm, $h_{EX} = 20$ mm, $\sigma = 0.1\ (\Omega m)^{-1}$, $\varepsilon_r = 80$, and $n_{EX} = n_G = n_T = 100$. d_{EX} was 30 mm for the sensors S-2 and S-3, whereas 20 mm was chosen for S-1 in order to keep the lower plane of the whole sensor at the same distance from the object. For the calculation of the S-1 sensitivity, we chose $R_L = R_0 = 5\Omega$, which represents a realistic value for a prototype coil at 50 kHz. The excitation current was set to 1 A; hence, V_0 becomes 5 V.

ΔZ in the EXC was calculated from the apparent power ΔP_{APP} in the whole object due to the eddy current density **S**:

$$\Delta Z = \frac{\Delta V}{I} = \frac{\Delta P_{APP}}{I^2}, \qquad (2)$$

$$\Delta P_{APP} = \int_{V_{OBJ}} \frac{1}{\kappa} \mathbf{S} \cdot \mathbf{S}^* dV, \qquad (3)$$

$$\mathbf{S} = -j\omega\mu\kappa\mathbf{A}. \qquad (4)$$

In cylinder coordinates, the vector potential **A** has only an angular component because of symmetry conditions. Within the object, this component $A(r,z)$ can be calculated according to reference 15 as

$$A(r, z) = \frac{2M\mu_0}{h_{EX}\pi r_{EX}} \int_0^\infty \left\{ J_1(\alpha r)J_1(\alpha r_{EX})e^{-\left(d_{EX} + \frac{h_{EX}}{2}\right)\alpha} \sinh\left(\frac{\alpha h_{EX}}{2}\right)\frac{Z(\alpha, z)}{N(\alpha)} \right\} d\alpha. \quad (5)$$

In the lower gradiometer coil ($z = d_G$), one obtains

$$A(r_G, d_G) = \frac{M}{h_{EX}\pi r_{EX}} \int_0^\infty \left(J_1(\alpha r_G)J_1(\alpha r_{EX})e^{-\left(d_{EX} + \frac{h_{EX}}{2}\right)\alpha} \sinh\left(\frac{\alpha h_{EX}}{2}\right) Q(\alpha, d_G) \right) \frac{d\alpha}{\alpha} \quad (6)$$

with

$$N(\alpha) = (\mu\alpha + \mu_0\beta)^2 e^{h_Z\beta} - (\mu\alpha - \mu_0\beta)^2 e^{-h_Z\beta},$$

$$Z(\alpha, z) = (\mu\alpha + \mu_0\beta)e^{(z+h_Z)\beta} - (\mu\alpha - \mu_0\beta)e^{-(z+h_Z)\beta},$$

$$U(\alpha) = [\mu_0^2 k^2 - \alpha^2(\mu^2 - \mu_0^2)](e^{-h_Z\beta} - e^{h_Z\beta}), \quad (7)$$

$$Q(\alpha, d_G) = e^{d_G\alpha} + \frac{U(\alpha)}{N(\alpha)}e^{-d_G\alpha},$$

$$\beta = \sqrt{k^2 + \alpha^2}, \quad k^2 = j\omega\mu\kappa, \quad M = n_{EX}I\pi r_{EX}^2.$$

In the receiver coil at the opposite side of the object ($z_T = -d_T - h_Z$), the vector potential is

$$A(r_G, d_T) = \frac{4M\mu\mu_0}{h_{EX}\pi r_{EX}} \int_0^\infty \left(J_1(\alpha r_G)J_1(\alpha r_{EX})e^{-\left(d_{EX} + d_T + \frac{h_{EX}}{2}\alpha\right)} \sinh\left(\frac{\alpha h_{EX}}{2}\right)\frac{\beta}{N(\alpha)} \right) d\alpha. \quad (8)$$

The induced voltage V_I in a circular receiver coil with n turns is calculated as

$$V_I(r, z) = n\mu_0 \oint \mathbf{A}(r, z) \cdot \mathbf{ds} = 2\pi r\mu_0 nA(r, z). \quad (9)$$

It is emphasized that the above equations are the solution of the full wave equation and are hence also applicable at wavelengths near the skin depth in the object. Equations 5, 6, and 8 were evaluated with an adaptive recursive Newton-Cotes algorithm. The infinite object volume V_{OBJ} in equation 3 was replaced by a finite "large" value. This value was chosen such that a further increase by a factor of two yielded a relative change of P_{APP} of less than 0.1%. The resulting accuracy was considered to be sufficient for a sensitivity estimation in the framework of this feasibility study. All computations were carried out with MATLAB (The Mathworks Incorporated, Natick, Massachusetts).

Measurement Electronics

The concept of the transceiver is shown in FIGURE 5. ΔV must be amplified with high gain in order to achieve a sufficient resolution. Hence, the residual offset voltage V_{OR} must be kept as low as possible so as not to exceed the dynamical input range (DIR) of the

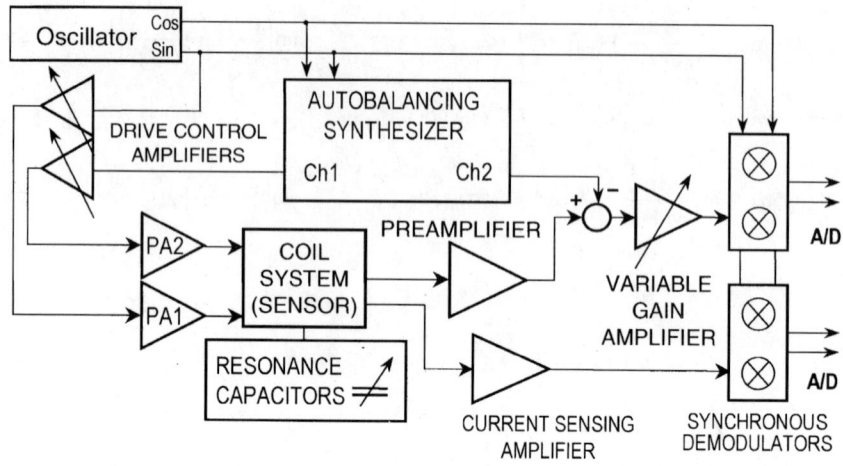

FIGURE 5. Schematic of the complete wideband transceiver.

amplifier. We have realized a two-stage compensation. The precompensation is carried out directly at the sensor output according to FIGURES 1–3. The excitation current is provided by one (S-2) or two (S-1, S-3) PAs.

The necessary compensation voltage V_C is provided by PA2, which is driven by channel 1 of the autobalancing synthesizer (ABS). V_C is automatically adjusted such that V_{OR} reaches a minimum in the undisturbed system (no conducting object). V_{OR} is preamplified (gain 225, manually adjustable) in two cascaded low-noise amplifiers. In the second compensation stage, the resulting signal is subtracted from a second compensation voltage, which is generated by channel 2 of the ABS in order to further suppress V_{OR}. The remaining signal is amplified (automatically adjustable gain of 0.5–50) and fed to a multiplying synchronous demodulator (MPY600, Burr Brown). The ABS generates voltages with variable amplitude and phase by adding two digitally adjustable sinusoidal voltages X and Y, which are 90° phase-shifted with respect to each other. It has been realized with an analog circuitry as depicted in FIGURE 6. The input signals (sine and cosine with identical amplitude) are fed to a network that can be switched into inverting or noninverting mode via a control signal ("sign X", "sign Y") in order to cover all four quadrants of the complex plane. The network consists of an inverting unity gain amplifier (OPA642, Burr Brown) and two fast video switches (MPC104, Burr Brown) that feed through either the original or the inverted signal. Then, the signals are amplified with adjustable gain amplifiers (AD603, Analog Devices), which are controlled via the analog inputs "magn X" and "magn Y" and summed together in order to form the output signal $Z = X + jY$. The reference signals are generated by two direct digital synthesizers (AD9850, Analog Devices). The power stages of the PAs have been realized with the EL2008 (Elantec), which is driven by gain adjustable amplifiers (AD603, Analog Devices). The whole transceiver electronics device is controlled via a PC by two commercial DAQ-cards (ACL8112,

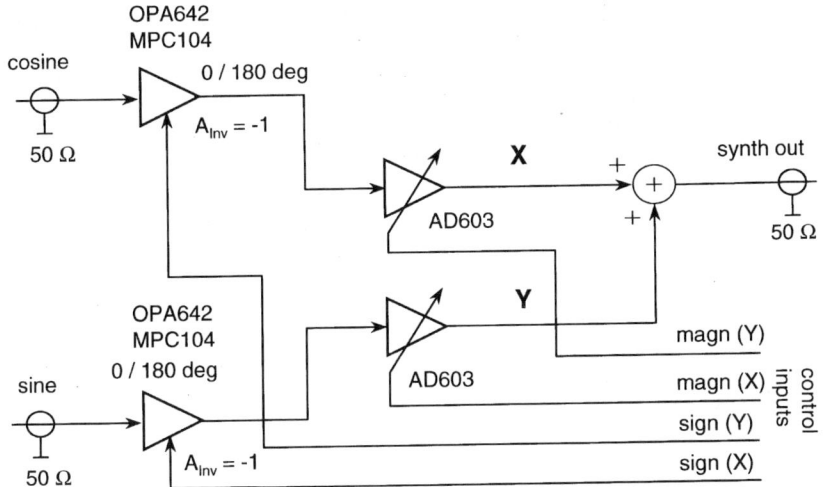

FIGURE 6. Schematic of the autobalancing synthesizer (only one channel is shown). The sine and cosine input signals are buffered, inverted if necessary, and amplified with variable gain in order to generate the 90° phase-shifted voltages X and Y. X and Y are then summed together. The control signals—magn (X), magn (Y), sign (X), and sign (Y)—determine the magnitude and sign of the two voltages, respectively.

ADLink Technology) and a program written under LABVIEW™ (National Instruments, Austin, Texas).

The suppression capability of the electronic balancing system was evaluated by feeding a current of 500 mA_{eff} into a circuit according to FIGURE 1, with the resonance circuit replaced by a resistor of 10 Ω. R_C was also set to 10 Ω.

RESULTS

Feasibility Study

The simulation results for 50–200 kHz are shown in FIGURE 7. The solid line is the resistivity change (real part of ΔZ) in the EXC of S-1; the dotted line is the corresponding real part of the sensitivity s if $R_C = R_0$; and the dashed line and the dash-dotted line represent the Re(s) of sensors S-2 and S-3, respectively. The imaginary parts of s and ΔZ are three orders of magnitude lower at low frequencies and thus have been disregarded. The s of all three coil configurations lies in the range of a few mV-Ωm at 50 kHz. Reduction of the distance d_{EX} to 10 mm increases the sensitivity. The values for s, V_0, and V_I at 50 kHz are given in TABLE 1.

From the values shown, it follows that a resolution of about 1 μV is necessary in order to resolve 10^{-3} (Ωm)$^{-1}$. The sensitivity increases with the square of the frequency. At 50

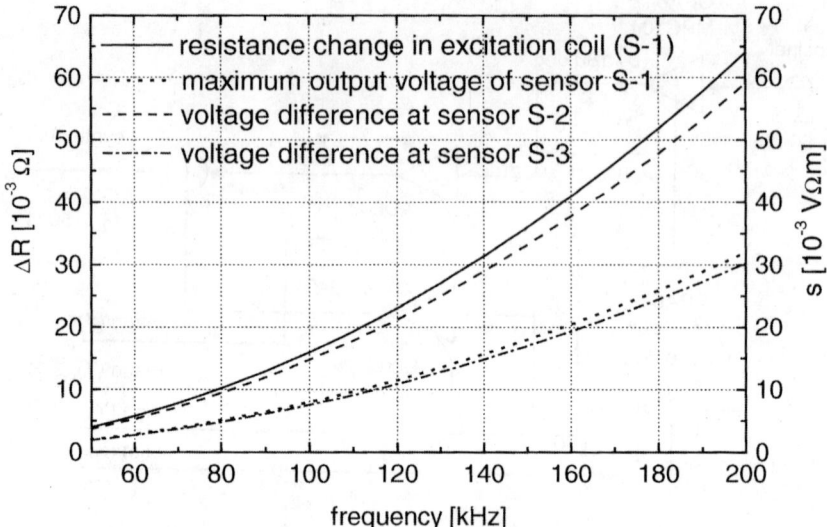

FIGURE 7. Simulation results for sensors S-1, S-2, and S-3.

kHz, a $|\Delta\kappa|$ of 1 $(\Omega m)^{-1}$ yields a signal of some few mV, which must fit into the DIR of the receiver.

Electronics

A wideband receiver (50 kHz–5 MHz) has been realized according to FIGURE 5. The DIR of the synchronous demodulator is 0.8 V, which requires an amplifier gain of at least 390 in order to discriminate 1 μV with 12-bit resolution of the A/D converter (including sign). This restricts the DIR of the amplifier to about 2 mV. It is reasonable to keep V_{OR} lower than 10% of ΔV; thus, V_{OR} should not exceed 200 μV. In consequence, V_0 (5 V) must be suppressed by at least 88 dB via compensation if sensor S-1 is applied, whereas for sensor S-2 ($V_I = 18.1$ V) suppression of approximately 100 dB is necessary. In the case of sen-

TABLE 1. Simulated Sensitivities and Induced Voltages of the Different Sensors

Sensor	s at 50 kHz [10^{-3} VΩm]	Voltage at the Undisturbed Sensor Output (V_0, V_I) [V]
S-1	max. 2.01	5.0
S-2	3.69	18.1
S-3	1.89	147.0[a]

[a]Voltage at one gradiometer coil; this voltage is essentially canceled out by the second coil.

TABLE 2. Suppression of V_0 or V_I by Electronic Compensation

Suppression	Frequency [MHz]					
	0.05	0.1	0.5	1	3	5
ABS channel 1 [dB]	97	98	109	110	129	102
ABS channels 1 and 2 [dB]	115	118	126	110	129	105

sor S-3, V_I (147 V) must be suppressed by about 120 dB. The induced voltages in the gradiometer coils theoretically cancel out mutually; however, according to reference 8, in practice a suppression of at most 40–50 dB can be reached by mechanical balancing of the magnetometer. Hence, the remaining 70–80 dB must be achieved with the compensation electronics. In practice, the gain should be higher than 390 for reducing the quantization error. This requires even better suppression of V_{OR}, so the two-stage concept is reasonable.

TABLE 2 shows the measured data for the suppression of V_0 and V_I by the compensation electronics. The first row corresponds to compensation with channel 1 of the ABS only (compensation stage 1 at the sensor output), whereas the second row shows the data when both compensation stages (channels 1 and 2) are active. It is seen that almost the full compensation can already be reached in stage 1. However, further improvement is possible by additional balancing with ABS channel 2 for lower frequencies.

The total harmonic distortion of the oscillator does not exceed 0.3% throughout the whole frequency range. The spectral noise voltage of the amplifier chain (full gain) is 11.7 nV/√Hz. The synchronous demodulator limits the bandwidth in the baseband to 40 Hz; hence, we obtain a signal-to-noise ratio (SNR) of 22 dB for a signal of 1 µV.

The magnitude error of the synchronous demodulator remains within 3% over the full frequency range at maximum output voltage; however, the phase shift becomes as high as 20° at 5 MHz. In response to a unit step, the output low-passes of the synchronous demodulators settle with an error of 0.02% within 65 ms.

DISCUSSION

General

Our approach is an extension of previous systems[5,8] to multifrequency operation. The electronics is specially optimized for measurements at low frequencies. According to the simulation results, it is possible to measure conductivities with a resolution of 10^{-3} $(\Omega m)^{-1}$ at frequencies down to 50 kHz. The sensitivity is limited by the following effects:

(1) s increases linearly with the excitation current, which is limited by the admissible thermal losses in the EXC. Furthermore, the admissible SAR in the tissue must not be exceeded.

(2) The inductivity and parasitic capacitances of the receiver coils determine the characteristic parallel resonance frequencies. The measurement frequency must always remain below the lowest resonance frequency.

(3) The SNR of the receiving amplifier limits the resolution. An SNR of 0 dB is expected for a signal of 100 nV, which can be resolved with a gain ≥ 3900. Depending on the geometry, 100 nV is expected at 10–20 kHz in response to a $\Delta\kappa$ of 10^{-3} $(\Omega m)^{-1}$. Thus, a fully optimized system may still operate at frequencies as low as 10 kHz.

From the simulation results, it follows that the largest sensitivity can be expected from an S-2 configuration. Moreover, S-2 is suitable for inductive impedance tomography, as has been shown in reference 12. However, this concept requires the highest effort for compensation. The S-1 configuration is the most simple one as it requires only a single coil. The most complex system is S-3. It can be satisfactorily balanced mechanically for a single frequency, but the balancing is extremely difficult for multifrequency operation. Any mismatch between the pickup coils will result in a frequency-dependent residual offset voltage V_{OR} due to asymmetric capacitive stray pathways. Hence, additional electronic balancing is necessary.

Electronics

Due to the large bandwidth of the amplifiers, errors in gain and phase are inevitable. Hence, our concept is only meaningful in combination with a calibration unit, for example, a coil that is terminated by reference impedances (not shown in FIGURE 5). The calibration procedure can be fully automated.

The performance of the system is significantly influenced by the noise voltage at the output of the power amplifiers. As this voltage can hardly be kept below some mV_{eff} in wideband operation, band-pass filtering of either the compensation voltage or the input signal is required. This can be best achieved by a tunable resonance circuit. We have not yet realized this filtering unit in our prototype; hence, we must reduce the noise by excessive averaging, which slows down the acquisition speed. This disadvantage shall be eliminated in future work.

Data Interpretation

The eddy current density is highest in a ring-shaped region near the surface of the observed tissue. Hence, the system is insensitive to structures deep inside the object and near the symmetry axis. An analytical solution for the relationship between conductivity and voltage is only obtainable for simple geometries and homogeneous tissue. Otherwise, the 3D eddy current problem must be solved numerically. Alternatively, parameters of the measured spectra can be correlated to underlying tissue properties, which is sufficient for event detection. Such an approach may be applicable, for example, for noninvasive monitoring of brain edema. Also, transplant rejection monitoring for subsurface organs (e.g., kidneys)[16] may become possible in a contactless way. For a more accurate assessment of the conductivity distribution, a tomographic approach with either a rotating arrangement or multicoil arrays must be employed.[12]

REFERENCES

1. KANAI, H. et al. 1987. Electrical measurement of fluid distribution in legs and arms. Med. Prog. Technol. **12:** 159–170.
2. VAN LOAN, M.D. et al. 1993. Use of bio-impedance spectroscopy (BIS) to determine extracellular fluid (ECF), intracellular fluid (ICF), total body water (TBW), and fat-free mass (FFM). In Human Body Composition: In Vivo Methods, Models, and Assessment. Plenum. New York.
3. LOZANO, A. et al. 1995. Segmental body fluid shift estimation during HDT positions by electrical impedance measurements. In Proceedings of the Ninth International Conference on Electrical Bio-Impedance, p. 233–236.
4. GERSING, E. 1982. Impedanzspektroskopie als Hilfe bei Herzoperationen. Elektronik **9:** 88.
5. NETZ, J. et al. 1993. Contactless impedance measurement by magnetic induction—a possible method for investigation of brain impedance. Physiol. Meas. **14:** 463–471.
6. LU, L. et al. 1996. Parametric modelling for electrical impedance spectroscopy system. Med. Biol. Eng. Comput. **34:** 122–126.
7. SCHARFETTER, H. et al. 1998. A model of artifacts produced by stray capacitance during whole body or segmental bioimpedance spectroscopy. Physiol. Meas. **19:** 247–261.
8. TARJAN, P.P. & R. MCFEE. 1968. Electrodeless measurements of the effective resistivity of the human torso and head by magnetic induction. IEEE Trans. Biomed. Eng. **15:** 266–278.
9. HART, L.W. et al. 1988. A noninvasive electromagnetic conductivity sensor for biomedical application. IEEE Trans. Biomed. Eng. **35:** 1011–1021.
10. AL-ZEIBAK, S. & H.N. SAUNDERS. 1993. A feasibility study of in vivo electromagnetic imaging. Phys. Med. Biol. **38:** 151–160.
11. GUARDO, R. et al. 1995. Contactless recording of cardiac related thoracic conductivity changes. In Proceedings of the Seventeenth Conference of the IEEE/EMBS, p. 1581–1582.
12. GRIFFITHS, H. et al. 1999. Magnetic induction tomography: a measurement system for biological tissues. This volume.
13. WAKAMATSU, H. 1997. A dielectric spectrometer for liquid using the electromagnetic induction method. Hewlett-Packard Journal, p. 37–44.
14. GEDDES, L.A. & L.E. BAKER. 1967. The specific resistance of biological material—a compendium of data for the biomedical engineer and physiologist. Med. Biol. Eng. **5:** 271–293.
15. WACH, P. 1979. Theoretische Untersuchung der Rückwirkung der Wirbelströme bei der kontaktlosen Leitfähigkeitsmessung. Elektrotech. Maschinenbau **96:** 505–509.
16. OLLMAR, S. 1997. Noninvasive monitoring of transplanted kidneys by impedance spectroscopy—a pilot study. Med. Biol. Eng. Comput. **35**(suppl. 1): 336.

APPENDIX

List of Variables

$\mathbf{A}$	magnetic vector potential [A]
$A(r,z)$	φ-component of $\mathbf{A}$ [A]
d_{EX}	distance between excitation coil and proximal object surface [m]
d_G	distance between lower gradiometer coil and proximal object surface [m]
d_T	distance between distal receiver coil and distal object surface [m]
h_{EX}	height of the excitation coil [m]
I	excitation current [A]
$J_1(...)$	Bessel function of first kind and first order
$n_\#$	number of turns of a coil (subscript #—EX: excitation coil, G: gradiometer coil, T: distal receiver coil; no subscript: general circular coil)
P_{APP}	apparent power [VA]

r	radius [m]
$r_\#$	radius of circular coil # [m] (subscript #—EX: excitation coil, G: receiver coil)
R_0	loss resistance of the undisturbed resonance circuit [Ω]
R_C	compensation resistor [Ω]
s	sensitivity [VΩm]
S	current density [Am^{-2}]
V_0	voltage drop along the undisturbed resonance circuit [V]
V_C	compensation voltage [V]
V_I	induced voltage in the receiver coil (undisturbed system) [V]
V_{OBJ}	object volume [m^3]
V_{OR}	residual offset voltage due to incomplete compensation [V]
z	axial coordinate [m]
ΔV	voltage change due to eddy currents [V]
ΔZ	impedance change in the excitation coil [Ω]
$\Delta \kappa$	change of the complex electrical conductivity [(Ωm)$^{-1}$]
ε_r	relative electrical permittivity
ε_0	electrical permittivity of the vacuum [As(Vm)$^{-1}$]
κ	complex electrical conductivity $\sigma + j\omega\varepsilon_0\varepsilon_r$ [(Ωm)$^{-1}$]
μ	relative magnetic permeability
μ_0	magnetic permeability of the vacuum [Vs(Am)$^{-1}$]
σ	electrical conductivity [(Ωm)$^{-1}$]
ω	radian frequency [s^{-1}]

Abbreviations

ABS	autobalancing synthesizer
BIS	bioimpedance spectroscopy
C	resonance capacitor
DIR	dynamical input range
EXC	excitation coil
IBIS	inductive bioimpedance spectroscopy
L_{ex}	excitation coil (EXC)
L_{rec}	receiving coil
PA1, PA2	driving power amplifiers
SAR	specific absorption rate
SNR	signal-to-noise ratio

Magnetic Induction Tomography

A Measuring System for Biological Tissues

H. GRIFFITHS,[a] W. R. STEWART,[a] AND W. GOUGH[b]

[a]*Department of Medical Physics and Clinical Engineering, University Hospital of Wales, Cardiff CF4 4XW, United Kingdom*

[b]*Department of Physics and Astronomy, University of Wales, Cardiff CF2 3YB, United Kingdom*

ABSTRACT: A single-channel magnetic induction system operating at 10 MHz has been constructed. The system consists of an excitation coil and a sensing coil, between which different objects can be scanned. The eddy currents induced in the object cause perturbations in the sensed magnetic field, which are measured with a phase-sensitive detector with backing off of the signal to improve sensitivity. Scans were obtained for saline solutions with conductivities ranging from 0.001 to 6 Sm^{-1}, encompassing the range for biological tissues. The imaginary part of the perturbation in the sensed magnetic field was found to be proportional to saline conductivity, consistent with theoretical prediction, and had a constant of proportionality of -1.2% per Sm^{-1}. A filtered back-projection algorithm was used to generate tomographic images from the scans.

INTRODUCTION

When a conductive body is placed in an oscillating magnetic field, eddy currents are induced in the body that perturb the magnetic field in the vicinity. This principle has been used extensively for the nondestructive testing of metals. It has also been used for tomographic imaging of various metallic and ferromagnetic objects, for the process industry, using arrays of coils operating at frequencies of up to 500 kHz.[1]

The idea of using a similar method for medical imaging is very attractive because direct contact with the tissue would not be necessary (traditional electrical impedance tomography requires the attachment of electrodes to the patient). Furthermore, as magnetic fields are not "blocked" by poorly conducting tissues such as bone, a magnetically coupled system might eventually prove more suitable for imaging the brain than traditional applied-electric-field techniques where the skull acts as a barrier. The difficulty in developing such a method for biological tissues is that their conductivities are much lower than those of metals and the perturbations in the sensed magnetic field are very small.

Systems consisting of an excitation coil and a sensing coil, with amplitude detection, operating at frequencies of 2 and 5.5 MHz, were shown capable of imaging various conducting objects.[2,3] However, no convincing results with conductivities in the range for biological tissues were obtained. In a recent publication, Korzhenevskii and Cherepenin[4] presented an excellent theoretical analysis of the two-coil arrangement and advocated the direct measurement of phase rather than amplitude to detect the small perturbations in the magnetic field predicted.

We have taken a different approach and have used phase-sensitive detection and a third coil to allow subtraction of the signal due to the magnetic field sensed in the absence of an object. Measurements with a 10-MHz single-channel system are presented for different saline solutions, with conductivities spanning the tissue range.

THEORY

Consider two coils positioned coaxially and spaced by a distance $2a$: a sinusoidal current, of angular frequency ω, flows in one coil and the other experiences a magnetic field B. Let a circular disk of dielectric of radius R, thickness t, conductivity σ, and relative permittivity ε_r be placed coaxially and centrally between the coils. The currents induced in the disk cause a perturbation, ΔB, in B. If the skin depth of the electromagnetic field in the dielectric is large compared with t (i.e., the interaction is weak), it can be shown (see APPENDIX) that

$$\frac{\Delta B}{B} = (\omega \varepsilon_0 \varepsilon_r - j\sigma)\left(\frac{ta^3 \omega \mu_0}{2}\right)\left\{\frac{1}{a^2} - \frac{a^2 + 2R^2}{(a^2 + R^2)^2}\right\} \quad (1)$$

where ε_0 and μ_0 are the permittivity and permeability of free space, respectively. Equation 1 shows that the conductivity of the disk affects the imaginary part of $\Delta B/B$, while its permittivity affects the real part.

METHODS AND MATERIALS

Measurement System

The single-channel system is shown schematically in FIGURE 1. A magnetic resonance imaging control console (Surrey Medical Imaging Systems, United Kingdom) was used as a signal source and phase-sensitive detector. The master waveform generator in the console provides a 10-MHz continuous sine wave of 1-V peak-to-peak amplitude. This signal was gated, phase-shifted, amplified, and used to drive an excitation coil. Inclusion of a 50-Ω impedance matching unit maximizes the current in the coil. The excitation coil consisted of three turns of miniature coaxial cable (RG179) wound on a 9-cm-diameter plastic former and connected as shielded turns, a configuration known to be insensitive to electric fields. The sensing coil was a single shielded turn of cable 1.5 cm in diameter. The two coils were mounted on Perspex brackets 17.5 cm apart. A third coil, 4 cm in diameter, consisting of three shielded turns, was used as a "back-off". This coil was mounted on a bracket that could be rotated, enabling it to be orientated so that the induced emf was in antiphase with and equal in amplitude to that induced in the sensing coil. These coils were connected to a 50-Ω combiner. This allowed the signal from the magnetic field sensed in the absence of an object to be nulled to improve the sensitivity of the measurements. The impedance matching unit on the back-off coil was used as a phase-shifter, allowing accurate nulling to be achieved. The use of a second field-sensing coil for backing off the signal means that the null should be unaffected by any variation of current in the excitation coil.

The output of the combiner was amplified and connected to the phase-sensitive detector. The MRI console produces a gating pulse at the start of each acquisition period; this

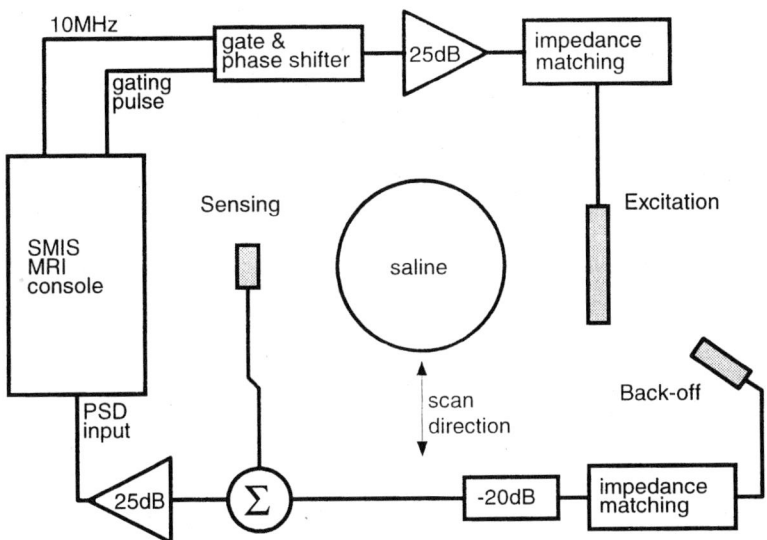

FIGURE 1. Schematic of the single-channel induction tomography system.

was used to trigger the gating circuit so that it admitted the waveform for only 30 ms of the 200-ms sampling period. In this way, the real and imaginary parts of the signal could be measured during excitation and for a period afterwards, enabling subtraction of dc offsets.

A sliding and rotating platform between the excitation and sensing coils allowed different objects to be translated and rotated to obtain profiles of $\Delta B/B$ for tomographic imaging. Before scanning an object, the back-off was adjusted to null the signal. The back-off was then partially removed, by rotating the coil, and the phase-shifter was adjusted so that the signal appeared entirely in the real part of the recording: the back-off was then reinstated.

Signal Amplitude as a Function of Conductivity

Saline solutions (500 mL) of different conductivities, ranging from 0.001 (deionized water) to 6 Sm^{-1} in glass beakers 9 cm in diameter, were scanned for displacements of up to 18 cm on either side of the central position (with no rotation). At 10 MHz, the conductivities of mammalian tissues range from about 0.02 Sm^{-1} for bone to just under 2 Sm^{-1} for CSF.[5]

Image Reconstruction

Images were reconstructed from the measured profiles by filtered back-projection along the axis of the coils.[6] The inherent assumptions in this process were as follows: because the interaction of the magnetic field with the conducting solution was weak, the field lines remained fixed in space and only the solution intersecting the central axis contributed to $\Delta B/B$.

Sensitivity as a Function of Position

To investigate how the sensitivity varied along the axis of the coils, a series of measurements were performed with a thin cylinder of strong saline solution (diameter 1.9 cm, height 11.5 cm, $\sigma = 24$ Sm^{-1}). Scans were performed along the line midway between the coils, as before, and along paths displaced by 4.5 cm towards each coil in turn.

RESULTS

Signal Amplitude as a Function of Conductivity

FIGURE 2 shows the apparent $\Delta B/B$ versus displacement of the 9-cm-diameter beaker recorded for four different saline conductivities. The values are expressed as a percentage of the signal recorded in the absence of an object and with the back-off disconnected, this being the total signal due to the magnetic field at the sensing coil.

FIGURE 3 shows the apparent $\Delta B/B$ versus saline conductivity for the beaker in the central position between the coils. The imaginary part was fitted by the straight line, Im($\Delta B/B$) $= -0.991\sigma$ (not drawn), with a multiple correlation coefficient, $R^2 = 0.996$.

Imaging

FIGURE 4 shows the image reconstructed from the imaginary part profile for a conductivity of 2 Sm^{-1}. Because of the time taken to acquire each profile and the symmetry of the arrangement, only the one profile was used and was back-projected through 65 angles.

Sensitivity as a Function of Position

FIGURE 5 shows the results of scans of the 1.9-cm-diameter cylinder taken at the three positions between the coils.

DISCUSSION

When the 9-cm-diameter beaker of solution was scanned between the coils, the imaginary part of the apparent $\Delta B/B$ was maximum in magnitude at the central position (FIGURE 2). It is useful to compare these values with those predicted by equation 1, setting the following values for the parameters: $a = 8.75$ cm, $t = 7.9$ cm (depth of saline), $R = 4.5$ cm, and $\varepsilon_r = 80$ (for water). The experimental arrangement did not exactly correspond to the theoretical model as the cylindrical volume of saline solution was not coaxial with the coils; its height was similar to its diameter, so the model is used nevertheless. Equation 1

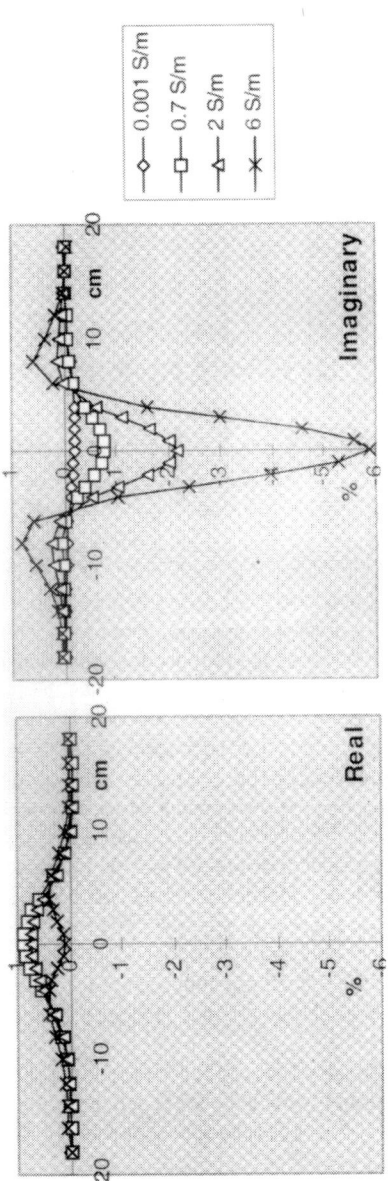

FIGURE 2. Apparent $\Delta B/B$ versus displacement of the 500-mL beaker for different saline conductivities. The standard error in the measurements was less than 0.01%.

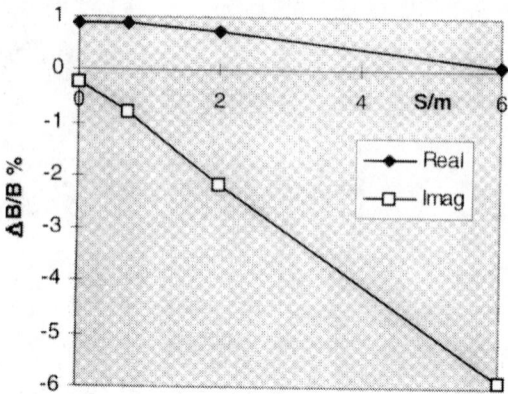

FIGURE 3. Apparent $\Delta B/B$ versus saline conductivity, for the central position.

reduces to $\Delta B/B = (0.052 - j1.2\sigma)\%$. Thus, the observed proportionality of the imaginary part of the apparent $\Delta B/B$ with conductivity is close to that predicted theoretically. For the real part, the correspondence is less good; the observed value, although correct in sign, is not constant at 0.05% (the theoretical value), but is up to 20 times larger. For the solution with conductivity of 6 Sm^{-1}, the magnitude was not maximum in the central position, but passed through a local minimum (FIG. 2). As the skin depth at this conductivity (6.5 cm) was no longer large compared with the dimensions of the volume, the theoretical model might be inapplicable.

Our interpretation of these observations is that the imaginary part of the apparent $\Delta B/B$ was accurately measuring the true $\Delta B/B$ due to the conduction eddy currents in the saline. The fact that the real part of the apparent $\Delta B/B$ was much larger than its theoretical value could be due to residual capacitive coupling between the excitation and sensing coils, even though they were screened. For the conductivity of 0.7 Sm^{-1}, typical of a high-water-content tissue, this error in the real part was comparable with the value of the imaginary part, the supposed true signal due to the conduction eddy currents (FIGURE 3). However, the two effects have been separated by the phase-sensitive detection. It is difficult totally to screen a coil, even as a shielded loop, because a small gap at the end of the screen is always necessary. Furthermore, in our system, the impedance matching units are at present unscreened and this needs to be remedied.

The reconstructed image (FIG. 4) is a reasonable representation of the 9-cm beaker of solution even though it involved the approximation of a "pencil beam" of sensitivity along the coil axis. Nevertheless, it suggests that this is an approach worthy of further investigation.

The scans of the 1.9-cm-diameter cylinder of solution (FIG. 5) show that the sensitivity varies along the axis, being greatest near the sensing coil; here, the maximum amplitude of the imaginary part of $\Delta B/B$ was –0.21% compared with only half this value for the other two scans. Such variations should be included in the image reconstruction as a weighting

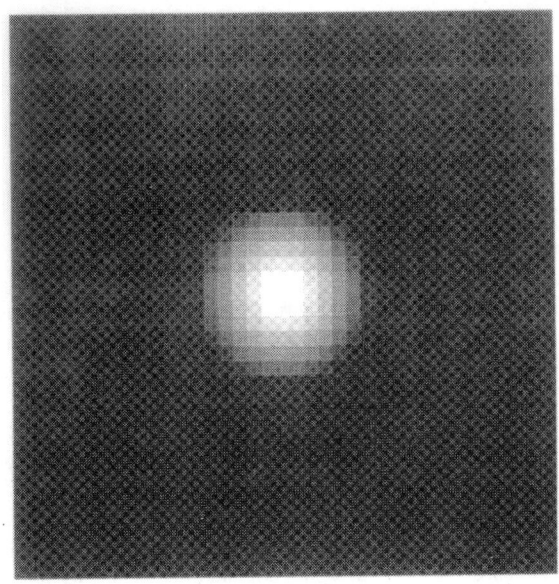

FIGURE 4. Image of the 9-cm-diameter beaker, containing 2 Sm^{-1} saline solution, reconstructed by filtered back-projection from the imaginary part profile (FIG. 2) for 65 orientations. The line diagram indicates the actual size and position of the beaker.

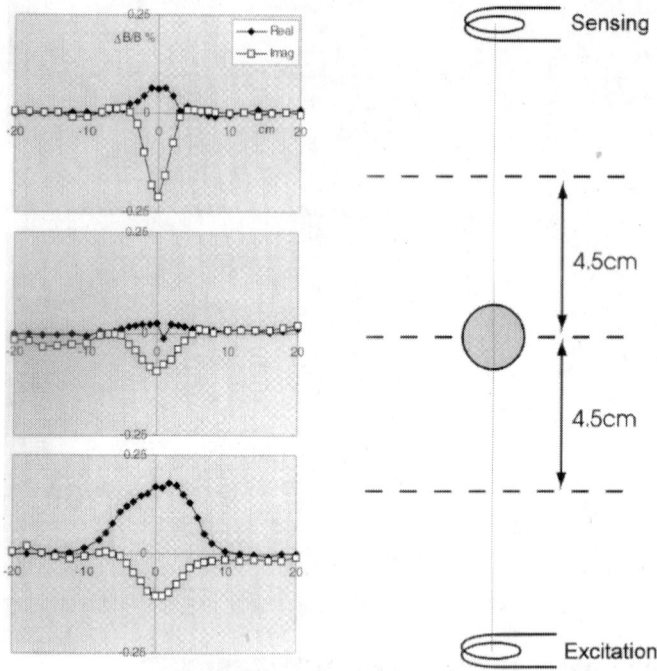

FIGURE 5. Profiles of $\Delta B/B$ obtained with a 1.9-cm-diameter cylinder of 24 Sm^{-1} saline solution scanned at three positions (dashed lines) between the two coils.

factor along the back-projection path, and these observations support theoretical arguments for the introduction of this factor.[4]

Consider the change in total signal amplitude that would be expected theoretically for a typical tissue conductivity, for instance, 1 Sm^{-1}, which corresponds to the saline concentration of 0.1 mol/L used by Al-Zeibak and Saunders.[2] For the 9-cm-diameter beaker, equation 1 predicts $\Delta B/B = (0.052 - j1.2)\%$ (see above), which amounts to a change in total amplitude of $(1.00052^2 + 0.012^2)^{1/2} - 1 = 0.00059$, that is, 0.06%. It is difficult, therefore, to understand why these authors observed a 73% increase in signal if only eddy currents were responsible; it is possible that capacitive coupling was still very significant in their system. The figure of 0.06% illustrates the unsuitability of amplitude detection for induction tomographic imaging of biological tissues. The change in phase angle required to be measured in the method proposed by Korzhenevskii and Cherepenin[4] would be $\tan^{-1}(0.012/1.00052) = 0.7°$. It should now be established whether direct phase measurement or the method used here, of back-off with phase-sensitive detection, will be the more practicable. In designing a system for clinical use, mechanical scanning will not be suitable and a fully electronic, multiple-coil system, similar to those used at lower frequencies,[1] will need to be developed.

REFERENCES

1. PEYTON, A.J., Z.Z. YU, G. LYON, S. AL-ZEIBAK, J. FERREIRA, J. VELEZ, F. LINHARES, A.R. BORGES, H.L. XIONG, N.H. SAUNDERS & M.S. BECK. 1996. An overview of electromagnetic inductance tomography: description of three different systems. Meas. Sci. Technol. **7:** 261–271.
2. AL-ZEIBAK, S. & N.H. SAUNDERS. 1993. A feasibility study of *in vivo* electromagnetic imaging. Phys. Med. Biol. **38:** 151–160.
3. AL-ZEIBAK, S., D. GOSS, G. LYON, Z.Z. YU, A.J. PEYTON & M.S. BECK. 1995. A feasibility study of electromagnetic inductance tomography. *In* Proceedings of the Ninth International Conference on Electrical Bio-Impedance, Heidelberg, p. 426–429.
4. KORZHENEVSKII, A.V. & V.A. CHEREPENIN. 1997. Magnetic induction tomography. J. Commun. Technol. Electron. **42**(no. 4): 469–474.
5. DUCK, F.A. 1990. Physical Properties of Tissue. Academic Press. New York/London.
6. BROOKS, R.A. & G. DI CHIRO. 1975. Theory of image reconstruction in computed tomography. Radiology **117:** 561–572.

APPENDIX

Consider a circular disk of radius R and thickness t, placed centrally and midway between a small excitation coil and a small sensing coil as shown. The coils are a distance $2a$ apart ($t \ll 2a$). The disk has conductivity σ and is nonmagnetic, so its permeability is μ_0. The skin depth δ is assumed to be much greater than t, which means that the attenuation produced by the disk is small. We use spherical polar coordinates (r, θ, ϕ) as shown (FIG. A1).

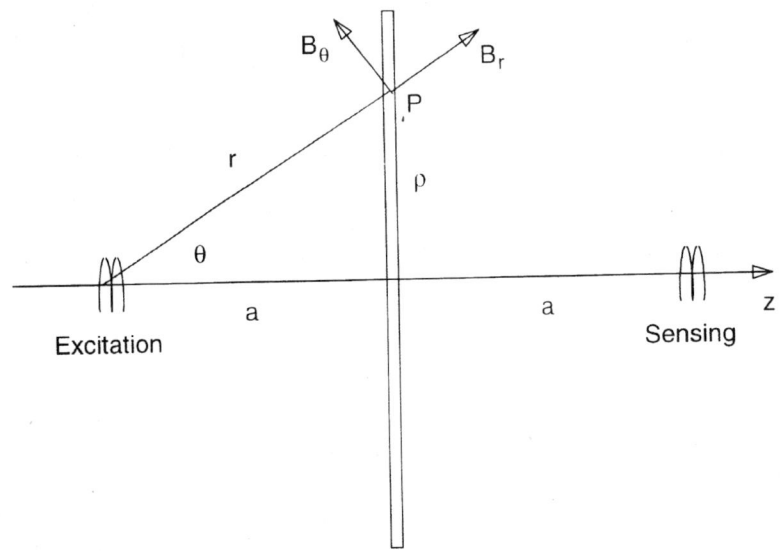

FIGURE A1. Magnetic field at a thin disk due to a small excitation coil.

At a point P on the disk, the magnetic B-field has components

$$B_r = \frac{\mu_0}{4\pi}\frac{2m\cos\theta}{r^3}, \qquad B_\theta = \frac{\mu_0}{4\pi}\frac{m\sin\theta}{r^3},$$

where m is the equivalent magnetic dipole moment of the coil. The longitudinal field is then

$$B_z = \frac{\mu_0 m}{4\pi r^3}(2\cos^2\theta - \sin^2\theta) = \frac{\mu_0 m}{4\pi}\left[\frac{2a^2 - \rho^2}{(a^2+\rho^2)^{5/2}}\right].$$

Hence, the flux threading a circular path of radius ρ centered on the axis is

$$\Phi = \int_0^\rho B_z(\rho')2\pi\rho'd\rho',$$

which is readily shown to be

$$\frac{\mu_0 m}{2}\frac{\rho^2}{(a^2+\rho^2)^{3/2}}.$$

The induced voltage around this path is $-j\omega\Phi$, and this also equals the line integral $2\pi\rho E_\phi$ of the induced electric field. The current density is given by $\mathbf{j} = \sigma\mathbf{E}$, so

$$J_\phi = \frac{-j\omega\sigma\mu_0 m}{4\pi}\frac{\rho}{(a^2+\rho^2)^{3/2}} = \frac{-jm}{2\pi\delta^2}\frac{\rho}{(a^2+\rho^2)^{3/2}}$$

where δ is the skin depth $(2/\omega\mu\sigma)^{1/2}$. Consider now a thin annulus of the disk, between ρ and $\rho+d\rho$. The current it carries is

$$dI = j_\phi t d\rho = \frac{-jmt}{2\pi\delta^2}\frac{\rho}{(a^2+\rho^2)^{3/2}}d\rho.$$

The field produced by this induced current at the sensing coil is given by the usual formula for a single-turn circular coil:

$$dB = \frac{\mu_0\rho^2 di}{2(a^2+\rho^2)^{3/2}} = \frac{-j\mu_0 mt}{4\pi\delta^2}\frac{\rho^3 d\rho}{(a^2+\rho^2)^3}.$$

Now, the field at the sensing coil due to the excitation coil is $B = \mu_0 m/(16\pi a^3)$, so

$$\frac{dB}{B} = \frac{-4jta^3}{\delta^2}\frac{\rho^3 d\rho}{(a^2+\rho^2)^3}.$$

The total field ΔB due to the induced currents in the entire disk is found by integrating this equation, which gives finally

$$\frac{\Delta B}{B} = \frac{-jta^3}{\delta^2}\left\{\frac{1}{a^2} - \frac{a^2 + 2R^2}{(a^2+R^2)^2}\right\}.$$

If the disk has significant relative permittivity ε_r, the imaginary term $j\omega\varepsilon_0\varepsilon_r$ must be added to the conductivity in the expression for δ, where ε_0 is the permittivity of free space.

Progress in Realization of Magnetic Induction Tomography

ALEXANDER V. KORJENEVSKY AND VLADIMIR A. CHEREPENIN

Institute of Radioengineering and Electronics, Russian Academy of Sciences, Moscow 103907, Russia

> **ABSTRACT:** The method enabling one to obtain tomographic images of an electrically conductive or dielectric object by the excitation of the variable magnetic field inside it and by measuring the resulting field around the object is described. The main equations and theoretical estimations are given. It is shown that phase-sensitive measurements should be used in magnetic induction tomography. The measuring system providing the data set necessary for the image reconstruction is discussed. Under the conditions of the measurements discussed in this paper, image reconstruction is possible with the use of a simple method of convolution and back-projection along magnetic lines. Computer simulation demonstrates the visualization of the conductivity distribution by the method of magnetic induction tomography with phase measurements.

INTRODUCTION

The use of the interaction of a variable magnetic field with conductive media can be used for visualization of internal structures of biological tissues and opens wide prospects in medical tomography. In references 1 and 2, the theoretical basics of such an approach were discussed and the need of phase measurements was shown. This is distinct from reference 3, where experimental research was described, but mainly an empirical approach was used, and results for the objects with conductivity corresponding to biological tissues were not obtained. In reference 4, ingenious experiments were presented to test the theoretical predictions, in particular, the relation between the conductivity of the object and the phase shift for initial and disturbed magnetic fields over a conductivity range of biological tissues. We consider in this report the theoretical model of the measuring system for induction tomography and describe a simple method of image reconstruction and our experimental setup.

Let the source and receiver of a variable magnetic field be separated in space. For example, this can consist of two identical coils: (1) the inductor, connected to the source of alternating voltage, $U_i = U_1 \cos(\omega t)$; (2) the detector, connected to the phase-sensitive receiver. In a quasi-stationary approximation, the system can be considered as a transformer without a core. The inductive connection means that the part of the magnetic flow created by the inductor penetrates a coil of the detector and evokes an electromotive force in it. The inductor and detector are connected only by the lines of the magnetic field threading both coils. If a conductive or magnetic object is placed between the coils, the magnetic field will change due to induced currents and displacement currents in the object or due to its magnetization. If the geometry of a magnetic field is kept constant, the signal of the detector would change only with crossing by an object of the magnetic bunch, threading both coils. The change will be an increase with the increase of the object's extent along this bunch. Thus, there is an analogy with X-ray tomography, where a rectilinear beam of X rays is replaced by a curved beam of magnetic lines. Of course, the situation in the case of a quasi-static electromagnetic field essentially differs from the situation with short-wave radiation. The equation $div\mathbf{B} = 0$ means that it is impossible to change the magnetic field in a local bunch of magnetic lines without changing the geometry and value of the field in space surrounding this bunch. Such a nonlocality of interaction limits the resolution of the system.

To have a possibility of image reconstruction by back-projection along the undisturbed magnetic lines, it is necessary that changes caused by the medium would be small; that is, the measurements should be carried out in conditions of weak skin effect: $\delta \gg l$, where δ is the thickness of skin for a magnetic field in the medium. On the other hand, the medium should have an effect on the magnetic field sufficient for registration by the detector. These conditions are the criteria for a choice of the tomograph's working frequency, ω. Thus, the working frequency of the system for visualization of the human body should be chosen in a range of 10–20 MHz.

BASIC EQUATIONS

The electromagnetic field in space filled with inhomogeneous medium is described by the Maxwell equations, which can be written down in the case of harmonic time dependencies in the following form:

$$\nabla^2 \varphi + \nabla \ln\left(\sigma + \frac{i\omega}{4\pi}\varepsilon\right) \cdot \left(\nabla\varphi + \frac{i\omega}{c}\mathbf{A}\right) = 0,$$

$$\nabla^2 \mathbf{A} + \nabla \ln\mu \times (\nabla \times \mathbf{A}) - \frac{4\pi\mu}{c}\left(\sigma + \frac{i\omega}{4\pi}\varepsilon\right)\left(\nabla\varphi + \frac{i\omega}{c}\mathbf{A}\right) = 0, \quad (1)$$

$$\nabla \cdot \mathbf{A} = 0,$$

$$\mathbf{B} = \nabla \times \mathbf{A}, \quad \mathbf{E} = -\nabla\varphi - \frac{i\omega}{c}\mathbf{A}.$$

Here, μ and ε are the magnetic permittivity and electrical permittivity, respectively, and σ is the conductivity of the medium. The first equation (for scalar potential) corresponds to electrical impedance tomography; the second (for vector potential) corresponds to induction tomography. If the inductor's field $\mathbf{A}_0$ is only slightly affected by the medium and $\mu = 1$, the system (equation 1) can be approximately replaced by the equation

$$\nabla^2 \mathbf{A} = \frac{4i\pi\omega}{c^2}\left(\sigma + \frac{i\omega}{4\pi}\varepsilon\right)\mathbf{A}_0. \quad (2)$$

It is visible from equation 2 that induced current caused by conductivity of the medium contributes to the imaginary part of the magnetic field, which is in quadrature to the inductor's field, and displacement current, proportional to permittivity, contributes to the in-phase field. Thus, measuring both quadratures of a detector's signal allows the independent determination of conductivity and permittivity of the medium.

Let us consider the equivalent circuit of the system, including inductor L_1 (connected to a source of current), detector L_2, and a low conductive object located between them (FIG-

URE 1). The model of the object here is the winding of the transformer L_3, loaded with connected-in-parallel active resistance $R \gg L_3\omega$ and capacity $C \leq 1/\omega R$ (we assume there the weak skin effect and that the displacement current in the object does not exceed a conduction current). From the Kirchhoff equations for this circuit, and neglecting the highest-degree terms of the small parameters $\omega L_3/R$ and $\omega^2 L_3 C$, we obtain a relation between a current in the inductor and voltage on the detector and between the voltages on inductor and detector:

$$U_2 = \left[\omega M_{13}M_{23}\left(\frac{1}{R} + i\omega C\right) + iM_{12}\right]\omega I_1$$

$$= \left[M_{12} - i\omega M_{13}M_{23}\left(1 - \frac{M_{12}M_{13}}{M_{23}L_1}\right)\left(\frac{1}{R} + i\omega C\right)\right]\frac{U_1}{L_1} \quad (3)$$

where U_i and I_i are the voltages and currents in the windings, respectively, and L_i and M_{ij} are the coefficients of self and mutual induction, respectively. From this equation, in approximation of small disturbances, as well as followed from equation 2, we notice that the amplitude of the signal of the detector does not depend on the conductivity, but does depend on the permittivity of the object. The influence of a conductive object manifests as a change of the phase of the registered signal. Use of only phase measurements for reconstruction of conductivity allows for the reduction of the influence of spurious capacitive couplings and the high permittivity of the object.

Let the shift of phases α between current in an inductor and voltage on the detector differ little from 90°: $\Delta\alpha = \alpha - \pi/2 \ll 1$, which is always possible to ensure by the appropriate choice of frequency ω. From equation 3 in the linear approximation, we obtain

$$\Delta\alpha = \frac{\omega M_{13}M_{23}}{M_{12}R}. \quad (4)$$

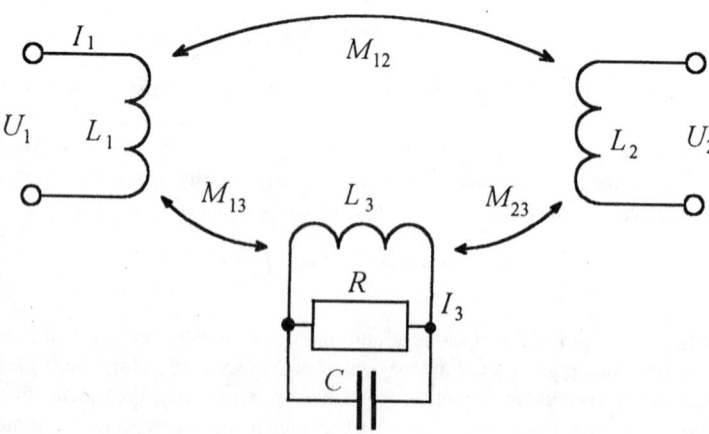

FIGURE 1. Equivalent circuit of the system.

The value of resistance R for a vortical current, induced by a magnetic field in the object, is inversely proportional to the cross-section area through which the current flows and to the conductivity of the object σ. If a small test object has an extent dl along a magnetic field and wholly crosses a common magnetic flow of the inductor and detector, expression 4 can be rewritten down as the following:

$$d\alpha = \omega W \sigma dl \qquad (5)$$

where W is a geometrical weight factor dependent on a mutual disposition of the inductor, object, and detector. Capacity C for the test object can be estimated from the same geometrical reasons as $\varepsilon_0 \varepsilon W dl$, which can be used for the reconstruction of the permittivity by results of measurements of the in-phase magnetic field component. For the whole change of the signal detector's signal in linear approximation, we obtain

$$dU_2 = -\omega^2 (\sigma + i\omega\varepsilon_0\varepsilon) W M_{12} I_1 dl.$$

For an extended conductive medium after integrations of equation 5 along a line of a magnetic field connecting the inductor and detector, we obtain that the measured phase shift $\Delta\alpha$ is proportional to the linear integral of the weighed conductivity:

$$\Delta\alpha = \omega \int_L W \sigma dl.$$

Having a set of such integrals for inductors and detectors located around the investigated object, it is possible to reconstruct the distribution of the conductivity in a cross section of the object.

RESULTS

The method of convolution and back-projection can be used for the reconstruction of conductivity in a cross section of an object. This method is widely used in electrical impedance tomography. However, for induction tomography, as is visible from equations 1 and 2, the measured data correspond to the distribution of the conductivity itself, instead of the gradient of conductivity in electrical impedance tomography, whose main equation is $\sigma \nabla^2 \varphi + \nabla \sigma \cdot \nabla \varphi = 0$. Thus, the stage of convolution (filtration) cannot be missed at reconstruction here. The possibility of the use of magnetic lines for back-projection during image reconstruction is illustrated in FIGURE 2. Coincidence of the zone of phase sensitivity (shaded in the picture), calculated by direct problem solving, with the magnetic line is demonstrated here. The reconstruction of the internal structure of conducting objects with a small internal variation of conductivity, such as a human body, requires using reference phase shifts corresponding to a body with homogeneous conductivity close to the average conductivity of the body. In other cases, total phase shifts, caused by the whole body, mask small variations caused by its internal structure. The reference data can be obtained, for example, from the measured data by the method used in electrical impedance tomography with static visualization[5] or by measurements on a different frequency or with a phantom.

For obtaining of the data required for reconstruction of the image, the tomograph must contain a set of inductors and detectors located in the plane of visualization. The obvious configuration is the arrangement of transmitting and receiving coils on a circle around the

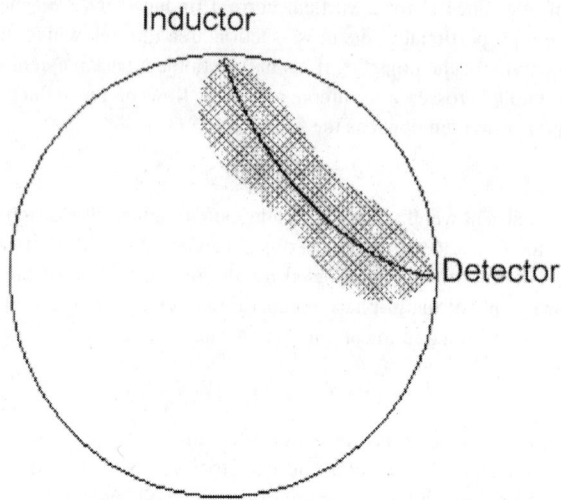

FIGURE 2. Phase-sensitivity zone (shaded) and magnetic line, connecting the detector and inductor coils.

object. As the lines of a magnetic field continue at both sides from a plane of the inductor, inductors and detectors should be placed inside the shield to avoid the influence of surrounding objects. On low frequencies (up to several MHz), the most suitable is a ferromagnetic shield. On higher frequencies, the conducting electromagnetic shield is more simple and effective. For many tasks, a system with a linear arrangement of inductors and detectors above a flat rectangular shield, providing subsurface visualization in the plane orthogonal to the coils, and a system with a two-dimensional array of the coils, providing three-dimensional visualization, will be useful.

The block diagram of the laboratory measuring unit operating at 20 MHz is shown in FIGURE 3. It consists of the current source, connected to the inductor coils, and a set of identical receivers with frequency converters and limiting amplifiers at the output. All receivers have a common heterodyne; the frequency of the output signals is 20 kHz. One of the receivers is connected to the field-detecting coils and the other measures the current in the inductors. The detection of phase shifts is performed at low frequency directly by a microprocessor with RISC architecture.

For illustration of the possibility of induction tomography, computer simulation of the measurement procedure was carried out for a tomograph with 32 inductors and detectors. The direct problem in linear approximation can be solved using the Green function for equation 2. Using the vector potential of the magnetic dipole as $\mathbf{A}_0$ and neglecting displacement currents, the amplitude of the magnetic field disturbance $\mathbf{B}_1$ caused by an object is

$$\mathbf{B}_1 = \frac{i\omega}{c^2} \int_V \sigma \frac{\mathbf{R} \times (\mathbf{m} \times \mathbf{R}_0)}{R_0^3 R^3} dV$$

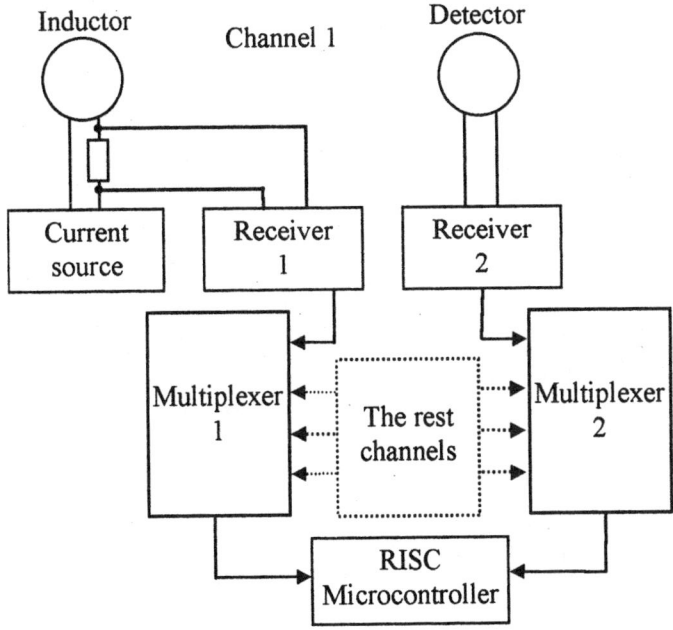

FIGURE 3. Block diagram of the measuring system.

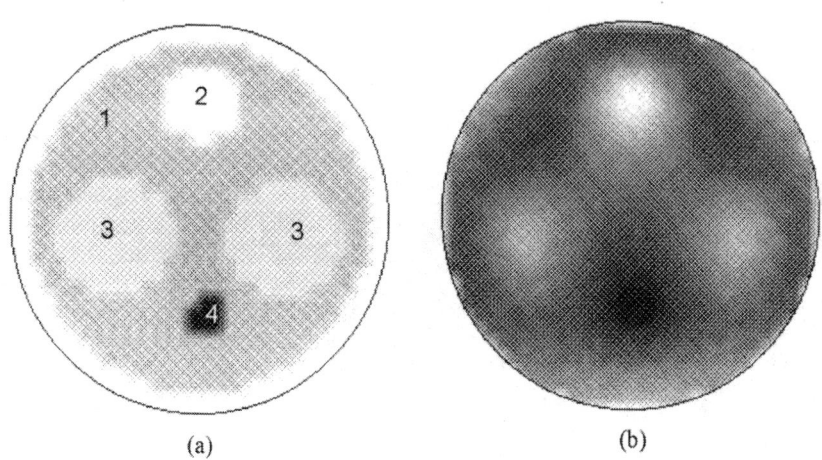

FIGURE 4. Initial distribution of conductivity, approximating a cross section of the human thorax (a) and its visualization by magnetic induction tomography (b). The areas marked in part a correspond to (1) skeletal muscles (0.1 S/m), (2) spine (0.007 S/m), (3) lungs (0.05 S/m), and (4) heart (0.5 S/m).

where **m** = amplitude of the magnetic moment of the inductor, **R** = radius-vector from the current point of the medium to the detector, and $\mathbf{R}_0$ = radius-vector from the inductor to the current point. Calculated disturbances determine the phase shifts of detected signals. These phase shifts were used as input data for reconstruction of conductivity by the method of convolution and back-projection along magnetic lines. The distribution of conductivity in a cross section of the object used in the simulation is shown in FIGURE 4a. This distribution approximates the cross section of a human chest. The result of reconstruction is shown in FIGURE 4b.

REFERENCES

1. KORZHENEVSKII, A.V. & V.A. CHEREPENIN. 1997. Magnetic induction tomography. J. Commun. Technol. Electron. **42:** 469–474.
2. KORJENEVSKY, A. & V. CHEREPENIN. 1997. Induction tomography: theory, computer simulation, and elements of measuring system. Med. Biol. Eng. Comput. **35**(suppl. 1): 330.
3. AL-ZEIBAK, S., D. GOSS, G. LYON, Z.Z. YU, A.J. PEYTON & M.S. BECK. 1995. A feasibility study of electromagnetic inductance tomography. *In* Proceedings of the Ninth International Conference on Electrical Bio-Impedance, Heidelberg, p. 426–429.
4. GRIFFITHS, H., W.R. STEWART & W. GOUGH. 1999. Magnetic induction tomography: a measuring system for biological tissues. This volume.
5. KORJENEVSKY, A.V. 1995. Reconstruction of absolute conductivity distribution in electrical impedance tomography. *In* Proceedings of the Ninth International Conference on Electrical Bio-Impedance, Heidelberg, p. 532–535.

Magnetic Impedance Tomography[a]

J. C. TOZER, R. H. IRELAND, D. C. BARBER,[b] AND A. T. BARKER

Department of Medical Physics and Clinical Engineering, University of Sheffield, Royal Hallamshire Hospital, Sheffield S10 2JF, United Kingdom

> ABSTRACT: Tissue can be characterized by its electrical impedance, especially if measurement can be extended over a range of frequencies. Recently, there has been a great deal of interest in imaging the distribution of electrical impedance through the technique of electrical impedance tomography (EIT). However, EIT has a number of practical problems relating to the placement of electrodes on the body. Such contacts are not required to collect magnetic field data around an object through which current is flowing and thus this approach may be more practical than EIT in the clinical environment. This paper describes the technique of magnetic impedance tomography (MIT), which allows reconstruction of the current distribution from magnetic field measurements. The reconstruction techniques used to generate the images and the prototype data collection system are described. Images produced using data collected from discrete and distributed current phantoms and the thorax during human respiration are presented.

INTRODUCTION

The ability to image the distribution of electrical impedance within a patient can provide useful clinical information. The principal existing technique for imaging electrical impedance is electrical impedance tomography (EIT). Current is introduced into the patient via surface electrodes, and the voltages developed as a result of the current flow are measured on the surface. From these measurements, the internal resistivity distribution can be reconstructed. EIT has a number of advantages over other medical imaging techniques; for example, it is harmless and relatively inexpensive, and data can be collected rapidly. It may also be useful for tissue characterization if the complex tissue impedance is measured. Such measurements require the application of injected currents in the range of 10 kHz to over 1 MHz.[1,2]

However, EIT suffers from a number of disadvantages, most of which are related to the placement of electrodes on the body, as discussed by Kolehmainen *et al.*[3] For example, incorrect or unknown positioning of electrodes results in a distorted image and precludes the generation of a single-frequency image of the absolute distribution of resistivity (known as a static image); consequently, difference images (images of a temporal change in resistivity) are commonly presented. High contact impedances attenuate the signal and mismatched contact impedances compromise the common-mode signal rejection. The resolution is also limited, in part, by the physical limitation of electrode area and the impracticality of applying a large number of electrodes to the body.

Magnetic impedance tomography (MIT), a technique proposed by Ahlfors and Ilmoniemi in 1992,[4] also uses two electrodes to inject current into a conducting object; however, rather than sensing surface potentials, the magnetic field generated by the current flow is detected outside the object. This makes all but two of the EIT electrodes redundant. In the

---

[a]This work was supported by the EPSRC (United Kingdom).
[b]To whom all correspondence should be addressed.

configuration that we have investigated, the geometry of these current injection electrodes is not critical, thus removing the errors associated with the use of electrodes. Any number of magnetic field measurements can be made outside the body and, since the position of the magnetic field detectors can be precisely determined, single-frequency static imaging should be possible. In EIT, the surface voltages are related directly to the resistivity distribution. This is an ill-conditioned, nonlinear relationship that requires a nonlinear image reconstruction algorithm. In MIT, the field is linearly related directly to the current pattern within the object, which makes reconstruction of the current patterns a linear, although ill-conditioned, problem. The subsequent reconstruction of the resistivity distribution from these patterns is nonlinear, but this is fairly well conditioned.

The rest of this paper outlines the imaging problem of MIT and explains the novel methodology that we have used to collect the MIT data. The first images produced from measurements on phantoms and the human thorax using this approach are presented.

THE IMAGING PROBLEM

The magnetic field generated by electrical current flow is given by the Biot-Savart Law:

$$B = \frac{\mu_0}{4\pi} \int \frac{J \times R}{|R|^3} \, dV \tag{1}$$

where B is the magnetic flux density generated by J, the current density, in a volume conductor V (R is the perpendicular distance between J and B, and μ_0 is the permeability of free space). A total of n vector magnetic field measurements and the discretization of the volume conductor with m voxels provide the matrix formulation

$$B = FJ \tag{2}$$

where B is the vector of size n containing the magnetic field measurements, F is an $n \times m$ sensitivity matrix specifying the relationship between the current and magnetic field, and J is a vector of size m of the unknown currents.

Calculation of the unknown currents from magnetic field measurements is an ill-posed problem with a nonunique solution,[5–7] and thus regularization is essential to produce a meaningful solution.[8] Tikhonov, damped, or truncated regularization methods can be typically applied to such ill-conditioned problems using a regularization parameter calculated from any of a number of methods, for example, Picard plots, L curves, or generalized cross-validation.[8]

However, regularization reduces the effects of high-frequency components of the data (such as noise and edges) and thus regularized solutions tend to be a smoother version of the true solution. Two basic types of current distribution were considered for imaging: a small number of discrete current-carrying conductors and a volume conductor with nonconducting regions. For the case of discrete conductors, improved resolution of the image was achieved when an iterative grid refinement technique was used. This technique is based on the work by Srebro,[9] where the "center of gravity" of the initial solution is calculated and an ellipse is formed that contains retained pixels. A new solution is then calculated based on this new grid and the process is iterated. The sum of all the iterative solutions is used to form a final grid from which the final solution is derived. A second iterative stage improved the resolution further, which involved taking the Srebro solution as the initial solution, refining the pixellation based on a selection criterion (such as rejecting those pixels having intensities of less than half the mean for the whole image), and solving for a new regularized solution based on the reduced pixel set. This process can be iterated until a minimum number of pixels is reached.

This iterative grid refinement method is suitable for a small number of discrete current-carrying conductors, but is inappropriate for a volume conductor. By considering the singular values and basis functions[10] of the sensitivity matrix F, it appears that the effect of regularization is to reduce or eliminate the small singular values that correspond to the basis functions that contribute to the central area of the image. Thus, in addition to the smoothing effect of regularization, the solution is dominated by the outer rings of pixels (those nearest to the magnetic field detectors). In order to compensate for this effect, column normalization[7,10] is used where F_0 replaces F in equation 2. F_0 is given by

$$F_0 = FG \quad \text{where} \quad G = diag\left[\frac{1}{\|F(:,1)\|, \ldots, \|F(:,m)\|}\right]. \quad (3)$$

This column normalization alters the singular values and basis functions and results in a regularized solution that retains greater information about the central region.

DATA COLLECTION SYSTEM

The majority of previous theoretical work and phantom studies in the field of MIT has involved the measurement of magnetic fields on a plane above the surface of the object under investigation, which is assumed to be 2D.[11,12] However, in order to generate a tomographic image, we applied axial currents to the object under investigation and measured the magnetic fields on a perpendicular plane encircling the object. FIGURE 1 shows the basic MIT measurement configuration.

The amplitude and frequency of the applied current that we have used are different from other MIT groups. Typical amplitudes of 100 mA have been used[12,13] at frequencies

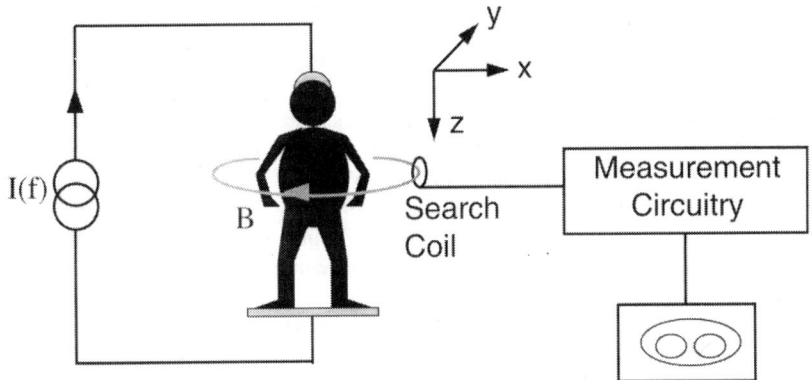

FIGURE 1. MIT measurement configuration.

of 16 Hz to 1 kHz.[4,12,13] These current amplitudes greatly exceed the maximum current stated in the European safety standard EN60601 that may be safely applied to the human body at the given frequencies. By analogy with EIT, it is likely to be useful to measure the complex tissue impedance exhibited by tissue at frequencies of over 10 kHz to allow tissue characterization. Hence, a frequency range of 10 kHz to 1 MHz was chosen for the injected current. At these frequencies, currents of 1–10 mA rms can be safely injected into the human body as specified by EN60601. Despite these relatively low current levels, it was found that search coils have sufficient sensitivity at these frequencies to measure the magnetic fields with an adequate signal-to-noise ratio to allow images to be generated. These are considerably cheaper and easier to use than the SQUIDs used by other MIT groups[4,11,13] and allow the possibility of parallel data collection from a large number of detectors on multiple planes surrounding the object under investigation.

SYSTEM DESCRIPTION

The current applied to the object under investigation is produced by an automatic gain-controlled voltage source with current amplitude feedback. This configuration behaves as a current source, although a time delay is built into the feedback circuit to stabilize the circuit for inductive loads (the nature of the injected current loop is inductive and this tends to cause instability with a conventional current source). The current delivered to the object under investigation is monitored throughout the measurement procedure, allowing compensation for any variation in drive current during the data collection. The search coil used to measure the magnetic field is placed on a platform perpendicular to the current flow, which defines the plane on which the measurements are made. Location marks on the measurement platform allow accurate positioning and orientation of the search coil. The object under investigation passes through a 20-cm-radius hole in the center of the measurement platform, which is large enough to allow the human thorax to be imaged. The vector magnetic field is measured at 15 points along 16 tangents, giving a total of 240 vector field measurements.

The size of the search coil is an important parameter; the induced voltage V is given by

$$V = -N\frac{d(BA)}{dt} \qquad (4)$$

where N is the number of turns, A is the area of the coil, B is the magnetic flux density, and t is time. A small coil will give an accurate point measurement of magnetic field, but the signal induced in the coil will be small. As the coil area increases, the induced signal increases, but the field measurement is an average measurement over the area of the coil. An 80-turn, 18-mm-diameter coil was found to be a suitable compromise between accuracy and signal size. The coil was wound to minimize interwinding capacitance and hence increase the resonant frequency to a value well above the measurement frequency range. The induced voltage in the coil is amplified by a low-noise, high-bandwidth amplifier and then passed through an integration stage that compensates for the frequency-dependent amplitude of the induced voltage in the coil. The signal is then synchronously detected, low-pass filtered, and sampled. The samples are averaged for 20 ms to reduce noise, and dc offsets are monitored throughout the data collection procedure to allow for compensation of drift in the detector stages.

The signal-to-noise ratio of the system is dependent upon the current distribution, but (for example) a 10 mA rms current passed down a single wire in the center of the target region results in an average magnetic field of 10 nT rms detected at a radius of 20 cm. Use of low-noise electronic components, synchronous detection, and averaging result in a signal-to-noise ratio of 89 dB at 100 kHz for 10 nT rms.

We have collected magnetic field data for a number of resistivity distributions. The image reconstruction techniques previously discussed in this paper assume a uniform current distribution in the axial direction and hence phantoms that approximate this ideal were used. First, up to five conducting rods of length 2 m were used to test the ability of the imaging system to distinguish between discrete sources. Second, a square cross-section plastic container of height 0.51 m and width 0.28 m filled with saline, with plate electrodes at top and bottom, was used as a phantom into which nonconducting inserts were placed. Finally, measurements were performed on two human volunteers. Electrodes were placed on the head and feet, and magnetic field measurements were made at chest height. Measurements were made at maximum inspiration and maximum expiration.

RESULTS

The images presented in this section are all generated from single-frequency measurements made with an injected current of 10 mA rms at 100 kHz.

FIGURE 2 shows a static image generated from data collected from three vertical rods carrying equal current. The iterative grid refinement method has been used to generate the image shown in FIGURE 2. The rods are clearly visible and their imaged position corresponds closely to their actual position in the phantom.

When simple noise-free simulated distributed current phantoms are imaged, the approximate current patterns can be seen in the static images. When similar images are reconstructed from measured data, the perturbation in the current pattern is evident, but difficult to interpret. The poorer resolution for the measured data image arises because the

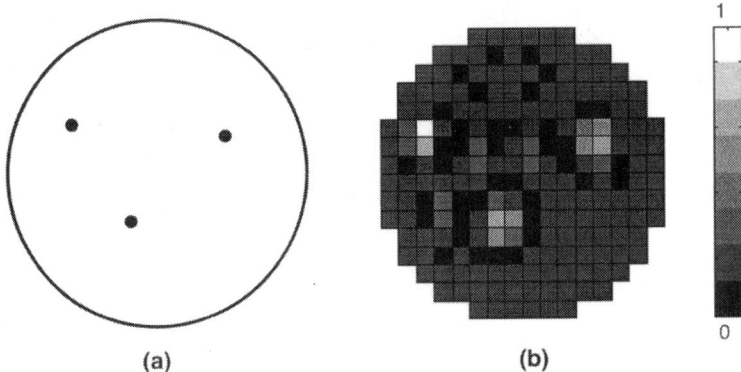

FIGURE 2. (a) Position of three thin equal-current-carrying rods. (b) Reconstructed image for data measured from the three-rod phantom.

reconstruction has to be constrained to prevent amplification of any noise present on the data. Consequently, difference images are presented in FIGURES 3 and 4.

FIGURE 3 shows a difference image generated from measurements made on the saline phantom (saline in a square container with a nonconducting object placed towards the top-left corner) using the column normalization technique described earlier. It can be seen that the current distribution has been modified as expected by the presence of the nonconducting object: there is an increase in current flow in the region surrounding the object and a decrease in current flow in the area of the object.

FIGURE 4 shows a differential image produced from data collected from a human thorax at full inspiration and full expiration showing structures consistent with the lungs (using the column normalization technique). As far as we are aware, these are the first MIT images of human subjects that have been produced.

CONCLUSIONS

We have demonstrated the feasibility of using magnetic field measurements to produce images of current distribution, at least in two dimensions, and have made the first steps towards developing MIT as a new medical imaging technique. A prototype data collection system has been developed, and image reconstruction techniques have been developed and evaluated. Three distinct cases have been investigated: discrete objects, distributed current patterns, and current passing through the human thorax. A repeatable and reliable method of reconstructing discrete objects has been developed that gives an accurate resolution of a small number of objects. For distributed current, the regularization required because of the ill-conditioned nature of the problem and the presence of even small levels of noise can lead to images with relatively poor resolution. Suitable constraints to improve the stability and noise susceptibility of the solution should be investigated.

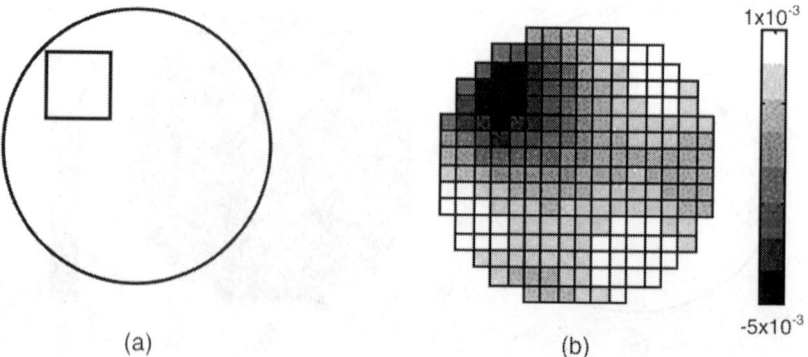

FIGURE 3. (a) Position of nonconducting object. (b) Reconstruction of current distribution from measured data. Difference image of a phantom with nonconducting object placed towards the top-left corner.

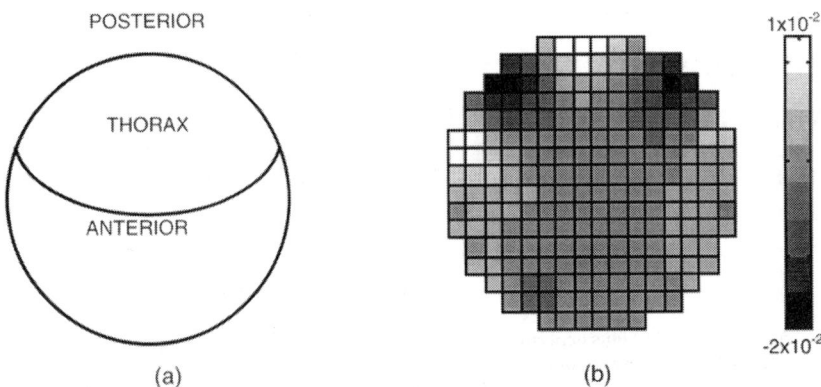

FIGURE 4. (a) Position of thorax. (b) Reconstruction of current distribution from measured human data. Difference image of full inspiration minus full expiration. The thorax filled approximately the top half of the imaged area.

REFERENCES

1. Brown, B.H. *et al.* 1994. Cardiac and respiratory related electrical impedance changes in the human thorax. IEEE Trans. Biomed. Eng. **41**(8): 729–734.
2. Osypka, M. & E. Gersing. 1995. Tissue impedance spectra and the appropriate frequencies for EIT. Physiol. Meas. **16**: A49–A55.
3. Kolehmainen, V. *et al.* 1997. Assessment of errors in static electrical impedance tomography with adjacent and trigonometric current patterns. Physiol. Meas. **18**: 289–303.
4. Ahlfors, S. & R.J. Ilmoniemi. 1992. Magnetic imaging of conductivity. *In* Proc. 14th Int. Conf. IEEE Eng. Med. Biol. Soc. (Paris), p. 1717–1718.
5. Sarvas, J. 1987. Basic mathematical and electromagnetic concepts of the biomagnetic inverse problem. Phys. Med. Biol. **32**: 11–22.
6. Williamson, S.J. & L. Kaufman. 1981. Biomagnetism topical review. J. Magnetism Magn. Mater. **22**: 129–201.
7. Gorodnitsky, I.F. *et al.* 1995. Neuromagnetic source imaging with FOCUSS: a recursive weighted minimum norm algorithm. Electroencephalogr. Clin. Neurophysiol. **95**: 231–251.
8. Hansen, P.C. 1994. Regularization tools: a Matlab package for analysis and solution of discrete ill-posed problems. Numerical Algorithms **6**: 1–35.
9. Srebro, R. 1996. Iterative refinement of the minimum norm solution of the bioelectric inverse problem. IEEE Trans. Biomed. Eng. **43**: 547–552.
10. Golub, G.H. & C.F. Van Loan. 1996. Matrix Computations. Third edition. Johns Hopkins University Press. Baltimore.
11. Birgul, O. & Y.Z. Ider. 1996. Electrical impedance tomography using the magnetic field generated by injected currents. *In* Proc. 18th Int. Conf. IEEE Eng. Med. Biol. Soc. (Amsterdam).
12. Hong, H.D. & M.D. Fox. 1995. Magnetic backprojection imaging of the vascular lumen. IEEE Trans. Biomed. Eng. **42**(1): 102–108.
13. Muftuler, L.T. & Y.Z. Ider. 1996. Measuring AC magnetic field distribution using MRI. *In* Proc. 18th Int. Conf. IEEE Eng. Med. Biol. Soc. (Amsterdam).

Evaluation of Impedance Technique for Detecting Breast Carcinoma Using a 2-D Numerical Model of the Torso

MICHAL M. RADAI,[a] SHIMON ABBOUD,[a] AND MOSHE ROSENFELD[b]

[a]*Department of Biomedical Engineering*

[b]*Department of Fluid Mechanics, Faculty of Engineering, Tel Aviv University, Tel Aviv, 69978 Israel*

ABSTRACT: Previous experimental studies showed that significant changes occur in the electrical properties of breast cancer tissue compared to the surrounding normal tissue. This phenomenon motivated studies on cancer detection using electrical impedance techniques. In the present study, a two-dimensional model of the torso and a numerical method were used to investigate the changes in the potential distribution as a result of a malignant tissue present in the breast. A transverse MRI image of the woman's torso was scanned. Noise reduction and contour-following algorithms were applied to differentiate between eight compartments in the torso. The extracted tissue types were lungs, blood, ribs, bone marrow of the cord, breast fat, skin, skeletal muscle, and heart muscle. Isotropic homogeneous conductivity was assigned to each one of these compartments. The volume conductor problem was solved numerically using the finite volume method to determine the potential distribution developed due to the dipole source. Cases without and with artificially inserted malignant region with realistic sizes were examined to investigate the sensitivity of impedance techniques to detect breast cancer. Significant changes were detected in the potential distribution inside the volume conductor as a result of the realistic size of breast tumors. A linear relation was found between the surface potential in the vicinity of the tumor region and the size of the tumor. For a small malignant area of 0.22 cm^2, the surface potential near the tumor region decreased only slightly from a value of 13.81 mV in the normal case to 13.67 mV (0.14 mV change; 1.0%). For a larger malignant area of 5.43 cm^2, the potential decrease was more pronounced, 11.29 mV (2.52 mV change; 18.3%), indicating that realistic sizes of breast tumor result in significant changes in the surface potential. Thus, impedance techniques employed in the present study show very good promise in detecting breast cancer.

INTRODUCTION

Breast cancer is the most commonly diagnosed cancer and a major leading cause of cancer death among women in the United States and Europe. The average incidence of breast cancer in the last years is approximately 110 per 100,000 women, and the death rate is approximately 27 per 100,000 women.[1] Early detection is essential for reducing the need for radical surgeries and for improving survival rates.

Existing breast cancer detection methods include ionizing invasive and noninvasive procedures (like X rays, ultrasound, thermography, diaphanoscopy, and palpation). Recently, several groups[2,3] investigated the possibility of detecting breast cancer by electrical impedance techniques that are based on changes in the electrical properties of the biological tissues. Measuring the surface potential distribution due to an induced current source can provide information about changes of the conductivity inside the volume conductor, as well as about the volume or location of internal organs. The use of impedance techniques for detecting breast cancer is based on the assumption that molecular changes affect the electrical properties of the tissue as a malignant tissue is developing. Surowiec et al.[4] found that there are significant differences in the electrical properties between cancerous and normal tissue. This change takes place quite early in the transition of the tissue from normal to malignant, giving hope for early detection of breast cancer employing electrical impedance techniques.

Kejariwal et al.[2] studied a two-dimensional impedance tomography system based on a simple array of RC components (resistive-capacitive circuits). Using Surowiec's findings,[4] concerning the changes in the breast cancer conductivity, they concluded that a tumor in a size of 1% of the torso area produces more than 4% change in the circumference potential magnitude compared to a model without a tumor. Piperno et al.[3] used an imaging device based on measuring the dielectric properties of the breast tissues and performed a clinical study on 6000 patients. Their findings showed that breast cancer can be detected reliably using impedance techniques.

Recently, studies from our laboratory used the finite volume method (FVM) to investigate the potential distribution inside the volume conductor due to internal current sources. Several aspects related to the influence of geometrical asymmetries on the surface potential, such as skull thickness on the scalp potential distribution[5] or ischemic brain on the left-right asymmetry of visual evoked potentials,[6] were examined. Another work investigated the effect of the location of the internal current source on the scalp potentials.[7]

These very same techniques can be employed for the theoretical study of the applicability of impedance methods to detect breast cancer. The aim of the present study is to evaluate the feasibility of using principles of impedance technique based on numerical simulation to detect breast cancer. The forward problem is solved numerically for realistic two-dimensional approximation of the torso using the finite volume method. The potential distribution inside the volume conductor due to an external current source is calculated for several imposed electrical properties of the malignant tissue. The changes in the surface potential distribution without and with artificially inserted malignant region of realistic sizes were examined to investigate the sensitivity of impedance techniques to detect breast cancer.

METHODS

Solution of the Potential due to a Current Source

The volume conductor problem is assumed to be linear and, for the frequencies used in bioimpedance techniques (~20 kHz), capacitive components of the electric impedance of the body tissues can be neglected.[8] The external current source is represented as a bipolar source on the torso surface (enclosing the two sides of the right breast). The distribution of the potential in the presence of a current source in a volume V with the surface S is given by the Gauss law:

$$\oint_S \sigma \nabla \psi \cdot d\vec{S} = -\int_V I d\vec{V} \tag{1}$$

where σ is the conductivity, ψ is the potential, and I is the current volume source density. In the initial stage of the present study, a two-dimensional approximation is used, reducing the Gauss law into its two-dimensional form:

$$\oint_l \sigma \nabla \psi \cdot \vec{dl} = -\iint_S I_s \cdot \vec{ds} \tag{2}$$

where $\vec{dl}$ is a length element, $\vec{ds}$ is the surface area element, and I_s is the current source density. The boundary conditions specify that no current flows into the air, that is, $\sigma \partial \psi / \partial n = 0$ (where n is the normal to the boundary).

Approximation of the Volume Conductor Equation by the FVM

In the 2-D FVM, the physical domain is divided into a large number of arbitrary quadrilateral polar cells, known also as the primary cells. The division is performed by generating an appropriate polar mesh. The indices i,j are assigned to the center of each quadrilateral cell, according to the r and θ polar coordinate system. The four faces are denoted by $i \pm \frac{1}{2}$, $j \pm \frac{1}{2}$. The length vectors of the cell sides are given by the normal length vectors l^r or l^θ (according to the direction). The discrete unknowns $\psi_{i,j}$ are defined at the center of the cells (not at the vertices as in most discretization methods) to simplify the calculation of the fluxes.

The integral conservation equation 1 is discretized for each primary cell. It is approximated by the second-order-accurate scheme:

$$\sum_{\text{four faces}} (\sigma \cdot \nabla \psi) \cdot \vec{\Delta l} = -I_s \cdot \vec{\Delta s} \tag{3}$$

or, in expanded form,

$$(\sigma \nabla \psi \cdot \Delta l^r)_{i+\frac{1}{2},j} - (\sigma \nabla \psi \cdot \Delta l^r)_{i-\frac{1}{2},j} + (\sigma \nabla \psi \cdot \Delta l^\theta)_{i,j+\frac{1}{2}} - (\sigma \nabla \psi \cdot \Delta l^\theta)_{i,j-\frac{1}{2}} \tag{4}$$

$$= -I_{i,j} \cdot \vec{\Delta s}.$$

Each term in the left-hand side represents the current flow through the relevant side, while the right-hand side stands for the current source inside the cell (if existent). The components of the length vector are computed from

$$\Delta l^r = r \cdot \Delta \theta \cdot \hat{r} \tag{5}$$

$$\Delta l^\theta = \Delta r \cdot \hat{\theta}$$

and the area of the cell is

$$\Delta s = r_{i,j} \cdot \Delta r \cdot \Delta \theta. \tag{6}$$

Equations 3 and 4 are the discrete equivalent of the Gauss law for each cell: the sum of the fluxes across the faces of each cell is equal to the current source inside the cell. The boundary condition (zero current flow) is applied by setting to zero the appropriate current flow term in equation 4.

The gradient operator for each face of the primary cell is given by

$$\nabla = \frac{\partial}{\partial r}\hat{r} + \frac{1}{r} \cdot \frac{\partial}{\partial \theta}\hat{\theta}. \tag{7}$$

Studies of the treatment of the singular points or the boundaries between regions with different conductivities are beyond the scope of the present article. Full details can be found in references 5–7 and 9. The FVM approximation yields a large set of sparse linear equations, which are solved iteratively by the successive line over relaxation method.

RESULTS

The 2-D Real Geometry Model of the Torso

An MRI image (FIGURE 1) of an axial section of the torso was used to define a 2-D model of the woman's torso.[10] The image was scanned by an HP ScanJet Plus scanner with 16 Gray levels and 150 dots per inch resolution. Noise reduction and contour-following algorithms were applied to differentiate between eight torso compartments (FIGURE 2). The extracted tissue types were lungs, blood (inside the heart cavities), ribs, bone marrow of the cord, breast fat, skin, skeletal muscle, and heart muscle. Isotropic homogeneous conductivity was assigned to each compartment. The conductivity magnitudes[11–16] were 0.046, 0.606, 0.00523, 0.097, 0.04, 0.1, 0.148, and 0.46 [ohm · m]$^{-1}$, respectively. A circle-

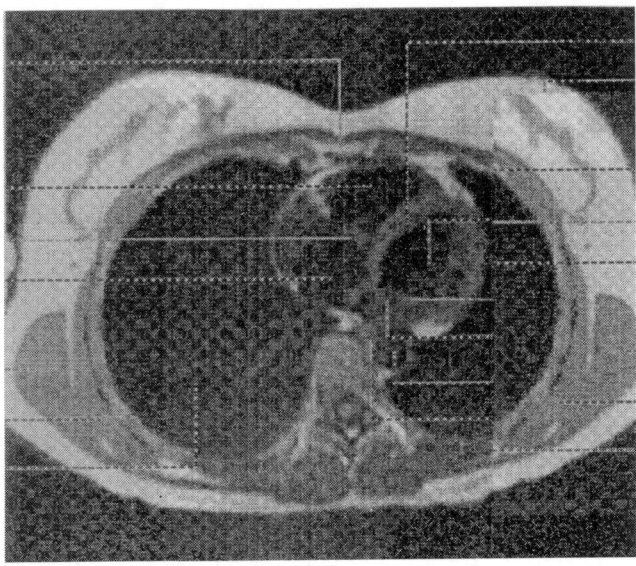

FIGURE 1. The original MRI image of a woman's torso.[10]

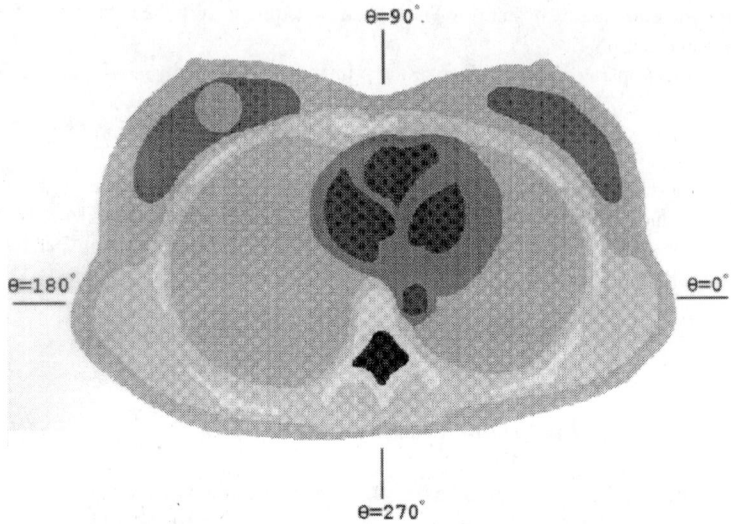

FIGURE 2. The segmented torso after image processing, with artificially inserted breast tumor.

shaped tumor tissue was added artificially to the right-side breast, with a conductivity of 0.714 ohm^{-1} · m^{-1}.[17]

Numerical Results

A polar coordinate system (r, θ) was employed on the segmented torso, with 70 × 140 mesh points, giving a total of 9800 points. This results in a resolution of approximately 2 mm in the radial direction (r) and 2.6° in the circumferential direction (θ). A bipolar current source of 1 mA, simulating the external current source, was located on the surface of the torso, at both sides of the right breast (the negative pole at $\theta = 90°$ above the sternum, and the positive pole at $\theta = 139°$). The discrete equations resulting from the finite volume method were solved by the iterative line successive over relaxation method. The convergence criterion of the total residual was set to 10^{-4}. The simulation was carried out on a Pentium-Pro PC, consuming several minutes of CPU time per solution. Simulations with different realistic sizes of the malignant tissue inside the right breast were performed (FIGURE 2). The largest tumor was placed at the circumferential angle of $126° \leq \theta \leq 136.3°$ with an area of 5.43 cm^2 (diameter of 2.63 cm).

FIGURES 3 and 4 show the equipotential lines in cases without and with the presence of the tumor tissue, respectively. There is a visible change in the behavior of the potential lines in the vicinity of the tumor area. Their density is lower in the case with the tumor tissue (FIGURE 4), suggesting a low potential difference over the tumor due to its higher conductivity. It should be emphasized that the potential distribution in the present numerical method is calculated for the entire region, not just for the boundary lines. This facilitates in the interpretation of the results and allows a deeper understanding of the surface distribution.

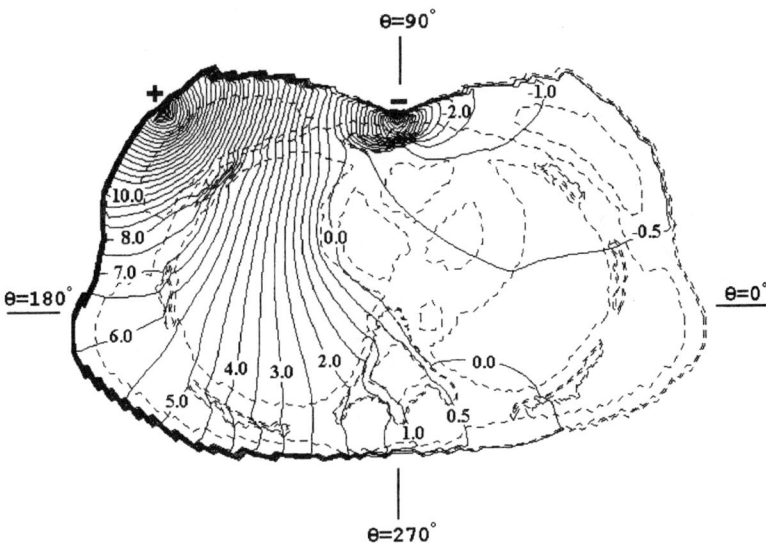

FIGURE 3. The potential distribution inside a normal torso.

FIGURE 5 presents the surface potentials over the right side of the breast for cases without and with malignant tissue of different sizes. Prominent decrease in the surface potential can be observed in the cases with the larger tumors. FIGURE 6 shows the percentage difference in the surface potential at $\theta = 136°$ (near the tumor) between the normal case

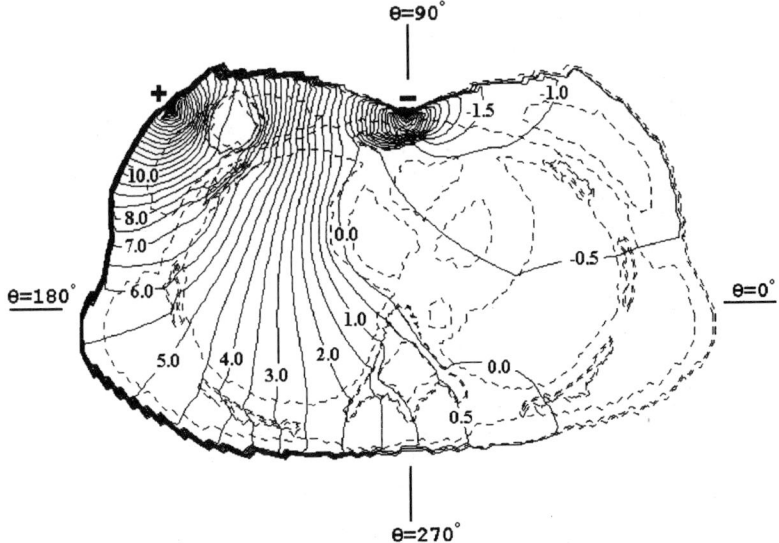

FIGURE 4. The potential distribution inside the torso in the presence of a malignant tissue.

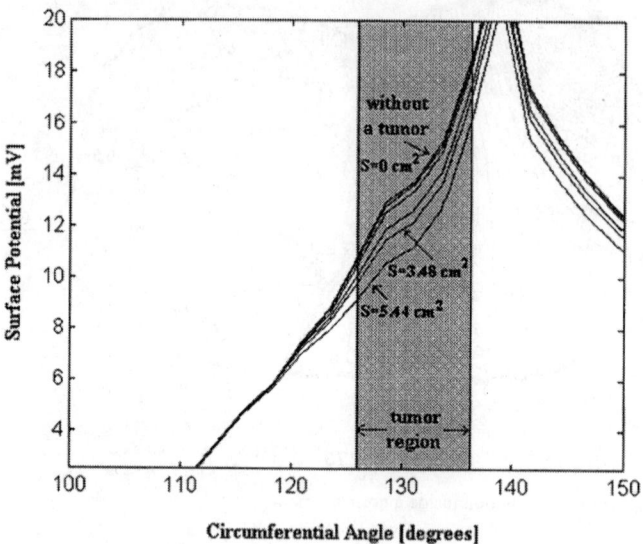

FIGURE 5. Surface potential distribution over the right-side breast in several cases with different tumor sizes.

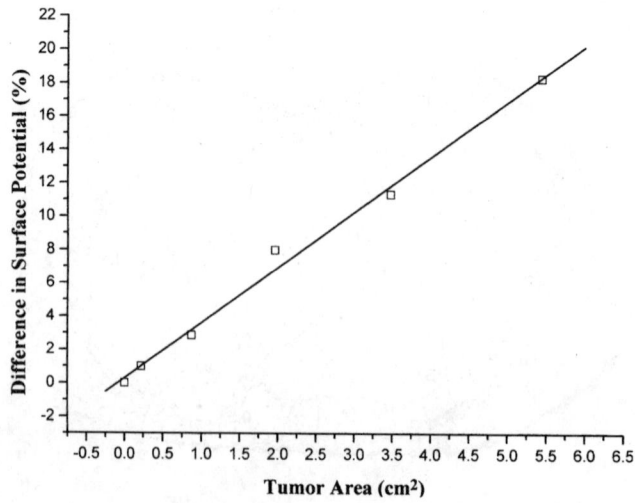

FIGURE 6. The percentage difference in the surface potential (for a single location over the tumor at $\theta = 136°$) between the normal case and cases with several realistic sizes of the tumor (0.22 to 5.43 cm^2). The presence of a tumor resulted in a reduction of up to 18% in the surface potential.

and cases with several sizes of the tumor ranging between 0.22 and 5.43 cm² in area. Strong linear correlation ($r = 0.996$) was obtained between the surface potential and the tumor size. The presence of the tumor resulted in reduction of up to 18% in surface potential. Note that the change in percent was calculated from

$$\left[\frac{(\Psi_{normal} - \Psi_{tumor})}{\Psi_{normal}}\right] \cdot 100.$$

FIGURE 7 shows the absolute difference in the circumferential surface potential distribution between the normal breast and the case with the largest tumor. The largest difference of 2.5 mV in the surface potential is observed in the region of the tumor (emphasized by the shaded area). This reflects a change of 18% compared to the normal case.

DISCUSSION AND CONCLUDING REMARKS

The impedance technique is a low cost and safe procedure in comparison to other imaging techniques. On the other hand, the spatial resolution of this technique is not as good and impedance images show significant intersubject variability.[18] As a result of these limitations, impedance techniques are not being used yet as a routine diagnostic tool. One area in which impedance techniques have been used for clinical purposes is breast cancer. Previous experimental studies demonstrated that significant changes of the electrical properties occur in the presence of cancer tissue. This observation motivated studies on cancer detection using impedance techniques. Piperno et al.[3] used an imaging device based on

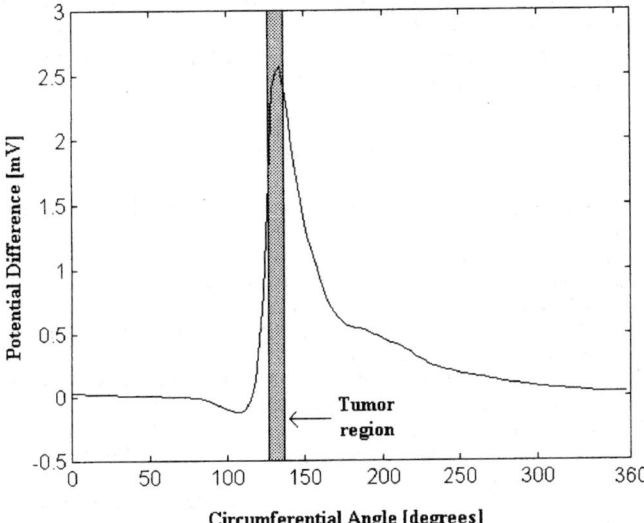

FIGURE 7. The difference in the circumferential surface potentials between the case of a normal breast and the case with the largest simulated tumor (5.43 cm² area; 2.63 cm diameter). The largest difference of 2.5 mV in the surface potential is observed in the region of the tumor (emphasized by the shaded area).

measuring the dielectric properties of the breast tissues and performed a clinical study on 6000 patients. They concluded that impedance techniques could indeed detect breast cancer with good reliability. In a study by Holder et al.,[19] however, only limited success was achieved in producing images of the breast using synthetic reference data.

These limitations and the difficulties encountered in applying impedance techniques to detect breast cancer motivated us to conduct a theoretical study to investigate the feasibility of using principles of impedance technique for this issue. A realistic 2-D geometry model of the torso taken from an MRI scan of a healthy female subject[10] was used to investigate the changes in the potential distribution as a result of variations in the volume conductor properties (the presence of the malignant tissue). Eight tissue types were used to describe the different compartments of the torso. The volume conductor problem was solved numerically using a finite volume method to determine the ability of impedance techniques to detect cancer.

It was found that significant changes occur in the potential distribution in the volume conductor in the presence of malignant tissues. The surface potential near the tumor region changes significantly for realistic size of the tumor. In the case of the largest tumor studied (5.43 cm^2 area; 2.63 cm diameter), a difference as large as 18% was found in the surface potential near the tumor. This finding is in disagreement with the work of Kejariwal et al.[2] that showed only 4% difference between the malignant and the normal breast. However, in their study, they used a two-dimensional RC components model, with only three compartments of the torso.

The present theoretical study is an additional step in the evaluation of impedance techniques to detect breast cancer. Although it was found that significant changes occur in the surface potential due to a current source when a malignant tissue is present, further study is needed to obtain more conclusive results. First, the model should be extended to more realistic three-dimensional cases to simulate accurately the volume conductor problem. Second, the sensitivity of the results to the source location as well as to the location and extent of the tumor should be tested.

REFERENCES

1. HULKA, B.S. 1997. Epidemiologic analysis of breast and gynecologic cancers. Prog. Clin. Biol. Res. **396:** 17–29.
2. KEJARIWAL, M., K. KASTER, J. JURIST & J. PAKANATI. 1993. Breast cancer detection using electrical impedance tomography: SPICE simulation. *In* Proceedings of the IEEE Engineering in Medicine and Biology Society Conference: paper no. 456.
3. PIPERNO, G., E.H. FREI & M. MOSHITZKY. 1990. Breast cancer screening by impedance measurements. Front. Med. Biol. Eng. **2**(2): 111–117.
4. SUROWIEC, A.J., S.S. STUCHLY, J.B. BARR & A. SWARUP. 1988. Dielectric properties of breast carcinoma and the surrounding tissues. IEEE Trans. Biomed. Eng. **35**(4): 257–263.
5. ESHEL, Y., S. WITMAN, M. ROSENFELD & S. ABBOUD. 1995. Correlation between skull thickness asymmetry and scalp potential estimated by a numerical model of the head. IEEE Trans. Biomed. Eng. **42**(3): 242–249.
6. ABBOUD, S., L. BAR, M. ROSENFELD, H. RING & I. GLASS. 1996. Left-right asymmetry of visual evoked potentials in brain-damaged patients: a mathematical model and experimental results. Ann. Biomed. Eng. **24**(1): 75–86.
7. ABBOUD, S., M. ROSENFELD & J. LUZON. 1996. Effect of source location on the scalp potential asymmetry in a numerical model of the head. IEEE Trans. Biomed. Eng. **43**(7): 690–696.
8. FREESTON, I.L. & R.C. TOZER. 1995. Impedance imaging using induced currents. Physiol. Meas. **16**(3): A257–A266.

9. ABBOUD, S., Y. ESHEL, S. LEVY & M. ROSENFELD. 1994. Numerical calculation of the potential distribution due to dipole sources in a spherical model of the head. Comput. Biomed. Res. **27**(6): 441–455.
10. EL-KHOURY, G.Y., R.A. BERGMAN & W.J. MONTGOMERY. 1995. Sectional Anatomy by MRI. Chapter 11, p. 392. Churchill Livingstone. New York.
11. YAMAMOTO, T. & Y. YAMAMOTO. 1976. Electrical properties of the epidermal stratum corneum. Med. Biol. Eng. **14**(2): 151–158.
12. GEDDES, L.A. & L.E. BAKER. 1967. The specific resistance of biological material—a compendium of data for the biomedical engineer and physiologist. Med. Biol. Eng. **5**(3): 271–293.
13. PFUTZNER, H. 1984. Dielectric analysis of blood by means of a raster-electrode technique. Med. Biol. Eng. Comput. **22**(2): 142–146.
14. SAHA, S. & P.A. WILLIAMS. 1989. Electric and dielectric properties of wet human cancellous bone as a function of frequency. Ann. Biomed. Eng. **17**(2): 143–158.
15. JOINES, W.T., Y. ZHANG, C. LI & R.L. JIRTLE. 1994. The measured electrical properties of normal and malignant human tissues from 50 to 900 MHz. Med. Phys. **21**(4): 547–550.
16. TAMURA, T., M. TENHUNEN, T.M. LAHTINEN, T. REPO & H.P. SCHWAN. 1994. Modelling of the dielectric properties of normal and irradiated skin. Phys. Med. Biol. **39**(6): 927–936.
17. SUROWIEC, A., S.S. STUCHLY, L. EIDUS & A. SWARUP. 1987. *In vitro* dielectric properties of human tissues at radiofrequencies. Phys. Med. Biol. **32**(5): 615–621.
18. BOONE, K., D. BARBER & B. BROWN. 1997. Imaging with electricity: report of the European concerted action on impedance tomography. J. Med. Eng. Technol. **21**(6): 201–232.
19. HOLDER, D.S., N. ANELLS & K.G. BOONE. 1994. *In vivo* images of the female breast obtained with the Sheffield Mark 1 electrical impedance tomography system. *In* Proceedings of the Third Meeting of the European Concerted Action on Impedance Tomography (Ankara, Turkey).

A Comparison of the Siconolfi and Cole-Cole Procedures for Multifrequency Impedance Data Analysis

LEIGH WARD,[a] NIGEL FULLER,[b] BRUCE CORNISH,[c] MARINOS ELIA,[b] AND BRIAN THOMAS[c]

[a]*Department of Biochemistry, University of Queensland, Brisbane QLD 4072, Australia*
[b]*Dunn Clinical Nutrition Center, Cambridge, United Kingdom*
[c]*Center for Medical and Health Physics, Queensland University of Technology, Brisbane, Australia*

ABSTRACT: The established Cole-Cole and newer Siconolfi methods for analysis of multifrequency impedance data were compared in a group of normal healthy individuals studied under bedside conditions. Impedance quotients derived from each procedure were similarly well correlated with independent dilutional estimates of total body water. Although both methods estimated resistance at zero frequency, were highly correlated, and provided impedance quotients with very similar correlations with extracellular water, these estimates were significantly different and thus may not be used interchangeably. The Siconolfi procedure demonstrated no significant advantage over the Cole-Cole method. In view of the sound theoretical basis for the latter, it is concluded that analysis of MFBIA data by the Cole-Cole method is to be preferred.

INTRODUCTION

Multiple frequency bioelectrical impedance analysis (MFBIA) has become a popular technique for the noninvasive quantitative analysis of body water compartments.[1-3] The technique is based on the theory that low-frequency current preferentially passes through the extracellular water space (ECW), while at high frequency an electrical current penetrates the cell membrane and thus is conducted through the total body water space (TBW). In order that this theory may be used to derive prediction equations for ECW and TBW, it is necessary to define appropriately low and high frequencies at which impedance should be measured.

While some authors, for example, Segal et al.,[4] have suggested that measurements at 5 and 100 kHz are adequate for this purpose, others, for example, Boulier et al.,[5] have reported that, for prediction of TBW in particular, measurement at much higher frequency (1 MHz) is required. An alternative approach is to avoid selecting single frequencies, within a practicable measurement range, assumed to represent optimal predictive frequencies for ECW and TBW and to model impedance data collected over many frequencies in order to estimate the impedance at both zero and infinite frequency, which are not experimentally determinable. Such modeling is typically performed by fitting data to the Cole-Cole function.[6] In practice, this is usually performed by plotting reactance versus resistance at each measured frequency and fitting the experimental data to the theoretical semicircular plot using nonlinear regression[7] or iterative curve fitting.[8]

More recently, Siconolfi and colleagues[8,9] have suggested an alternative approach in which the start of the impedance plateau of an impedance-frequency response curve is identified and the resistance at this frequency, defined as the total circuit resistance (RT), is used to predict TBW. The intercept of the regression of resistance versus frequency on the resistance axis provides an estimate of ECW resistance ($R2$). Although high correlations of impedance quotients, $H^2/R2$ and H^2/RT (H = height), with tracer dilutional estimates of ECW and TBW were obtained in their study, there was no direct comparison of the performance of their procedure to that of the commonly used Cole-Cole method.

We report here a comparison of the Cole-Cole and Siconolfi methods when applied to a cross-sectional group of normal subjects measured under typical bedside conditions.

METHODS

Fifteen subjects (6 males and 9 females) participated in the study. Subject characteristics were as follows: weight, 79.8 ± 18.0 kg; height, 173.1 ± 7.8 cm; age, 50.1 ± 5.4 years; BMI, 26.5 ± 5.1 kg-m^{-2}. TBW and ECW were determined using tracer dilution techniques described elsewhere.[10] Briefly, these were NaBr dilution for ECW (actually determined as corrected bromide space) and D_2O dilution for TBW.

MFBIA data were obtained for 248 frequencies, logarithmically spaced in the range of 4 to 1012 kHz, using an SEAC SFB2.3 impedance monitor. Impedance and phase angle were measured, and resistance and reactance were calculated for each frequency. Data were fitted to the Cole-Cole model by regression as previously described[7] using all frequencies and $R2$ computed by extrapolation to zero frequency and RT by extrapolation to infinite frequency. $R2$ and RT were also estimated using the procedures of Siconolfi et al.[8,9] and as described above. Third-order least-squares regressions were used with RT at the start of the impedance plateau, being defined as the resistance at the frequency at which impedance changed by 1% for a 25-kHz increase in frequency.[8,9] This procedure is, de facto, estimating the "inflection point" in the regression where the change in impedance is asymptotically approaching a pseudoplateau.[5] This inflection point may be determined, assuming a two-process model, by nonlinear regression using a technique described previously.[11] An advantage of this method is that the inflection point is evaluated with a set of goodness-of-fit statistics (correlations, covariances, and residuals). The methods were compared by consideration of the correlations and SEE (standard errors of estimates) associated with regressions of the various estimates of $R2$ and RT with the independent dilutional estimates of ECW and TBW, respectively.

RESULTS

As noted by Siconolfi et al.[8,9] the estimates of $R2$ obtained by the different methods were highly correlated (e.g., $r = 0.995$; $R2_{Cole} = 1.04 \times R2_{Sic} + 54.5$), but there was a highly significant bias ($p < 0.00001$) between the two sets of data: mean $R2_{Cole} = 687$ ohm and $R2_{Sic} = 607$ ohm with limits of agreement of 57 to 104 ohm. These differences are unlikely to be due to errors associated with poor data fitting by one or both methods since the SEE values of $R2$ were 0.32 ± 0.05% and 0.36 ± 0.11% for the Siconolfi and Cole-Cole methods, respectively. The magnitudes of the correlation coefficients and the SEE for

TABLE 1. Correlation Coefficients (r) and Standard Errors of Estimates (SEE) for TBW and ECW Assessed by Siconolfi and Cole-Cole Models

Model	Quotient	r	SEE (L)
	TBW		
Cole-Cole	H^2/Z_c	0.72	6.05
Cole-Cole	H^2/R_∞	0.68	7.00
Siconolfi	H^2/RT	0.70	6.41
Inflection point	H^2/RT	0.73	5.92
	ECW		
Cole-Cole	$H^2/R2$	0.63	3.90
Siconolfi	$H^2/R2$	0.66	3.75
Inflection point	$H^2/R2$	0.63	3.88

regression of $H^2/R2$ against ECW were similar to those of the Siconolfi procedure, providing the best correlation and the lowest SEE (TABLE 1).

There was no significant difference between the Siconolfi and inflection point estimates of RT, 464 ± 92 and 510 ± 91 ohm, respectively, although for one subject the 1% change in impedance required by the Siconolfi method did not occur within the frequency range of the data. Regression of H^2/RT against TBW, measured by D$_2$O dilution, yielded correlations of 0.70 and 0.73 and SEE values of 6.41 L and 5.92 L for the Siconolfi and inflection point methods, respectively (TABLE 1). These may be compared with correlations of 0.72 and 0.62 and SEE values of 6.05 L and 7.4 L obtained using the impedance quotients, H^2/Z_c and H^2/R_∞, respectively, obtained from Cole-Cole analysis.

DISCUSSION

Although Siconolfi et al.[9] found that their procedure provided marginally better estimates of TBW and ECW than previously published methods (N.B.: only single-frequency BIA methods were compared), the key comparison with the Cole-Cole MFBIA method was not performed as in the present study.

Typically, TBW is predicted using the Cole-Cole model by either the resistance at infinite frequency (R_∞) or the impedance at maximal reactance (Z_c), as here. In the absence of a second-validation subject group, we were only able to compare the Siconolfi and Cole-Cole methods on the basis of the correlation coefficients and SEE. However, these data suggest that any advantage of Siconolfi modeling is indeed marginal (TABLE 1). This is not unexpected since, as observed previously,[10] in normally hydrated individuals, TBW is equally well predicted by any frequency. ECW is slightly better predicted by a low frequency.

An advantage claimed for the method by Siconolfi and colleagues is that data for all frequencies are used in the analysis, unlike in the Cole-Cole method in which up to 25% of frequency data points are rejected.[9] This need not be the case. The Cole-Cole data analysis method, as employed above, used all data points. In fact, repeating the above analysis by removing data outliers or constraining the frequency window did not significantly alter the results.

In conclusion, Siconolfi modeling is a method that may have some advantages, for example, stability of estimates during fluid shifts,[9] which we were not able to test here. However, until it has been more extensively validated, our observations indicate that the continued use of Cole-Cole modeling is to be preferred.

REFERENCES

1. KUSHNER, R.F. 1992. Bioelectrical impedance analysis: a review of principles and applications. J. Am. Coll. Nutr. **11:** 199–209.
2. THOMAS, B.J., B.H. CORNISH & L.C. WARD. 1992. Bioelectrical impedance analysis for measurement of body fluid volumes: a review. J. Clin. Eng. **17:** 505–511.
3. LUKASKI, H.C. 1996. Biological indexes considered in the derivation of the bioelectrical impedance analysis. Am. J. Clin. Nutr. **64:** 397S–404S.
4. SEGAL, K.R., S. BURASTO, A. CHUN, P. CORONEL, R.N. PIERSON & J. WANG. 1991. Estimation of extracellular and total body water by multiple frequency bioelectrical impedance measurement. Am. J. Clin. Nutr. **54:** 26–29.
5. BOULIER, A., A.L. THOMASSET & A. APFELBAUM. 1992. Bioelectrical-impedance measurement of body water. Am. J. Clin. Nutr. **55:** 761–762.
6. COLE, K.S. 1968. Membranes, Ions, and Impulses: A Chapter of Classical Biophysics. UCLA Press. Los Angeles.
7. CORNISH, B.H., B.J. THOMAS & L.C. WARD. 1993. Improved prediction of extracellular and total body water using impedance loci generated by multiple frequency bioelectrical impedance analysis. Phys. Med. Biol. **38:** 337–346.
8. SICONOLFI, S.F., M.L. NUSYNOWITZ, S.S. SUIRE, A.D. MOORE & J. LEIG. 1996. Determining blood and plasma volumes using bioelectrical response spectroscopy. Med. Sci. Sports Exercise **28:** 1510–1516.
9. SICONOLFI, S.F., R.J. GRETEBECK, W.W. WONG, R.A. PIETRZYK & S.S. SUIRE. 1997. Assessing total body and extracellular water from bioelectrical response spectroscopy. J. Appl. Physiol. **82:** 704–710.
10. CORNISH, B.H., L.C. WARD, B.J. THOMAS, S.A. JEBB & M. ELIA. 1995. Evaluation of body water volumes in humans by multiple frequency bioelectrical impedance analysis (MFBIA). Eur. J. Clin. Nutr. **50:** 159–164.
11. DUGGLEBY, R.G. & L.C. WARD. 1990. Analysis of physiological data characterized by two regimes separated by an abrupt transition. Physiol. Zool. **64:** 885–890.

Practical Limits of the Kramers-Kronig Relationships Applied to Experimental Bioimpedance Data

PERE J. RIU AND CRISTINA LAPAZ

Department of Electronic Engineering, Universitat Politècnica de Catalunya, 08034 Barcelona, Spain

ABSTRACT: Use of the Kramers-Kronig integral relationships has been proposed by several authors as a means to qualify the validity of experimental impedance data or to obtain the imaginary part of the impedance (or the permittivity) when only the real part is available. Few works are found in the literature where these relationships are applied. The goal of the present work is to investigate the practical limits on the applicability of these mathematical expressions when real factors such as a limited number of measurement frequencies or instrumentation errors are taken into account. We use simulated and real data to perform calculations and conclude that those expressions are practically applicable in almost every experimental situation, including the detection of measurement errors.

INTRODUCTION

The frequency-domain integral relationships known as Kramers-Kronig (KK) transforms relate the permittivity and conductivity of a material[1] or the real and imaginary part of a measured impedance,[2] provided that the material is linear, causal, and stable and that the value of the impedance is finite in the whole frequency range. These transforms have been widely used in the passive network theory,[3] but their reported use in analyzing biological materials or electrochemical data is very scarce.

Two main uses have been devised for KK transforms: calculation of the imaginary part (or the phase) when only the real part (or the magnitude) of an impedance is known, provided that the measurement of the real part, or the magnitude, is usually less prone to errors than the imaginary part; also, KK transforms can be used in assessing the validity of a measured impedance when both components are experimentally obtained.

As KK transforms are analytical expressions, they can be used when the impedance functions are known in analytical form. However, this is never the case in experimental procedures. Also, they assume that the impedance values are known for $f = 0, \ldots, \infty$ and again this is not the case. Moreover, some of the errors introduced by the measuring system will produce effects that can be identified by the KK transforms, while other errors will not.

Theoretical limits to the KK transforms applied to impedance data have been already established,[4] but practical limitations such as the minimum number of frequency points needed, the effects of the numerical integration method chosen, the effect of the frequency range, and the effect of measurement errors and noise have never been reported.

METHODS

Kramers-Kronig Equations

Although KK transforms can take several mathematical forms, depending on the immittance functions being used, we only worked with those relating the real and the imaginary parts of the impedance $Z(\omega) = R(\omega) + jX(\omega)$:

$$R(\omega_a) = R(\infty) + \frac{2}{\pi} \int_0^\infty \frac{\omega X(\omega) - \omega_a X(\omega_a)}{\omega^2 - \omega_a^2} d\omega, \qquad (1)$$

$$X(\omega_a) = \frac{2\omega_a}{\pi} \int_0^\infty \frac{R(\omega) - R(\omega_a)}{\omega^2 - \omega_a^2} d\omega. \qquad (2)$$

Even if we have an analytical expression that describes our impedance, these integrals cannot be solved for any arbitrarily chosen function. In addition, if we have a function describing our data, use of KK transforms may not be necessary. Thus, in general, numerical integration methods are required even with simulated data.

Effect of the Number of Points and Frequency Range

In order to analyze the effect of the number of points and the frequency range used in the numerical integrations, we simulated experimental data by constructing impedance functions according to the widely used Cole-Cole model:

$$Z(\omega) = R_\infty + \frac{R_S - R_\infty}{1 + \left(j\dfrac{\omega}{\omega_c}\right)^{1-\alpha}}. \qquad (3)$$

Functions constructed this way are consistent with the conditions of stability and finite values for the impedances and allowed us to make comparisons with the theoretically correct value.

Effect of the Integration Method

In order to investigate the possible effect of the integration method, we used two different integration methods: trapezoidal and eighth-order Newton-Cotes. Newton-Cotes is a recursive method, so the function to be integrated must be known at any point. Obviously, this method cannot be used with experimental data, so we used it here as a gold standard. All the calculations were performed using Matlab 5.1 (The MathWorks Incorporated, Natick, Massachusetts).

TABLE 1. Relative Errors when Recursive Integration Methods Are Used

Frequency Range	$\alpha = 0$	$\alpha = 0.3$	$\alpha = 0.5$
1 Hz–100 MHz	0.1%	0.1%	0.15%
10 Hz–10 MHz	0.12%	0.14%	0.28%
100 Hz–1 MHz	1.3%	2%	2.5%
1 kHz–100 kHz	12%	19%	22%

Effect of Measurement Errors

Both random and systematic errors are considered. For random errors, measurements are supposed to be contaminated with Gaussian incorrelated noise. For systematic errors, a measurement channel according to reference 5 was built using a Spice simulator. Different kinds of errors in the measurement channel were tested, including current-generation to voltage-detection cross talk, finite CMRR of the amplifiers, and electrode mismatch with finite input impedance in the amplifiers.

RESULTS

Integration Method, Number of Points, and Frequency Range

Recursive integration methods yield errors that depend only on the frequency range used and on the shape of the real part. Taking a wide enough frequency range, the resulting errors are those of the integration method itself, generally under 0.1% in the area around the maximum value of Im[$Z(f)$]. Relative errors tend to increase in the regions where Im[$Z(f)$] is theoretically zero (for obvious reasons), so all the values presented in this paper correspond to the relative errors in the area near the maximum of the imaginary part. TABLE 1 summarizes the errors calculated using different frequency ranges and different shapes. All the frequency ranges were selected to be symmetrical around the relaxation frequency (f_C=10 kHz). The shape was changed by selecting different values of α (0, 0.3, and 0.5). It must be noted that describing an actual biological tissue using a Cole-Cole model with a single dispersion in the frequency range of 1 Hz to 100 MHz is unrealistic, but the goal here was to assess the errors arising from a finite frequency range.

When nonrecursive methods are used, the number of points used in the integrations becomes relevant. Results for the error as a function of the point density (points/decade) are shown in FIGURE 1 for three frequency ranges. When the number of points is large enough (>50 points/decade), the results roughly correspond to those of TABLE 1. Surprisingly, when the number of points decreases, the error decreases too and finally becomes negative; thus, theoretically, there is a value for the number of points that would produce a null error. FIGURE 1 shows the absolute value of the error because logarithmic coordinates were used, but the singularity is clearly observed. Further decreasing the number of points produces a sharp increase of the magnitude of the error.

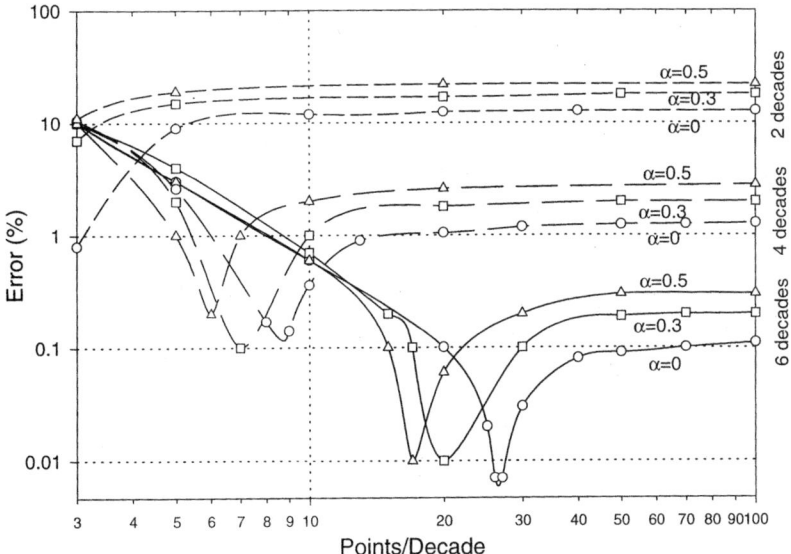

FIGURE 1. Absolute value of the relative error when the number of points, the frequency range, and the shape are changed, using trapezoidal integration.

The integration points were spaced logarithmically for these calculations, which is usual in experimental procedures. Other calculations using linearly spaced points showed no significant differences.

Random Errors

To study the effect of random errors (noise), we considered that each measurement was contaminated with additive random noise. Thus,

$$\text{Re}[Z(\omega_i)] = R_0(\omega_i) + n_i \qquad (4)$$

with n_i being random variables having Gaussian distribution and being independent from each other. Under that hypothesis, it is possible to estimate the variance of the error in the calculated imaginary part using error propagation theory. If linearly spaced points in the frequency axis are considered, then

$$\hat{\sigma}^2\{\text{Im}[Z(k \cdot \Delta\omega)]\} = \frac{4}{\pi^2}\sigma_{\text{Re}[Z]}^2 \sum_{\substack{i=0 \\ i \neq k}}^{M} \frac{k^2}{(i^2 - k^2)^2} \qquad (5)$$

where $k \cdot \Delta\omega = \omega_a$.

For M finite, this summation involves Euler gamma functions and their derivatives. When the number of points used becomes infinite ($M \to \infty$), then

$$\hat{\sigma}^2\{\text{Im}[Z]\} = \frac{1}{3}\sigma^2_{\text{Re}[Z]}. \quad (6)$$

If logarithmically spaced points are used, the expression for the variance of the error is then

$$\hat{\sigma}^2\{\text{Im}[Z(10^{k/d} \cdot \omega_1)]\} = \frac{4}{\pi^2} 10^{\frac{2k}{d}} \left(10^{\frac{1}{d}} - 1\right)^2 \sigma^2_{\text{Re}[Z]} \sum_{\substack{i=0 \\ i \neq k}}^{M} \frac{10^{\frac{2i}{d}}}{\left(10^{\frac{2i}{d}} - 10^{\frac{2k}{d}}\right)^2} \quad (7)$$

where

$10^{k/d} \cdot \omega_1 = \omega_a$,
d: number of points per decade,
ω_1: initial frequency of the frequency range used.

No closed form could be found for equation 7, so only numerical evaluations for particular cases were performed.

FIGURE 2 shows the estimated variance simulating the noise by using the random number generator of Matlab, with Gaussian distribution, applied to 500 realizations of the KK transform on the same data. Noise was set to have $\sigma^2\{n_i\} = 1$ for the sake of simplicity. Also shown are the numerical evaluations of equation 5, using 10^4 linearly spaced points, and equation 7, using 40 logarithmically spaced points (same as the points used in the simulation), as well as the 1/3 value. Results, at least for the central part of the frequency

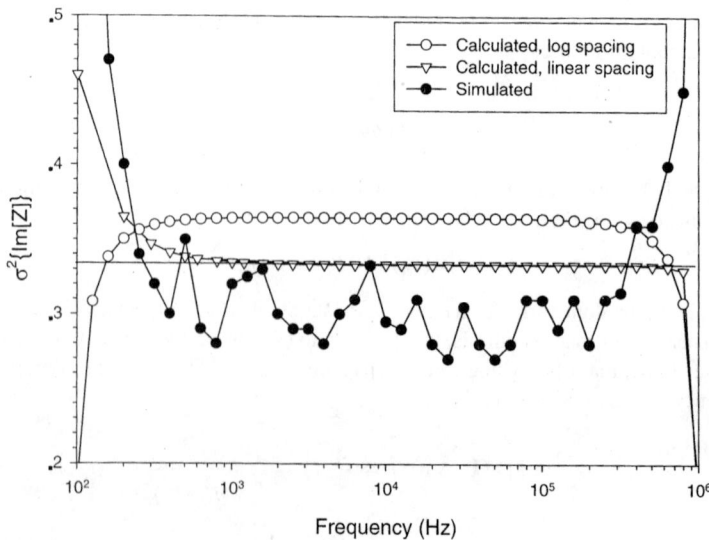

FIGURE 2. Estimation of the variance using 500 realizations with trapezoidal integration and 10 points/decade (●), compared with the calculations using linear (▽) and logarithmically (○) spaced intervals. The theoretical value of 1/3 is also shown.

range used, are independent of the number of points, the frequency range, and the shape of the real part.

Systematic Errors

Two kinds of systematic errors can be expected. Type one errors are caused by parasitic impedances in series or parallel (or combination) with the expected one. In those cases, the resulting measured value will not be the actual wanted value, but it will have all the properties of an impedance function; thus, KK transforms will treat it as a regular impedance.

The second type are errors produced by noncalibrable causes, such as a finite CMRR of the amplifiers or a cross talk between the injection and detection sides. In those cases, KK transforms may be able, at least, to identify that the real and imaginary parts are not in agreement. FIGURE 3 shows the measurement channel used to simulate CMRR errors. A detailed description of this circuit as well as the meaning of the values of the components can be found in reference 5. Results are shown in FIGURE 4. The actual value corresponds to an RC circuit standing for a biological impedance. The *measured* value is the imaginary part obtained by the simulated measurement system, and the KK transform is the imaginary part recovered from the *measured* real part. Note that the recovered part is not exactly equal to the actual value. Errors may arise from the implementation of the KK transforms, as seen above, and also because CMRR affects the measurement of the real part as well as the imaginary part.[5]

DISCUSSION AND CONCLUSIONS

From the above analysis, we conclude that KK transforms are suitable to be used in almost every experimental situation, even with a small number of points if errors about 1% can be tolerated. The actual accuracy for a given situation should be investigated for that particular situation because factors like the frequency range can produce large effects

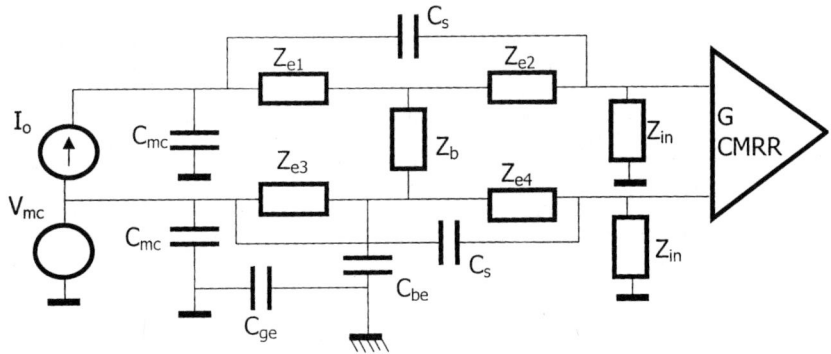

FIGURE 3. Circuit used to simulate systematic errors in the measurement channel. A detailed description of the elements can be found in reference 5.

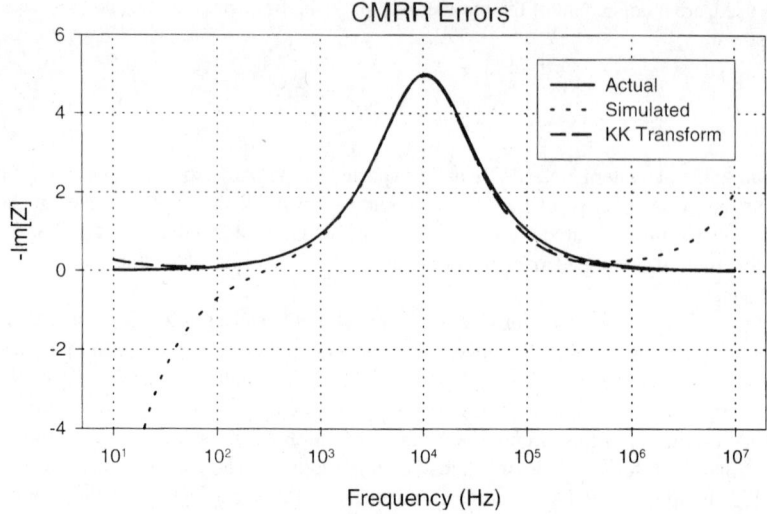

FIGURE 4. Imaginary part calculated from the KK transforms when CMRR errors are present in the measurement system. This is compared with the measured one and the actual value.

depending on the shape of the impedance. In our study, only frequency ranges symmetrical to the relaxation frequency and only one relaxation frequency have been considered.

Noise contaminating the measurements is somewhat reduced by the KK transforms, assuming that it is incorrelated. This may or may not be the case in experimental situations, depending on the measurement method employed.

When applied to data contaminated with systematic errors, those transforms are able to identify the kinds of errors that produce non-impedance-like results, even when the real part has errors too.

REFERENCES

1. FOSTER, K.R. & H.P. SCHWAN. 1995. Dielectric properties of tissues. *In* Handbook of Biological Effects of Electromagnetic Fields, p. 25–102. CRC Press. Boca Raton, Florida.
2. MACDONALD, J.R. 1987. Impedance Spectroscopy. Wiley. New York.
3. BODE, H.W. 1954. Network Analysis and Feedback Amplifier Design. Van Nostrand. New York.
4. URQUIDI-MACDONALD, M., S. REAL & D.D. MACDONALD. 1986. Application of Kramers-Kronig transforms in the analysis of electrochemical impedance data. II. Transformations in the complex plane. J. Electrochem. Soc. **133:** 2018–2024.
5. RIU, P.J., J. ROSELL, A. LOZANO & R. PALLAS-ARENY. 1995. Multifrequency static imaging in electrical impedance tomography. Part 1. Instrumentation requirements. Med. Biol. Eng. Comput. **33:** 784–792.

Experimental Assessment of Phase Magnitude Imaging in Multifrequency EIT by Simulation and Saline Tank Studies

ANTHONY FITZGERALD,[a] DAVID HOLDER,[a] AND HUW GRIFFITHS[b]

[a]*Department of Clinical Neurophysiology, University College London, Middlesex Hospital, London W1N 8AA, United Kingdom*

[b]*Department of Medical Physics, University of Wales College of Medicine, Cardiff CF4 4XW, South Glamorgan, United Kingdom*

ABSTRACT: Multifrequency EIT (MFEIT) data can be used to form dual-frequency images that display the change of complex resistivity with frequency relative to a selected reference frequency. It has only been possible to calculate the complex resistivity at the image frequency from MFEIT images by assuming some a priori information, such as a homogeneous, resistive reference or a resistivity described by a single dispersion Cole model. The purpose of this paper is to introduce an alternative method of image formation, referred to as "phase magnitude imaging", which enables the complex resistivity of tissue to be obtained independently of the tissue model and without the need for a homogeneous reference. It was expected that the major obstacle to practical application of this technique would be instrumentation errors that affect the measurement of phase. To assess these effects, a cucumber cortex was imaged in a saline-filled tank using an HP4284A impedance analyzer. Cole parameters determined from the phase magnitude images differed by up to 300% from results of the simulation. These errors were reduced to less than 15% by using reciprocity data to partially correct for the influence of stray capacitance on the voltage measurement.

INTRODUCTION

Background

Tetrapolar impedance measurements on the body and on *ex vivo* samples of tissue have demonstrated measurable and distinctive quadrature components in the complex resistivity.[1–3] The quadrature component has been largely ignored in multifrequency EIT (MFEIT) for two reasons. First, because of the unknown complex resistivity at the reference frequency, attempts to determine the quadrature component from MFEIT data have required assumptions that are not always true when imaging on the body. The method of Griffiths and Jossinet[4] assumed a reference distribution that was homogeneous and purely resistive. Fitzgerald *et al.*[5] assumed that the resistivity is modeled by a single Cole-type dispersion. Both of these assumptions may be false *in vivo*. The second reason that the quadrature component has been ignored is that it is smaller in magnitude, but is subject to larger measurement errors, than the in-phase component of resistivity.[6,7]

Purpose

The purpose of this paper is to introduce and experimentally assess the accuracy of a new image formation technique that allows the in-phase and quadrature components of the complex resistivity to be determined from MFEIT data without requiring any assumptions.

Design

The image formation method, termed "phase magnitude imaging", is a modification of the method of Griffiths and Jossinet.[4] Rather than back-project the difference in phase between the reference and image frequencies as Griffiths and Jossinet do, phase magnitude images are formed by the back-projection of the phase value recorded at the image frequency.

The influence of measurement errors on this technique is investigated by computer simulations and by practical recordings on a saline-filled tank containing cucumber test objects previously described by Holder et al.[8] (see FIG. 1).

Reciprocal data were collected in the practical experiments and used in a correction intended to reduce the effects of instrumentation errors on the technique.

THEORY

Phase Magnitude Imaging

Dual-frequency images are formed by back-projecting the logarithm of the ratio of perturbed to reference complex boundary potentials.[9] The real and imaginary images obtained display the ratio of the logarithm of the resistivity modulus and phase difference

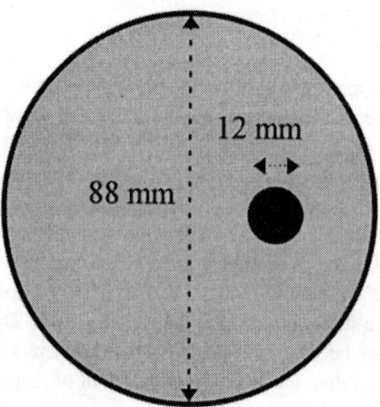

FIGURE 1. Cucumber section (dark) in 0.03% potassium chloride solution. This arrangement was used in the practical experiment and modeled using the finite difference method.

relative to the reference frequency, with pixel values s' and s'', respectively. The complex resistivity at the image frequency [$\rho_2^* = |\rho_2|\exp(j\phi_2)$] can be calculated from the pixel values s' and s'' according to

$$|\rho_2| = |\rho_1|\exp(s') \tag{1}$$

$$\phi_2 = s'' + \phi_1 \tag{2}$$

where $\rho_1^* = |\rho_1|\exp(j\phi_1)$ is the complex resistivity at the reference frequency. It is clear from equations 1 and 2 that the complex resistivity cannot be calculated directly from the pixel values of the dual-frequency images without prior knowledge of the resistivity and phase at the reference frequency. The example that Griffiths and Jossinet[4] discuss is when a homogeneous, resistive reference is available. Then, $|\rho_1|$ can be measured and ϕ_1 will be zero since the medium is purely resistive. When this type of reference is not available, for example, *in vivo* imaging, a normalized resistivity, relative to that at the reference frequency, can be determined for each pixel from equation 1. However, it is not possible to calculate the phase angle ϕ_2 in equation 2 because of the unknown phase angle ϕ_1 associated with the reactance at the reference frequency. The method proposed in this paper to overcome this problem is to form the second set of images by back-projecting the phase of the boundary potentials at the image frequency only, rather than the phase difference between the image and reference frequencies. The phase angle of the tissue resistivity at the image frequency is then given by

$$\phi_2 = s''. \tag{3}$$

The advantage of this technique, referred to as phase magnitude imaging, is that no reference set is required to form the phase images. A reference frequency is needed only for the purposes of determining the resistivity modulus. If the value $|\rho_1|$ is known, then $|\rho_2|$ can be determined from equation 1. If not, the normalized value $|\rho_2|/|\rho_1|$ will be obtained. An expected problem that could limit the practical application of this technique is the fact that the quadrature component of the signal is subject to measurement errors due to undesired capacitances.

Correction Using Reciprocity Data

The complex voltage $V_1^* = V_1\exp(\theta_1)$ generated between a given pair of electrodes when current is injected between another pair is theoretically identical to the voltage V_2^* recorded when the current is driven and the voltage measured between the reciprocal pairs of electrodes. This principle is employed in some EIT systems to improve the accuracy of measurement by hardware adjustment of a phase offset to minimize differences in the real component of the voltage between reciprocal pairs. A software implementation of this technique is proposed as a means to reduce errors related to stray capacitance and phase delays in the instrumentation in the case that a hardware phase offset adjustment is not available, for example, a multiplexed impedance analyzer. A phase offset, θ_{offset}, given by

$$\theta_{\text{offset}} = a\tan\{[V_1\cos(\theta_1) - V_2\cos(\theta_2)]/[V_1\sin(\theta_1) - V_2\sin(\theta_2)]\} \tag{4}$$

was added to the recorded phase angles so that the difference in the real component of the reciprocal pairs V_1^* and V_2^* was set to zero. θ_{offset} was restricted to between ±90° so that only one angle was selected.

METHODS

Direct Measurement of Impedance of Saline and Cucumber

Transverse (radial) sections were bored from the cortex of a large cucumber using a cork boring tool. The complex resistivity of several lengths of cucumber section was calculated from data recorded at eight frequencies in a geometric progression from 1 kHz to 20 kHz using an HP4284A impedance analyzer according to the method of Holder et al.[8] Electrode impedance was not more than 10% of the total impedance for the frequencies used. Cole parameters determined from the averaged complex resistivity of the transverse sections are given in TABLE 1. These were used for the simulations described in the next subsection, and the normalized Cole plot is shown in FIGURE 2. Using the method for determining the resistivity of liquids described by Holder et al.,[8] the resistivity of a 0.03% potassium chloride solution was determined to be 16.0 Ωm at a temperature of 19 °C.

Simulated MFEIT

A finite difference model, using data from the direct measurements, was used to simulate the arrangement shown in FIGURE 1. Two sets of images were formed from the results of the simulation. The set of difference images was obtained by using the data from the simulated homogeneous, resistive saline solution of resistivity 16.0 Ωm as the reference. The set of phase magnitude images was formed at the eight frequencies using 1 kHz as the reference for the resistivity modulus images. Cole plots were determined from the central pixel within the cucumber region and these are shown in FIGURE 2. Parameters for these plots are presented in TABLE 1.

TABLE 1. Cole Parameters Derived from the Resistivity Plots for Direct Measurements, Simulations, and Saline Tank Images of Cucumber Cortex

Cole Plot from:	ρ_∞/ρ_0	F_c (kHz)	α
cucumber cortex (direct measurement)	0.050	3.96	0.189
simulated difference images	0.507	12.3	0.194
simulated phase magnitude images	0.507	12.3	0.194
saline tank difference images	0.339	17.4	0.278
saline tank phase magnitude images	−1.265	54.6	0.239
saline tank phase magnitude images after reciprocity correction[a]	0.388	18.1	0.272

[a]Parameters determined by fitting the real component of resistivity.

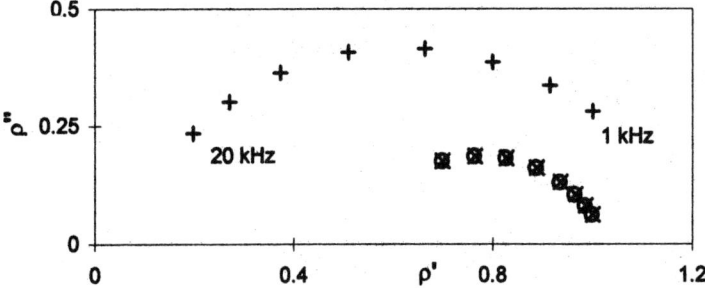

FIGURE 2. Cole plots from direct measurements on cucumber (+) and from difference images (○) and phase magnitude images (×) from data generated by the finite difference model. ρ' and ρ'' are the real and imaginary components of resistivity normalized to the real part at 1 kHz.

Practical MFEIT

A cylindrical tank, 2 cm deep, with 16 equally spaced electrodes around the circumference, was filled with 0.03% potassium chloride solution at 19 °C and a longitudinal section of cucumber cortex was placed as in FIGURE 1. The HP4284A impedance analyzer, multiplexed to drive current and measure voltage between selected pairs of electrodes,[10] was used to record reciprocal MFEIT data with an adjacent configuration. Images were formed as in the simulations. Cole plots are compared in FIGURE 3 and parameters from these plots are presented in TABLE 1.

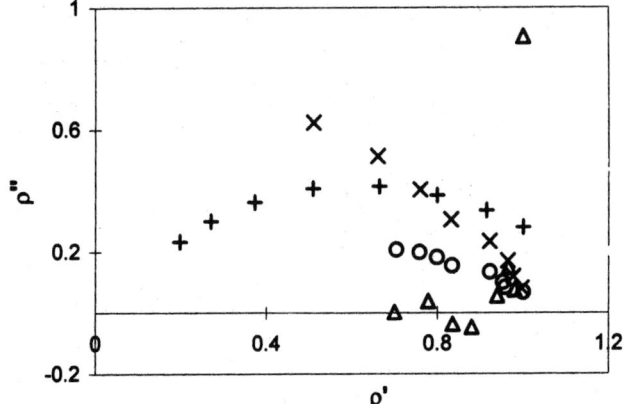

FIGURE 3. Cole plots for cucumber cortex from direct measurements (+), difference images (○), phase magnitude images (×), and phase magnitude images after reciprocity correction (Δ).

A second set of phase magnitude images were formed subsequent to the application of a correction, implemented in software, to the voltage measurements using the reciprocity data as outlined earlier in this paper.

RESULTS AND DISCUSSION

Simulated MFEIT

The Cole plot calculated from the simulated difference images differs markedly from the actual Cole plot for the cucumber (FIG. 2). This is due to the finite resolution of the EIT technique and the nonlinear response to resistivity change: the simulated cucumber region occupied less than 2% of the total volume and had a resistivity that was 240% greater than the saline at the lowest frequency and 40% greater at the highest frequency. The second point apparent from FIGURE 2, which is illustrated by the results in TABLE 1, is that the Cole parameters obtained from the phase magnitude images agree (within rounding errors from the simulation) with the parameters from the difference images.

Practical MFEIT

The Cole plots from the saline tank difference images do not correspond to the actual plot for the cucumber section (FIG. 3). This is again due to the finite resolution and nonlinear response to resistivity change of the EIT technique itself. Therefore, the Cole parameters from the saline tank images should be compared to those from the simulated difference images, rather than those from the direct measurements on the cucumber. TABLE 1 shows that parameters derived from the difference images of the simulated and saline tank studies are reasonably consistent with the results from the simulation, differing by between 30% (ratio of low frequency and high frequency limiting resistivities, ρ_∞/ρ_0) and 40% (α).

It was expected that errors, such as those arising from stray capacitances in the multiplexer and unshielded cables of the modified HP4284A, would cause problems in the accurate measurement of voltage, particularly the imaginary component. This is evident in the results from the phase magnitude images of the saline tank. FIGURE 3 shows that the imaginary component of resistivity continues to increase beyond the expected turning point of 17 kHz (characteristic frequency, F_c) and TABLE 1 shows that parameters from the phase magnitude images differ by up to 300% from those of the difference images. Following correction using the reciprocity data, the imaginary component determined from the phase magnitude images is clearly made worse (FIG. 3) and the data cannot be fitted by a circular arc. Interestingly, however, errors in the real component of resistivity, which the correction is designed to improve, are significantly reduced to less than 15% (see TABLE 1).

CONCLUSIONS

Simulations demonstrate that it is theoretically feasible to use phase magnitude imaging to determine the complex resistivity of tissue from MFEIT data. The technique is independent of the tissue model and does not need a homogeneous, resistive reference. However, practical application of phase magnitude imaging requires accurate measurement of the phase and magnitude of voltage, which is difficult to achieve with current multifrequency EIT systems. The measurement of phase may be useful, though, for the correction based on reciprocity, which was shown to improve the calculation of the real component of resistivity from phase magnitude images. Further work is required to determine the best use of the reciprocity data to correct general errors in MFEIT.

REFERENCES

1. GERSING, E., F. BACH, C. BROCKHOFF, M.M. GEBHARD, G. KEHRER, A. MEIBNER & H.J. BRETSCHNEIDER. 1991. Messung der elektrischen impedanz von organen—methodische grundlagen. Biomed. Tech. **36**(4): 70–77.
2. RIGAUD, B., L. HAMAOUI, M.R. FRIKHA, N. CHAUVEAU & J-P. MORUCCI. 1995. *In vitro* tissue characterization and modelling using electrical impedance measurements in the 100 Hz–10 MHz frequency range. Physiol. Meas. **16**(3): A15–A28.
3. CORNISH, B.H. 1994. Swept frequency bioimpedance analysis for the determination of body water compartments. Ph.D. thesis, Queensland University of Technology, Queensland, Australia.
4. GRIFFITHS, H. & J. JOSSINET. 1994. Bioelectrical spectroscopy from multi-frequency EIT. Physiol. Meas. **15**(2A): 59–64.
5. FITZGERALD, A.J., B.J. THOMAS, B.H. CORNISH, G.J. MICHAEL & L.C. WARD. 1997. Extraction of electrical characteristics from pixels of multi-frequency EIT images. Physiol. Meas. **18**: 107–118.
6. BROWN, B.H., D.C. BARBER, W. WANG, L. LIQIN, A.D. LEATHARD, R.H. SMALLWOOD, A.R. HAMPSHIRE, R. MACKAY & K. HATZIGALANIS. 1994. Multifrequency imaging and modelling of respiratory related electrical impedance changes. Physiol. Meas. **15A**: 1–12.
7. WEBSTER, J.G. 1990. Electrical Impedance Tomography. IOP Pub. Bristol, United Kingdom.
8. HOLDER, D., Y. HANQUAN & A. RAO. 1996. Some practical biological phantoms for calibrating multifrequency electrical impedance tomography. Physiol. Meas. **17A**: 167–177.
9. GRIFFITHS, H., H.T.L. LEUNG & R.J. WILLIAMS. 1992. Imaging the complex impedance of the thorax. Clin. Phys. Physiol. Meas. **13A**: 77–81.
10. BAYFORD, R.H., K.G. BOONE, Y. HANQUAN & D.S. HOLDER. 1996. Improvement of the positional accuracy of EIT images of the head using a Lagrange multiplier reconstruction algorithm with diametric excitation. Physiol. Meas. **17A**: 49–57.

Some Design Concepts for Electrical Impedance Measurement

H. G. GOOVAERTS, TH. J. C. FAES, E. RAAIJMAKERS, AND R. M. HEETHAAR

Department of Clinical Physics and Informatics, Institute for Cardiovascular Research ICarVU, University Hospital Vrije Universiteit, 1007 MB Amsterdam, the Netherlands

ABSTRACT: Design concepts for the implementation of two basic functions for measurement of electrical impedance are presented: current injection and voltage measurement. At relatively high frequencies, the application of an alternating current through the body or a body segment results in electromagnetic stray fields that reduce the amount of current actually injected into the tissue under study. It is shown that electrical isolation and small dimensions of the isolated section are indispensable in order to substantially reduce these stray currents. The paper describes a new wideband current source configuration driven by direct digital sine wave synthesis (DDS) presenting very low stray currents due to a symmetrical layout. Two implementations of the actual current source circuit are presented: (1) a voltage-controlled system and (2) a current conveyor-based circuit.

A wideband input amplifier with transformer coupling is described. The current source, amplifier, and (in case of tomography) multiplexer are also situated on an electrically isolated front end. The presented concepts are applied in a new electrical impedance tomograph (EIT) presently under construction in our department.

INTRODUCTION

Measurement of tissue impedance is a well-known technique that can be applied in various fields of investigation. In general, volume conduction in the body is governed by two pathways: (1) a conduction through extracellular fluid and (2) an intracellular conduction path. Multifrequency measurements enable estimation of the ratio between these pathways. From such measurements, corner frequencies can be estimated that are related to fluid volumes in intra- and extracellular compartments and that enable discrimination between different types of tissue. Since the electrical properties of various types of tissue differ largely, depending on their structure, these corner frequencies may cover a relatively wide frequency range from approximately 4 kHz to over 1000 kHz. The current source should be capable of delivering a current of constant amplitude over the whole frequency range. Furthermore, an accurate determination of the magnitude and phase angle or the real and imaginary part of the measured impedance is required. This requires a measuring channel consisting of a wideband input amplifier with a coherent demodulator.

The configurations as described in this paper are presently subject to international patent application.[1]

SYSTEM CONCEPTS AND DESIGN

For reasons of patient safety, the current source and input amplifier should be electrically isolated from the instrument ground. This isolation, however, should be obtained not only for relatively low frequencies, but over the whole frequency range in which the system is to be operated. It follows that the layout of the isolated section must be such that stray capacitances are kept small, which restricts the physical size of the floating or isolated part of the circuit. We opted for transformer coupling of the signal exciting the current source as well as for the signal from the output of the input amplifier.[2,3]

Current Source

The application of an alternating current through the body or a body segment results in electromagnetic stray fields that reduce the amount of current actually injected into the tissue under study. This radiation effect can be reduced substantially by application of electrical isolation and a symmetrical configuration of the current source. Due to such a configuration, common-mode voltages at the input amplifier of the measuring system are also diminished. In FIGURE 1, the effect of electrical isolation is elucidated. Transformer T1 provides for such isolation and transfers the excitation signal from generator G onto a current source circuit CS, which produces a current i to pass through impedance Z. However, as shown in the figure, a portion i_2 of the applied current will leak through the stray capacitance C_s to ground and is returned to the current source through the isolation gap capacitance C_i. In the case that C_i can be made small compared to C_s, the amount of leakage current is mainly determined by this isolation gap capacitance C_i.

It would be very convenient if the current source was configured in such a way that common-mode voltages presented to the measuring input could be substantially reduced. This would require a symmetrical layout of the current source. Moreover, a symmetrical layout will provide for an additional reduction of stray currents, especially in an electrically isolated configuration. The symmetry of the output circuit will produce a zero refer-

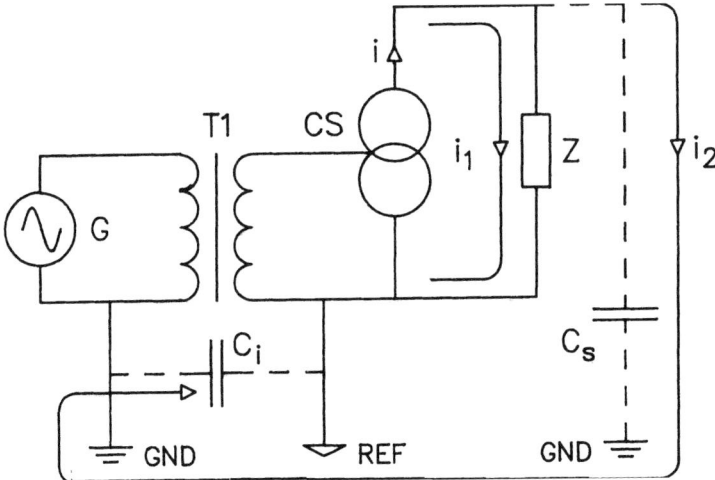

FIGURE 1. Diagram to illustrate the effect of electrical isolation to reduce stray currents.

ence that is centered in the load impedance under study and stray currents will only be generated with respect to this reference.

Among various approaches, we decided on the two following options to obtain a constant current source on the isolated section shown in FIGURE 1:

(a) The voltage-controlled output type circuit, where the actual current is measured and compared to a reference set point. The frequency range in which such a system behaves as a current source is determined by the bandwidth of the control loop.

(b) The current conveyor or transconductance-based circuit, which inherently presents a high output impedance over a relatively large frequency range. In addition, the actual current can be measured and controlled as discussed in option (a) so as to improve accuracy.

In FIGURE 2, the block diagram representation of the developed current source is shown. Both options are implemented and shown in sections (a) and (b) of the figure, respectively. The actual current source is divided into a control section having a driving output D and a sensing input S, to which one of the aforementioned current source options is connected.

The operation can be described as follows. A sine wave obtained, for example, from a 10-bit DDS (AD7008) is inductively coupled onto the floating part of the current source by means of transformer T1. The signal at the output of this transformer is passed onto a wideband amplifier, the gain of which is determined by the output of a control circuit (labeled 8). The configuration of the control circuit depends on the bandwidth in which the current source should operate. In general, it consists of a peak detector and an integrating

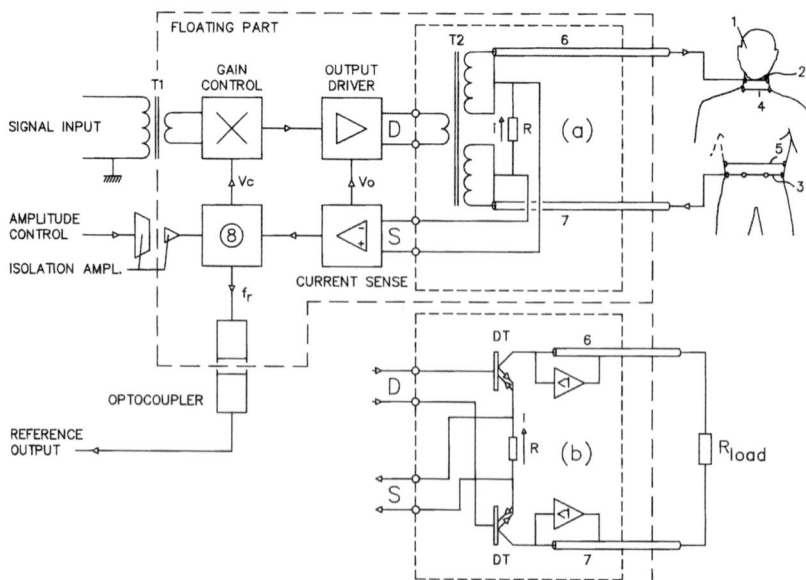

FIGURE 2. Block diagram of the presented current source with two output options: (a) a voltage-controlled current source and (b) a current conveyor circuit. See text for further explanation.

circuit, which form a conventional control loop. The set point of this loop can be controlled by the output of the isolation amplifier, but may as well be established on the floating part by means of a reference voltage. The output of the gain-controlled amplifier is entered into an output driver. In option (a), the driver's output is transferred through transformer T2 to current injection electrode arrays 2 and 3 placed on patient 1. In option (b), the output driver excites two current conveyor circuits or voltage-controlled current sources (Diamond Transistors or DT) in a bridge configuration.

In both situations, the output current i is monitored through a precision resistor R. Although the given configuration shows a thoracic impedance cardiography (TIC) application, the setup has been validated for total body impedance analysis (BIA) as well as for *in vitro* measurement involving small volumes of suspensions. The shielding of the current-carrying cables might cause a problem because an increased current resulting from the capacity of these cables will be drawn from the outputs of the transformer with increasing frequency. In the arrangement of version (a), only the current flowing through the patient is determined. In version (b), the shields of the current-carrying cables (labeled 6 and 7) are separately driven so as to minimize the current due to the capacity of these cables.

From the current sensing circuit, an auxiliary output can be obtained to produce a control voltage V_o for elimination of DC offsets in case option (b) is applied. Finally, an optocoupling device provides for a timing reference related to the injected current for phase measurement.

Input Amplifier

Commonly, input stages are composed of wideband operational amplifiers configured as a differential or instrumentation amplifier. In that setup, common-mode rejection decreases due to parasitic capacitances, which cause an imbalance of the symmetrical arrangement increasing with frequency. Hence, common-mode rejection at 1 MHz will be substantially reduced. Electrical isolation combined with a symmetrical layout of the isolated section will improve the suppression of common-mode signals at high frequencies.[4,5] This again requires a small physical layout of the isolated section.

Generally, coaxially screened leads are used to connect the measuring electrodes to the input stage. Unfortunately, the cable's capacitance is then placed directly across the inputs of the amplifier. The effective cable capacitance can be largely reduced by active shielding or "bootstrapping". This method can be implemented with a simple op-amp circuit. Unfortunately, every op-amp that is in use today shows extra poles, and sometimes zeros, in the open-loop gain curve caused by the load interaction with the output impedance of the amplifier. This output impedance interacts with reactive loads to change the single-pole response into a multipole response. Hence, instabilities can occur in the aforementioned configuration. We therefore decided to use an input stage with a moderate open loop gain and a closed loop gain of <1. In FIGURE 3, the simplified diagram of the input amplifier is given in a setup for TIC. The floating part contains a pair of amplifiers constructed from a junction FET and a PNP transistor in a symmetrical configuration and a transformer-coupled wideband amplifier. Since the voltage gain presented by the input stage is inherently <1, the circuit acts as a stable differential source follower connected to a transformer. For frequencies above approximately 1 kHz, the circuit serves as an input impedance transformer to pass the high-frequency signal measured at electrodes 4 and 5 to T1. Guarding is

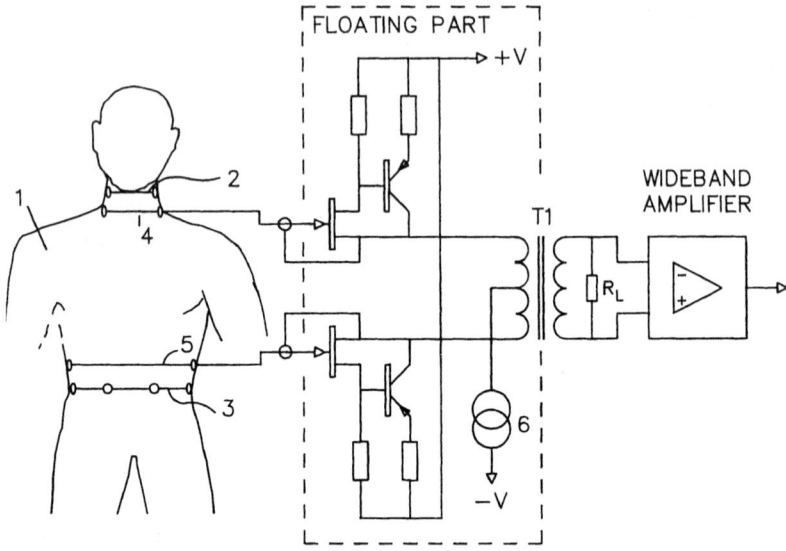

FIGURE 3. Simplified diagram of the electrically isolated and transformer-coupled input amplifier.

achieved in a conventional way by connecting the cable shielding to the output of the source follower.

The transformer passes the signal over the isolation barrier and, at the same time, realizes impedance matching. The arrangement of the current source 6 in combination with the floating input stage results in an improved rejection of common-mode signals acquired at the measuring electrodes. Separation of primary and secondary windings into different chambers will largely reduce the isolation gap capacitance. Consequently, high-frequency common-mode signals presented at the primary winding will also be suppressed.

Demodulator

Determination of the magnitude and phase of the impedance under study is commonly achieved by means of lock-in amplifiers.[6] In FIGURE 4, the block diagram of our approach for lock-in measurement is given. The reference or carrier insertion signal is reconstructed from the measuring input. A phase-locked loop (PLL) is used for this purpose as it will lock onto the input signal with zero phase shift. In this way, the output of the demodulator is directly related to the magnitude of the measured impedance, |Z|, and phase measurements can be performed with respect to a quadrature channel obtained from the excitation source through a 90° phase-shifter. An advantage of this approach is that magnitude and phase angle are directly available as analogous signals and require no further processing. Noise in the measuring channel is mainly effective on the determination of |Z|; for the determination of phase angle, the noise will be substantially reduced through the averaging that occurs in the PLL. In this way, errors in phase measurement are reduced with

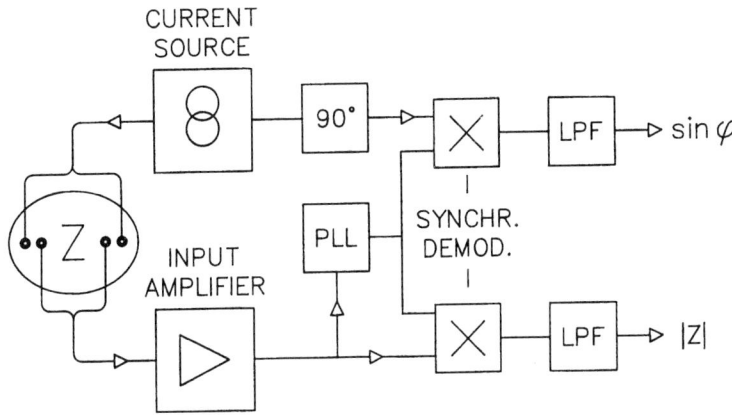

FIGURE 4. PLL-demodulator as applied in a system for thoracic impedance cardiography.

respect to the former approach. The bandwidth of the loop can be controlled independently from the bandwidth of the input signal for optimum acquisition and noise suppression characteristics. This type of system is capable of producing a stable and noise-free reference signal that tracks any variations in frequency and phase of the input signal.[7]

PERFORMANCE OF CIRCUITS

Current Source

The impedance range of the current source for proper operation is limited by supply voltage and current amplitude. The presented arrangement is capable of delivering 2.5 mA_{rms} into a load impedance, R_{load}, of 2 kΩ. In our systems, we apply an excitation current of 300 μA_{rms}. We measured the following performance:

	Version (a)	Version (b)
Output impedance @ 1 MHz:	>64 kΩ	>75 kΩ
Bandwidth (−3 dB, R_{load} = 2 kΩ):	1 kHz–3 MHz	1 kHz–6.3 MHz
Accuracy (2 kHz–1 MHz):	<±1.0%	<±0.5%
Stability:	<±0.2%	<±0.1%.

Input Amplifier

The input amplifier including the coupling transformer has been applied in a substantial number of units for TIC. We established the following specifications:

Input impedance: 200 kΩ (AC guarding)
Bandwidth: 3 kHz–1 MHz (±0.1%)
Noise (2 kHz–1 MHz; R_{el} = 10 kΩ): <20 nV/√Hz
Isolation mode rejection ratio (IMRR) ($V_i \leq 8$ V$_{pp}$): >150 dB @ 4 kHz,
>110 dB @ 64 kHz,
>40 dB @ 1024 kHz.

It should be noted that all measurements, except IMRR @ 1024 kHz, have been performed with cables of 1 m length attached to the system. This is of major importance since changes in the position and conduct of cables introduce slight differences in the measured impedance, especially at high frequencies.

Transformer Coupling

We used a Siemens potcore N26/18-11 with a primary inductance of 33 mH. The transformation ratio was 5:1. The signal transfer of the isolation transformer was measured with matched termination (R_L = 660 Ω). The value of the termination resistance was determined by adjustment so as to obtain a flat square-wave response at 64 kHz. The transformer was driven from a voltage source. Changes in the transfer ratio were $<\pm 10^{-3}$ in the frequency range between 3 kHz and 1 MHz. Phase shift was <1.1° at 300 kHz and <3.6° at 1 MHz.

Demodulator

The demodulator is applied in a system for TIC with a dynamic range of 50 Ω. Full-scale Z_0 demodulator output is 2.0 V. The overall gain between the demodulator and dZ/dt output is 78·10³. The resulting noise at the dZ/dt output in the bandwidth of interest (0–10 Hz) is approximately 40 mV$_{p-p}$, equivalent to 0.13 mΩ$_{p-p}$. This establishes a maximum signal-to-noise ratio of 385,000:1 or 112 dB. In the situation of TIC, measurement values of Z_0 are within 20–40 Ω, reducing the effective signal-to-noise ratio to around 106 dB.

DISCUSSION AND CONCLUSIONS

The basic consideration in the presented design is the electrical isolation of current source and input amplifier so as to reduce stray capacitances with respect to the object under study and the surrounding equipment. Of course, isolation is inevitable for *in vivo* application on the basis of safety regulations; in order to comply with these, though, there is a choice between a number of other alternatives: for example, isolation of the total impedance meter. Then, however, stray capacitances will remain relatively large since the complete isolated system still presents a substantial capacitance with respect to surrounding conductors. A further improvement is the symmetrical configuration of the current source that reduces stray effects occurring at the object under study. Proper isolation introduces some further constraints as regards the transfer of the excitation signal onto the isolated section. Transformer coupling performs well in a frequency range between a few kHz and some MHz. Two versions of the current source have been presented. The voltage-controlled option, (a), has an advantage as regards patient safety. The current-carrying electrodes are connected with each other by a very low impedance path: two secondary windings of the transformer and the small precision resistor, R. In this setup, it is very unlikely that large currents will be injected through the electrodes in a fault condition. The current conveyor option, (b), does not prevent the drawing of large currents from the floating power supply in an overload condition. However, this could be taken care of to a certain extent by introducing a capacitor in both output lines.

The input amplifier is configured as a low-gain differential follower circuit. Due to this approach, we did not encounter any major stability problems with guarding of the input cables.

In conclusion, it can be stated that new configurations of a current source and input amplifier for bioimpedance measurement perform very well in the frequency range of our measurements: 4 kHz–1024 kHz. The operational impedance range of version (a) is 0–2 kΩ, whereas version (b) shows an operational range of 0–15 kΩ. This makes both current sources suitable for application in various fields of bioimpedance measurement, including thoracic impedance cardiography as well as *in vitro* studies on small subjects or preparations. The input amplifier is stable and shows a good IMRR.

REFERENCES

1. HEETHAAR, R.M. & H.G. GOOVAERTS (inventors); GRANULAB PROJECT BV (assignee). 1996. International patent appl. no. 96932860.8-2305. Date of application: September 25, 1996.
2. GOOVAERTS, H.G. *et al.* 1998. An electrically isolated balanced wideband current source: basic considerations and design. Med. Biol. Eng. Comput. **36:** 598–603.
3. GOOVAERTS, H.G. *et al.* 1998. A wideband high-CMRR input amplifier and PLL-demodulator for multi-frequency impedance measurement. Med. Biol. Eng. Comput. **36:** 761–767.
4. GOOVAERTS, H.G. & J.W. METSELAAR. 1987. An isolated microelectrode amplifier for measurements on papillary muscle subject to a rapid temperature step. Med. Biol. Eng. Comput. **25:** 324–328.
5. TRILLAUD, C. & J. JOSSINET. 1992. An improved design of voltmeter for semi-parallel data acquisition. Clin. Phys. Physiol. Meas. **13**(suppl. A): 5–10.
6. MIN, M. *et al.* 1992. Design concepts of instruments for vector parameter identification. IEEE Trans. Instrum. Meas. **41:** 50–53.
7. GIACOLETTO, L.J. 1977. Electronic's Designers Handbook. Second edition. McGraw–Hill. New York.

Impedance Modulation by Pulsed Ultrasound

JACQUES JOSSINET, BERNARD LAVANDIER, AND DOMINIQUE CATHIGNOL

Institut National de la Santé et de la Recherche Médicale, INSERM U281, 69424 Lyon Cedex 03, France

ABSTRACT: The propagation of an acoustic wave in an electrolyte solution produces local and periodic conductivity changes. This acousto-electrical interaction is due to the variations of the parameters controlling ionic conductivity against pressure and temperature. The overall effect is about 10^{-7} % Pa^{-1} for solutions of physiological ions and is practically independent of the ionic species involved. The bulk compressibility of the medium is responsible for about 47% of the effect, the change in viscosity due to pressure changes is responsible for about 18%, and the changes of ionic mobility against temperature are responsible for about 35%. Detectable impedance changes were produced in the focal zone of a 500-kHz focused transducer using moderate intensity ultrasound (peak pressure < 1 MPa). This technique potentially enables the association of the spatial resolution of pulsed ultrasound and impedance measurement, although technical improvements and feasibility studies are still needed prior to practical applications.

INTRODUCTION

The spatial resolution of impedance techniques is intrinsically limited by the properties of the state equation governing the potential within a conductor (Laplace equation in a not charged conductor of isotropic and homogeneous conductivity). The current injected using two electrodes spreads within the conductor and, at a given point, the current density, $\vec{J}$, depends on the distribution of the conductivity within the medium and the boundary conditions (shape of the conducting body, size, and locations of injection electrodes). The ratio of the voltage difference between two measuring electrodes, $\psi_A - \psi_B$, to the current, I_ϕ, injected using another pair of electrodes, ϕ_C and ϕ_D, is termed the mutual impedance of the object and is denoted Z. When the conductivity of a volume element, ΔV, is uniformly changed by $\Delta\sigma$, the potential, ϕ, created by the source electrodes becomes $\phi + \Delta\phi$, and the impedance is changed by ΔZ, according to equation 1, derived by Geselowitz[1] using Green's theorem:

$$\Delta Z = \Delta\sigma \int_{\Delta v} \frac{\nabla(\phi + \Delta\phi)\nabla(\psi)}{I_\phi I_\psi} dv = \Delta\sigma \int_{\Delta v} s(x, y, z) dv \qquad (1)$$

where ψ is the potential distribution that would be created if the measuring electrodes were used to pass a current I_ψ. The quantity $s(x,y,z)$ is the sensitivity per unit volume at point $M(x,y,z)$ for the electrode system used. Hence, the local and periodic conductivity changes produced by an acoustic wave propagating in a body result in corresponding changes in this body's impedance. The purpose of the present study was to investigate the origin and the magnitude of this interaction effect.

THEORY

Experimental Evidence

It can be experimentally observed that pressure affects the conductivity of electrolyte solutions. For instance, a decrease in the resistance of samples of a range of electrolytes submitted to isothermal compression has been reported by Körber.[2] At constant temperature, the conductivity of seawater increases with static pressure.[3] It can therefore be expected that the periodic pressure changes due to the propagation of an acoustic wave through a given volume element would also affect the conductivity of the medium. However, the compression resulting from the propagation of an acoustic wave is not isothermal and the associated temperature changes also affect the conductivity of the medium.[4] As appreciable effects can be expected, certain authors have considered the possible application of the dc signal resulting from the interaction between an electric current and a sound wave at the same frequency for the transcutaneous stimulation of brain.[5,6] In the present study, a constant current was used.

The Propagation of Ultrasound in an Aqueous Solution

Aqueous solutions of electrolytes were taken as conduction models of biological substances. In such solutions, the attenuation of ultrasound waves is negligible, which canceled, in the present study, the influence of the absorption of ultrasound by the medium. The propagation of an acoustic wave consists of pressure changes traveling in the medium at velocity c. A given volume element submitted to such a wave experiences a periodic displacement, ξ, and a periodic compression/expansion cycle.[7] Assuming that the wave propagates along the z-axis, the propagation equation is written under the form of equation 2:

$$\frac{\partial^2 \xi}{\partial t^2} = \frac{1}{\rho \beta_s} \frac{\partial^2 \xi}{\partial^2 z} \quad \text{with} \quad c^2 = \frac{1}{\beta_s \rho} \tag{2}$$

where ρ is the density (kg m^{-3}) of the medium and β_s is its adiabatic compressibility (reciprocal of its adiabatic bulk compressibility modulus, E).

During a period of the acoustic wave, the mechanical work applied to a given volume element is converted into heat. As the time constant of heat transfer between a given volume element and the surrounding medium is generally much longer than an acoustic wave's period, no appreciable heat transfer can take place and the compression/expansion cycle is adiabatic. The following sections describe how the conductivity of an electrolyte solution is affected by these pressure and temperature changes.

Involved Phenomena

The phenomena involved in the acousto-electric interaction are summarized in FIGURE 1. The conductivity of an electrolyte solution essentially depends on the concentration of dissolved ions and their mobilities. The conductivity, σ, of a binary electrolyte is given by equation 3:

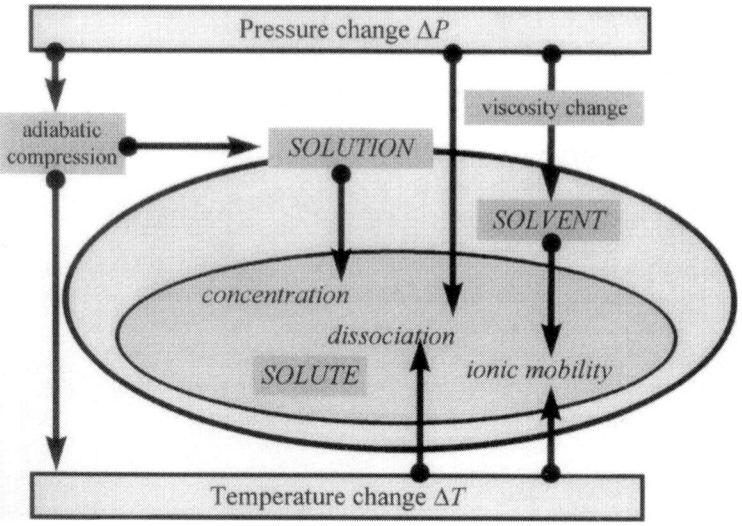

FIGURE 1. The phenomena responsible for the modulation of conductivity by an acoustic wave in an aqueous solution of electrolyte. These phenomena affect the solution (bulk compressibility), the solvent (viscosity), and the solute (dissociation). The changes in the solvent mobility affect the mobilities of the dissolved ions.

$$\sigma = F k_{\pm} \alpha C (z_+ u_+ + z_- u_-) \tag{3}$$

where

σ: conductivity of the solution (S m^{-1}),
F: faraday ($\approx$96,487 C mol^{-1}),
$k_{\pm}$: mean ionic activity ($\gamma_{\pm} \leq 1$),
α: dissociation coefficient,
C: volume concentration (mol m^{-3}),
z_+, z_-: number of charges of the cation and anion, respectively,
u_+, u_-: mobilities of the cation and anion, respectively (m^2 volt^{-1} s^{-1}).

The pressure and temperature affect differently the variables in equation 3. The activity coefficient, $k_{\pm}$, accounts for the conductivity deficiency as ionic concentration increases. This is due to the coulombic forces exerted by all the ions dissolved in the solution on each of them. This coefficient differs appreciably from 1 for high values of ionic concentration. It can be seen that $\gamma_{\pm}$ is not affected by the propagation of an acoustic wave in a solution as the effect is intrinsically small at usual concentrations ($k_{\pm} \approx 1$) and only a limited region of the solution is modified by the pressure burst at a given time,[8] so the total influence exerted is practically unchanged. Therefore, the changes in conductivity are only due to the effect of pressure and temperature upon the molality (volume concentration) C, the dissociation coefficient α, and the ionic mobilities u_+ and u_-.

Both temperature and pressure affect the dissociation constant, α, in partially dissociated weak electrolytes. In the present study, only strong (totally dissociated) electrolytes were used. The dissociation coefficient was thus equal to unity and independent of pressure and temperature. Hence, the remaining relevant variables in equation 3 were molality C and the ionic mobilities u_+ and u_-. The differentiation of equation 3 with these variables gives equation 4:

$$\frac{\Delta \sigma}{\sigma} \approx \frac{\Delta C}{C} + \frac{\Delta(z_+ u_+ + z_- u_-)}{z_+ u_+ + z_- u_-}. \tag{4}$$

Effect of Pressure and Temperature upon the Molality

As the total number of ions present in the solution is constant, the molality (volume concentration) of the solution is affected by changes in the solution's specific volume, V, against pressure and temperature. Under adiabatic conditions, the compression and the thermal expansion of the medium take place simultaneously and have opposite effects. The adiabatic compressibility, β_S (Pa^{-1}), is defined by equation 5:

$$\beta_S = -\frac{1}{V}\frac{\partial V}{\partial P} \tag{5}$$

where P is the pressure and V is the specific volume of the medium (m^3 kg^{-1}). Finally, the changes in molality are expressed by equation 6:

$$\frac{\Delta C}{C} \approx \frac{1}{C}\frac{\partial c}{\partial P}dP = -\frac{1}{V}\frac{\partial V}{\partial P} = \beta_S \Delta P. \tag{6}$$

Effect on Ionic Mobility

Ion mobility is the limit speed reached by an ion in solution in the presence of a constant and uniform unity electric field. Assuming that ions are spheres and using Stokes' law for viscosity forces, ionic mobility can be expressed by equation 7:

$$u = \frac{z_i q_e}{6\pi \eta r R} \tag{7}$$

where q_e is the electron charge and R is the radius of the ion. Both temperature and pressure affect the viscosity, η, of the solvent. Above 4 °C, the viscosity of water decreases with pressure with a coefficient, H_P, of about $-17.3 \cdot 10^{-11}$ Pa^{-1} at 20 °C according to Warburg and Sachs, reported by Partington.[9] At a constant pressure, ionic mobilities increase with temperature by about 2% K^{-1} (TABLE 1). This effect is responsible for the ≈2% K^{-1} change in the conductivity of biological substances against temperature.[10] Finally, the change in ionic mobility is given by equation 8:

$$du = \frac{\partial u}{\partial T}dT - H_P dP. \tag{8}$$

TABLE 1. Ion Mobilities[a]

Ions	u (10^{-8} m^2 s^{-1} V^{-1})	m_T (%K^{-1})
Na$^+$	5.19	2.48
K$^+$	7.62	2.17
Ca^{2+}	6.2	2.55
Cl$^-$	7.91	2.48
I$^-$	7.7	2.17
F$^-$	5.4	2.55

[a] Values of ionic mobilities, u, at 25 °C and thermal coefficients, m_T, for some physiological ions from Pethig[10] and Kohlrausch.[13]

Adiabatic Temperature Changes

The volume changes during the adiabatic compression/expansion cycle can be considered as the sum of a volume change at a constant temperature under the effect of pressure change and a volume change due to the thermal effect. Using the isothermal compressibility β_T and the cubic thermal expansion coefficient θ (K^{-1}) yields equation 9:

$$\beta_T \Delta p + \theta \Delta T = \beta_S \Delta p. \tag{9}$$

Using thermodynamic equations [$\beta_S/\beta_T = \gamma = C_P/C_V$, $\Delta W = Pd(1/\rho)$], one may derive several equivalent expressions of the rate of the induced temperature change against pressure change:[7]

$$\Theta = \frac{\Delta T}{\Delta P} = \frac{T\theta}{\rho C_P} = \frac{\beta_S(1-\gamma)}{\theta} = \frac{(1-\gamma)}{\theta \rho c^2} \tag{10}$$

where T is the absolute temperature and C_P is the specific heat capacity of the solution (J kg^{-1} K^{-1}).

Finally, the conductivity change can be expressed by equation 11, which defines the interaction coefficient K_I:

$$\Delta \sigma = \sigma \left[\beta_S - H_P + \Theta \frac{(z_+ u_+ m_{T+} + z_- u_- m_{T-})}{z_+ u_+ + z_- u_-} \right] \Delta P = \sigma K_I \Delta P. \tag{11}$$

At a given time, the change ΔZ of the measured impedance results from the conductivity changes produced in the whole medium by the pressure field:

$$\Delta Z(t) \approx \iiint_{medium} s(x, y, z) K_I \sigma \Delta P(t) dv. \tag{12}$$

If focused ultrasound is used, the pressure appreciably varies only within the acoustic beam, of width $w(z)$, and the influence of the medium not passed by the wave can be neglected. Assuming that the interaction coefficient K_I is constant in the medium, equation 12 can be transformed into equation 13:

$$\Delta Z(t) \approx K_I \int\limits_{\text{path}} \int\limits_{\text{width}} s(x, y, z)\sigma(x, y, z)\Delta P(t)dv. \tag{13}$$

If pulsed ultrasound is used, only a limited portion of the path is submitted to pressure changes at a given time. The length of this portion is the product of the burst length and the velocity of ultrasound in the considered medium. This gives the longitudinal spatial resolution of the acousto-electric modulation effect. The transverse spatial resolution is determined by the width of the sound beam and thus depends on the characteristics of the acoustic transducer used.

NUMERICAL APPLICATION

The purpose of this section is to give values illustrating the magnitude of the effects. The temperature change associated with the adiabatic pressure change was calculated using equation 10. With the numerical values given in TABLE 2, one obtains about $1.4 \cdot 10^{-8}$ KPa^{-1}. The interaction coefficient K_I is the sum of three terms (terms in brackets in equation 11). The first term is the bulk compressibility, the value of which is about $46 \cdot 10^{-11}$ Pa^{-1} (TABLE 2). The second term is the pressure coefficient of the solvent viscosity. The numerical value is about $17.3 \cdot 10^{-11}$ Pa^{-1} (cf. subsection entitled "Effect on Ionic Mobility"). The last term, the change of ionic mobility against temperature, was calculated using the values found in TABLE 1. The values of the three terms of the interaction coefficient calculated for NaCl, KCl, and CaCl$_2$ solutions are given in TABLE 3.

EXPERIMENTAL MEASUREMENT

Experimental Setup

The detectability of the interaction effect was checked in saline. The measurements were carried out in a measurement chamber, consisting of a 20-mm-long Lucite cylinder

TABLE 2. Thermodynamic Data Used in the Present Study

Parameter	Value	Units
Density[7]	998.2	kg m^{-3} (water)
Density[7]	1004.6	kg m^{-3} (saline)
Compressibility β_T[7]	$45.86 \cdot 10^{-11}$	Pa^{-1} (water)
Cubic expansion θ[12]	$20.7 \cdot 10^{-5}$	K^{-1} (water)
Cubic expansion θ[7]	23.9	K^{-1} (saline)
Specific heat C_p[14]	4181.8	J kg^{-1} K^{-1} (water)
$\gamma = C_p/C_V$[7]	1.00656	(water)
Sound velocity[15]	1480	ms^{-1} (water)

TABLE 3. Calculated Values[a]

	Bulk Compressibility	Water Viscosity against Pressure	Ionic Mobility against Temperature	Total
NaCl	46.2	17.3	33.5	$97.0 \cdot 10^{-11}$ Pa^{-1}
KCl	46.2	17.3	31.7	$95.2 \cdot 10^{-11}$ Pa^{-1}
$CaCl_2$	46.2	17.3	35.0	$98.5 \cdot 10^{-11}$ Pa^{-1}

[a]Calculated contributions of the bulk compressibility, the pressure effect on viscosity, and the temperature effect upon ion mobility to the conductivity changes produced the propagation of an acoustic wave in aqueous solutions of physiological ions.

of 85-mm inner diameter, closed by two acoustically transparent membranes perpendicular to the beam axis. This chamber was immersed in a larger tank filled with degassed water and was positioned using three orthogonal micromanipulators.

In the present study, a single pair of electrodes, located inside the above chamber, was used to inject the current and to measure the interaction signal. The electrodes consisted of two vertical, parallel, 1-mm-in-diameter stainless steel rods covered by an insulating sheath, so only a 3-mm-long portion was active in the middle of each electrode (FIG. 2).

The ultrasonic field was generated by a focused transducer, 50 mm in diameter, and fed with 20-µs-long bursts (10 periods of a 500-kHz sine wave) at a repetition frequency of 10 Hz, synchronized with the current (FIG. 3). The maximum peak pressure was 1 MPa in the focal zone, where the electrodes were placed. The current was injected using a purpose-built balanced voltage-to-current convertor of less than 0.1 mS output conductance. The

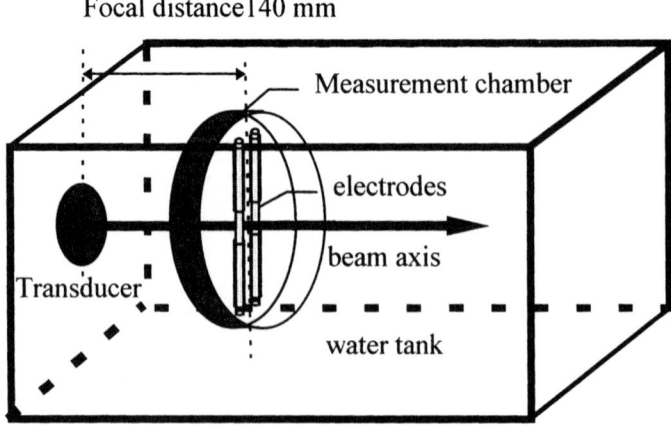

FIGURE 2. Representation of the experimental setup. The positioning system is not drawn for clarity. An acoustically transparent membrane was pasted on each side of the measurement chamber, so only a limited quantity of the tested liquid was used for each experiment.

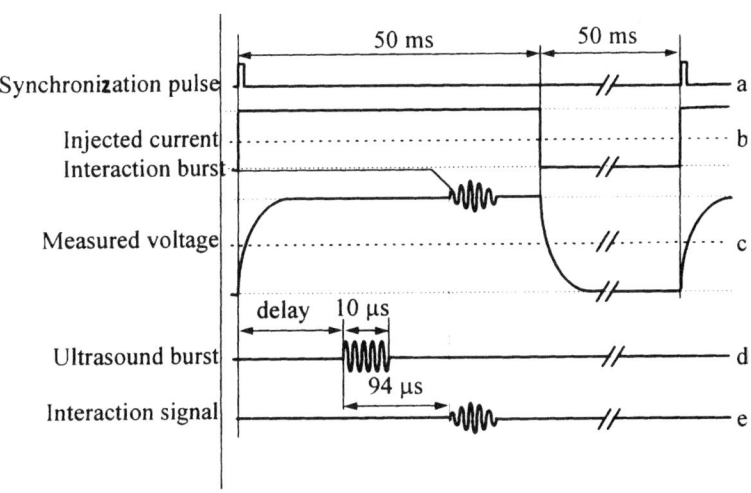

FIGURE 3. Signal timing. For clarity, the time scales are distorted. The injected current (b) and the acoustic burst (d) were synchronized. The electric signal (c) was sensed by the electrode after 94 μs, representing the propagation time of the acoustic wave from the transducer to the focal zone, where the electrodes were placed. According to the settings, the acoustic burst could be sent on either the positive or negative half-wave of the injected current.

current consisted of symmetrical square waves (up to ±12 mA) to ensure a constant current during the propagation of the sound burst and to avoid dc electrode polarization.

The voltage difference between the electrodes was amplified by a differential amplifier with a 670-kΩ input impedance, a gain of 100, and a passband from 20 kHz to 2 MHz. A Tektronix 2430 digital oscilloscope was used to display, digitalize, and transmit the data to a PC-compatible microcomputer.

Results

Measurements were carried out in various electrolyte solutions, especially in isotonic saline for the purpose of the present study. A voltage difference was observed when the sound wave was passing near the electrodes. The signal consisted of bursts at the ultrasound frequency. A signal of smaller magnitude, denoted V_0, was also observed in the absence of any injected current. The signal—so-called "Ultrasonic Vibrational Potential" (UVP)—is due to the Debye effect.[11] UVP results from the displacement of the ions in the solution by the frictional forces produced by the periodic displacement of the surrounding liquid. As the masses and frictional coefficients of the positive and negative ions are not equal, this results in a periodic separation of charges. In the present study, the relevant signal was obtained by systematically subtracting V_0 from the signal measured in the presence of an injected current. A sample of the interaction signal is shown in FIGURE 4.

The peak value, V_X, of the signal was automatically calculated from the recorded waveforms. The results obtained in physiological saline are shown in FIGURE 5. The measured signal was an increasing function of the applied acoustic peak pressure and current. How-

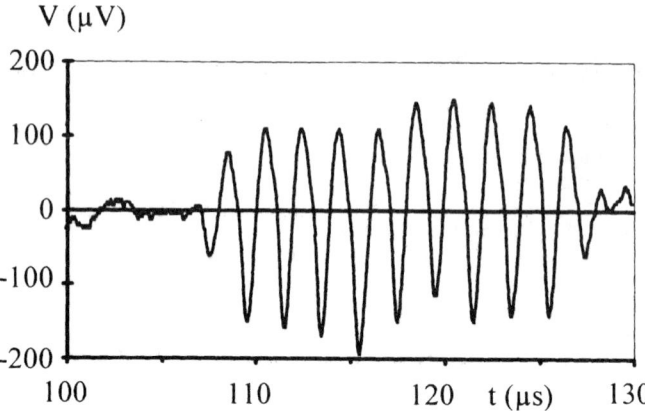

FIGURE 4. Typical interaction signal (after subtraction of V_0) at the output of the $G = 100$ amplifier.

ever, it was not possible to relate the value of the measured signal to the theoretically expected magnitude of the interaction signal. The reasons were (i) the use of the two-electrode technique in which the medium impedance and the electrode contact impedances add, (ii) the nonuniform sensitivity distribution of a pair of electrodes, and (iii) the production of conductivity changes of opposite polarities (thus tending to cancel each other) by the used sinusoidal acoustic wave. Thus, the measured signal was presumably much smaller than the theoretical value.

DISCUSSION

An appreciable interaction signal was observed in experimental conditions *in vitro*. A larger magnitude signal can be expected if the effect of a bipolar acoustic wave could be avoided. The advantage of the interaction signal is that it only exists where and when the pressure field affects a volume region passed by a current. Hence, there is no baseline at the frequency of the relevant signal, and the amplifier gain is only limited by the signal-to-noise ratio. Furthermore, with a constant current, the interaction signal is at the same frequency as the transmitted acoustic wave, which enables coherent demodulation. The volume producing the signal depends on the width of the beam and the length of the burst (30 mm for a 20-μs burst and a sound velocity[12] of 1480 ms^{-1}). This resolution can be improved using shorter acoustic signals and, possibly, processing the signal using proper deconvolution techniques.

From equation 13, it can be seen that the impedance modulation is proportional to the conductivity and sensitivity at a given volume element. It can be observed in TABLE 3 that two of the three phenomena involved in the interaction only depend on the physical properties of the solvent (compressibility and effect of pressure upon the solvent viscosity). The effect of the induced temperature changes upon ionic mobilities (TABLE 3) depends on the ion species. However, the numerical values of ion mobilities and their temperature coefficients result in a relatively constant effect. This can be understood considering that

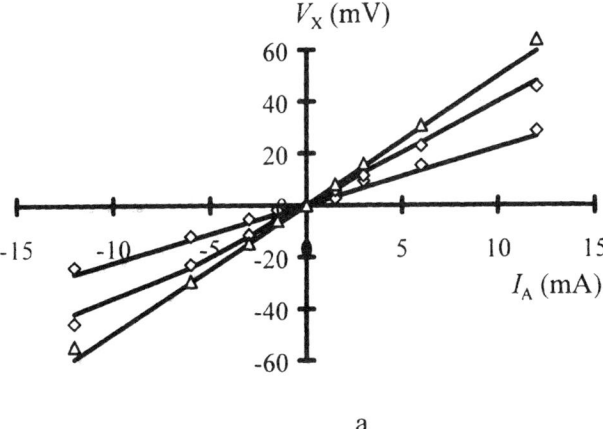

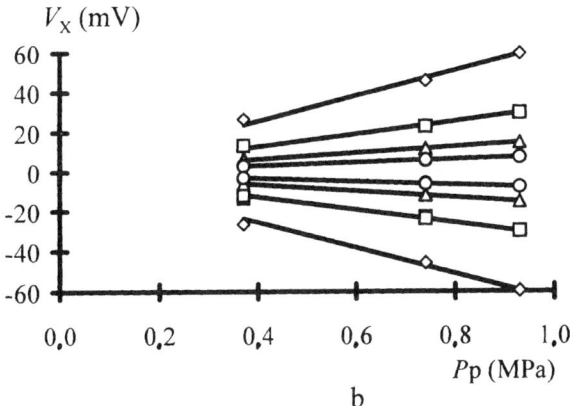

FIGURE 5. (a) Plots of the magnitude V_X of the interaction signal measured in isotonic saline against the injected current I_A for three values (0.37, 0.74, and 0.93 MPa) of the peak pressure. (b) The same data plotted against the peak pressure, P_P, for four pairs of symmetrical values of the injected current (±1.5, ±3, ±6, ±12 mA).

(i) the major effect of temperature upon ion mobility is the change in solvent viscosity and (ii) the physical differences between ion species are relatively small. Finally, the values obtained for physiological ions (TABLE 3) show that the acousto-electric interaction effect depends very little on the ion species ensuring the conduction.

CONCLUSIONS

The present study enabled the theoretical calculation of the magnitude of the acousto-electric interaction. The experimental measurements showed that the signal produced by moderate intensity ultrasound is detectable in electrolyte solutions, at least in the focal zone of the transducer. Improved experimental setup is needed for practical applications of this signal. The major advantage is that only the region affected by the sound wave creates a signal at a given time, so this modality potentially enables impedance measurement with the spatial resolution of pulsed ultrasound. However, prior to practical applications, technical improvements and feasibility studies are still needed, including the design of hardware systems combining impedance measurement and time windowing techniques, the optimization of the acoustic signal, and measurements in absorbing (cellular) media.

ACKNOWLEDGMENTS

We acknowledge A. Matias and R. Jarry for the fabrication of the water tank, the measurement chamber, and the mechanical elements; and Y. Theillère for the construction of the voltage-to-current convertor and differential amplifier.

REFERENCES

1. GESELOWITZ, D.B. 1971. An application of electrocardiographic lead theory to impedance plethysmography. IEEE Trans. Biomed. Eng. **BME-18:** 38–41.
2. KÖRBER, F. 1909. Über den Einfluss des Druckes auf das elektrolytische Leitvermögen von Lösungen. Z. Phys. Chem. **67:** 212–248.
3. SHILLING, C.W., M.F. WERTS & N.R. SCHANDELMEIER. 1976. Physical and chemical properties of sea water. *In* The Underwater Handbook, p. 45–84. Wiley. New York.
4. FOX, F., K.F. HERZFELD & G.D. ROCK. 1946. The effect of ultrasonic waves on the conductivity of salt solutions. Physiol. Rev. **70:** 329–339.
5. FRY, W. 1968. Electrical stimulation of brain localized without probes—theoretical analysis of a proposed method. J. Acoust. Soc. Am. **44:** 919–931.
6. RABAH, H., G. PRIEUR, A. ROUANÉ, D. KOURTICHE, A. HEDJIEDJ & L. BARRITAULT. 1994. Interaction des champs électriques et acoustiques: approche mathématique et premiers résultats expérimentaux pour une application éventuelle en stimulation transcutanée. Innov. Technol. Biol. Med. **15:** 49–59.
7. DUNN, F., P.D. EDMONDS & W.J. FRY. 1969. Absorption and dispersion of ultrasound in biological media. *In* Biological Engineering, p. 205–332. McGraw-Hill. New York.
8. JOSSINET, J., B. LAVANDIER & D. CATHIGNOL. 1998. The phenomenology of acousto-electric interaction signals in aqueous solutions of electrolytes. Ultrasonics **36:** 607–613.
9. PARTINGTON, J.R. 1955. Effect of pressure on the viscosity of liquids. *In* An Advanced Treatise on Physical Chemistry. Vol. 2, p. 89. Longmans, Green. New York.
10. PETHIG, R. 1984. Dielectric properties of biological materials: biophysical and medical applications. IEEE Trans. Electr. Insul. **EI-19:** 453–474.

11. DEBYE, P. 1933. A method for the determination of the mass of electrolytic ions. J. Chem. Phys. **1:** 13–16.
12. WELLS, P.N.T. 1977. Longitudinal waves. *In* Biomedical Ultrasonics. Chapter I. Wave Fundamentals, p. 3–25. Academic Press. New York/London.
13. KOHLRAUSCH, F. 1956. Tabellen. *In* Praktische Physik, p. 670–673. Teubner. Stuttgart.
14. PERRY, R.H., D.W. GREEN & J.O. MALONEY. 1984. Cubical expansion of liquids. *In* Perry's Chemical Engineers' Handbook, p. 3–106. McGraw–Hill. New York.
15. LIDE, D.R. 1994. Properties of water in the range 0–100°. *In* CRC Handbook of Chemistry and Physics. CRC Press. Boca Raton, Florida.

Focused Impedance Measurement (FIM)

A New Technique with Improved Zone Localization

K. S. RABBANI, M. SARKER, M. H. R. AKOND, AND T. AKTER

Biomedical Physics Group, Department of Physics, University of Dhaka, Dhaka-1000, Bangladesh

ABSTRACT: Conventional four-electrode impedance measurements (FEIM) cannot localize a zone of interest in a volume conductor. On the other hand, the recently developed electrical impedance tomography (EIT) system offers an image with reasonable resolution, but is complex and needs many electrodes. By placing two FEIM systems perpendicular to each other over a common zone at the center and combining the two results, it is possible to obtain enhanced sensitivity over this central zone. This is the basis of the proposed new method of focused impedance measurement (FIM). Sensitivity maps in both 2D and 3D show the desired improvement. A comparison of stomach-emptying studies also indicates the improvement achieved. This new method may be useful for impedance measurements of large organs like stomach, heart, and lungs. Being much simpler in comparison to EIT, multifrequency systems can be simply built for FIM. Besides, FIM may have utility in other fields like geology where impedance measurements are performed.

INTRODUCTION

Conventional four-electrode impedance measurement (FEIM) is a simple technique and has been the subject of many studies with applications in different branches of science including physiological measurements. However, the measurements suffer as the zone of sensitivity is not well defined and may include organs other than those of interest, thus making the interpretations difficult and unreliable.[1] A significant leap in impedance measurements was the introduction of electrical impedance tomography (EIT), which provides images of tissue impedance distribution, enabling the possibility of looking into body organs in an effective way.[2,3] Although the resolution offered by EIT is still poor compared with other imaging modalities (about 10% for a 16-electrode system), even such degree of resolution is often not required for studies of large organs like heart, lungs, and stomach. In practice, a region of interest is usually marked out in EIT consisting of many pixels and the temporal behavior of the whole region is analyzed. Therefore, it appears that a technology bridging the intermediate region may have useful applications. With this in mind, the new focused impedance measurement (FIM) technique was proposed[4–8] and developed at the Biomedical Physics Laboratory of the University of Dhaka. Necessary instrumentation has been designed and fabricated in the laboratory and the performance of the system has been studied on 2D and 3D phantoms. A gastric-emptying study was also performed *in vivo* and the results have been compared with those obtained using EIT.

METHODS

Fundamentals

The new FIM is basically a combination of two orthogonal sets of four-electrode measurements. With reference to FIGURE 1, ApqB are the electrodes in a conventional four-electrode measurement, while CrsD form another similar set perpendicular to the former, with the zone bounded by p, r, q, and s forming the common zone of interest. Potential measuring electrodes p and q work for the current drive pair AB, while r and s similarly work for the pair CD. A conventional four-electrode measurement through ApqB gives the effective impedance of the zone bounded by equipotentials aa′ and bb′ (shown shaded) with sensitivity falling away from the center. Similarly, measurement through electrodes CrsD gives the effective impedance between the equipotentials cc′ and dd′ (shown shaded) with sensitivity varying in a similar way. If these two perpendicular measurements are combined, the impedance of the central common zone gets an enhanced weight, thus offering some degree of focusing. The combination may be done through simple algebraic addition of admittance or of impedance when an enhanced sensitivity for the central zone can be expected.[7]

A simplified admittance model is shown in FIGURE 2 for an equally spaced electrode system where the curved equipotentials have been replaced by straight lines. The square zone bounded by the current electrodes and divided into nine squares is assumed to be the total sensitive zone. Each of the small nine zones is labeled with an admittance value (Y_{11}, Y_{12}, ..., etc.). It is assumed that the admittance of a zone is the same if measured along any

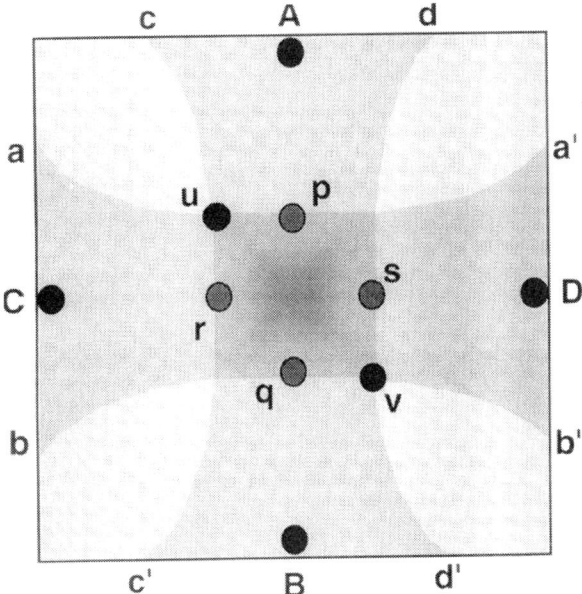

FIGURE 1. The sensitive zones in FEIM and FIM in a volume conductor.

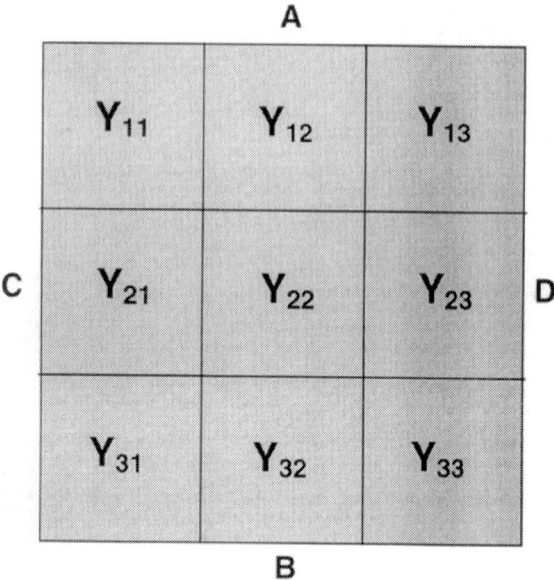

FIGURE 2. Simplified admittance model of the zone of interest.

direction. When current is driven through AB and potential is measured across pq, the measured admittance is thus the parallel combination $(kY_{21} + Y_{22} + kY_{23})$, where k is a constant factor, usually less than 1, which takes care of the sensitivity differences between the central zone and the outer ones. Similarly, for the perpendicular measurement through electrodes CrsD, the admittance is $(kY_{12} + Y_{22} + kY_{32})$. An algebraic addition of the two measurements gives the total measured admittance as

$$Y_T = 2Y_{22} + k(Y_{21} + Y_{23} + Y_{12} + Y_{32}). \tag{1}$$

Therefore,

$$\delta Y_T/\delta Y_{22} = 2 \tag{2}$$

and

$$\delta Y_T/\delta Y_{ij} = k \tag{3}$$

where i and j stand for the other subscripts in the above equation.

These two derivatives present a simple picture of the sensitivity differences of the outer zones from the central one. Since $k < 1$, the central zone has more than twice the sensitivity of the outer ones. Thus, in this description, the central zone may be said to be "focused".

For impedance, the algebraic addition of the two perpendicular impedance measurements would be, using the same subscripts as before,

$$Z_T = \frac{Z_{21}Z_{22}Z_{23}}{Z_{21}Z_{23} + kZ_{21}Z_{22} + kZ_{22}Z_{23}} + \frac{Z_{12}Z_{22}Z_{32}}{Z_{12}Z_{32} + kZ_{12}Z_{22} + kZ_{22}Z_{32}} \tag{4}$$

and the sensitivity may not be so easily obtained. However, intuitively, it may be inferred that the impedance of the central zone (Z_{22}) would have more contribution compared to the outer zones.

Practically, the equipotentials would change shape and location if there are objects of various conductivities in the active region. However, assuming that the conductivities do not differ much from a case of uniform conductivity throughout, this model would provide a simple approach.

From an experimental point of view, impedance measurement is usually preferred over a measurement of admittance because of its simplicity. In a four-electrode system, by driving the outer electrodes with a constant current, the potential measured between the two central electrodes is directly proportional to the desired impedance. Therefore, such measurements were chosen for the present work and a system was accordingly designed and fabricated.

As mentioned before, the focused system basically involves two independent four-electrode measurements, which need eight electrodes in all. However, through some modified placement of the measuring electrodes and by electrically isolating the two current drives so that they do not interact, it was possible to reduce the number of electrodes to six and to obtain the desired combined impedance through a single measurement as described below.

In FIGURE 1, electrode u can replace electrodes p and r for measurements in either of the perpendicular directions as it falls on the appropriate equipotentials aa' and cc', respectively. Similarly, electrode v can replace electrodes q and s for similar measurements. Now, if the alternating currents through electrodes AB and CD can be made to have the same frequency, magnitude, and phase, but be electrically isolated, the potential measured across uv will be directly proportional to the sum of the individual four-electrode impedances. The prototype was designed and fabricated following this concept as described below.

Instrumentation

A block diagram of necessary instrumentation developed for the FIM technique is shown in FIGURE 3. A sinusoidal signal at about 30 kHz is generated using a Wien Bridge oscillator. This is branched out to two isolated current drives (AB and CD) through appropriate voltage-to-current convertors and isolating transformers. The necessary electrode connections are shown on a circular body. The current drives may be set in the same phase or in the opposite phase by simply reversing the electrode connections from one of the two isolating transformers. Since the two isolating transformers may not be exactly equal, two amplitude adjusting circuits as shown were introduced to make the two perpendicular driving currents the same. The combined impedance measurement (sum) is carried out through measuring the potentials between electrodes u and v. The measured potential is amplified, filtered, rectified, and smoothed out to obtain a dc voltage that is proportional to the combined impedance. This dc output voltage may be measured using a digital voltmeter for manual work or may be fed to a computer for automated data acquisition.

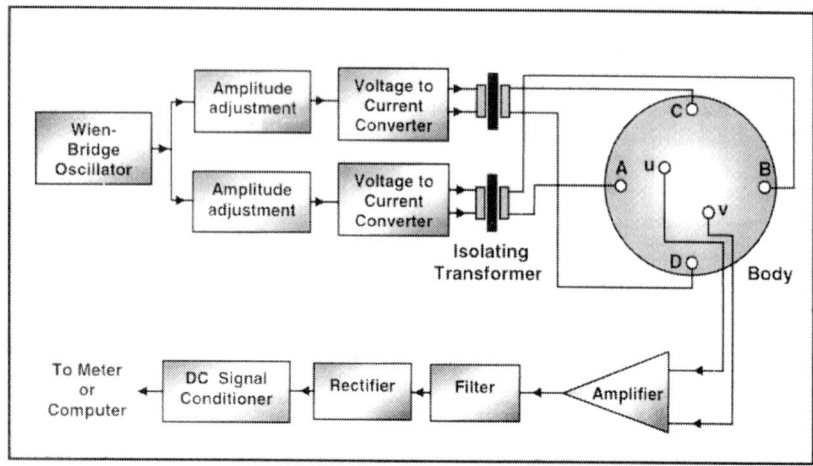

FIGURE 3. A block diagram of the six-electrode FIM system.

Sensitivity Mapping

For sensitivity measurements in 2D, a phantom was made of a deep plastic container containing saline. The dimensions of the liquid volume were about 30 cm × 30 cm × 30 cm. Thin, long, tinned copper wires were suspended vertically using insulating weights to form the electrodes. The current drive electrodes almost touched the walls of the phantom, while the potential electrodes were fixed centrally (viewed from the top) according to the new scheme (u and v in FIGURE 1, diagonally). The separation between these potential electrodes measured along either of the drive electrode pairs was 8 cm. Impedance measurements were carried out with uniform conductivity first (i.e., only with the saline) and then with a cylindrical insulating or conducting object introduced vertically at different positions. The percentage changes in impedance with respect to the uniform conductivity value were determined and were then plotted against position in different directions in order to obtain the requisite sensitivity variations.

The 2D sensitivity was also mapped using a shallow phantom (saline depth: 1.5 cm) where carbon electrodes were employed. The features were found to be similar.

For sensitivity measurement in 3D, the deep plastic container as used for the above mentioned 2D work was used, but small button-type electrodes were attached in a vertical plane near the center of one of the vertical sides, again according to the scheme shown in FIGURE 1 (viewed from a side). Spherical insulating and conducting objects of varying diameters were suspended with thin cotton threads from the open top at desired positions. Sensitivity maps were made on planes parallel to the electrode plane at different distances from it. Values shown in this paper are for a spherical insulating object about 3.5 cm in diameter.

Stomach-Emptying Study

The change in impedance was measured around the stomach region of a subject using both the FEIM and FIM techniques on different days after similar drinks of saline. The electrode placement is indicated in FIGURE 4. For the FEIM current drive, the electrodes AB were used and the central two worked as the potential electrodes. A similar stomach-emptying study was performed earlier using the EIT technique. The result obtained using EIT[3] was taken as the standard as the stomach can be easily outlined from the image to make up a region of interest (see FIGURE 11 later) and the temporal change in impedance over this region can then be plotted out.

RESULTS AND OBSERVATIONS

Sensitivity Plotting

Typical sensitivity plots for both FIM and FEIM obtained for 2D (using the deep phantom) along two perpendicular directions are shown in FIGURES 5 and 6. FIGURE 5 is for the direction in which electrodes for FEIM are arranged (AB in FIGURE 1), while FIGURE 6 is for the direction perpendicular to it (CD). In both cases, the sensitivity falls off away from the central zone and, apparently, the peak sensitivity of the FEIM system is more than that for FIM. However, a significant negative value for FEIM can be seen towards the right in FIGURE 5 corresponding to the region between the potential measuring electrode and the current drive electrode. Due to this negative sensitivity, erroneous interpretations may be made while measurements are performed on the human body using surface electrodes. There is no negativity in FIM along these two directions of current drive. However, some negativity has been observed along the diagonals, but the degree is much less as can be seen in the map shown in FIGURE 7 obtained using the 2D shallow phantom.

In order to obtain the 2D sensitivity map as shown in FIGURE 7, measurements were made only on the two top quadrants. Since there is a symmetry, these values were appro-

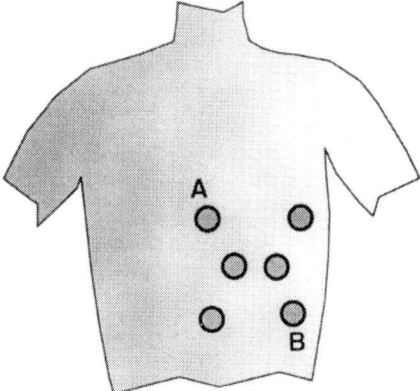

FIGURE 4. Arrangement of surface electrodes for the gastric-emptying study.

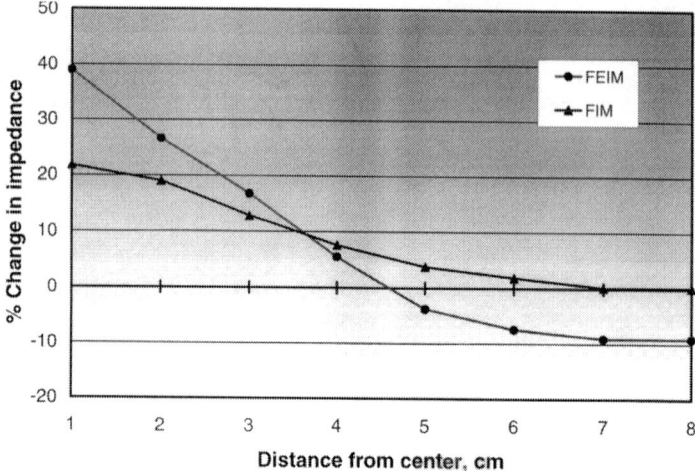

FIGURE 5. 2D sensitivity plots along the direction in which the FEIM electrodes are arranged. The potential electrode is located between 4 and 5 on the horizontal axis. Note the negative sensitivity at the right for FEIM.

priately reflected to represent the two lower quadrants. Here, XA, XB, XC, and XD show the positions of the current drive electrodes, while XU and XV are the positions of the potential electrodes. The percentage changes in impedances are displayed together with an approximate gray shading. The negatively sensitive zones are partially shaded from a corner. Although measurements could not be made at XU and XV because of the electrodes, they have been shaded at the value of the other two corners of the square formed by them. The two plots and the map show the focusing effect quite clearly.

It can also be seen in FIGURES 5 and 6 that, in the case of FEIM, the slope is too steep and slight uncertainties in the position of an object, even within the central zone, will change the results significantly. On the other hand, the sensitivity in the case of the proposed FIM varies less within the central zone, which is more desirable from a practical point of view. This is because the position of a physical organ in the human body may not be precisely located or it may change slightly during measurement due to physiological movements within.

Measurements were carried out using objects of different diameters, both conducting and insulating. The sensitivity distributions were similar, except for the reduced percentage changes in impedance for smaller objects, which are expected.

For sensitivity studies in 3D for electrodes fixed in a vertical plane, FIGURE 8 shows a plot along the horizontal axis starting from the center and on a plane at a depth of 2.5 cm from the electrode plane. FIGURE 9 shows the depth sensitivity at the center (away from the electrode plane). It can be seen by comparing FIGURES 6 and 8 that the sensitivity of FIM is significantly greater than that of FEIM in 3D, which is in contrast to the 2D results mentioned above.

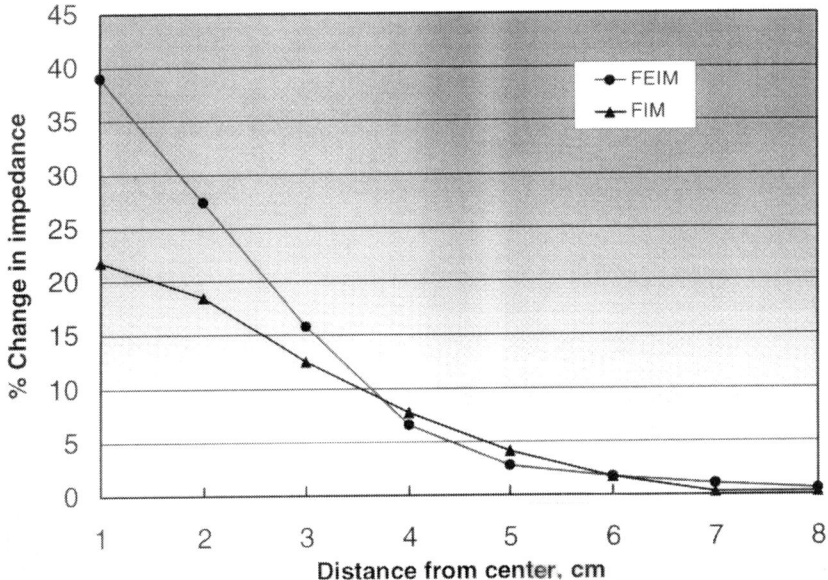

FIGURE 6. 2D sensitivity plots perpendicular to the direction in which the FEIM electrodes are arranged. Note the absence of negative sensitivity for both.

0	0	0	0.17	0.3	2.6	2.1	1.7	0
0	0	0	-1.7	XA	3.4	2.6	1.7	0
0	0	-1.7	-4.3	-0.3	6.6	4.8	2.6	2.1
0	-0.9	-4.3	XU	14.7	10.7	6.4	3.4	2.6
1.3	XC	-0.3	14.7	20.3	15.2	-0.3	XD	0.3
2.6	3.4	6.4	10.7	14.7	XV	-4.3	-0.9	0
2.1	2.6	4.8	6.6	-0.3	-4.3	-1.7	0	0
0	1.7	2.6	3.4	XB	-1.7	0	0	0
0	1.7	2.1	2.6	0.3	0.17	0	0	0

FIGURE 7. 2D sensitivity (% change in impedance) map for FIM. The focusing is clear, although there is some spread along one diagonal and some negativity along the other diagonal.

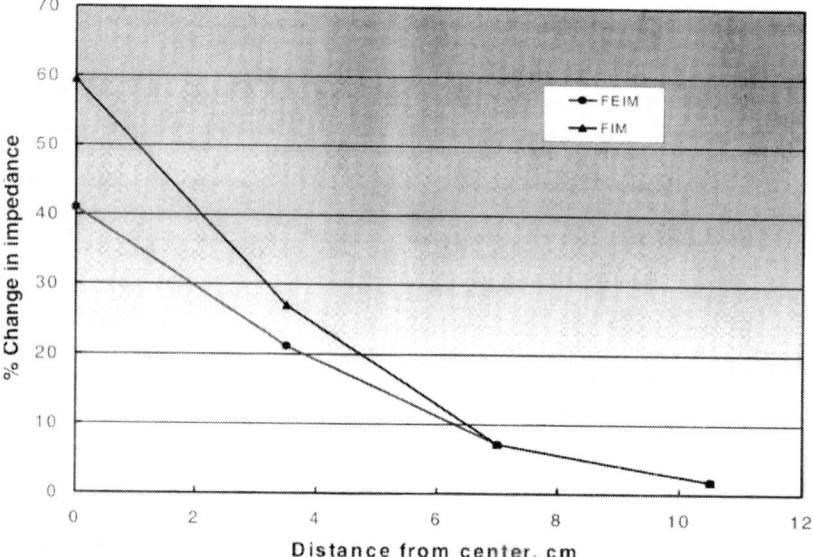

FIGURE 8. 3D sensitivity along the horizontal axis on a plane at a depth of 2.5 cm from the electrode plane. Note that FIM has greater value in contrast to the 2D figures.

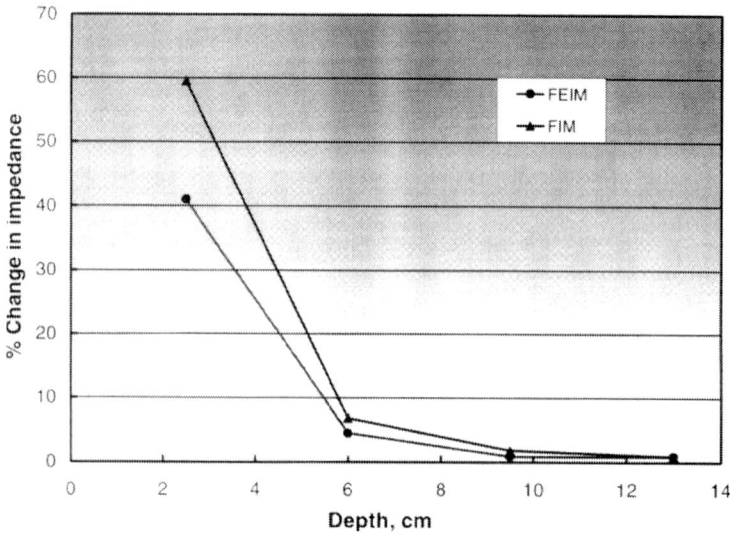

FIGURE 9. 3D sensitivity along depth for a central location. Again note the greater sensitivity for FIM.

Stomach Emptying

Stomach-emptying studies using EIT were performed in the laboratory earlier and four representative images of changed resistance in the frontal plane from a sequence of 30 images (one every minute) are shown in FIGURE 10. These images in the frontal plane were obtained using a reusable spring-loaded ring electrode system developed in the Biomedical Physics Laboratory of the University of Dhaka[3] and depend on the 3D effect of EIT. The electrode ring, of about 15 cm in diameter, was strapped in the front of the stomach region. Initial readings taken in an empty stomach served as the reference. Just after a drink of 500 mL of saline, the resistance in the stomach region goes down, which is shown by the white zone (within the black-outlined box) in sequence 1 of FIGURE 10. This region is marked as the region of interest and the variation of the sum of the pixels over this region was studied over time and is shown in FIGURE 11. It can be seen that the value returns back almost to the predrink level in about 15 to 20 minutes. This is because water is gradually pushed out of the stomach. However, as can be seen in FIGURE 10, as the resistance in the stomach region builds up (due to emptying out), resistance in another zone slightly to the lower right of the stomach gradually goes down. This is possibly the region of the duodenum where the saline is pushed out from the stomach. Similar behaviors were reported in the transverse plane.[2]

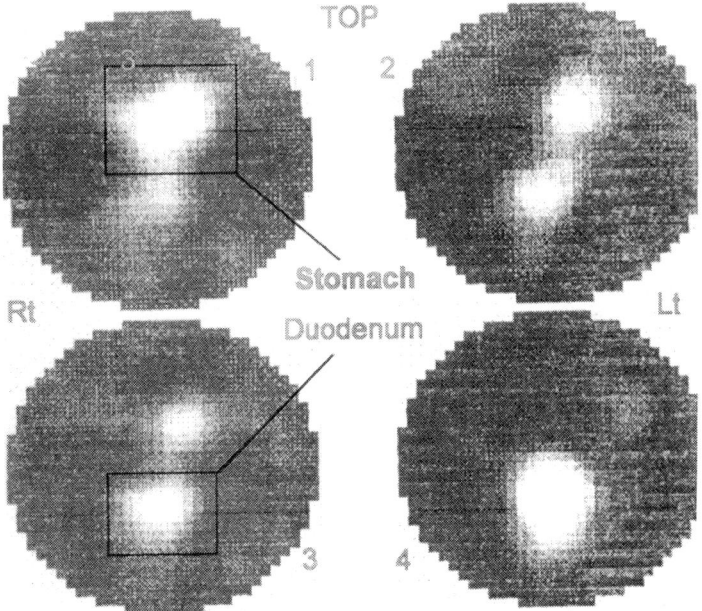

FIGURE 10. Frontal plane EIT images of the stomach region after a drink of saline: 1, 2, 3, and 4 indicate representative frames taken from a sequence of 30 frames at one per minute. Outlined regions indicate the locations of stomach and duodenum.

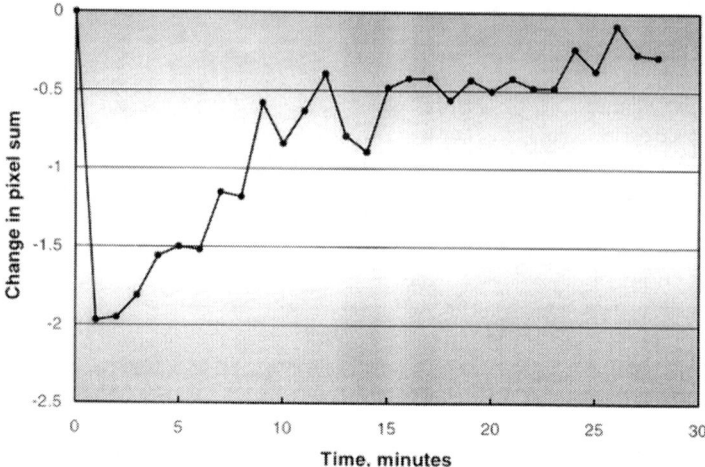

FIGURE 11. Stomach emptying as obtained by region-of-interest analysis over the marked stomach region in FIGURE 10.

Using conventional FEIM, it was quite difficult to find a suitable configuration of electrodes on the human body in order to obtain a gastric-emptying curve as obtained from EIT. Mostly, they looked different and it appears that the contribution from the duodenum made the behavior complicated. However, FIM gave a behavior (FIGURE 12) very close to what was anticipated on the basis of EIT. This means that FIM was successful in isolating the stomach from the duodenum. The objects of interest in this measurement are in 3D

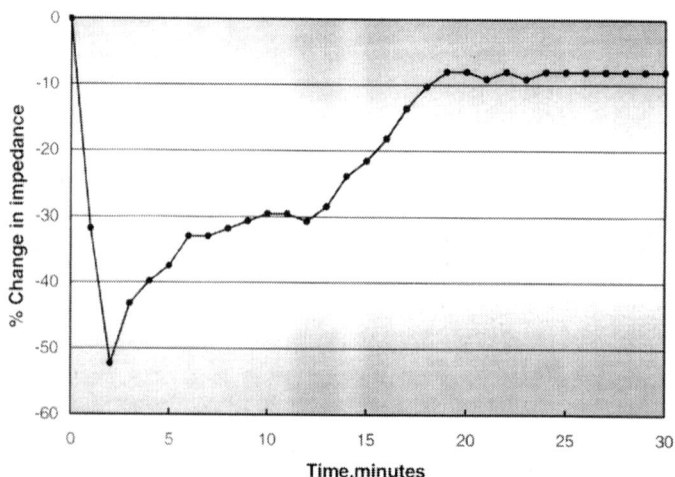

FIGURE 12. Stomach emptying as obtained by the new FIM technique. Note the agreement with that for EIT.

with respect to the electrode plane and they show the success in focusing obtained using the new FIM method.

DISCUSSION

Any electrical measurement suffers from the inherent problem that current paths are not predefined in a volume conductor. Depending on the distribution of conductivity, they will change and adapt accordingly. However, with simplifying assumptions of near-uniform conductivity distribution, some useful information may be obtained and this is the basis of all impedance measurements. For cases with large isolated objects whose positions and behaviors are approximately known, such as for organs in the human body, useful information may be obtained even in cases with significant changes in conductivity. Obviously, these techniques will be useful if the information sought for does not need to be very precise.

The present work uses 30 kHz for the current drive; this choice is arbitrary as below 100 kHz body tissues are well known to behave in a resistive manner. To keep the system simple, phase detection was not employed. However, improvement in these areas will definitely improve the sensitivity and dynamic range of the system. Reversing the phase to one of the current drives in this system will make it possible to measure the difference of the two perpendicular impedances or of the admittances. A combination of the sum and the difference may provide further information.

The area and volume of the zone of interest may be changed by changing the separation of the electrodes. The separation of the drive electrodes will affect the depth of the sensitive region. On the other hand, the separation of the potential measuring electrodes will change the dimensions of the focused zone. Of course, the presence of a highly conducting or insulating object in the neighborhood will alter the sensitivity distribution significantly and has to be remembered in any interpretation.

Furthermore, by replacing the two potential measuring electrodes in FIM by a number of electrodes placed diagonally, and combining the potentials measured between different pairs for the two current drives separately, an image with a low resolution may be obtained. This has been named pigeon hole imaging (PHI).[7]

To sum up, FIM may be a technique of choice for many *in vivo* measurements as it offers a significant improvement over the conventional four-electrode technique (FEIM) without much increase in complexity. FIM forms a bridge between the techniques of four-electrode measurement and the more complex and sophisticated tomography (EIT). For the functional studies of large organs like stomach, heart, lungs, etc., the resolution of 10% offered by a 16-electrode EIT is often not required and FIM may be a suitable alternative. Besides, for multiple frequency measurements separating resistive and capacitive components at different frequencies, FIM would offer a much simpler and low-cost alternative compared to EIT and will increase the scope of the measurement further.

REFERENCES

1. RAHMAN, M. 1994. Development of a four-electrode impedance measurement system for gastric emptying and gastric acid secretion studies. M.Sc. thesis, University of Dhaka, Bangladesh.

2. BARBER, D.C. & B.H. BROWN. 1984. Applied potential tomography. J. Phys. E Sci. Instrum. **17:** 723–733.
3. RABBANI, K.S., M. HASAN, A.B.M.H. KABIR, M. AHMED & S. NAHAR. 1995. Electrical impedance tomography (EIT) in the frontal plane using ring electrode configuration. *In* Proceedings of the Regional Conference of the IEEE Engineering in Medicine and Biology Society and the Fourteenth Annual Conference of the Biomedical Engineering Society of India, New Delhi, India, p. 1.43–1.44.
4. SARKER, M. 1995. Development of a new technique of electrical impedance measurement with enhanced zone focusing for physiological investigations. M.Sc. thesis, University of Dhaka, Bangladesh.
5. AKOND, M.H.R. 1996. Development of a focused impedance measurement technique based on a new orthogonal electrode placement system for physiological investigation. M.Sc. thesis, University of Dhaka, Bangladesh.
6. AKTER, T. 1997. Two-dimensional sensitivity mapping of focused impedance measurement technique. M.Sc. thesis, University of Dhaka, Bangladesh.
7. RABBANI, K.S. 1997. Focused impedance measurement (FIM) and pigeon hole imaging (PHI), two new electrical impedance modalities for biomedical and other applications. Dhaka Univ. J. Sci. Submitted.
8. RABBANI, K.S., M. SARKER, M.H.R. AKOND, T. AKTER & M. RAHMAN. 1999. Focused impedance measurement using six electrodes, a new technique for localizing objects under the surface in a volume conductor. Submitted for Bangladesh patent.

Impedance Parameter Characterizing Apple Bruise

ESZTER VOZÁRY, PÉTER LÁSZLÓ, AND GÁBOR ZSIVÁNOVITS

Department of Physics and Control, University of Horticulture and Food Industry, H-1118 Budapest, Hungary

ABSTRACT: The electrical impedance spectra of Jonathan apples exposed to different pressing force were measured in the frequency range from 1 kHz to 1 MHz with an HP 4284A precision RLC meter. The apoplasmic resistance (R_a), the symplasmic resistance (R_s), and the R_a/R_s ratio were determined as a function of the force and the deformation. Below the bioyield deformation, there was no observable change in the value of R_a/R_s. Above the bioyield, the R_a/R_s ratio markedly decreased in consequence of the R_a decrease due to both the increased ion concentration in the apoplasmic part and the decrease of cell membrane resistance as a result of cell membrane rupture.

INTRODUCTION

Recently, several studies were published in the field of electrical impedance spectroscopy of plant tissues.[1-3] Analyzing impedance spectra, the different cellular structures—as outer (apoplasmic) and inner (symplasmic) electrolyte systems, which are separated by plasma membrane—can be represented by elements of a linear equivalent electrical circuit.[1,3,4] In this way, both the resistance and the capacity of the cellular structures can be evaluated.[1-4]

Various environmental effects may strongly influence the physiological status of plants and, in consequence, may change the electrical properties of plant tissues—for example, a decrease of impedance at 60 Hz was observed after watering plants.[1] The ratio between the symplasmic and apoplasmic resistance was changed during dehydration of potato and carrot pieces.[4] In experiments where sprouting of potato tuber was inhibited by gamma radiation, the ratio of the impedance measured at 50 kHz to the impedance at 5 kHz as well as the ratio of the phase angle at 15 kHz to the phase angle at 80 kHz were strongly dependent on the absorbed dose.[5] Nutrition status like phosphorus and potassium deficiencies in *Trifolium subterraneum* had definite influence on various electrical parameters.[6] In contrast, by monitoring the value of electrical impedance parameters under the effect of different environmental factors, the changes of condition in the cellular structure can be followed.

There are several models of equivalent electrical circuits approaching the measured impedance spectra with different accuracy. The simplest one is the Hayden model, in which only the apoplasmic and symplasmic resistance can be calculated.[1] The modified Hayden model also considers the phase angle and the capacity of the cell membrane.[4] The "double-shell model" calculates the extracellular and intracellular resistance together with the interior resistance of vacuoles, as well as the capacity of the plasma membrane and the tonoplast membrane.[3] For highly differentiated tissues, for example, wood tissues, the impedance spectrum can be satisfactorily described by a distributed circuit.[2]

The ripening process of various fruits can be followed by the changes of some impedance parameters, such as the resistance of the extracellular part or the resistance and capacity of the cell membrane.[7,8] A decrease of apoplasmic resistance can be observed during the ripening and storage of apple tissues.[8] The changes in the cell wall, the vacuole, and the membranes detected by impedance spectroscopy can be monitored in the ripening process of nectarine fruits.[7]

The impedance spectrum of homogeneous and sound (unbruised) apple tissue can be approached in a relatively simple way by the modified Hayden model.[8] The resistance of the apoplasmic (extracellular) and symplasmic (intracellular) part of the tissue and the capacity of the cell membrane can be determined by this model.

The modulus of the impedance at 1 kHz, which has a high value for unbruised and a low value for bruised apple tissues, can be used for characterizing the degree of the mechanical damage of apples.[9]

During loading and transport, apple tissues directly under the skin can be bruised without visible signs by relatively low stress, causing the cell membrane to rupture. The ion content can be changed in the apoplasmic part of the tissue, and the resistance of the cell membrane can be decreased because of the cell membrane rupture. These changes in the extracellular and intracellular part in bruised apple tissue probably can be determined from the locus curve approached by the modified Hayden model. The degree of apple tissue bruise presumably can be characterized by the ratio of the apoplasmic resistance to the symplasmic resistance.

The objective of this work was to measure the hysteresis loop of apple tissue under different pressing force and to measure the electrical impedance spectrum of the apple tissue at the same place where the pressing force was applied. On the basis of the modified Hayden model, the apoplasmic resistance and the symplasmic resistance from the measured impedance spectra were determined for different pressing force, for different deformation, and for different hysteresis loop. The connection of both electrical resistances with the degree of tissue bruise was also investigated.

MATERIALS AND METHODS

Materials

Fresh Jonathan apples of good quality purchased on the local market were used for the measurements. Care was taken to select apples that were free from bruises. The fruits were given 24 h to equilibrate to room temperature before any measurement was made. All measurements were made at room temperature.

Methods

Mechanical Measurements

An Instron-type texture analyzer, SMS TA-XT2, was used to cause mechanical compression stress on the skin of the whole apple along the equator of the fruit. The velocity of the penetrating cylinder of 6-mm diameter was 0.1 mm/s. The value of the forces was varied by steps of 1.5 N from 0 N up to 24 N. The bioyield and the skin rupture force for this apple variety were about 8–12 N and 21–25 N, respectively,[10,11] at these conditions. The force, the deformation, and the hysteresis loop—loading-unloading cycle—were determined for all measurements.

Impedance Measurements

The impedance spectra in the frequency range of 1 kHz–1 MHz were determined with an HP 4284A precision RLC meter connected by an HIPB interface to an IBM computer.[5] The measuring device was calibrated by using OPEN and SHORT corrections. The magnitude ($|Z|$) and the phase angle (ϕ) of the complex impedance were measured, when the voltage on the sample was 1 V. The electrodes—gold-plated copper wires—were 0.6 mm in diameter and 4 mm long. The distance between the two electrodes was 2 mm. The two electrodes were punctured into the same place on the surface of the whole apples where the press by the texture analyzer was taken.

There also were impedance measurements performed on thin apple slices cut out from the apple flesh under the skin in depths of 1 cm. The impedance of the apple tissue was calculated from the impedance spectra measured on slices of 3.5 mm × 3.5 mm × 30 mm at interelectrode distances of 2 mm, 5 mm, 10 mm, and 20 mm as described earlier in the literature[3] and by us.[8] There were unbruised (sound) and bruised apple slices used for the measurements. Bruise was made by pressing forces above the bioyield on the surface of the slices. The impedance spectrum of apple puree was also determined in the same way as the impedance of slices.

The real part $R = |Z|\cos\phi$ and the imaginary part $X = |Z|\sin\phi$ of the measured complex impedance were calculated, and the locus curves were plotted in the case of whole apples. For the apple slices and puree, the real and imaginary parts of the calculated tissue impedance were plotted.

A circle arc was fitted to the locus curve and, from the parameters of the circle arc, the R_a and R_s values were calculated from the modified Hayden model.[4] The modified Hayden model[4] contains the intracellular or symplasmic resistance (R_s), the extracellular or apoplasmic resistance (R_a), and the plasma membrane impedance (Z_m) with constant phase angle (ψ)[12] as can be seen in FIGURE 1. The resultant impedance is

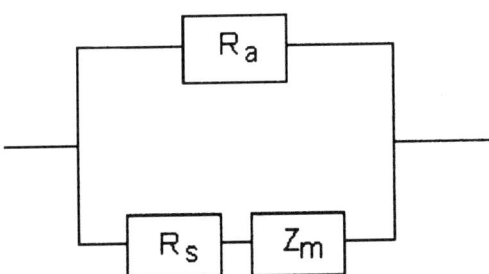

FIGURE 1. The modified Hayden model contains the symplasmic resistance (R_s), the apoplasmic resistance (R_a), and the plasma membrane impedance (Z_m) with constant phase angle.

$$Z = \cfrac{1}{\cfrac{1}{R_a} + \cfrac{1}{R_s + Z_m}} \quad (1)$$

and

$$Z_m = \frac{\cos\psi + j\sin\psi}{C_m \omega} \quad (2)$$

where $j = \sqrt{-1}$, $\omega = 2\pi f$, f is the frequency, and C_m is the cell membrane capacity. The R_a and R_s values were determined from the locus curve of the spectrum.

RESULTS AND DISCUSSION

Mechanical Measurements

The loading-unloading curve with different pressing force was measured for every sample. In FIGURE 2, the hysteresis loops of apple tissue for pressing forces of 3, 6, 12, 16.5, and 21 N can be seen. These force-deformation plots were selected as typical ones from measured curves. It can be observed that the bioyield values are indeed in the range of 9–13 N for pressing force and 0.7–1 mm for deformation.

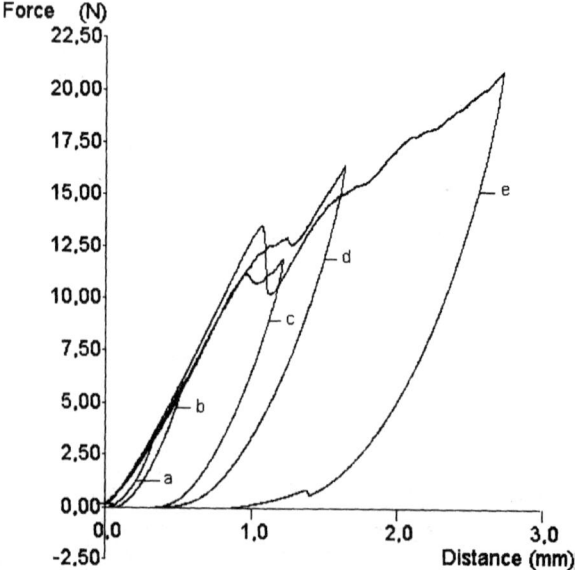

FIGURE 2. The loading-unloading cycle of whole apples measured on the equator. The pressing forces on the skin were 3, 6, 12, 16.5, and 21 N, as denoted by a, b, c, d, and e, respectively.

The bioyield point on the force-deformation curve occurs when there is an increase in deformation with a decrease or no change of force. In some agricultural products, for example, in apple, the presence of this bioyield point is an indication of initial cell rupture in the cellular structure of the material. The bioyield point may occur at any point beyond the point where the curve deviates from the initial straight line portion.[11]

The hysteresis loop, the area between the loading and unloading curves, is the energy absorbed by apple tissue during one cycle. The area of the hysteresis loop has very low value under the bioyield point in comparison to the values above the bioyield point. This means that there is no significant absorbed energy used for cell rupture below the bioyield point. Above the bioyield point, considerable increase of the area of the loading-unloading loop indicates the increasing work performed for cell rupture.

Probably, under mechanical stress, ruptured cell substances have different electrical properties from those of normal apple tissue; therefore, the impedance spectra of sound and bruised (pressed on the surface) apple slices and apple puree were determined.

Electrical Measurements

Apple Slices and Puree

In FIGURE 3, curves a, b, and c represent the locus curves of sound apple slices, bruised apple slices, and apple puree, respectively. For bruised slice, the radius of the locus curve is smaller than the radius of that for sound slice, in good agreement with the result for the bruised apple.[9]

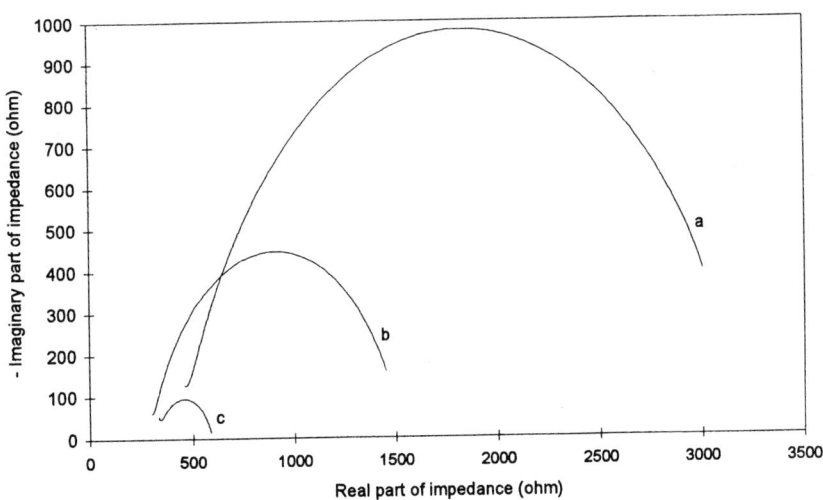

FIGURE 3. The locus curves of apple slices and apple puree. The curves of sound (unbruised) and bruised (under mechanical stress) apple slices and of apple puree are denoted by a, b, and c, respectively.

The locus curve of the puree has very little radius. This decrease in the radius of the locus curve—if the modified Hayden model is used for analysis of the locus curve—can be explained by the decrease in the apoplasmic resistance. R_a, the resistance of the apoplasmic (extracellular) part, can be decreased by increasing the number of charged particles as a consequence of the rupture of cells; that is, several charges from the symplasmic (inner) part of the cells can come out into the extracellular part. A circular arc was fitted to the locus curves in FIGURE 3, and the R_a and R_s values were evaluated from the circular arc parameters. The values of the R_a/R_s ratio were 10, 4, and 1 for the locus curves of the sound slices, the bruised slices, and the puree, respectively. Thus, in the puree state, there is no difference between the apoplasmic and symplasmic resistance. The locus curve of c in FIGURE 3 represents the capacity of the membrane fragments of totally ruptured cells.

On the basis of these results, a decreasing R_a/R_s ratio can be expected with increasing bruise of apple flesh.

Whole Apples

The locus curves of impedance spectra measured on the surface of whole apples after pressing stress with forces of 0, 3, 6, 12, 16.5, and 21 N are displayed in FIGURE 4. A remarkable contraction and a slight increase of the radius of the locus curves can be observed after pressing the apple, in accordance with the forces being higher or lower than the bioyield threshold.

For each measured impedance spectrum, the locus curve was approached by the modified Hayden model and the R_a and R_s resistance were evaluated. The values of the apoplas-

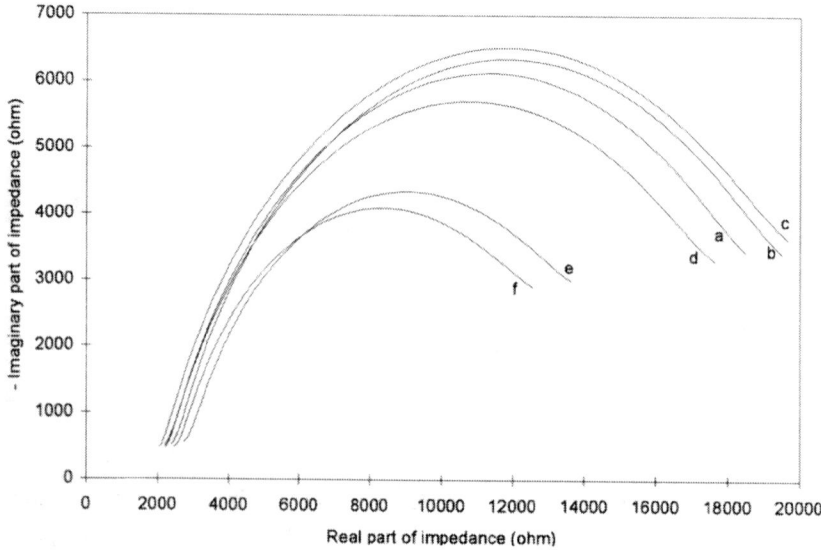

FIGURE 4. The locus curves measured on the surface of whole apples. The surface of the apple skin before the impedance measurements was pressed by forces of 0, 3, 6, 12, 16.5, and 21 N, as denoted by a, b, c, d, e, and f, respectively.

mic and symplasmic resistance (with the standard deviation) as a function of pressing force can be seen in FIGURE 5. Practically, there is no change in the value of R_s, but there is a significant decrease in the value of R_a when the pressing force exceeds the bioyield point. R_a can be decreased by the increase of the concentration of charged particles in the extracellular part of the apple tissue as a result of mixing the extracellular and intracellular fluids after pressing the apple flesh with a force destructing the cells.

In some cases, a slight increase in the radius of the locus curve was observed for low values of the pressing force, as presented in FIGURE 3. This higher value of R_a for weakly stressed apple flesh can be explained by the flow of the extracellular fluids from the part directly under the apple skin into the other extracellular part far from the skin. This flow is allowed by the elastic motion of the cell membranes.

The relatively high standard deviation for the pressing force of 9 N can be explained by the fact that a 9-N force may be below the bioyield for some apples, while above the bioyield for other apples.

The R_a/R_s ratio was calculated for each measurement and plotted as a function of pressing force (not shown) and deformation (FIGURE 6). It can be seen that the decrease of the value of this ratio appears at deformations greater than the bioyield point.

The ratio of R_a to R_s was also plotted against the area of the hysteresis loop (FIGURE 7). A decrease was observable above the bioyield point.

Generally, the values of both R_a and R_a/R_s were significantly decreased above the bioyield point and the value of R_s was not changed in the investigated range of pressing forces. The degree of the decrease of the R_a/R_s ratio depends on the degree of the bruise.

The lowest value of the R_a/R_s ratio calculated for the locus curves measured on whole apples cannot reach the very low R_a/R_s value of apple puree partly because of the impedance of the apple skin and partly because forces higher than 24 N will rupture the apple

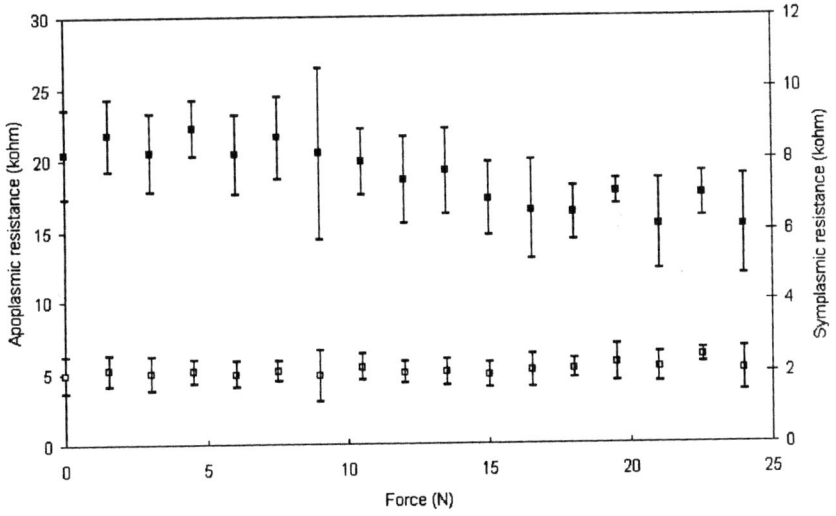

FIGURE 5. R_a, the apoplasmic resistance (denoted by ■), and R_s, the symplasmic resistance (denoted by □), with the standard deviations as a function of the pressing forces.

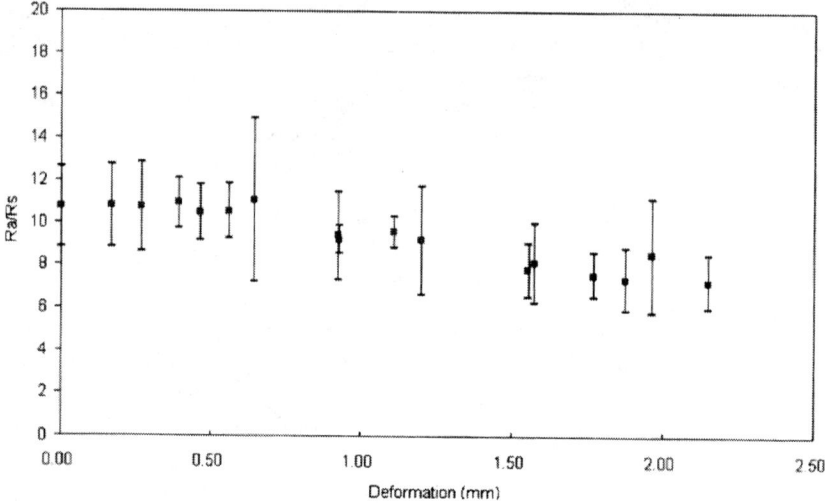

FIGURE 6. The ratio of the apoplasmic resistance to the symplasmic resistance (R_a/R_s) with the standard deviations as a function of the deformation.

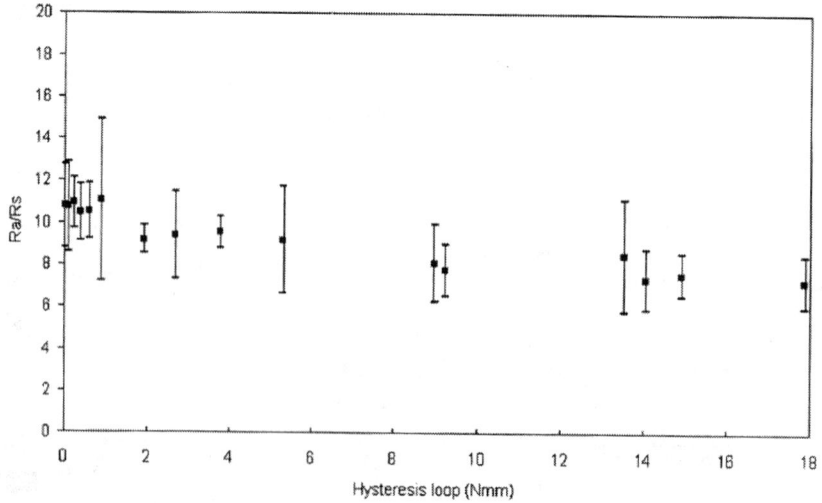

FIGURE 7. The ratio of the apoplasmic resistance to the symplasmic resistance (R_a/R_s) with the standard deviations as a function of the hysteresis loop.

skin and will not cause more bruise. The deformation at 24-N pressing force is no higher than 2–3 mm—that is, between the measuring electrodes, there is bruised tissue at a depth of about 2 mm and unbruised tissue at lower depth.

These results are in good agreement with the impedance spectra measured in ripening nectarine[7] when the reduction of the radius of the locus curve is caused by the degradation of the cell wall.

The R_a/R_s ratio, instead of the R_a resistance, is better for characterizing the apple bruise because the standard deviation of R_a was higher than that of R_a/R_s. The measured resistance depends on the magnitude of the cells, that is, on the magnitude of the apple, but the R_a/R_s value does not; the ratio depends on the apple bruise only.

In conclusion, the described impedance measurement can give information about the invisible bruise—as cell rupture—of apple tissue under the apple skin. The value of R_a/R_s in bruised tissue decreases by 30% versus the value of this ratio in normal, unbruised tissue. More measurements are necessary to obtain mathematical formulae of the change of R_a/R_s as a function of pressing force and deformation.

REFERENCES

1. HAYDEN, R.I., C.A. MOYSE, F.W. CALDER, D.P. CRAWFORD & D.S. FENSOM. 1969. Electrical impedance studies on potato and alfalfa tissue. J. Exp. Bot. **20:** 177–200.
2. REPO, T. & M.I.N. ZHANG. 1993. Modeling woody plant tissues using a distributed electrical circuit. J. Exp. Bot. **44:** 977–982.
3. ZHANG, M.I.N. & J.H.M. WILLISON. 1991. Electrical impedance analysis in plant tissues: a double shell model. J. Exp. Bot. **42:** 1465–1475.
4. TOYODA, K. 1994. Impedance spectroscopic analysis in agricultural products. *In* Developments in Food Engineering. Part I, p. 143–145. Blackie. Glasgow/London.
5. FELFÖLDI, J., P. LÁSZLÓ, S. BARABÁSSY & J. FARKAS. 1993. Dielectric method for detection of irradiation treatment of potatoes. Radiat. Phys. Chem. **41:** 471–480.
6. GREENHAM, C.G., P.J. RANDALL & W.J. MÜLLER. 1982. Studies of phosphorus and potassium deficiencies in *Trifolium subterraneum* based on electrical measurements. Can. J. Bot. **60:** 634–644.
7. HARKER, F.R. & J.H. MAINDONALD. 1994. Ripening of nectarine fruit: changes in the cell wall, vacuole and membranes detected using electrical impedance measurements. Plant Physiol. **106:** 165–171.
8. VOZÁRY, E., B. KRIZSAINÉ NIEMIROW, P. LÁSZLÓ & P. SASS. 1996. Electrical impedance of apple tissues during ripening [abstract]. Prog. Biophys. Mol. Biol. **65**(suppl. 1): 213.
9. COX, M.A., M.I.N. ZHANG & J.H.M. WILLISON. 1993. Apple bruise assessment through electrical impedance measurements. J. Hortic. Sci. **68:** 393–398.
10. LÁSZLÓ, P. & J. ZANA. 1993. Characterizing the quality of apple varieties by rheological properties [abstract]. *In* Postharvest '93 Conference (Kecskemét, Hungary): 17.
11. MOHSENIN, N.N. 1986. Physical Properties of Plant and Animal Materials. Gordon & Breach. New York.
12. MACDONALD, J.R. 1987. Impedance Spectroscopy. Wiley–Interscience. New York.

State Estimation in Time-Varying Electrical Impedance Tomography

JARI P. KAIPIO,[a] PASI A. KARJALAINEN,[a] ERKKI SOMERSALO,[b] AND MARKO VAUHKONEN[a]

[a]*Department of Applied Physics, University of Kuopio, 70211 Kuopio, Finland*

[b]*Department of Mathematics, Helsinki University of Technology, Espoo, Finland*

> ABSTRACT: In electrical impedance tomography (EIT), an estimate for the cross-sectional impedance distribution is obtained from the body by using current and voltage measurements made from the boundary. All well-known reconstruction algorithms use a full set of independent current patterns for each reconstruction. In some applications, the impedance changes may be so fast that information on the time evolution of the impedance distribution is either lost or severely blurred. We have recently proposed the formulation of EIT as a state estimation problem and the recursive estimation of the state with the aid of the Kalman filter. In this paper, we study the so-called smoothing extension of the Kalman filter in the estimation of the time-varying impedance distribution. We will also discuss how to implement prior spatial information on the solution to the state space formalism. The enhanced performance of the proposed approach is verified with the aid of a simulation.

INTRODUCTION

In electrical impedance tomography (EIT), current patterns are applied to electrodes on the surface of the body and the resulting voltages are measured. An approximation to the resistivity (impedance) distribution inside the body is then made based on these boundary measurements. Impedance tomography is seldom used in anatomical imaging. The advantage of EIT over, for example, CT and MRI, however, is the good temporal resolution that makes it possible to track relatively fast impedance changes in the human body. The impedance changes caused by cardiac activity serve as an example of the need for fast tracking.[1,2]

During exercise, the heart rate might be near 200 beats per minute. In the traditional approach, fast tracking usually necessitates the use of either few current patterns, which limit the spatial resolution, or short integration/demodulation times, which in turn yield noisy measurement data. Another problem in the traditional approach is that the impedance distributions at each time are not statistically independent, although we assume that the impedances in each pixel inside the volume change relatively fast. It would then not be appropriate to consider each reconstruction separately since we can lose much of the time-sequential information if the successive reconstructions are carried out independently.

Current hardware systems that are based on parallel architecture are commonly thought to be capable of such a frame rate that the impedance distribution can be thought to be reasonably steady within the acquisition of a single frame. However, this applies only to two-dimensional modeling, in which there are usually 16 or 32 electrodes. In three-dimensional modeling, no less than 3 electrode layers, each with 16 or 32 electrodes, should be used.[3] For example, in a 4-layer setup, we could have 128 measurement instants with a parallel system. Considering a high-demand situation with a heart rate of 150 beats/min and 24 frames/s, we are left with 0.13 ms for the demodulation. It is likely to turn out that the resulting noise levels are intolerable in such a case. In a nonparallel system, we would be far beyond reasonable performance.

We have recently proposed the formulation of EIT as a state estimation problem and the recursive estimation of the state with the aid of the Kalman filter.[4] The Kalman filter can be interpreted as a temporal regularization of the time-varying EIT problem. In this approach, the impedance distribution was preintegrated into regions of interest (ROI). The impedances of these ROIs were then tracked with the Kalman filter. The use of ROIs renders many of the computational problems inherent with the Kalman filter insignificant. However, the ROI method is not always appropriate since it presupposes that the boundaries of the ROIs do not change, which is often the case in reality. On the other hand, defining the discretized impedance distribution as the state causes severe stability and tracking problems that are due to the large-dimensional representation of the unknown variable, in this case the impedance/conductivity values in each pixel. These problems have been largely solved by us with the embedding of spatial regularization into the Kalman filter equations.[5,6]

The Kalman filter suffers from a delay in the estimates that is due to the fact that the Kalman filter is a causal filter and thus uses only information from the past. If the impedance estimates are not used in real-time controlling, which is usually the case, the computations can be done off-line. In this case, it is reasonable to demand that the estimates for the impedance distribution at each time instant are based on all measurements at all times. The solution to this problem is called the Kalman smoother.

In this paper, we study the applicability of the smoothing extension of the Kalman filter in the estimation of the time-varying impedance distribution. The Kalman smoother is an off-line procedure in which all acquired data are used in the estimation of the state at each time. The Kalman smoother does not exhibit such delays as the Kalman filter. After introducing the temporal and spatial regularization formulation, we evaluate the proposed approach by a simulation that shows the differences in using the Kalman filter and smoother and also the effect and necessity of the addition of the spatial regularization.

METHODS

Temporal Regularization: The Kalman Estimators

In this paper, we discuss only the linearized EIT problem. The exact nonlinear problem is discussed in a later section of the paper. We will also only consider a parallel measurement system—that is, all potential measurements that correspond to a single current pattern are measured simultaneously. Consider first the time-invariant case. Let U be the vector containing the voltage measurements corresponding to all current patterns. The linearization of the mapping $U = U(\rho)$ at $\bar{\rho}$ is

$$U(\rho) = U_0 + J(\bar{\rho})(\rho - \bar{\rho}) \qquad (1)$$

where $\rho \in \mathbb{R}^N$ is the impedance distribution that is set to a constant value in each (FEM) discretization element and the Jacobian $J = J(\bar{\rho})$ is also obtained from the FEM discretization. With K current patterns $I_k \in \mathbb{R}^M$, we would then have $U \in \mathbb{R}^{KM}$ corresponding to the classical frame. We can write equation 1 in the block form

$$U = \begin{pmatrix} U_1 \\ \vdots \\ U_K \end{pmatrix} = \begin{pmatrix} U_{0,1} \\ \vdots \\ U_{0,K} \end{pmatrix} + \begin{pmatrix} J_1 \\ \vdots \\ J_K \end{pmatrix} (\rho - \bar{\rho}) \tag{2}$$

so that the k-th blocks correspond to the current pattern I_k. In a time-varying situation, the measurements $U_1,...,U_K$ do not correspond to the same impedance distribution since the distribution changes over time during the measurement cycle. Let the current pattern at time t be $I(t)$ so that it is one of the patterns $I_1,...,I_K$ and denote the measurements at this time by U_t. Let $k(t)$ indicate which of the patterns is used at time t.

The so-called observation equation that is associated with the measurements is thus

$$U_t = U_{0,k(t)} + J_{k(t)}[\rho(t) - \bar{\rho}] + w(t) \tag{3}$$

where $\rho(t)$ is the impedance distribution at time t and $w(t)$ values are the measurement errors.

If nothing is known or assumed about the time evolution of the impedance distribution, very little can be done. Another problem is to derive the optimal estimator even when a feasible model would be determined. However, it turns out that there are classes of stochastic evolution models that cover a wide range of physically sound evolution models and for which there are feasible recursive solutions when related to observation equations such as equation 3. These classes are called the first-order (continuous-valued) Markov processes, which can be defined on either continuous or discrete time-index sets. We will discuss only the discrete time-index sets in this paper. See, for example, reference 6 for a treatment of an originally continuous time-index set problem of a similar type as the one discussed in this paper. We note especially that if the time evolution can be described with a stochastic parabolic partial differential equation, such as the diffusion equation, the corresponding discrete time evolution model can in principle be derived.

However, with no better evolution model available, one usually chooses the Brownian motion, or the random walk, process. In this paper, we will also select this model, although it is clearly seen that there must be more feasible models. The evolution of $\rho(t)$ will thus be assumed to be of the form

$$\rho(t+1) = \rho(t) + v(t) \tag{4}$$

where $v(t) \in \mathbb{R}^N$ is the state noise process. Equation 4 is called *the state equation*.

Equations 3 and 4 constitute a so-called *state space* representation of the linearized EIT system. The mathematical problem is now to estimate the *state* $\rho(t)$ based on a subset of the observations $\{U(1),...,U(T)\}$ at each time t, where T indicates the total number of measurements. Normally, we have $T \gg K$, that is, each current pattern is employed several times. Denote the estimate of $\rho(t)$ that is based on the observations $\{U(1),...,U(k)\}$ by $\rho_{t|k}$. The most common recursive estimators of the state $\rho(t)$ are called the Kalman predictor ($\rho_{t|t-1}$), filter ($\rho_{t|t}$), and smoother ($\rho_{t|T}$). In the case of the above-defined state space representation (random walk), the Kalman recursions for the predictor and the filter take the form

$$\tilde{\rho}_t = U_t - U_{0,k(t)} - J_{k(t)}(\rho_{t|t-1} - \bar{\rho}) \tag{5}$$

$$K_t = \Gamma_{t|t-1} J_{k(t)}^T [J_{k(t)} \Gamma_{t|t-1} J_{k(t)}^T + \Gamma_w(t)]^\dagger \tag{6}$$

$$\rho_{t|t} = \rho_{t-1|t} + K_t \tilde{\rho}_t \tag{7}$$

$$\Gamma_{t|t} = \Gamma_{t|t-1} - K_t J_{k(t)}^T \Gamma_{t|t-1} \tag{8}$$

$$\rho_{t+1|t} = \rho_{t|t-1} + K_t \tilde{\rho}_t \tag{9}$$

$$\Gamma_{t+1|t} = \Gamma_{t|t} + \Gamma_v(t) \tag{10}$$

where $\tilde{\rho}_t$ is the prediction error, $\Gamma_{(\cdot)}$ are certain covariance matrices, and $(\cdot)^\dagger$ denotes the (pseudo)inverse. Of major interest in this problem are the observation noise covariance $\Gamma_w(t)$, which is determined by the analysis of the measurement system, and especially the state noise covariance $\Gamma_v(t)$, which is discussed later in this section. Details and explanations of the application of the Kalman filter to the time-varying EIT estimation problem can be found in references 4, 5, and 7. The recursive smoothing equations (the backward run) are

$$\rho_{t-1|T} = \rho_{t-1|t-1} + A_{t-1}(\rho_{t|T} - \rho_{t|t-1}) \tag{11}$$

$$A_{t-1} = \Gamma_{t-1|t-1} F_{t-1}^T \Gamma_{t|t-1}. \tag{12}$$

This means that the calculation of the smoothing estimates requires a forward run that yields the estimates $\rho_{t|t}$ and $\rho_{t|t-1}$ (both the predictor and the filter) and also the backward gain matrices A_t.[8]

If both noise processes $w(t)$ and $v(t)$ are Gaussian, it is worth noting that the Kalman estimators exhibit several optimality properties—in particular, they yield the minimum mean square estimates for the associated statistical estimation problems.[9] Also, even when the processes are not Gaussian, the Kalman estimators yield the best *linear* estimates for the associated problems.

The temporal regularization is achieved easily with the adjustment of a single state space model parameter: the covariance of the state noise process $\Gamma_v(t)$. While this parameter is in principle time-varying and matrix-valued, it is very often sufficient to assume that it is of the form

$$\Gamma_v(t) = \gamma I \tag{13}$$

where $\gamma > 0$ is a scalar parameter and I is the identity matrix. The rate at which the Kalman estimators can track the changes in the state variable is controlled by adjusting the parameter γ. The faster that changes are allowed, the larger we should set γ. However, a too large γ will produce unstable estimates.

Spatial Regularization: The Augmented Observation Equations

The estimation of a large-dimensional state space is often practically infeasible since the estimates either are very noisy (large γ) or cannot track the changes adequately fast (small γ), with no acceptable trade-off. In the ROI restriction,[4] the problem was solved by reducing the dimension of the state variable to approximately three (the heart and both lungs separately) by performing a so-called preintegration of the state. In the following, we discuss the modification of the observation equations so that it is possible also to track a large-dimensional state space. However, this necessitates a model for the (statistical) spatial properties of the state.

Consider, as before, first the time-invariant problem. Spatial regularization is most commonly implemented with the aid of Tikhonov regularization, which in the linearized EIT case amounts to the minimization of the functional

$$F_\alpha(\rho) = \|U - U_0 - J(\rho - \bar{\rho})\|^2 + \alpha \|L(\rho - \rho_*)\|^2 \qquad (14)$$

with respect to ρ, where α is the regularization parameter and L is the regularization matrix.[10] The Tikhonov regularization (equation 14) can be interpreted as the least-squares solution of the augmented (overdetermined) system of equations[11]

$$\min_\rho \left\{ \begin{pmatrix} U - U_0 + J\bar{\rho} \\ \sqrt{\alpha} L \rho_* \end{pmatrix} - \begin{pmatrix} J \\ \sqrt{\alpha} L \end{pmatrix} \rho \right\}. \qquad (15)$$

If the null spaces of the matrices J and L intersect only trivially, the matrix in equation 15 has full column rank and thus the problem (equation 15) has a unique solution.

The key idea in the approach to be proposed is to interpret the lower matrix and vector blocks in equation 15 as "virtual observations", whereas the upper blocks correspond to actual observations.

We will thus identify equation 3 with the time-indexed version of equation 15 to obtain the augmented (spatially regularized) observation equations

$$\begin{pmatrix} U_t - U_{0,k(t)} + J_{k(t)}\bar{\rho} \\ \sqrt{\alpha} L \rho_* \end{pmatrix} = \begin{pmatrix} J_{k(t)} \\ \sqrt{\alpha} L \end{pmatrix} \rho(t) + w(t) \qquad (16)$$

that are used in the computation of the prediction errors $\tilde{\rho}_{t|t-1}$. Spatial regularization has previously been combined with Kalman filtering in EIT[5] and dynamical wire tomography.[6]

The assumptions on the spatial properties of the state are coded in the parameters α, L, and ρ_*. The usual choice is to fix $L = I$ and $\rho_* = 0$ and to adjust the regularization parameter α. In some cases, the impedance distribution can be assumed to be smooth, thus suggesting the construction of L to approximate some two- (or three-) dimensional equivalent to a one-dimensional difference matrix. Such a matrix is, for example, the Jacobian of the discrete approximation of the nowadays fashionable total variation functional.[12] Other possibilities include more elaborate constructions that can model various types of nonhomogeneously correlated smoothness properties.[7,13]

RESULTS

We constructed a simple time-varying impedance distribution and calculated the measurements assuming that all potentials that correspond to a single current pattern are measured simultaneously. A 16-electrode 2D configuration with trigonometric current patterns

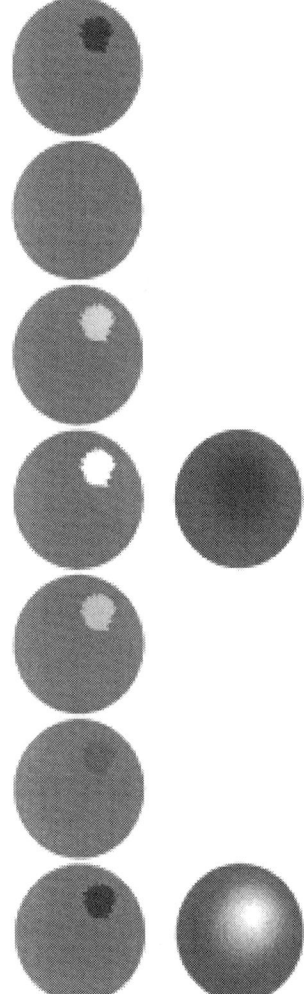

FIGURE 1. Left column: The true time-varying impedance distribution—7 samples from a set of 36 distributions (2 frames). Right column: The corresponding traditional estimates shown at the locations that correspond to the time instants when a full set of measurements have been acquired.

was used. The time-varying impedance distribution with reconstructions that conform to the traditional observation hypothesis is shown in FIGURE 1. With traditional, we mean that the measurements corresponding to a full set of current patterns are used as if they were from the same impedance distribution. The whole stack in FIGURE 1 corresponds to two classical frames. It is clearly seen that the only thing that can be stated on the basis of these reconstructions is that something happens in the upper right-hand corner of the domain.

The corresponding estimates with the Kalman filter with three different regularization parameters are shown in FIGURE 2. The other relevant parameters were

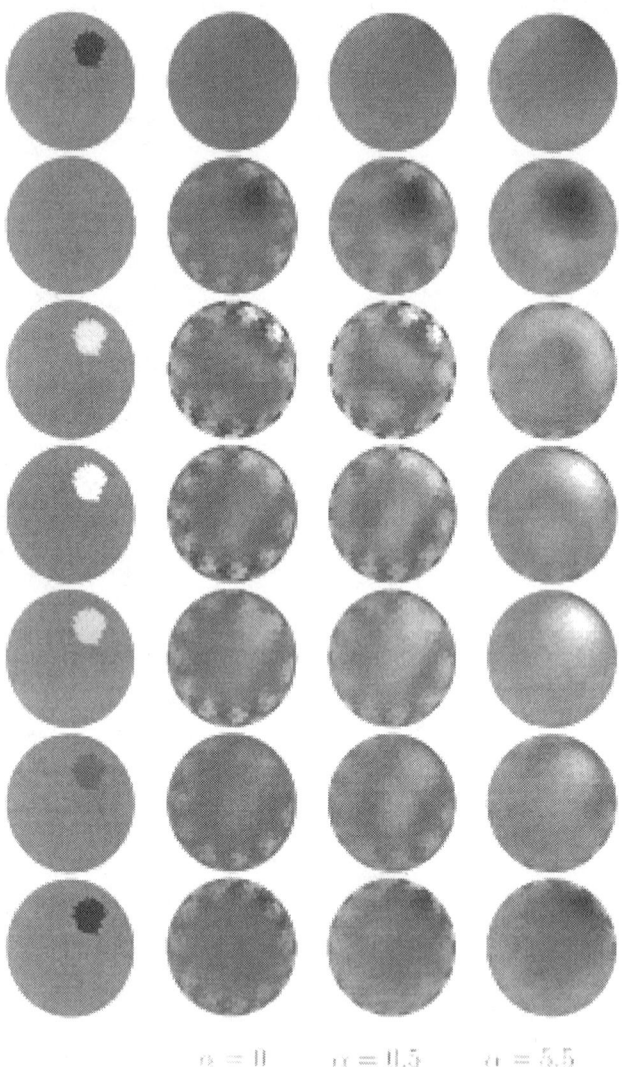

FIGURE 2. Left column: The true time-varying impedance distribution. The other three columns: Kalman filtering estimates with different regularization parameters.

$$\Gamma_w(t) \equiv \begin{pmatrix} 10^{-3}I & 0 \\ 0 & I \end{pmatrix} \qquad (17)$$

and $\Gamma_v(t) = \gamma I$, with $\gamma = 10^{-3}$. The regularization matrix L corresponded to the Jacobian of the total variation functional. The state dimension (number of FEM elements) was $N =$

100. It is also obvious that the estimates are useless when spatial regularization is not used ($\alpha = 0$). Note especially the electrode artifacts. Thus, the Kalman filter does not solve the problem by itself. However, with proper spatial regularization ($\alpha > 0$), meaningful estimates can be obtained. The Kalman filtering estimates are based on the current and past observations only, which induces a slight delay (approximately 1/3 frame) in the estimates. Although not shown in this paper, a closer inspection also shows that the tracking speed of the Kalman filter depends on which of the current patterns is used at each time. This behavior is similar as in the reduced state (ROI) estimation.[4]

The corresponding results with the Kalman smoother are shown in FIGURE 3. The results are qualitatively the same as with the Kalman filter, except for the following. The delay that is inherent in the filtering result is avoided when the smoother is employed. The other difference is that the tracking speed of the Kalman smoothing estimate does not depend considerably on the currently employed current pattern. Also, note that the first and the last estimates in FIGURE 3 are clearly inferior to the other estimates. This follows from the simple fact that the first estimate is based only on the future (no measurements before $t = 0$) and the last is based only on the past (no measurements after $t = T$), whereas the other estimates are based on both past and future observations.

The main problem, though, in the implementation of the smoother is that the additional computational and storage requirements are large. The qualitative nature of the estimates, such as the smoothness, the distortions, and the trade-off between the tracking speed and noisiness of the estimates, is controlled by the choices of the parameter α and the matrices $\Gamma_v(t)$, $\Gamma_w(t)$, and L. Unfortunately, there do not seem to be simple selection rules for α and the matrices.

CONCLUSIONS

We have demonstrated the applicability of the Kalman filtering and smoothing approach to the time-varying EIT reconstruction problem. We have also shown that a simple application of the Kalman recursive estimators does not yield meaningful estimates in the large-dimensional state problem without the proposed spatial regularization. While the performance difference in many applications in system theory between the Kalman filter and smoother is negligible, thus suggesting the use of the computationally much less demanding Kalman filter, the results shown in this paper indicate that in this case the difference is significant enough to warrant the use of the Kalman smoother.

The Kalman filter approach was earlier shown to work well when ROIs were used as the state parameters instead of the impedances of the FEM element. In this case, spatial regularization was not necessary due to the small number of state variables. A more thorough assessment of the applicability in real situations requires further studies, especially with respect to the relevant temporal and spatial regularization parameters. Also, if there is a more complex first-order Markov model for the impedance evolution than the random walk, it can be used with only a small increase in the complexity of the recursive equations.

438   ANNALS NEW YORK ACADEMY OF SCIENCES

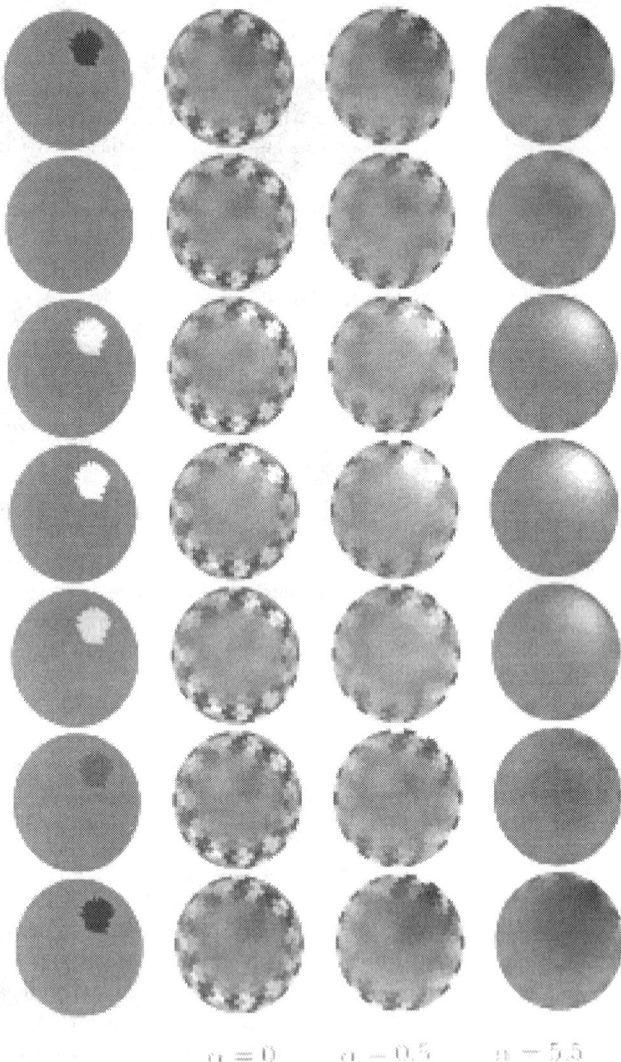

FIGURE 3. Left column: The true time-varying impedance distribution. The other three columns: Kalman smoothing estimates with different regularization parameters.

REFERENCES

1. BROWN, B., D. BARBER & A. SEAGAR. 1985. Applied potential tomography: possible clinical applications. Clin. Phys. Physiol. Meas. **6:** 109–121.
2. EYÜBOGLU, B., B. BROWN & D. BARBER. 1989. *In vivo* imaging of cardiac related impedance changes. IEEE Eng. Med. Biol. Mag. **8:** 39–45.

3. VAUHKONEN, P., M. VAUHKONEN, T. SAVOLAINEN & J. KAIPIO. 1997. Three-dimensional electrical impedance tomography based on the complete electrode model. IEEE Trans. Biomed. Eng. Submitted.
4. VAUHKONEN, M., P. KARJALAINEN & J. KAIPIO. 1998. A Kalman filter approach to track fast impedance changes in electrical impedance tomography. IEEE Trans. Biomed. Eng. **45:** 486–493.
5. KAIPIO, J., E. SOMERSALO, P. KARJALAINEN & M. VAUHKONEN. 1997. Recursive estimation of fast impedance changes in electrical impedance tomography and a related problem. *In* Proceedings of SPIE's 42nd Annual Meeting on Computational, Experimental, and Numerical Methods for Solving Ill-Posed Inverse Imaging Problems: Medical and Nonmedical Applications, p. 208–216. SPIE. San Diego.
6. BAROUDI, D., J. KAIPIO & E. SOMERSALO. 1998. Dynamical electric wire tomography: time series approach. Inverse Probl. In press.
7. VAUHKONEN, M., J. KAIPIO, E. SOMERSALO & P. KARJALAINEN. 1997. Electrical impedance tomography with basis constraints. Inverse Probl. **13:** 523–530.
8. ANDERSON, B. & J. MOORE. 1979. Optimal Filtering. Prentice–Hall. Englewood Cliffs, New Jersey.
9. MELSA, J. & D. COHN. 1978. Decision and Estimation Theory. McGraw–Hill. New York.
10. GROETSCH, C.W., 1993. Inverse Problems in the Mathematical Sciences. Vieweg. Braunschweig.
11. HANSEN, P. 1998. Rank-Deficient and Discrete Ill-Posed Problems: Numerical Aspects of Linear Inversion. SIAM. Philadelphia.
12. DOBSON, D. & F. SANTOSA. 1994. An image enhancement technique for electrical impedance tomography. Inverse Probl. **10:** 317–334.
13. VAUHKONEN, M., D. VADÁSZ, J. KAIPIO & P. KARJALAINEN. 1998. Tikhonov regularization and prior information in electrical impedance tomography. IEEE Trans. Med. Imaging. **17:** 285–293.

A Parametric Method to Resolve the Ill-Posed Nature of the EIT Reconstruction Problem

A Simulation Study

J. C. DE MUNCK,[a] TH. J. C. FAES,[a] A. J. HERMANS,[b] AND R. M. HEETHAAR[a]

[a]*Laboratory of Clinical Physics and Informatics, Institute of Cardiovascular Research ICaR-VU, University Hospital Vrije Universiteit, 1007 MB Amsterdam, the Netherlands*

[b]*Section of Applied Mathematics, Faculty of Information Technology and Systems, Delft University of Technology, Delft, the Netherlands*

ABSTRACT: The reconstruction problem of electrical impedance tomography (EIT) is to estimate the distribution of the conductivity inside an object from measured potential distributions on the circumference caused by injected current patterns. Mathematically, this reconstruction problem is an ill-posed nonlinear inverse problem, with many unknowns. In this paper, the ill-posed nature is demonstrated by analyzing the condition of the sensitivity matrix; the associated inverse problem can only be solved on a very coarse grid. To circumvent the ill-posed nature of the EIT reconstruction problem, we present a new parametric formulation. In this formulation, it is assumed that the object consists of compartments with homogeneous conductivity. The position, orientation, size, and conductivity of these compartments are treated as unknown parameters, which are determined by solving the forward problem (using the boundary element method) and optimizing the parameters (using Powell's or the simplex method) in order to fit the parameters to the EIT data. Simulations show that the parametric method is stable and adequately solves the EIT problem.

INTRODUCTION

Electrical impedance tomography (EIT) is a technique to derive the distribution of the conductivity inside an object by injecting electric currents into the object and measuring the resulting potential distributions. This technique has applications in geophysics,[1,2] industry,[3] and biomedical engineering.[4] From a mathematical point of view, the EIT reconstruction problem is a rather difficult one. It is a *nonlinear, ill-posed* inverse problem with *many unknowns*. In a 2D image, the number of unknowns equals the number of pixels of the EIT image, typically on the order of 100 to 400.

Various EIT reconstruction techniques have been proposed and applied in the literature.[5] There is the more or less heuristic approach of Barber and Brown,[6,7] which was later given a firm mathematical basis in reference 8. This algorithm is very fast, but it is restricted to objects with a circular geometry. Another class of solution methods is based on an iterative application of the finite element method (FEM).[9] Here, the FEM is used to solve the forward problem (predicting the potentials for a given conductor geometry), and the differences between the predicted and measured potentials are minimized using a Newton-like algorithm. This "brute force" approach can be applied without a priori restrictions on the geometry, but is very time-consuming.

A completely different approach is to linearize the nonlinear problem, starting from a homogeneous conductor.[10] In this approach, the dependence of the measured potential distribution on the unknown impedance distribution is approximated by using a series expansion that is truncated at linear order. In this way, conductivity corrections to the homogeneous approximation can be found by solving a linear system of equations. The corresponding system matrix is usually called the *sensitivity matrix*. In the first part of this paper, we investigate the practical usefulness of this method by analyzing the condition of the sensitivity matrix for different discretizations of the conductivity.[11]

In the second part of the paper, we present a new formulation of the EIT reconstruction problem. Instead of trying to reconstruct the individual pixels of the image, we put as a priori information into the model that the object consists of compartments with constant (homogeneous) conductivity. The sizes, positions, and orientations of these compartments are treated as unknown parameters, whose values have to be estimated from the data using a parameter fitting procedure. The model predictions, that is, the computed potentials for a given conductor geometry, can be efficiently obtained using the boundary element method.[12] Simulations with our parametric formulation show that the EIT reconstruction problem transforms from an ill-posed nonlinear problem with many unknowns into a stable nonlinear parameter estimation problem with only a few unknowns.

THE SENSITIVITY MATRIX METHOD

The core equation of EIT, which describes the relationship between the conductivity $\sigma(\mathbf{x})$, the potential ψ, and the applied current density j, is here stated as

$$\begin{cases} \nabla \cdot (\sigma \nabla \psi) = 0, & \mathbf{x} \in \Omega \\ \sigma \nabla \psi \cdot \hat{\mathbf{n}} = j, & \mathbf{x} \in \partial\Omega. \end{cases} \quad (1)$$

Here, Ω represents a 2D cross section of the object, $\partial\Omega$ represents its circumference, and $\hat{\mathbf{n}}$ represents its outside normal. The current j is assumed to be zero, except at two points representing the injection electrodes. In this paper, we only consider the 2D version of the EIT problem. Therefore, we ignore the fact that, in practice, the currents may flow in three dimensions.

When ψ_A and ψ_B are two solutions of equation 1 with boundary conditions, j_A and j_B, the following identity can be derived:[13]

$$U_{AB}I_B = \int_\Omega \sigma \nabla \psi_A \cdot \nabla \psi_B d\Omega. \quad (2)$$

Here, I_B is the total current flowing through electrode pair B. Furthermore, U_{AB} is the potential difference measured by electrode pair B caused by a current injection of I_A through electrode pair A. In other words, U_{AB} is identical to the potential $\psi_A(\mathbf{x})$ evaluated at electrode pair B.

In a perturbation analysis, the conductivity and the potentials are expanded as follows:

$$\begin{cases} \sigma(\mathbf{x}) &= \sigma^{(0)} + \sigma^{(1)}(\mathbf{x}) + \sigma^{(2)}(\mathbf{x}) + \ldots \\ \psi_A(\mathbf{x}) &= \psi_A^{(0)}(\mathbf{x}) + \psi_A^{(1)}(\mathbf{x}) + \psi_A^{(2)}(\mathbf{x}) + \ldots \\ U_{AB} &= U_{AB}^{(0)} + U_{AB}^{(1)} + U_{AB}^{(2)} + \ldots \\ \psi_B(\mathbf{x}) &= \psi_B^{(0)}(\mathbf{x}) + \psi_B^{(1)}(\mathbf{x}) + \psi_B^{(2)}(\mathbf{x}) + \ldots \end{cases} \quad (3)$$

It is assumed that these series converge rapidly, so higher order terms are significantly smaller than lower order terms. Furthermore, it is assumed that $\sigma^{(0)}$ is constant in Ω. When the series expansions of equation 3 are substituted into equation 2 and terms of equal order in U_{AB} are collected, one finds after some manipulations (of which the details are described in a forthcoming paper[14]) that

$$U_{AB}^{(0)} I_B = \int_\Omega \sigma^{(0)} \nabla \psi_A^{(0)} \cdot \nabla \psi_B^{(0)} d\Omega \quad (4)$$

and

$$U_{AB}^{(1)} I_B = -\int_\Omega \sigma^{(1)} \nabla \psi_A^{(0)} \cdot \nabla \psi_B^{(0)} d\Omega. \quad (5)$$

When the potential is approximated to first order, that is, $U_{AB} \cong U_{AB}^{(0)} + U_{AB}^{(1)}$, the following linear relation between the measured potentials and the conductivity correction $\delta\sigma \equiv \sigma^{(0)} - \sigma^{(1)}$ is found:

$$U_{AB} \cong \frac{\int_\Omega \delta\sigma \nabla \psi_A^{(0)} \cdot \nabla \psi_B^{(0)} d\Omega}{I_B}. \quad (6)$$

In the reconstruction algorithm, this equation will be applied as follows. First, an initial guess $\sigma^{(0)}$ of the conductivity distribution is made. Using this guess, the potentials $\psi_A^{(0)}(\mathbf{x})$ and $\psi_B^{(0)}(\mathbf{x})$ are computed. Then, equation 6 gives a linear integral relationship between the measured potentials U_{AB} and the correction $\delta\sigma(\mathbf{x})$ of the initial guess $\sigma^{(0)}$. Since the measurements U_{AB} form a discrete set, the correction $\delta\sigma(\mathbf{x})$ has to be discretized too. This discretization is obtained by expanding $\delta\sigma(\mathbf{x})$ in a set of hat-shaped base functions $h_n(\mathbf{x})$, derived from a triangular grid (see FIGURE 1):

$$\delta\sigma(\mathbf{x}) \cong \sum_{n=0}^{N-1} \delta\sigma_n h_n(\mathbf{x}). \quad (7)$$

In this way, a piecewise linear approximation of the conductivity distribution is obtained, with $\delta\sigma = \delta\sigma_n$ on the n-th node. When the indices A and B, representing the applied current and voltage pairs, run over all noncoinciding and independent electrode pairs, equations 6 and 7 transform into a linear system of equations with the $\delta\sigma_n$ as unknowns:

$$U_k = \sum_{n=0}^{N-1} S_{kn} \delta\sigma_n, \quad k = 0, \ldots, K-1. \quad (8)$$

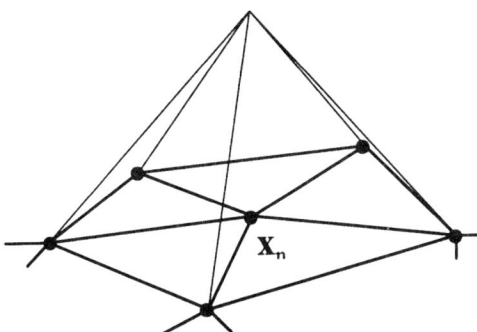

FIGURE 1. The discretization of the conductivity profile is obtained by expanding the conductivity in a series of hat-shaped functions, which are derived from a triangular grid. Here, the base function $h_n(\mathbf{x})$ is shown, which equals 1 at node $\mathbf{x}_n$ and falls off linearly to zero at the neighboring nodes.

Here, the combinations of A and B are referred to by the index k. The matrix S_{kn} is the so-called *sensitivity matrix*, which can be expressed as

$$S_{kn} \equiv \frac{\int_\Omega h_n(\mathbf{x}) \nabla \psi_A^{(0)}(\mathbf{x}) \cdot \nabla \psi_B^{(0)}(\mathbf{x}) d\Omega}{I_B}. \tag{9}$$

In theory, the number of discretization points N can be chosen equal to the number of independent measurements. In the case that neighboring electrodes are used, this number is $K \equiv (1/2)N_e(N_e - 3)$, with N_e being the number of electrodes. In FIGURE 2A, a discretization is shown, with $N_e = 16$ electrodes and $K = 104$ nodes. However, in practice, the number of discretization points that can be reconstructed may be much smaller because many of the equations in equation 8 may be (almost) linearly dependent. When this is the case, the solution of equation 8 becomes unstable and highly sensitive to modeling errors and to noise in the measurements. The problem can be simply solved by taking less discretization points than the number of independent measurements ($N < K$) and finding the least-squares solution of the overdetermined system of equations. In FIGURES 2B and 2C, such discretizations are depicted, with $N = 48$ and $N = 28$ nodes.

A least-squares solution can be found by performing a singular value decomposition (SVD) on the matrix S:[15]

$$S_{kn} = \sum_{i=0}^{N-1} \lambda_i \mathbf{u}_i \mathbf{v}_i^T, \quad \text{with} \quad \lambda_0 \geq \lambda_1 \geq \lambda_2 \geq \ldots \geq \lambda_{N-1} \geq 0, \tag{10}$$

where the sets of vectors $\mathbf{u}_i$ and $\mathbf{v}_i$ are the orthonormal sets of dimensions K and N, respectively. When N is chosen so small that all singular values λ_i are positive, the least-squares solution of equation 7 can be expressed as

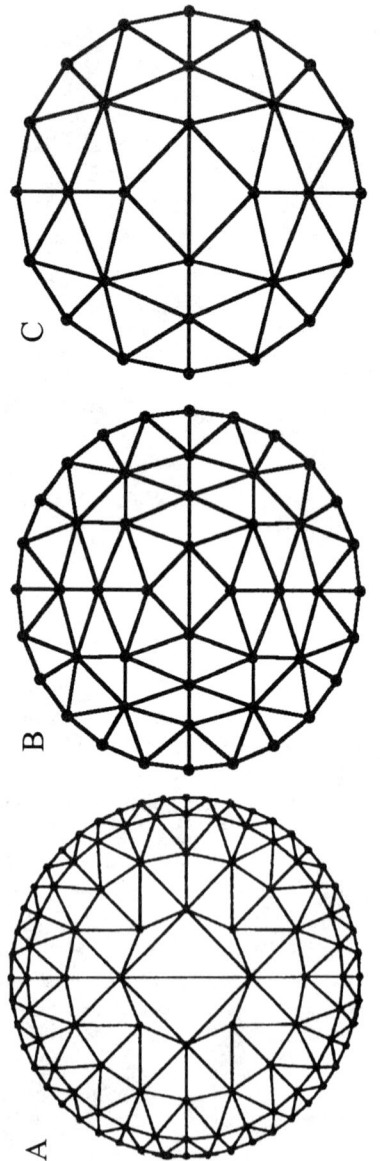

FIGURE 2. (A) An example of a grid on which the conductivity distribution is discretized. Here, the number of electrodes is 16. The number of discretization points N is maximum (104). The number of discretization points is reduced to 48 in part B and to 28 in part C.

$$\delta\sigma = \sum_{i=0}^{N-1} \frac{(\mathbf{u}_i^T \mathbf{U})}{\lambda_i} \mathbf{v}_i \tag{11}$$

where $\delta\sigma$ and $\mathbf{U}$ represent the vectors of the unknowns and the measurements, respectively. Equation 11 nicely demonstrates the instability of the solution when the equations become almost linearly dependent. In that case, the smallest singular values tend to zero and blow up the reconstruction when $\mathbf{U}$ contains measurement errors.

RESULTS: THE SENSITIVITY MATRIX

To investigate the practical possibilities of the sensitivity matrix method, we assumed that the object had a circular shape. In this case, the potentials $\psi_A^{(0)}$ and $\psi_B^{(0)}$ can be computed analytically. However, the integrations in equation 9 have to be performed numerically. We furthermore assumed that all currents are injected through neighboring electrodes and that they are equal in magnitude. Finally, it is assumed that the potentials are also measured by neighboring electrodes and that the number of electrodes equals 16. For this case, the sensitivity matrix (equation 9), its singular values (equation 10), and its conductivity distribution (equation 11) were computed.

FIGURE 3 shows the singular values as a function of the index i. Obviously, the singular values range over 16 orders of magnitude, indicating the instability of the solution of the inverse problem. One way to deal with this problem is to smooth the inverse solution by truncating the series in equation 11 or to add a positive constant to all λ_i terms. However, the quality of the inverse solution so obtained is highly dependent on the exact way that the smoothing is obtained (e.g., see reference 11). Therefore, we choose to reduce the number of unknowns instead, using the grids depicted in FIGURES 2B and 2C.

To demonstrate the performance of the method, we show here the result of a simulation study. A set of measurements was simulated by assuming a circular conductor with conductivity 1 (in arbitrary units) and two circular holes with conductivities 0.9 and 0.8; see FIGURE 4. The conductivities were chosen close to 1 because only then we may assume that the series in equation 3 will converge fast enough.

For the initial guess, the correct value of 1 was chosen. The sensitivity matrix was determined and the conductivity distribution was estimated using equation 11. FIGURE 5 shows the results on a grid of 48 points (A) and on a grid of 28 points (B). It appears that the main characteristics of the true impedance image are well estimated. However, the sizes of the smaller circles are hard to estimate from the reconstructed images. Other simulations, not shown here, also demonstrate that the main characteristics are estimated well with both the 48- and 28-point grids.

Our conclusion about the sensitivity method is that, when no noise is present, it is capable of reconstructing the low spatial frequencies, but only when the reconstruction is performed on a coarse grid. Detailed information of the object cannot be retrieved. Although, in principle, the number of pixels that can be reconstructed equals $(1/2)N_e(N_e - 3)$, in practice this upper bound is far too optimistic. Furthermore, the method is based on the assumptions that a good first guess of $\sigma^{(0)}$ is available and that the true conductivity distribution does not deviate too much from this constant.

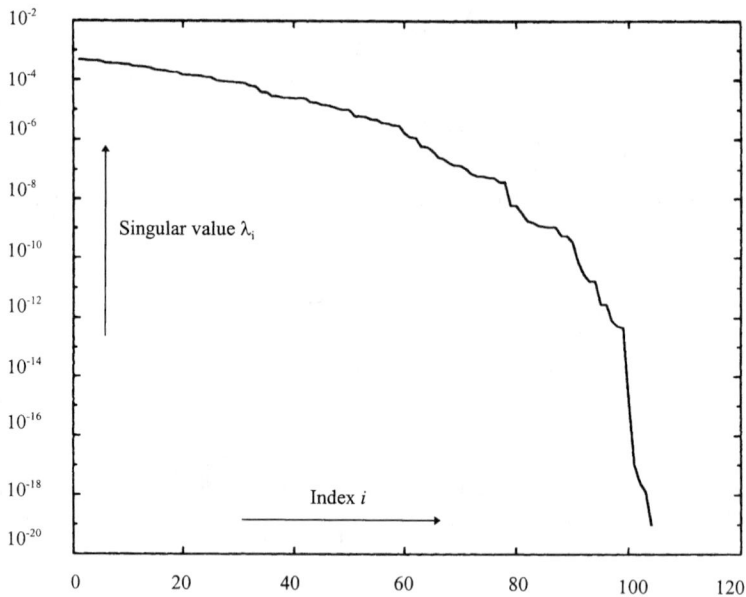

FIGURE 3. The distribution of the singular values of the sensitivity matrix S for the case of a circular cross section with 16 electrodes attached to the circumference. It follows that the singular values are within a range of 16 orders of magnitude, indicating that the full system of equations contains many linear dependencies and hence that the reconstruction is highly unstable.

THE PARAMETRIC METHOD

To overcome the difficulties of the sensitivity matrix method, we propose a reconstruction method in which the number of parameters that have to be estimated is limited and in which no linearization assumptions are required. In this proposed method, we assume that the object consists of compartments with constant conductivity, with unknown positions, orientations, sizes, and conductivities. With such a method, it is also very simple to use a priori information in the reconstruction, by simply setting some parameters to a known constant. The inverse problem is to determine that set of parameters giving the best description of the measurements.

For the application of the parametric method, two problems have to be solved—the forward and the inverse problem. The forward problem is to determine the potential distribution at the measuring electrode for a given set of current injection electrodes and a given conductor geometry. The inverse problem—the geometry of the conductor—is adapted iteratively in such a way that the deviation between the measured and the predicted potentials is minimum. Since we assume a piecewise constant conductivity profile, we can use the boundary element method (BEM)[12] in the forward computations. The BEM is based on the discretization of an integral equation that gives an implicit relationship between the potentials on the surfaces of a conductor with a piecewise constant conductivity. When a current density $j_0(\mathbf{x})$ is injected into the surface Γ_0 of an isolated 2D conductor (FIGURE 6),

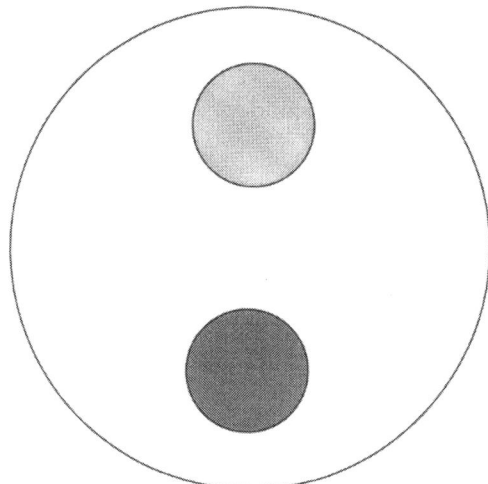

FIGURE 4. The conductor used for the simulation study to test the performance of the sensitivity method. The conductivity equals 1 (in arbitrary units), except at two circular parts. The conductivity of the upper circle equals 0.9, whereas the conductivity of the lower circle equals 0.8.

which consists of a set of J nested contours Γ_j ($j = 0, \ldots, J - 1$) with inner conductivity σ_j^- and outer conductivity σ_j^+, the following system of integral equations is valid for the potential $\psi(\mathbf{x})$ on the contours:

$$\pi[\omega^-(\mathbf{x}) + \omega^+(\mathbf{x})]\psi(\mathbf{x}) = \oint_{\Gamma_0} \log(R^{-1}) j_0 d\gamma' + \sum_{j=0}^{J-1} (\sigma_k^- - \sigma_k^+) \oint_{\Gamma_j} \psi \nabla' \log(R^{-1}) \otimes d\gamma \quad (12)$$

where $R \equiv |\mathbf{x} - \mathbf{x}'|$, $\mathbf{x} \in \Gamma_k$, and $k = 0, \ldots, J - 1$.

Here, ∇' is the gradient operator with respect to the integration point $\mathbf{x}'$, $d\gamma'$ is a line element along the contour, and the operator $\otimes$ yields the determinant of the vectors $\nabla' \log(R^{-1})$ and $d\gamma'$. Equation 12 can be obtained in a way very similar to reference 16, where an integral equation for the potential distribution caused by a current source inside a piecewise constant conductor is derived. Instead of the infinite medium potential that appears in references 12 and 16, we here have the first integral on the right-hand side playing the role of the source term.

Equation 12 can be discretized by expanding the potential in a set of hat-shaped base functions $h_n(\mathbf{x})$,

$$\psi(\mathbf{x}) \cong \sum_{n=0}^{N-1} \psi_n h_n(\mathbf{x}), \quad (13)$$

and subdividing the contours into a set of segments ranging from $\mathbf{x}_0$ to $\mathbf{x}_1$, $\mathbf{x}_1$ to $\mathbf{x}_2$, ..., $\mathbf{x}_{N-2}$ to $\mathbf{x}_{N-1}$. The base functions are chosen such that they equal 1 at the point $\mathbf{x}_n$ and linearly fall off to zero for points before and after the point $\mathbf{x}_n$ (FIGURE 7).

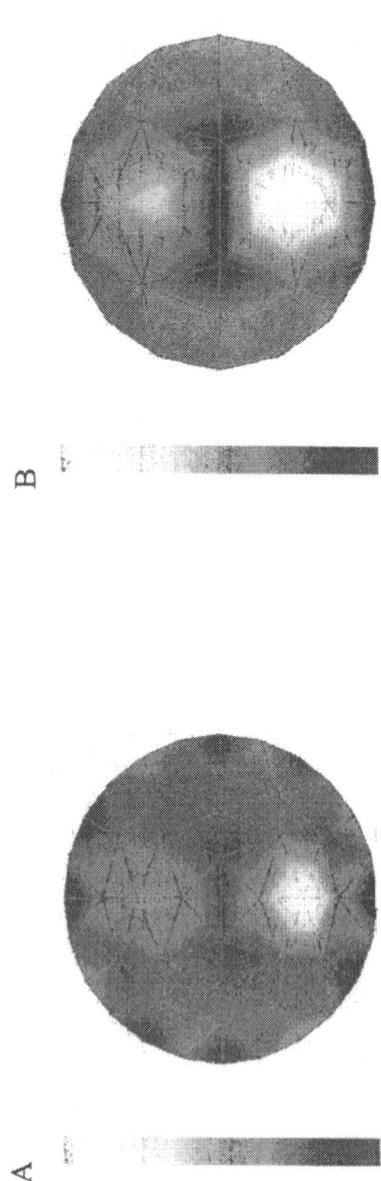

FIGURE 5. The reconstructed conductivity distribution using the sensitivity method. As input, the potentials simulated with the conductor of FIGURE 4 were used: (A) reconstruction on a grid of 48 points; (B) reconstruction on a grid of 28 points.

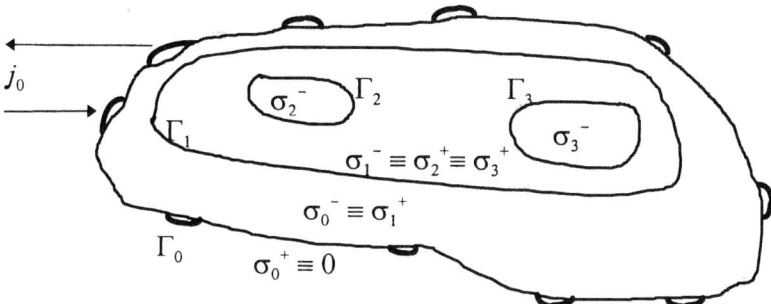

FIGURE 6. Graphical presentation of the geometry of the problem and the meaning of the symbols. The outer conductivity of a contour is the inner conductivity of another contour. In the example presented here, we have $\sigma_1^- \equiv \sigma_2^+ \equiv \sigma_3^+$ and $\sigma_0^- \equiv \sigma_1^+$. The conductor is completely characterized by the shapes of the contours and their inner conductivities.

Similar to the derivation of the system of equations in the sensitivity matrix method, we obtain a linear system of equations when equation 13 is substituted into equation 12:

$$\sum_{n=0}^{N-1} a_{mn} \psi_n = b_m \tag{14}$$

where the matrix elements a_{mn} and the right-hand side b_m can be computed analytically.[17] The system itself can be solved using a standard LU decomposition. By nature of the boundary element method and contrary to the sensitivity matrix method, the potential at the boundaries is discretized instead of the (unknown) conductivity inside the complete object. Therefore, in both discretizations, different types of base functions are involved.

The inverse problem is to find that combination of parameters for which the difference between the measured and predicted is minimum. This difference can be expressed in the cost function E:

$$E = \sum_A \frac{\sum_B |\tilde{U}_{AB} - U_{AB}|}{\sum_B |U_{AB}|} \cdot 100\% \tag{15}$$

where U_{AB} denotes the measured potential difference on electrode pair B caused by a current injection on electrode pair A, and $\tilde{U}_{AB}$ denotes the corresponding model prediction. The index A runs over all pairs of current injection electrodes that are used in the data acquisition and B runs over all voltage-measuring electrode pairs, except those that coincide with one of the current injection electrodes.

The predicted potentials $\tilde{U}_{AB}$ depend on the positions, shapes, and inner conductivities of the contours representing the conductor. In the inverse algorithm that we are proposing, a conductor is chosen as a starting value and next the contours are shifted, rotated, and stretched,

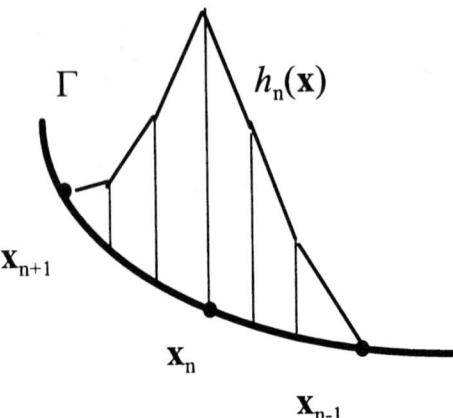

FIGURE 7. The base functions used to expand the potential. These functions are defined for **x** on a contour. They equal unity at one of the vertices and gradually fall off to zero at the next and the previous vertex on the contour.

$$\begin{pmatrix} \xi' \\ \eta' \end{pmatrix} = \begin{pmatrix} s\cos\varphi & -s\sin\varphi \\ s\sin\varphi & s\cos\varphi \end{pmatrix} \begin{pmatrix} \xi \\ \eta \end{pmatrix} + \begin{pmatrix} t_\xi \\ t_\eta \end{pmatrix}, \qquad (16)$$

in order to minimize the cost function. Here $(t_\xi, t_\eta)^T$ is the translation vector, φ is the rotation angle, and s is the stretching parameter. These transformations are separately applied for each contour. With this parameterization, there are four unknowns per contour, excluding the inner conductivity.

The minimization of the cost function is a nonlinear problem that can only be solved by iterative methods. For a proper functioning of nonlinear minimization methods, the parameters should be scaled such that a fixed step in each of the scaled parameters roughly has the same effect on the cost function. Furthermore, the parameters s and σ^- are kept positive by optimizing their logarithms. Each time that the minimization algorithm computes the next step, it uses the scaled parameters; and each time that this algorithm requires a cost function evaluation, the parameters are transformed back into their unscaled versions. We used either the simplex method or Powell's method[15] to minimize the cost function.

RESULTS: THE PARAMETRIC METHOD

To test the efficiency and robustness of our proposed inverse algorithm, we used a standard conductor shown in FIGURE 8. This conductor has a conductivity $\sigma^- = 1$, and it contains two large structures with a low conductivity ($\sigma^- = 0.1$) and a small good-conducting structure ($\sigma^- = 10$). Because of the resemblance between the standard geometry and the 2D cross section of the torso, the inner structures of the conductor will hereafter be referred to as lungs and aorta. It is assumed that the standard conductor has 32 equally spaced electrodes mounted on its outer contour.

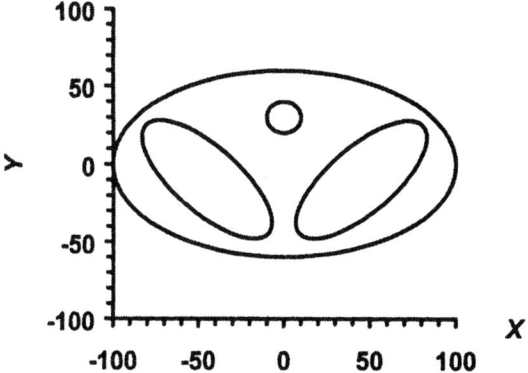

FIGURE 8. "Standard" conductor from which simulations are performed. The outer ellipse has a conductivity of $\sigma^- = 1$, the two big elliptical structures are relatively poor conducting ($\sigma^- = 0.1$), and the small circle is good conducting ($\sigma^- = 10$).

We studied the behavior of the simplex and Powell's minimization algorithms. In a simulation study, the standard geometry was distorted by moving, rotating, and scaling the lungs and keeping the other contours constant. Twenty-five random distortions were applied and, for each of these distortions, it was attempted to find back the standard geometry using the distorted geometry as a starting value and the potentials U_{AB} of the standard geometry as simulated data. The *success rate* and the number of BEM evaluations were determined. The success rate is defined as the relative number of reconstructions, for which the *average distance* between the standard conductor and the reconstructed conductor is less than 1% of the conductor's diameter. Here, the average distance is computed by averaging all distances between corresponding points (of the free contours). The number of BEM evaluations is proportional to the total computation time of the inverse algorithm.

It appears from TABLE 1 that the success rate of Powell's algorithm is 88% and that for the simplex method is 100%. The number of BEM evaluations is of the same order of magnitude.

TABLE 1. A Comparison of the Performance between the (Modified) Simplex and Powell's Minimization Method

Minimization Method	Success Rate	Number of BEM Evaluations
Powell's	88%	820
Simplex	100%	1024

DISCUSSION

Comparing the sensitivity matrix method and the parametric method from a theoretical point of view, we note that the applicability of the parametric method is much less restricted. With the sensitivity matrix method, a first guess of the conductivity is required, from which the true conductivity distribution must not deviate too much. Otherwise, the linear approximation becomes invalid. One could attempt to circumvent this disadvantage by deriving higher order approximations or by starting from an inhomogeneous distribution $\sigma^{(0)}(x)$ as a first guess. However, whether such variants would yield practical reconstruction methods is questionable because the derivation of equation 6 is based on the assumption that $\sigma^{(0)}$ is constant.

One could object that the comparison between both methods is not fair because the number of electrodes was 32 in the simulations with the parametric method and this number was only 16 with the sensitivity matrix method. Moreover, the number of unknowns was 8 with the parametric method and it was minimally 28 with the sensitivity matrix method. The reason why we used only 16 electrodes with the sensitivity matrix method is that, because of the piecewise linear approximation of the conductivity, with a larger number of electrodes, more triangles would have to be chosen at the boundary. This would decrease the resolution at the center still further. Furthermore, we consider the fact that the number of unknowns in the parametric method was only 8 as a special advantage of this method. With the sensitivity matrix method, the use of a grid with 8 nodes would have no practical meaning because the resolution would be too low.

The main theoretical restriction of the parametric method is the assumption that the object consists of nested compartments with constant conductivity. In principle, one could avoid this restriction by taking a sufficient number of small compartments. Practical limitations of this approach are that the method could become unstable and that the computation time would increase enormously. With the simulations presented in the previous section, where the number of compartments is limited, on average 1000 BEM evaluations were required, taking about 30 minutes on a fast PC.

Currently, the computation time is the main drawback of the parametric method. There are various possibilities to speed up the algorithm. First, one could use iterative methods to solve equation 14 instead of a full LU decomposition. Good initial guesses are available from previous cost function evaluations. Second, one could use the method described in reference 18 to solve a series of boundary element problems, in which only one or two compartments are different. Third, one could investigate whether our modifications of the simplex and Powell's method could be improved. However, we do not expect that these improvements will ever make the parametric method faster than the sensitivity matrix method, where each image reconstruction only requires a simple matrix vector multiplication.

The parametric method and the sensitivity matrix method also differ in the way that a priori knowledge is used in the reconstruction and in the amount of a priori knowledge used. For this reason, we will continue to explore both methods not only from a theoretical point of view, but also from a clinical point of view. In some cases, where one is interested in extracting detailed physical quantities from the data, and sufficient a priori information is available, the parametric method would be the most favorable algorithm. In other cases, where one is interested in fast changes in gross anatomy, the sensitivity matrix method is the method of choice.

ACKNOWLEDGMENTS

The part of this paper dealing with the sensitivity matrix is based on the master's thesis of Ir. L. Riemens. We wish to thank her for all the work she did.

REFERENCES

1. CHERKAEVA, E. & A.C. TRIPP. 1996. Inverse conductivity problem for inaccurate measurements. Inverse Probl. **12:** 869–883.
2. BORCEA, L., J.G. BERRYMAN & G.C. PAPANICOLAOU. 1996. High-contrast impedance tomography. Inverse Probl. **12:** 835–858.
3. PLASKOWSKI, A., M.S. BEEK, R. THORN & J. PYAKOWSKI. 1995. Imaging Industrial Flows: Applications of Electrical Process Tomography. Inst. Phys. Pub. Bristol/Philadelphia.
4. BROWN, B.H., D.C. BARBER & A.D. SEAGAR. 1985. Applied potential tomography: possible clinical application. Clin. Phys. Physiol. Meas. **6:** 109–121.
5. WEBSTER, J.G., Ed. 1990. Electrical Impedance Tomography. Adam Hilger. Bristol/New York.
6. BARBER, D.C. & B.H. BROWN. 1984. Applied potential tomography. J. Phys. E. Sci. Instrum. **37:** 723–732.
7. BARBER, D.C. & A.D. SEAGAR. 1987. Fast reconstruction of resistance images. Clin. Phys. Physiol. Meas. **8**(suppl. A): 47–54.
8. SANTOSA, F. & M. VOGELIUS. 1990. A backprojection algorithm for electrical impedance imaging. SIAM J. Appl. Math. **50:** 216–243.
9. YORKEY, T.J., J.G. WEBSTER & W.J. TOMPKINS. 1987. Comparing reconstruction algorithms for electrical impedance tomography. IEEE Trans. Biomed. Eng. **BME-34:** 843–851.
10. CALDERON, A.P. 1980. On an inverse boundary value problem. Seminar on Numerical Analysis and Its Application to Continuum Mechanics (Soc. Brasileira de Mathematica, Rio de Janeiro), p. 65–73.
11. DE MUNCK, J.C. 1997. A comparison of methods to determine mass transports from hydrographic measurements. J. Phys. Oceanogr. **27:** 1635–1653.
12. DE MUNCK, J.C. 1992. A linear discretization of the volume conductor boundary integral equation using analytically integrated elements. IEEE Trans. Biomed. Eng. **BME-39:** 986–989.
13. BRECKON, W.R. & M.K. PIDCOCK. 1987. Mathematical aspects of impedance imaging. Clin. Phys. Physiol. Meas. **8**(suppl. A): 77–84.
14. FAES, TH. J.C. et al. 1998. In preparation.
15. PRESS, W.H., B.P. FLANNERY, S.A. TEUKOLSKY & W.T. VETTERLING. 1988. Numerical Recipes in C. Cambridge University Press. London/New York.
16. BARNARD, A.C.L., J.M. DUCK, M.S. LYNN & W.P. TIMLAKE. 1967. The application of electromagnetic theory to electrocardiology II. Biophys. J. **7:** 463–491.
17. DE MUNCK, J.C., TH. J.C. FAES & R.M. HEETHAAR. 1998. The use of the boundary element method in electrical impedance tomography. *In* Boundary Element Research in Europe, p. 115–125. Computational Mechanics Pub. Southampton.
18. LOBRY, J. 1998. A new fast method for solving problems with moving boundary. *In* Boundary Element Research in Europe, p. 167–178. Computational Mechanics Pub. Southampton.

EIT Reconstruction of Static Images by a Genetic Algorithm Approach

R. OLMI, M. BINI, S. MANETTA, AND S. PRIORI

IROE-CNR (National Research Council), 50127 Firenze, Italy

ABSTRACT: A genetic algorithm (GA) approach is proposed for the reconstruction of static images in electrical impedance tomography (EIT). Genetic algorithms can be demonstrated to possess several advantages over more conventional "gradient-based" techniques. In particular, they are implicitly parallel and realize a good compromise between "exploration" and "exploitation", thus being more robust against the problem of false minima. The results of GA-EIT in numerical experiments are presented, compared to those obtained by other, more established inversion methods, such as the modified Newton-Raphson method and the double-constraint method. The GA approach is relatively expensive in terms of computation time and resources, requiring (for example) from several minutes to tens of minutes on a Pentium Pro 200–based machine for normal-size EIT problems. This currently limits the applicability of GA-EIT to the field of static imaging. However, in light of the development trend in the field of computing, an extension to real-time dynamic imaging applications is not inconceivable in the near future.

INTRODUCTION

The inverse problem of electrical impedance tomography (EIT) consists essentially of finding the coordinates of a point in an N-dimensional hyperspace, where N is the number of discrete elements whose union constitutes the tomographic section (TS) under consideration. The potentials measured on the boundary ∂TS are related to the currents injected through the boundary and to the N unknown conductivity values by a matrix equation like

$$\underline{\underline{S}}\phi = \underline{I} \qquad (1)$$

where $\underline{\underline{S}}$ is a matrix (usually coming from a finite element discretization procedure) implicitly containing the conductivity values, ϕ is the node potential vector (including potentials measured on ∂TS and unknown values inside TS), and $\underline{I}$ is the node current vector.

Rejecting the possibility of an inverse approach, that is, a "direct" solution of equation 1 with respect to the unknown quantities (element conductivities and internal node potentials), the problem is usually tackled in a direct way by the following:

(1) Guessing an N-tuple of coordinates (e.g., N conductivity or resistivity values).

(2) Solving the Laplace equation for the electric potential in TS, subjected to the suitable boundary conditions (injected current patterns and measured potential differences on the contour of the section), in the inhomogeneous medium where the conductivity was computed in the previous step.

(3) Computing some sort of error (or residue) involving measured and estimated potentials on the boundary of the region of interest. A possible choice is the sum of the squared differences between the two quantities.

(4) Finally, if the error is below a given acceptable value, the procedure terminates and the last computed N-tuple is taken as the problem solution. Otherwise, steps 1 to 3 are repeated.

It is well known that EIT reconstruction is an ill-posed problem and, as such, it is exposed to the problem of false minima. The "error" function is multimodal, that is, it presents several relative minima, and the reconstruction highly depends on the starting point (the initially guessed conductivity distribution).

The procedure outlined above converges to the "true" solution only in very rare cases. In general, reconstruction algorithms (especially those based on gradient methods) have a relevant probability to be trapped into a local minimum and, sometimes, the best solution of a "static" EIT problem is rather unsatisfactory.

These considerations suggest the possibility of usefully employing genetic algorithms (GAs) for the solution of the EIT problem. The notable characteristics of GAs can be summarized as follows:

- robustness, generality, and nonspecialization;
- no evaluation of function derivatives is needed;
- no assumption on function continuity is made—this makes GAs capable of optimizing either continuous or discontinuous functions.

GAs have been proved to be particularly suitable for the solution of multimodal problems because of their implicit parallelism.[1] The GA procedure used for EIT reconstruction is outlined in the following section.

METHODS

A genetic algorithm is a stochastic, adaptive method used in the solution of search and optimization problems,[1] inspired by Darwin's evolution theory. The method is applicable to all sorts of problems in which the solution can be represented as a set of parameters, called *genes*. A set of genes, that is, a possible solution, constitutes a *chromosome*. An objective function must also be defined for the problem (in GA lingo, it is called the *fitness* function), allowing the computation of a "figure of merit" for each guessed solution. The solution of a problem by a GA involves the generation of a *population* of guessed solutions, which are then evolved according to a "selection and reproduction" scheme based on the concept of "survival of the fittest", as described in detail in the next subsection.

The GA procedure is based on the sequential application of three operators:

(1) reproduction, which involves the selection of individuals from a population and their insertion in a "mating pool" that is used to produce the offspring generation;

(2) crossover, consisting of the exchange of genetic material between two tentative solutions (*parents*);

(3) mutation, consisting of the alteration of a single chromosome.

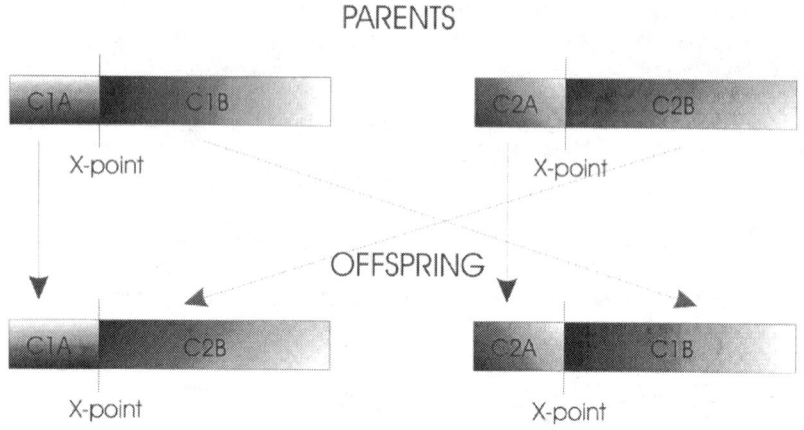

FIGURE 1. Principle of operation of single-point crossover.

Representing a chromosome by a string of binary digits, the simplest type of crossover (single-point crossover) is performed according to FIGURE 1. After a crossover point (X-point) is randomly chosen in the two parents (C_1 and C_2) selected for mating, two offspring are generated by exchanging the right-hand substrings (C_{1B} and C_{2B}) between the parents. More complex crossover procedures are commonly adopted in practical GAs (e.g., involving multiple X-points), but the principle of operation does not change.

The mutation operator acts on a single chromosome, as shown in FIGURE 2. Single mutation consists of randomly selecting a mutation point (M-point) and of complementing the chosen bit. As for crossover, other mutation procedures are sometimes used, essentially differing from that described here in the number of selected mutation points.

The crossover operator is used to produce new points in the search space starting from the "genetic" material present in the parent population, but it is not capable of building

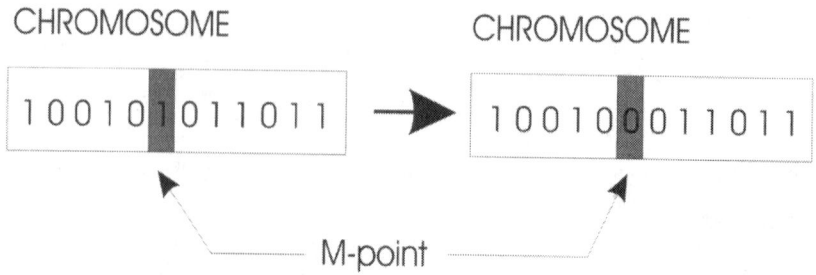

FIGURE 2. Principle of operation of single mutation.

new genetic material "from scratch", which is the task of the mutation operator. The former operator is usually applied on a large fraction of individuals, while the latter should be employed on a small fraction of individuals to avoid the degeneration of GA to a random search algorithm.

The Genetic Algorithm Approach to EIT

The flowchart of FIGURE 3 shows the principle of operation of GA. In the simplest implementation, a set (population) of tentative solutions (individuals) is generated, usually at random. For each individual, consisting of a sequence of N conductivity values (N is the number of elements discretizing the section under measurement), a *fitness* value is computed. The sequence of N conductivities characterizing an individual constitutes the *chromosome* or *genome*. In EIT applications, the fitness function is usually a function of the difference between the measured and computed potentials on the object boundary.

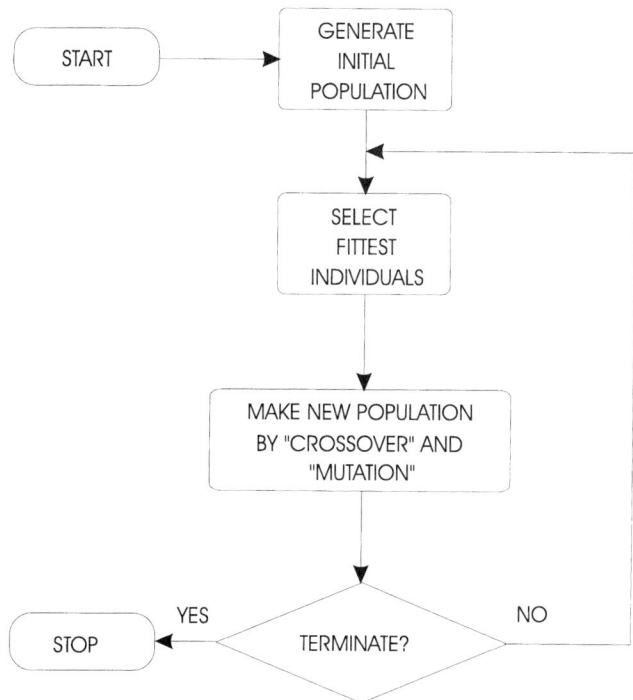

FIGURE 3. Flowchart of a simple genetic algorithm.

The next step is to rank the individuals according to their fitness value, giving to the fitter ones more chances to contribute to the successive iteration (generation). New individuals are then created by crossover (combination of couples of conductivity sequences) and mutation (low-probability random change of some conductivity value in the genome). After this step, the chosen termination criterion is applied, that is, we see if convergence has been reached (the residue is below a given value) or if the maximum number of generations has been exceeded. If the convergence test fails, the whole *selection + crossover + mutation* procedure is applied to the current population; otherwise, the fittest individual is assumed to be the solution of the EIT problem.

FIGURE 4 shows the representation chosen for the GA-EIT problem. Modeling, as usual, the cross section of the object under measurement by finite elements, a chromosome con-

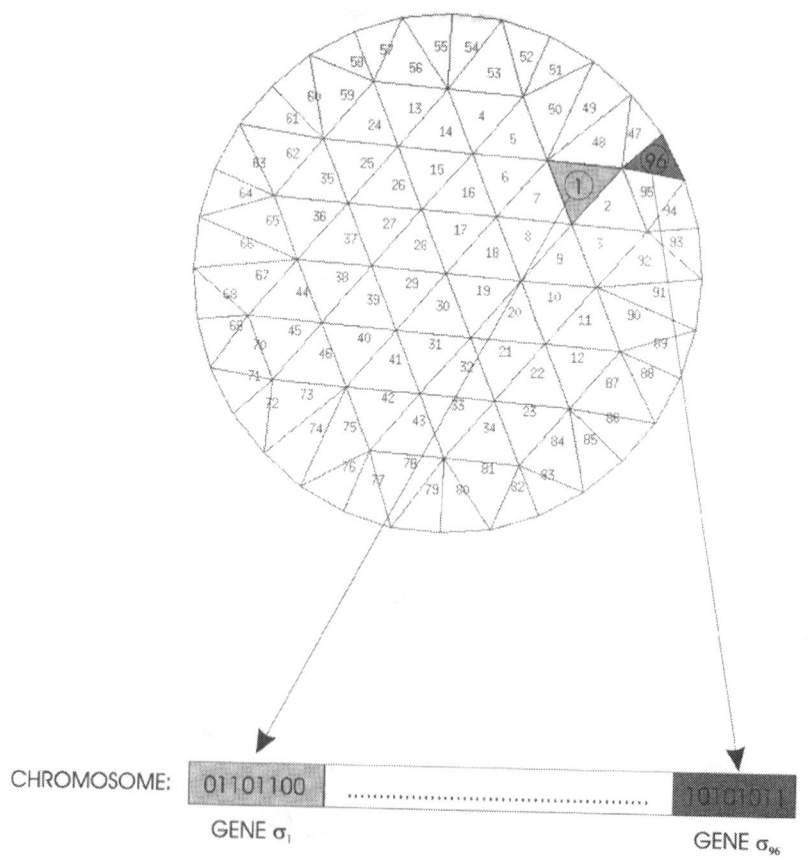

FIGURE 4. GA representation of the EIT problem.

sists of the sequence of conductivity values of the elements (i.e., in a tomographic image). The fitness function chosen for the problem involves the relative differences between the measured and computed potentials (respectively denoted by ϕ_{comp} and ϕ_{meas}):

$$fitness = N_c N_m \left[\sum_{j=1}^{N_c} \sum_{i=1}^{N_m} \left| \frac{\phi_{comp} - \phi_{meas}}{\phi_{meas}} \right| \right]^{-1} \quad (2)$$

where N_c is the number of current configurations (or projections) used and N_m is the number of measurements per configuration.

The actual GA-EIT reconstruction procedure consists of three nested algorithms. The first step serves to determine the best minimum and maximum conductivity values in the cross section. In this first GA, the chromosome consists of two real genes, representing the minimum (σ_{min}) and maximum (σ_{max}) values of the unknown conductivity distribution. The fitness function for this first problem is computed by equation 2 on a reduced population of tomographic images, randomly generated between σ_{min} and σ_{max} and evolved for a small number of generations.

The second step has the objective of determining a good starting value (σ_{start}) for the conductivity distribution. Here, the chromosome consists of a single real parameter and the fitness function is computed as in the first step.

In the third step, the actual EIT problem is solved by generating a full-size population of tomographic images, where the chromosome consists of an N-tuple of real genes (the N conductivity values in the cross section). In this last GA procedure, the initial population is

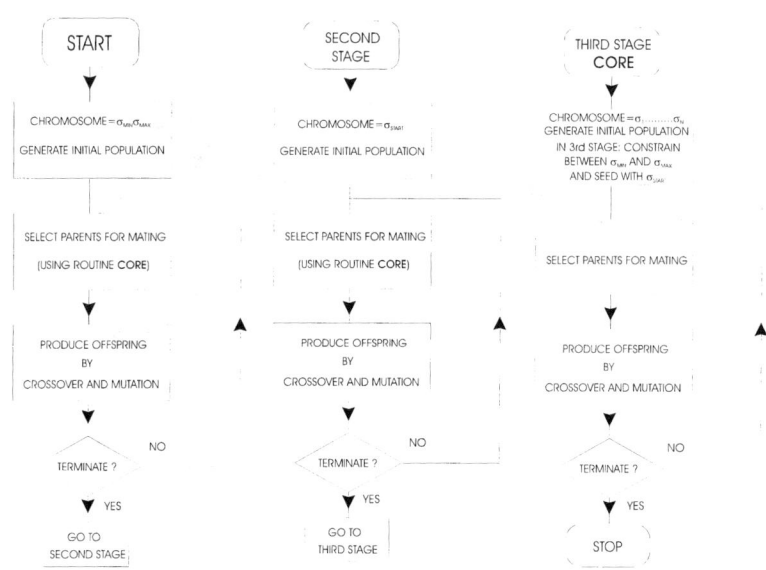

FIGURE 5. Three-step GA-EIT procedure.

constrained between σ_{min} and σ_{max} and seeded with σ_{start} (by imposing a couple of uniform tomographic images having a σ_{start} value). The entire three-step procedure is summarized in FIGURE 5.

Our implementation of GA-EIT uses overlapping populations, in which the best individuals of the "parent" generation survive to the detriment of the worst members of the "offspring" generation.

RESULTS

Comparison with Other Methods

GA-EIT has been tested by comparing the results obtained on numerical simulations with those obtained with two other methods: the modified Newton-Raphson method[2] and the double-constraint method.[3] As our attention is focused on "static" imaging, no method based on the back-projection between equipotential lines[4,5] has been used for the comparisons.

As an example of the results that can be obtained by GA-EIT, two simulations are presented:

- a square region (FIGURE 6a)—subdivided into 98 elements—having a conductivity value of 1 S/m and containing a rectangular conductivity region of 3 S/m;

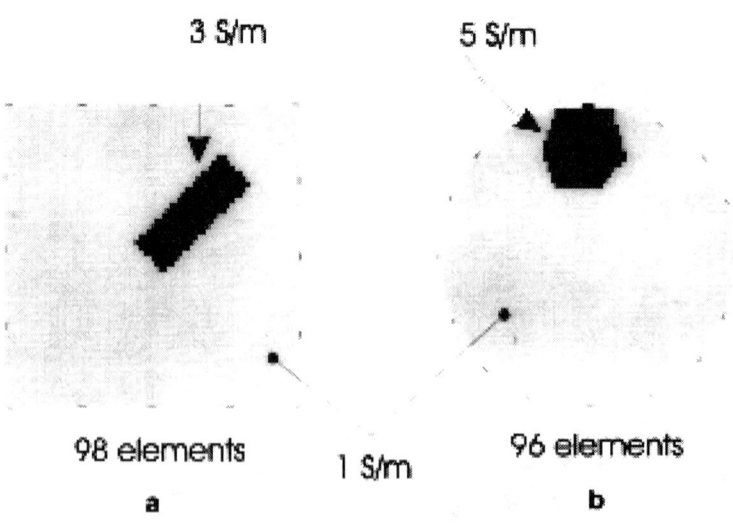

FIGURE 6. Rectangular (a) and circular (b) regions used for the simulations.

- a circular region (FIGURE 6b)—subdivided into 96 elements—presenting a circular conductivity region of 5 S/m in a background of 1 S/m.

Both cases assume 16 equispaced electrodes on the region boundary and data collection performed according to the neighboring method—with currents injected between adjacent pairs, a voltage reference electrode adjacent to the injection pair, and potential differences measured between the other 13 electrodes and the reference one. The neighboring method allows 16 different current configurations, for a total of 208 measurements.

The results of the comparison between GA-EIT and the other methods are shown in FIGURES 7 and 8. FIGURES 7a and 7b show the results obtained by GA-EIT on the square region with a population size of 16 and 32 individuals, respectively. FIGURE 7c shows the results obtained with the double-constraint method (which in this case performed better than Newton-Raphson). The faster reconstruction (FIGURE 7a) is good, but the slower one (FIGURE 7b) is practically perfect.

FIGURES 8a and 8b show the results obtained by GA-EIT on the circular region, with a population size of 16 and 32 individuals, respectively. FIGURE 8c shows the results obtained with the modified Newton-Raphson method with Marquardt regularization (which in this case performed better than double-constraint). As before, the 32-individual GA reconstruction (FIGURE 8b) is practically perfect. Also, for smaller population sizes (which means faster reconstruction), GA-EIT appears to reconstruct the object at least as well as the other methods.

Performance Analysis of GA-EIT

The dependence of the reconstruction error—the reciprocal of fitness computed by equation 2—on the number of generations and on the population size has been investigated for both problems described in the previous subsection. The results for the square problem are discussed here, with those for the circle problem being quite similar.

The error decreases with increasing generation, as shown in FIGURE 9 for population sizes ranging between 4 and 40 individuals. The error at a given generation generally decreases when population size is increased. However, it can be seen that the error does not depend linearly on the population size due to the stochastic nature of GAs: the error value at generation 490 for a population size of 8 is lower than that at generation 1000 for a population size of 40.

The dependence of the computation time on the population size has also been investigated. FIGURE 10 shows the time required to perform the computation on a workstation based on a Pentium Pro 200, with a termination condition of the following type:

$$if\ (1000\ generations)\ OR\ (error < 10^{-3}),\ then\ stop\ GA.$$

Three different computations were conducted for each population size, corresponding to the three bars of population size in FIGURE 10. The dependence of the computation time on the population size is almost linear, but again the stochastic nature of GAs reveals itself in a sharp deviation from linearity: in the third computation for a size of 24 individuals, for example, a time of 11 minutes was observed, while 24 minutes was needed in the first two computations for the same population size.

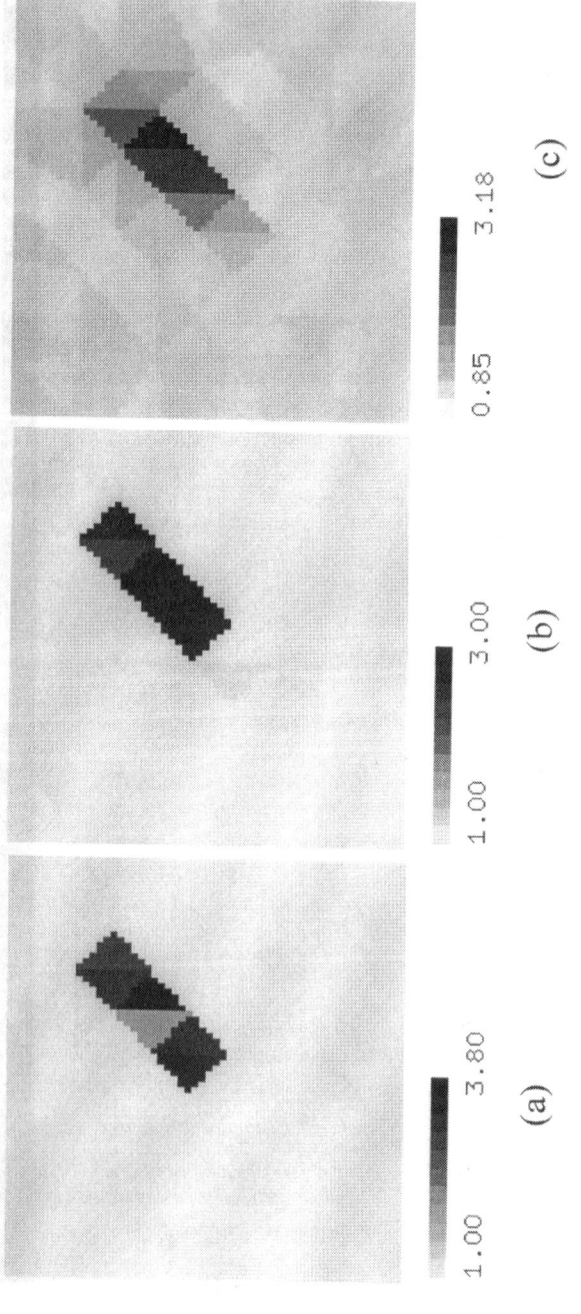

FIGURE 7. Output of reconstruction algorithms: (a) GA-EIT with 16 individuals; (b) GA-EIT with 32 individuals; (c) double-constraint.

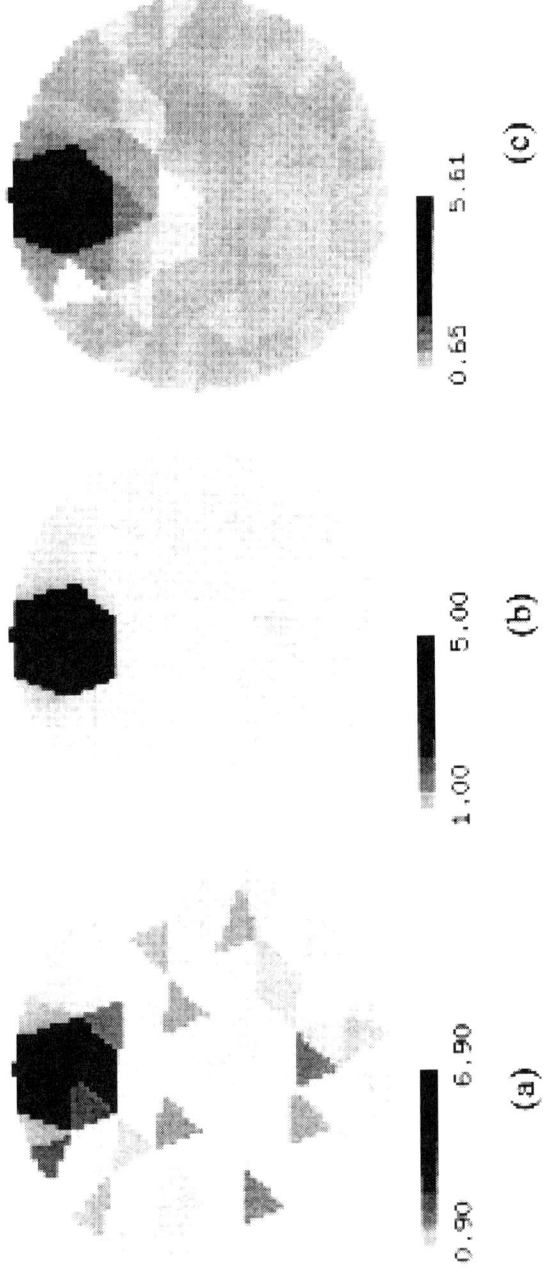

FIGURE 8. Output of reconstruction algorithms: (a) GA-EIT with 16 individuals; (b) GA-EIT with 32 individuals; (c) Newton-Raphson with Marquardt regularization.

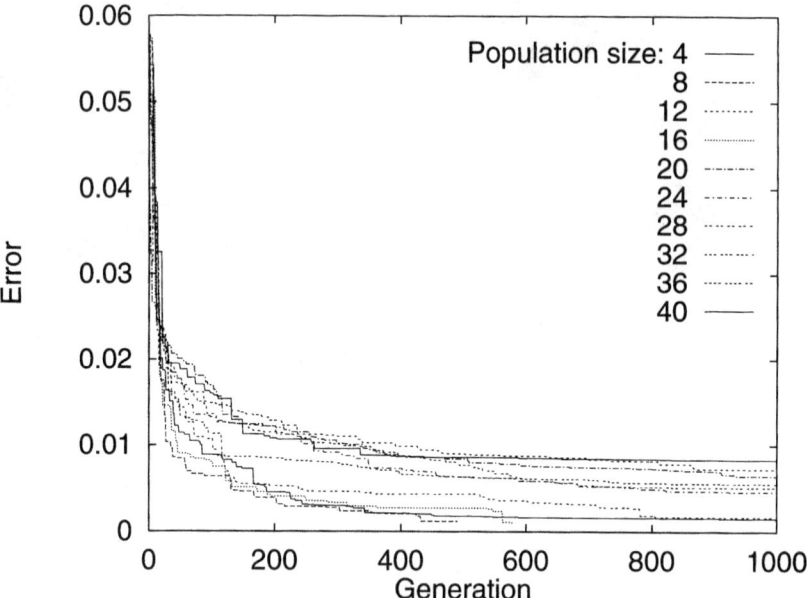

FIGURE 9. Dependence of the reconstruction error on the number of generations.

CONCLUSIONS

Genetic algorithms appear to be a promising tool for the solution of the EIT problem. Although rather expensive in terms of computation time and resources, which renders them presently unsuitable for real-time tomographic applications, GAs often outperform other more conventional techniques, converging to a "good" solution with practically no a priori knowledge.

With a suitable design of the reconstruction algorithm (we have employed a nested three-step GA), the probability of false convergence has been shown to be reduced to negligible levels, at least for the two-region problems developed so far.

In principle, the exploitation of a priori knowledge (concerning, for example, the range of conductivities in the EIT image) should allow one to obtain very good reconstructions and should substantially reduce the computation time. A faster procedure, combining the exploration power of GAs with the exploitation of knowledge typical of gradient-based techniques, is currently under development.

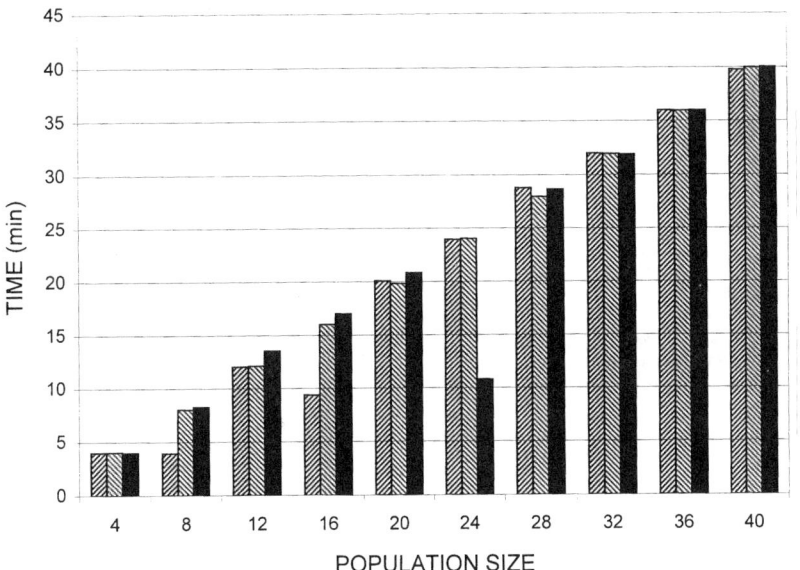

FIGURE 10. Dependence of the computation time on the population size.

REFERENCES

1. GOLDBERG, D.E. 1989. Genetic Algorithms in Search, Optimization, and Machine Learning. Addison–Wesley. Reading, Massachusetts.
2. WEXLER, A., B. FRY & M.R. NEUMAN. 1985. Impedance-computed tomography algorithm and system. Appl. Optics **24**(no. 3): 3985–3992.
3. YORKEY, T.J., J.G. WEBSTER & W.J. TOMPKINS. 1987. Comparing reconstruction algorithms for electrical impedance tomography. IEEE Trans. Biomed. Eng. **BME-34**(no. 11): 843–852.
4. BARBER, D.C. & A.D. SEAGAR. 1987. Fast reconstruction of resistance images. Clin. Phys. Physiol. Meas. **8**(suppl. 2A): 47–54.
5. HUA, P. & E.J. WOO. 1990. Reconstruction algorithms. *In* Electrical Impedance Tomography, p. 97–137. Adam Hilger. Bristol/New York.

Uniqueness, Shape, and Dimension in EIT

WILLIAM R. B. LIONHEART

Electrical Impedance Tomography Research Group, School of Computing and Mathematical Sciences, Oxford Brookes University, Oxford OX3 0BP, United Kingdom

ABSTRACT: We briefly review the known mathematical results on uniqueness of solution in electrical impedance tomography (EIT). Generally, a real or complex conductivity is determined uniquely by complete boundary data. Uniqueness results are also known for planar resistor networks. However, it is common to make gross errors in the forward modeling of the electrical fields and this may result in no consistent solution. In particular, a two-dimensional model is often used when data are collected from a three-dimensional domain. The boundary shape is often inaccurately known, and commonly modeled by a circle. No model conductivity consistent with measured data exists when the dimension or the boundary shape is wrong.

UNIQUENESS OF SOLUTION

Electrical impedance tomography seeks to recover the interior conductivity from measurements of current and voltage on the boundary of a body. It is important to ask from the start if the inverse problem of recovering the unknown conductivity from boundary data has a unique solution. This has been an active area of mathematical research since the early 1980s. There are many useful results as well as some unanswered questions. For the direct current case, Maxwell's equations reduce to

$$\nabla \cdot (\sigma \nabla \phi) = 0 \qquad (1)$$

which is the continuum version of Kirchhoff's and Ohm's law. Suppose the potential ϕ is known on the boundary for every possible pattern of injected current $j = \sigma \partial \phi / \partial \mathbf{n}$ (here, $\mathbf{n}$ is the unit outward normal to the boundary). There is only one conductivity $\sigma(x,y,z)$ that results in this complete set of boundary data, provided that the conductivity satisfies certain smoothness conditions. Most of the known uniqueness results are summarized by Isakov,[1] to whom we refer the reader for uniqueness results quoted without references. For the three-dimensional case, a conductivity with at least two bounded derivatives is uniquely determined by complete data. In the two-dimensional case, two derivatives (in the generalized sense) that are square-integrable are sufficient. Less is known about the more realistic case of discontinuous conductivities; however, in the case where the conductivity is piecewise analytic (possibly discontinuous on analytic curves), uniqueness holds.

If only the internal boundaries of a piecewise constant conductivity need to be recovered, there are some useful results in the two-dimensional case. In particular, certain simply connected domains can be uniquely identified by a single set of boundary voltage and current data. For recent results on reconstructing unknown internal boundaries, see reference 2.

Of course, real EIT systems use a finite number of electrodes to inject current and measure voltage. Very little is known about uniqueness in this case, although it is obvious that one cannot recover more unknown parameters of the conductivity than the number of independent measurements. If one models the body by a planar resistor network with sufficient connections and only $N(N-1)/2$ resistors, where N is the number of electrodes, then it is known that the resistor values, and the topology of the resistor network up to star-delta transformations, can be determined from current and voltage measurements at these electrodes.[3] In the bioimpedance case, we would prefer this result to extend to RC networks, but it is not known if that is the case.

When an alternating current is used, neglecting transient effects, the time-harmonic Maxwell's equations can be assumed to apply:

$$\nabla \times \mathbf{E} = j\omega\mu\mathbf{H}$$
$$\nabla \times \mathbf{H} = -j(\sigma + j\omega\varepsilon)\mathbf{E}. \qquad (2)$$

In this case, we have three unknown inhomogeneous scalar fields—σ, ε, and μ. If these are three times differentiable, then Ola et al.[4] have proved that they are uniquely determined from complete measurements of tangential electric and magnetic fields at the boundary, for a single fixed (nonresonant) frequency ω. However, in the bioimpedance case at sufficiently low frequencies, we can neglect $\omega\mu$, in which case we have the same equation as the direct current case with the conductivity replaced by the complex admittivity $\sigma + j\omega\varepsilon$. In this case, a complete knowledge of the complex current and voltage data at the boundary is sufficient to uniquely determine the admittivity.

THE ANISOTROPIC CASE

Biological tissue often has anisotropic electrical properties. In this case, the conductivity is replaced by a symmetric matrix. This means that we have six unknowns—σ_{11}, σ_{22}, σ_{33}, σ_{12}, σ_{23}, and σ_{13}—at each point. In this case, the conductivity matrix is not uniquely determined by boundary data. It is easy to construct two matrix-valued conductivity functions that give rise to the same data—one simply chooses them to be related by a coordinate change that preserves coordinates on the boundary. One cannot tell if the conductivity in the interior has been distorted, provided that distortion does not change the boundary. At least for analytical conductivities in three dimensions, this is the only ambiguity and we can recover the six unknown functions with an ambiguity of three functions. In two dimensions, essentially the same result is true for conductivities that are three times differentiable. Furthermore, if accurate *in vivo* conductivity measurements of anisotropic tissue are required, one must obtain information in addition to the boundary electrical measurements. One option is to estimate the principal directions of the conductivity matrix at each point using anatomical data, such as the alignment of muscle fibers, from magnetic resonance images. Some uniqueness results for the anisotropic uniqueness problem with additional data are given in reference 5. No results are known for the anisotropic full Maxwell's equations.

MODELING ERRORS

In electrical impedance tomography, some forward model must be used to solve for the electrical fields, given some assumed conductivity distribution. This may take the form of an analytical or semianalytical solution where a simple linear algorithm is used with simple geometry and a homogeneous background, or a finite element model where more general geometry or an inhomogeneous initial conductivity is used.

Often for reasons of simplicity or speed, a two-dimensional forward model is used for a three-dimensional domain. Similarly, a simple circular geometry is often assumed for the boundary when in fact the boundary has an irregular shape.

A reconstruction algorithm attempts to find a conductivity in the forward model that best fits the measured current and voltage data. If the model is wrong, it is interesting to know if there is some model conductivity that will exactly match the measured data. If there is not, then the algorithm will not converge; if there is, it may converge to a misleading result. Usually, the former case would be preferable.

ERRORS IN DIMENSION

Zero Height Electrodes

Let us suppose that we collect EIT data on some three-dimensional body, but restrict our measurements to some plane. Let us make the idealized assumption that our current drive electrodes are points and we can make point voltage measurements on the specified plane. If a point source of current is applied to the surface of a three-dimensional domain, even one of smoothly varying conductivity, the resulting potential will be of order $1/r$ as the distance r from the source tends to zero. By contrast, a point source applied to the surface of a two-dimensional domain will result in a potential with a singularity of order $\log r$. We see from this argument that it is possible to determine if one has a two- or a three-dimensional domain provided that one can measure sufficiently close to a drive electrode. Consequently, one cannot find a two-dimensional model conductivity consistent with the data collected from a three-dimensional domain with zero height electrodes.

The Separable Case

If the conductivity separates in some coordinate system, such as $\sigma(x,y,z) = s(x,y)\zeta(z)$, then it is possible to use the separation of variables in the solution of the forward problem $\nabla \cdot \sigma \nabla \phi = 0$. The particular case of $\zeta = 1$ of the translation invariant conductivity was analyzed by Ider et al.[6] Let us assume for simplicity, following reference 6, that the domain is the cylinder $x^2 + y^2 \leq R^2$, $-a \leq z \leq a$. Measurements will be made on the plane $z = 0$.

It is easy to check that the potential has the form

$$\phi(x, y, z) = \sum_{k=0}^{\infty} V_k(x, y) \cos\left(\frac{k\pi}{a}\right) z \qquad (3)$$

where each V_k satisfies the two-dimensional partial differential equation

$$\nabla \cdot s \nabla V_k - s(k\pi/a)^2 V_k = 0. \qquad (4)$$

Now suppose that the current density on the boundary satisfies $J(\theta,z) = f(\theta)g(z)$, where

$$g(z) = \sum_{k=0}^{\infty} c_k \cos\left(\frac{k\pi}{a}\right) z.$$

Then, the boundary condition for V_k is

$$s\frac{\partial V_k}{\partial n} = c_k f(\theta).$$

Suppose that we apply our current using electrodes of height h so that $g(z) = 1/h$ for $|z| < h/2$ and $g(z) = 0$ elsewhere. Hence,

$$c_0 = h/a \quad \text{and} \quad c_k = \left(\frac{2}{kh\pi}\right)\sin\left(\frac{k\pi h}{2a}\right) \quad \text{for} \quad k > 0.$$

In the extreme case, $h = a$ electrodes run the full height of the cylinder and we have a genuinely two-dimensional problem. Here, $V_k = 0$, except for $k = 0$, and we can solve the usual conductivity equation for two dimensions. As h/a becomes smaller, the series (3) for ϕ converges more slowly and we will have to solve more two-dimensional forward problems (4) to get the same accuracy. In the other extreme case where $h \to 0$, we have $g(z) = \delta(z)/a$ and $c_k = 1/a$. Here, the series (3) for ϕ is divergent at $z = 0$ because the potential will generally have a log $|z|$ singularity where $f(\theta) \neq 0$.

This analysis gives a clue as to why EIT reconstruction algorithms that use two-dimensional models of three-dimensional domains work to some extent. If the conductivity is approximately translation invariant (this is only a very crude approximation in the thorax for example, but perhaps better on a limb), then the error in assuming a two-dimensional model is the error in truncating the series (3) at the first term. This error diminishes as the height of the electrode increases.

As yet, no uniqueness results are known for the recovery of a translationally invariant conductivity from EIT data in the plane. However, the inverse problem has been solved numerically by Ider et al.[6] and by Butler and Bonnecaze.[7]

INCORRECT BOUNDARY SHAPE

The Two-Dimensional Case

As we have seen, it is unwise to model a three-dimensional region using a two-dimensional model, unless the conductivity and the current drive electrodes are translationally invariant. Let us suppose that we are in this situation, in which case the model and the body can be assumed to be two-dimensional. We will also assume that the conductivity is isotropic.

The two-dimensional case is special in that there is a rich variety of conformal mappings that can transform any smooth simply connected domain to any other. Conformal mappings are smooth invertible transformations that preserve angle, but not length. Suppose that σ and ϕ are conductivity and potential fields satisfying the two-dimensional conductivity equation $\nabla \cdot \sigma \nabla \phi = 0$. A conformal mapping transforms $\sigma \to \tilde{\sigma}$ and $\phi \to \tilde{\phi}$, where $\nabla \cdot \tilde{\sigma} \nabla \tilde{\phi} = 0$. The boundary current density $\sigma(\partial \phi/\partial \mathbf{n})ds$, where s is the arc length coordinate on the boundary of the domain, is invariant under conformal mappings.

Suppose now that we do not know the shape of the boundary, but we measure all current and voltage data with respect to some coordinate on the boundary. This corresponds roughly to knowing the electrode numbering, but not their spacing. To make the current measurement independent of the length scale, we assume that the cumulative current

$$I(s) = \int_0^s \sigma \partial \phi / \partial \mathbf{n} \, ds \tag{5}$$

is known together with the corresponding potential φ(s). Assuming some shape for the boundary, suppose that we reconstruct a conductivity consistent with these data. If we apply any conformal mapping to this domain and conductivity, the result will still be consistent with the measured data. As a consequence, we would expect to be able to reconstruct a consistent conductivity using the wrong boundary shape, and our image would be a conformal distortion of the true image.

However, this model of measurement may be unrealistic. For example, if the length scale on the boundary were known—imagine, for example, the electrodes were placed with the aid of a tape measure—then these data would not be invariant under conformal mappings, except for rotations and translations. In this case, only a model with the correct boundary shape and size would fit the measured data.

The Three-Dimensional Case

Conformal mappings are well known in two dimensions from complex analysis. Among the well-known conformal mappings are the Möbius transformations that correspond to inversions with respect to a circle. In three-dimensional space, the situation is very different. The only conformal mappings that are not similarities (combinations of translations, rotations, reflections, and dilations) are the three-dimensional Möbius transformations. Like their counterparts in two dimensions, these Möbius transformations preserve parts of circles and, of course, parts of spheres too. Here, we treat straight lines and planes as circles and spheres of infinite radius. See FIGURE 1 for an example.

For an isotropic three-dimensional body, boundary potential and current are invariant under conformal mappings. As in the two-dimensional case, this is the only ambiguity in the boundary shape.

Hence, the shape of our model must be related to the true boundary shape by a conformal mapping. Unlike the two-dimensional case where any two simply connected domains are so related, this is quite a rare occurrence in three dimensions. The set of conformal mappings can be described by 10 parameters. Of these, 7 come from the group of similari-

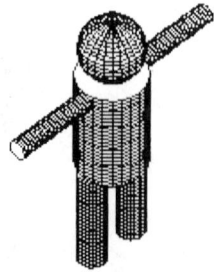 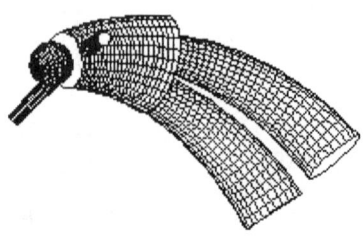

FIGURE 1. A Möbius transformation applied to a simple geometric figure. Note the preservation of circles and spheres.

ties, which simply means that one cannot determine position, orientation, and overall size by EIT measurement. Three suitably chosen measurements of the geometry of the boundary together with complete EIT data determine both the shape and the conductivity of the body. An example of such a set of measurements is found in reference 8, where further mathematical details of the above arguments are given.

Therefore, it can be seen that EIT data contain information about both the shape and conductivity and that it is unlikely that a consistent conductivity will be found if one gets the shape wrong.

CONCLUSIONS

The ideal when imaging three-dimensional bodies with irregular shape is to use a three-dimensional model with measured boundary shape. If the model shape is incorrect and the conductivity is isotropic, then there is no consistent conductivity for the model that will fit the data. This will be observed as a large residual voltage error, so any image produced will be known to be unreliable.

If measurements are taken in the plane, and the conductivity has approximate translational invariance perpendicular to the plane, then one must either use very tall drive electrodes if using a two-dimensional model or use the correct forward model as described by Ider et al.[6] If a length scale on the boundary is fixed in the two-dimensional case, then (as in the three-dimensional case) no consistent conductivity can be found when the model has incorrect boundary shape.

REFERENCES

1. ISAKOV, V. 1998. Inverse problems for partial differential equations. *In* Applied Mathematical Sciences, p. 127. Springer Pub. New York.
2. FRANK, H. & W. RUNDELL. 1998. The determination of a discontinuity in a conductivity from a single boundary measurement. Inverse Probl. **14:** 67–82.
3. COLIN DE VERDIERE, Y., I. GITLER & D. VERTIGAN. 1996. Reseaux electriques planaires II. Comment. Math. Helv. **71:** 144–167.
4. OLA, P., L. PAEIVAERINTA & E. SOMERSALO. 1993. An inverse boundary value problem in electrodynamics. Duke Math. J. **70**(no. 3): 617–653.
5. LIONHEART, W.R.B. 1997. Conformal uniqueness results in anisotropic electrical impedance imaging. Inverse Probl. **13:** 125–134.
6. IDER, Y.Z., N.G. GENCER, E. ATALAR & H. TOSUN. 1990. Electrical-impedance tomography of translationally uniform cylindrical objects with general cross-sectional boundaries. IEEE Trans. Med. Imaging **9**(no. 1): 49–59.
7. BUTLER, J.E. & R.T. BONNECAZE. 1997. Imaging of particle shear migration with electrical impedance tomography. American Institute of Chemical Engineers Annual Meeting.
8. LIONHEART, W.R.B. 1998. Boundary shape and electrical impedance tomography. Inverse Probl. **14:** 139–147.

Static Three-Dimensional Electrical Impedance Tomography

PÄIVI J. VAUHKONEN, MARKO VAUHKONEN, TUOMO SAVOLAINEN, AND JARI P. KAIPIO

Department of Applied Physics, University of Kuopio, 70211 Kuopio, Finland

ABSTRACT: In electrical impedance tomography, an approximation for the internal resistivity distribution is computed based on the knowledge of the voltages and currents on the surface of the body. Usually, it is assumed that the injected currents stay at the two-dimensional (2D) electrode plane and the reconstruction is based on 2D assumptions. However, the currents spread out in three dimensions (3D) and therefore the structures out of the current injection plane may have significant effect on the reconstructed images. We have studied possibilities of a finite element–based method to reconstruct static 3D images from real measurements made on a saline-filled tank. We show that the 3D static images obtained from simple experiments are better than the 2D difference images obtained from the same object. We further show that the static images obtained with 2D calculations are much worse than the images obtained with 3D calculations. We also discuss the effects of the boundary shape error on the reconstructed static 3D images.

INTRODUCTION

In electrical impedance tomography (EIT), images are produced by approximating the resistivity distribution within the subject. Currents are applied to the object using electrodes and the resulting voltages on the electrodes are measured. The internal resistivity distribution is computed based on these boundary data. There are many applications of this technology in medical and industrial use.[1]

In 2D EIT, currents are injected using an array of electrodes attached around an object. The images are reconstructed based on the assumption that the injected currents are confined to the two-dimensional electrode plane. However, the electric current spreads out in three dimensions and, if this is not considered in the reconstruction, off-plane structures may cause many errors, especially in static electrical impedance tomography.

Three-dimensional EIT methods have been discussed earlier, for example, in references 2–7. However, all these methods are based on simplified electrode models and they have shown results only for difference imaging. Quite often, also, the geometry has been fixed in order to be able to compute analytical solutions for the forward model. This approach is suitable for situations in which we are only interested in the dynamical behavior of the object. However, if absolute (static) resistivity values and images are needed, a more accurate approach has to be taken.

In this paper, we discuss the estimation of static 3D resistivity distributions. We use the so-called complete electrode model to describe the EIT measurements. The finite element method (FEM) is used to obtain a discretization of the governing equations. The FEM is suitable for complicated geometries and boundary conditions that exist in EIT when a real measurement situation is considered. The solution of the static 3D resistivity estimation problem is based on the generalized Tikhonov regularization.[8] We evaluate the proposed method with the real measurements made from a cylindrical saline-filled tank. We further show a difference between 2D and 3D static reconstructions. Also, effects of the boundary shape error are discussed.

METHODS

The methods for the reconstruction of impedance images are based on mathematical models that connect the internal resistivity distribution to the measurements made on the surface of the object. In this study, we have used the so-called complete electrode model because it is the most accurate model for the EIT since it can take into account the effects of the electrodes and the contact impedances between the object and the electrodes.[9–13] For the numerical solution of the complete electrode model, we have used finite element discretization and tetrahedral (triangular in the 2D case) elements with the second-order FEM basis (shape functions) in both 2D and 3D cases.

Difference Imaging

In difference imaging, two different data sets are used and the reconstruction is based on the voltage difference δU between these measurements. It is well known that the systematic and geometric errors are canceled in difference imaging.

The reconstruction of the resistivity distribution based on the surface measurements is a nonlinear problem. However, if we can assume that the resistivity distribution is a small perturbation from some assumed distribution (usually uniform), it is often adequate to solve only a linearized version of the problem.

Because of the ill-posedness of the problem, regularization methods have to be used. We used the generalized Tikhonov regularization in order to obtain stable solutions.[8] If we assume that the measured voltages can be approximated as (linearization)

$$U_{meas} \approx U(\rho_0) + J\rho - J\rho_0, \qquad (1)$$

the regularized version of the linearized EIT reconstruction problem can be written in the form

$$\min_{\rho} \{ \|\tilde{U} - J\rho\|^2 + \|L(\rho - \rho_0)\|^2 \} \qquad (2)$$

where J is the Jacobian of $U(\rho)$ with respect to ρ, $\tilde{U} = U_{meas} - U(\rho_0) + J\rho_0$, and L is a regularization matrix. The solution for equation 2 is

$$\delta\rho = (J^T J + L^T L)^{-1} (J^T \delta U) \qquad (3)$$

where $\delta\rho = \rho - \rho_0$ is the estimated resistivity change and $\delta U = U_{meas} - U(\rho_0)$ is the measured voltage change. The Jacobian is calculated in a reference distribution ρ_0 (usually a uniform distribution) with the aid of the so-called standard method.[14] The regularization matrix

$$L = \begin{bmatrix} \alpha_1 L_1 \\ \alpha_2 L_2 \end{bmatrix} \qquad (4)$$

that we used in the reconstruction approximates the directional derivatives in three dimensions. The parameters α_1 and α_2 are the regularization parameters. In L_1, we take into account ten nearest elements from the horizontal plane; in L_2, we take into account two nearest elements from the vertical plane, except on the bottom and on the top of the discretized image where we take into account only one nearest element. The chosen elements are weighted by the inverse of the distances between the centers of the elements. The regularization parameters were adjusted *a posteriori* by visual examination. In 2D cases, we used $L = \alpha_1 L_1$ as a regularization matrix. It should be noted that this type of regularization may not be the optimal one and we should use, for example, a total variation approach in the regularization (e.g., see references 15–17).

Static Imaging

In static imaging, we have one set of voltage measurements and even in the solution of the linearized problem only we need to calculate the measurements $U(\rho_0, z_0)$ that correspond to the linearization distribution ρ_0 with great accuracy. If the original nonlinear problem is to be solved, these measurements have to be solved in each iteration step. The solution to equation 2 can be written in the form

$$\rho = \rho_0 + (J^T J + L^T L)^{-1}(J^T[U_{meas} - U(\rho_0, z_0)]). \tag{5}$$

The linearization point (or the initial guess if the nonlinear problem is to be solved) ρ_0 has been chosen in the following way. By investigating the formula for U_l, we obtain[18]

$$U(\rho_0, z_0) = \rho_0 U(1, \tau) \tag{6}$$

where $\tau = z_0/\rho_0$, and ρ_0 and z_0 are constants. If we fix τ to some value, we could solve the homogeneous resistivity distribution $\rho \equiv \rho_0$. However, due to the systematic errors in the difference voltage measurements caused, for example, by the signal coupling in the multiplexers and input circuits, we found it better to model these errors with an additional constant function. Therefore, we modeled the measurements as

$$U_{meas} = H\tilde{\rho}. \tag{7}$$

Here,

$$H = [\mathbf{1}\ U(1, \tau)] \quad \text{and} \quad \tilde{\rho} = \begin{pmatrix} c \\ \rho_0 \end{pmatrix} \tag{8}$$

where $\mathbf{1} = (1, 1, \ldots, 1)^T$ and c is a constant. Now, the minimization problem becomes

$$\min_{\rho} \|U_{meas} - H\tilde{\rho}\| \tag{9}$$

and the solution is

$$\tilde{\rho}_{est} = (H^T H)^{-1} H^T U_{meas}, \tag{10}$$

from which the reference voltages can be computed as

$$U(\rho_0, z_0) = H\tilde{\rho}_{\text{est}}. \tag{11}$$

A similar approach has also been used in reference 19.

For the 3D inverse computations, we grouped the tetrahedra that were used in the forward calculations so that the union of three tetrahedra composed one element for the inverse calculations.

RESULTS

In this study, we have used real measurements made from a cylindrical tank (radius 15 cm and height 30 cm) with 48 electrodes, having 16 electrodes in three planes; see FIGURE 1. The measurements were carried out with a measurement system that is based on a PC computer, commercial data acquisition board and software, and an external current generation and switching board.[20] The tank was filled up to 20 cm from the bottom with the saline. On the bottom of the tank, halfway from the center to the edge, there was an agar target having a radius of 3 cm and a height of approximately 8 cm. The resistivity of the target in two experiments was either 81 Ωcm or 161 Ωcm and the resistivity of the saline was approximately 430 Ωcm. We injected currents and measured voltages between adjacent electrodes so that the measurements or current injections between the adjacent or between the lowest and the highest electrode planes were not used. Voltages measured on the current-carrying electrodes were not used in the reconstructions.

Results from the 3D static reconstructions with the second-order FEM basis are shown in FIGURES 2–5. The reconstructed mean resistivity was 171 Ωcm or 226 Ωcm on the target area, while the true resistivity was 81 Ωcm or 161 Ωcm, respectively. As one can notice, the calculated values are too high. This is because we have used only one step reconstructor, which is capable of estimating only small resistivity changes. Another reason is the regularization that assumes that the resistivity distributions are smooth.[13]

As a comparison, we reconstructed 2D static and difference images from the same objects. As a regularization matrix, we used the horizontal part of L, that is, the matrix $\alpha_1 L_1$. Static 2D reconstructions from the first experiment are shown in FIGURE 6. As one can see, the cross-sectional images are qualitatively much worse than the 3D static images. The reference voltage was computed in a mesh of 1192 elements and 2513 nodes.

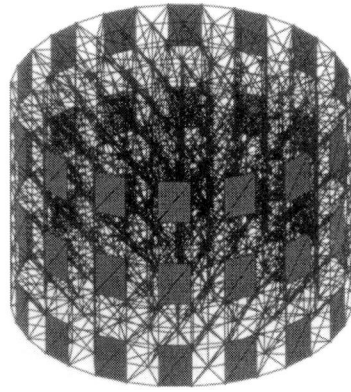

FIGURE 1. An example of the finite element mesh used in the calculations. Darkened elements are located under the electrodes.

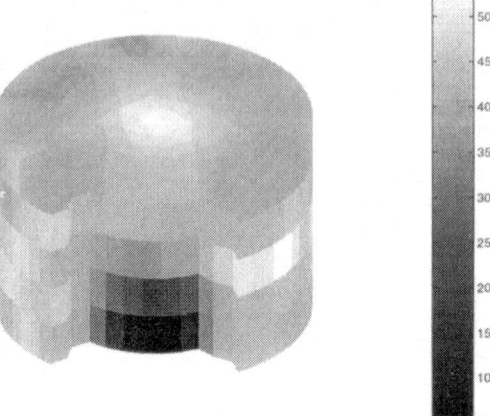

FIGURE 2. A static reconstruction from real measurements. The reference voltage has been calculated in a mesh of 6180 elements and 9779 nodes with second-order basis functions. Reconstruction with 2060 parameters. The true (measured) resistivity of the target was 81 Ωcm and the resistivity of the saline was 430 Ωcm. The mean resistivity of the target was 171 Ωcm.

From the difference images shown in FIGURES 7 and 8, there is a more distinct "shadow" of the target on the middle electrode plane (electrode plane 2) than in the 3D cases in FIGURES 3 and 5, on plane 3. Also, the reconstruction from the measurements of the first electrode plane is qualitatively worse in the 2D case than in fully 3D reconstruction.

We also tested the effect of the boundary shape error on the static reconstruction (FIGURE 9). In the reconstruction, we assumed the boundary shape to be slightly elliptic instead of being circular. The maximum error in the radius was 1%. As can be seen, even a small error in the forward model causes errors in the reconstructed image. If we increased the shape error to 3%, we could not reconstruct the static image.

CONCLUSIONS

In static imaging, the accuracy requirement of the computed potentials on the electrodes that correspond to the (initial) distribution ρ_0 is very high. It was found that the required accuracy (with the size of the mesh that was used) can be obtained with the 3D FEM when second-order basis functions are used. In principle, this required accuracy could also be obtained with the first-order basis, but this would necessitate the construction of another much more dense mesh.

When 2D calculations were applied to the 3D situation, a quite evident result was found. Static images could not be reconstructed from 3D data, at least not with high accuracy. If we wish to obtain static images from humans, we should carefully consider the boundary conditions in the "cutting planes", or the termination boundaries, of the FEM mesh. In this study, we were able to proceed with accurate boundary conditions (no cur-

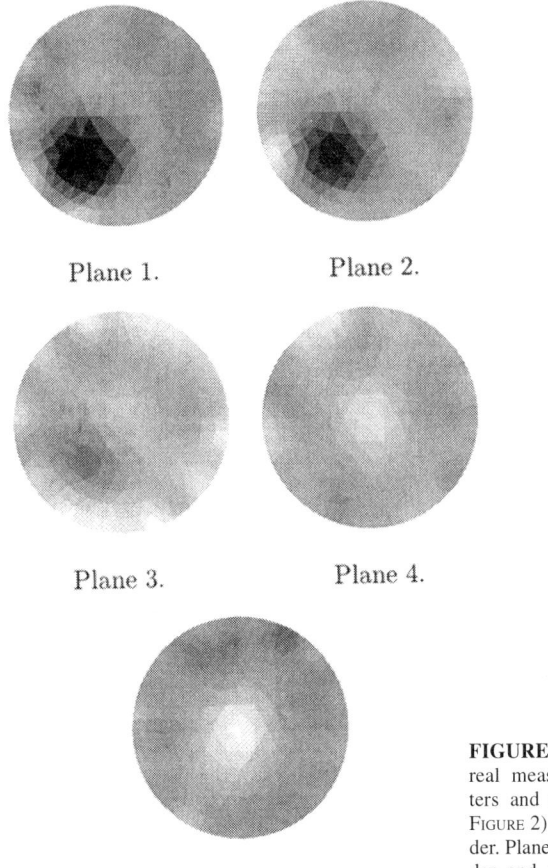

FIGURE 3. Static reconstruction from real measurements with 2060 parameters and the second-order FEM (as in FIGURE 2) in different planes of the cylinder. Plane 1 is on the bottom of the cylinder and plane 5 is on the top of the cylinder.

rent flow out from the bottom or top of the saline-filled cylinder), but in practice this would not be the case. Also, the boundary shape should be known accurately since even small errors in the boundary shape were shown to cause large errors in the reconstruction.

The proposed approach does not impose any restrictions on the geometry of the object (boundary) and therefore it is also possible to reconstruct images from humans without simplifying the geometry. This is especially important if static images are considered.

In order to obtain more accurate images, it is possible to increase somewhat the quality of the estimate by increasing the number of electrodes and the reconstructed parameters. However, it is as yet not clear to which task one should direct the effort—for example, the increase of the number of electrodes, the improvement of the regularization, the estimation of feasible conditions for the termination boundary, or the accuracy of the geometrical modeling of the object boundary. Also, due to the practical aspects in the human experiments, a certain limit in the number of electrodes is evident.

478 ANNALS NEW YORK ACADEMY OF SCIENCES

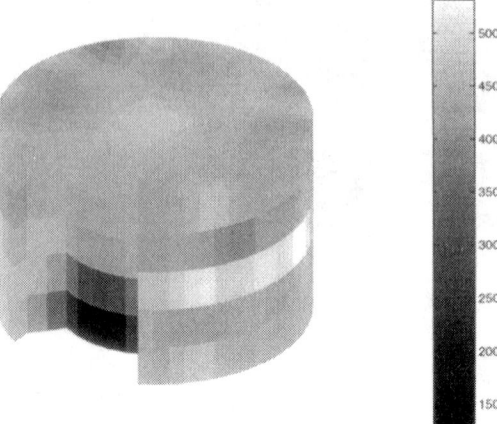

FIGURE 4. Same as in FIGURE 2, but the resistivity of the target was 161 Ωcm and the resistivity of the saline was 432 Ωcm. The mean resistivity of the target was 226 Ωcm.

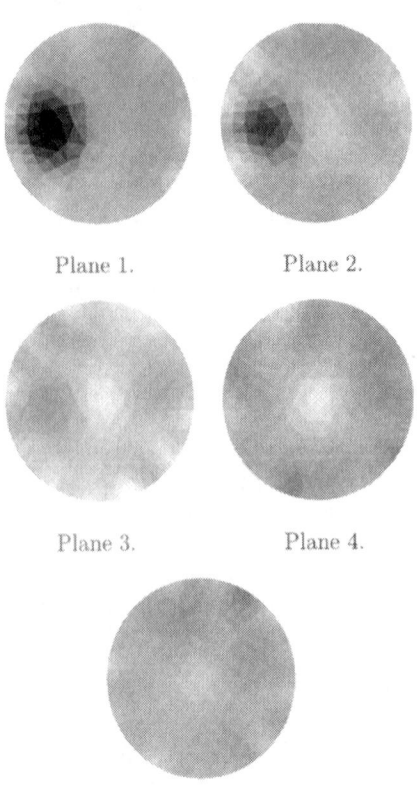

FIGURE 5. Static reconstruction from real measurements with 2060 parameters and the second-order FEM (as in FIGURE 4) in different planes of the cylinder. Plane 1 is on the bottom of the cylinder and plane 5 is on the top of the cylinder.

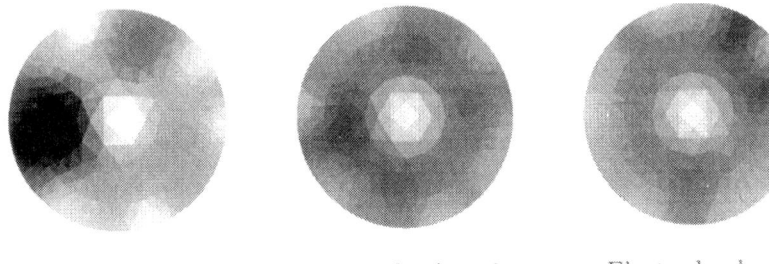

Electrode plane 1.   Electrode plane 2.   Electrode plane 3.

FIGURE 6. The 2D static reconstructions in each electrode plane from the same data as in FIGURE 4. The reference voltage has been calculated in a 2D mesh of 1192 elements and 2513 nodes with second-order basis functions. Reconstruction with 412 parameters.

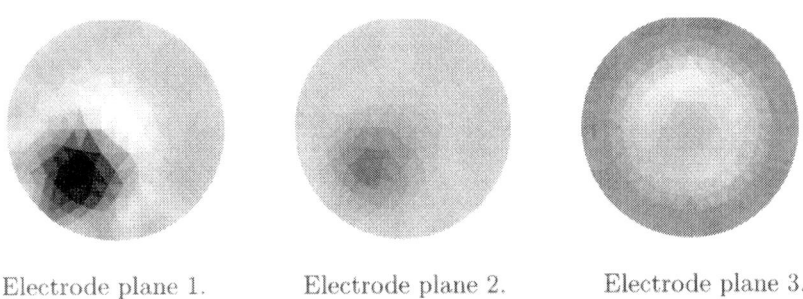

Electrode plane 1.   Electrode plane 2.   Electrode plane 3.

FIGURE 7. A 2D difference reconstruction in each electrode plane from the same data as in FIGURE 2.

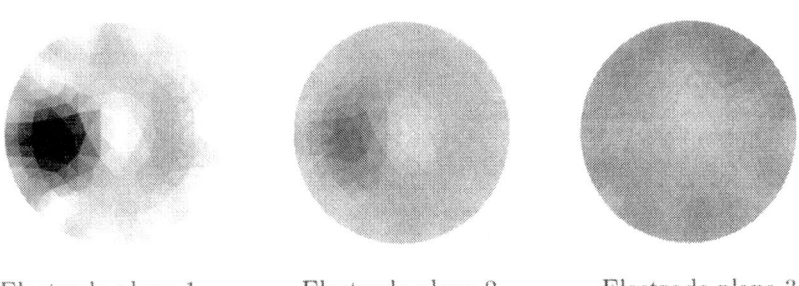

Electrode plane 1.   Electrode plane 2.   Electrode plane 3.

FIGURE 8. A 2D difference reconstruction in each electrode plane from the same data as in FIGURE 4.

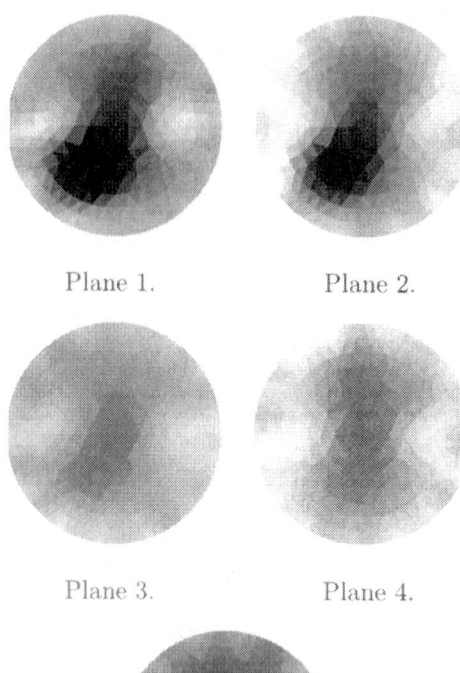

Plane 1. Plane 2.

Plane 3. Plane 4.

Plane 5.

FIGURE 9. Static reconstruction from real measurements with 2060 parameters (as in FIGURE 3) in different planes of the cylinder. The reference voltage and the Jacobian were calculated in a mesh with a maximum error of 1% in the boundary shape. Plane 1 is on the bottom of the cylinder and plane 5 is on the top of the cylinder. The mean resistivity of the target was 242 Ωcm.

REFERENCES

1. WEBSTER, J. 1990. Electrical Impedance Tomography. Adam Hilger. Bristol.
2. WEXLER, A. 1988. Electrical impedance imaging in two and three dimensions. Clin. Phys. Physiol. Meas. **9**(suppl. A): 29–33.
3. GOBLE, J., M. CHENEY & D. ISAACSON. 1992. Electrical impedance tomography in three dimensions. Appl. Comput. Electromagn. Soc. J. **7**: 128–147.
4. METHERALL, P., D. BARBER & R. SMALLWOOD. 1995. Three dimensional electrical impedance tomography. In Proc. IX Int. Conf. Electrical Bio-Impedance, Heidelberg, Germany, p. 510–511.
5. METHERALL, P., D. BARBER, R. SMALLWOOD & B. BROWN. 1996. Three-dimensional electrical impedance tomography. Nature **380**: 509–512.
6. METHERALL, P., R. SMALLWOOD & D. BARBER. 1996. Three dimensional electrical impedance tomography of the human thorax. In Proc. 18th Int. Conf. IEEE Eng. Med. Biol. Soc.
7. MORUCCI, J., M. GRANIE, M. LEI, M. CHABERT & P. MARSILI. 1995. 3D reconstruction in electrical impedance imaging using a direct sensitivity matrix approach. Physiol. Meas. **16**: A123–A128.
8. GROETSCH, C.W. 1993. Inverse Problems in the Mathematical Sciences. Vieweg. Braunschweig.

9. Cheng, K-S., D. Isaacson, J. Newell & D. Gisser. 1989. Electrode models for electric current computed tomography. IEEE Trans. Biomed. Eng. **36:** 918–924.
10. Somersalo, E., M. Cheney & D. Isaacson. 1992. Existence and uniqueness for electrode models for electric current computed tomography. SIAM J. Appl. Math. **52:** 1023–1040.
11. Paulson, K., W. Breckon & M. Pidcock. 1992. Electrode modelling in electrical impedance tomography. SIAM J. Appl. Math. **52:** 1012–1022.
12. Hua, P., E. Woo, J. Webster & W. Tompkins. 1993. Finite element modeling of electrode-skin contact impedance in electrical impedance tomography. IEEE Trans. Biomed. Eng. **40:** 335–343.
13. Vauhkonen, P., M. Vauhkonen, T. Savolainen & J. Kaipio. 1997. Three-dimensional electrical impedance tomography based on the complete electrode model. IEEE Trans. Biomed. Eng. In press.
14. Yorkey, T. & J. Webster. 1987. A comparison of impedance tomographic reconstruction algorithms. Clin. Phys. Physiol. Meas. **8**(suppl. A): 55–62.
15. Dobson, D. & F. Santosa. 1994. An image enhancement technique for electrical impedance tomography. Inverse Probl. **10:** 317–334.
16. Kolehmainen, V., E. Somersalo, P. Vauhkonen, M. Vauhkonen & J. Kaipio. 1998. A Bayesian approach and total variation priors in 3D electrical impedance tomography. In IEEE EMBS '98, p. 1028–1031.
17. Kolehmainen, V., M. Vauhkonen, P. Karjalainen & J. Kaipio. 1997. Spatial inhomogeneity and regularization in EIT. In Proc. 19th Int. Conf. IEEE Eng. Med. Biol. Soc., Chicago, p. 449–452.
18. Järvenpää, S. 1995. A finite element model for the inverse conductivity problem. Philos. Lic. thesis, University of Helsinki, Finland.
19. Korjenevsky, A. 1995. Reconstruction of absolute conductivity distribution in electrical impedance tomography. In Proc. IX Int. Conf. Electrical Bio-Impedance, Heidelberg, Germany, p. 532–535.
20. Savolainen, T., J. Kaipio, M. Vauhkonen & P. Karjalainen. 1996. An EIT measurement system for experimental use. Rev. Sci. Instrum. **67:** 3605–3609.

Development of a Reconstruction Algorithm for Imaging Impedance Changes in the Human Head

A. GIBSON,[a] R. H. BAYFORD,[b] AND D. S. HOLDER[a]

[a]*University College London, Middlesex Hospital, London W1N 8AA, United Kingdom*
[b]*Middlesex University, London N11 2NQ, United Kingdom*

> ABSTRACT: Accurate imaging of impedance changes in the brain with EIT using scalp electrodes ideally requires an algorithm designed for a 3D hemispherical object that is capable of imaging through the skull. A 2D algorithm is presented, intended as the first step towards a full 3D version. It is based on a sensitivity matrix approach and allows images to be reconstructed from any electrode positions. Its performance was assessed using a 2D circular tank with a simulated skull. The findings suggested the following: if polar current drive was used with no explicit skull compensation, a feature in the image would be placed 25% closer to the center and would be around one-third the amplitude of an identical perturbation in a homogeneous medium.

INTRODUCTION

Background

The imaging of impedance changes in the head provides a unique challenge for electrical impedance tomography (EIT). First, the impedance changes are small, of the order of 5% for evoked responses[1] and 10% for epilepsy.[2] Second, there is a discontinuity in impedance due to the skull, which has approximately 30 times the impedance of the scalp or brain. This has the dual effect of reducing the sensitivity of scalp measurements to a central impedance change and distorting the current flow within the head. Finally, the head presents an inherently three-dimensional geometry.

Much of the published work on EIT of the human head has concentrated on nonmetabolic impedance changes such as the displacement of cerebrospinal fluid and brain tissue by blood that occurs in intraventricular hemorrhage,[3] and blood flow changes related to the cardiac cycle.[4] The aim of our work is to image impedance changes associated with metabolic changes in the brain such as cell swelling during epilepsy,[2] changing blood flow during physiological evoked responses,[1] and ultimately the resistance decrease as ion channels open during the passage of an action potential.[5]

The first stage in this work is to answer the following question: Can physiological impedance changes be imaged noninvasively through the human skull? For this, we require a reconstruction algorithm with certain properties:

- The characteristics of the impedance change associated with evoked responses are not well understood. The time course is uncertain and, although the impedance is expected to decrease (due to an increase in blood flow), it is conceivable that there will be an increase (due to cell swelling). Increases and decreases may occur simultaneously. Because of this, it is desirable that the algorithm does not introduce unexpected or poorly understood artifacts that could be misinterpreted as a physiological impedance change.

- The first test of the method will be to image evoked responses, particularly visual evoked responses that are known to occur at the back of the head. Hence, in the first instance, the resolution is not important—to validate the method, it is only necessary to find out from which quarter of the brain the signal comes. Similarly, the nonlinearity in sensitivity and the resolution across the image are not important as evoked responses occur in the cortex, the extreme outer surface of the brain.

- The algorithm should be flexible with respect to electrode position. If current is driven on a pair of electrodes, it has been shown[6] using a 2D finite element model of the head that the sensitivity is 5 times greater if the current drive electrodes are on opposite sides of the head than if they are adjacent. It is not obvious what the most sensitive electrode positions will be on a 3D hemisphere and it will be necessary to optimize the electrode positions and combinations by trial and error.

- The algorithm should be capable of imaging through the skull and should include the full 3D geometry of the head.

Two reconstruction algorithms designed for imaging the head have been published, but neither one appears to fulfill all the properties listed above. Morucci et al.[7] used a sensitivity matrix to reconstruct images of test data from a model of a hemispherical head. While being a fully 3D algorithm, it was designed for adjacent current drive only and it has been shown that sensitivity is reduced when imaging through the skull using adjacent drive.[8]

Bayford et al.[9] back-projected Lagrange multipliers as a weighted average of the measured voltages instead of the measured voltages directly. This technique has been successfully used to reconstruct images from a 2D saline-filled tank using a ring of plaster of Paris to simulate the skull. A priori information such as the shape and conductivity of tissues in the head can be included in the calculation of the Lagrange multipliers. However, the method was not designed to allow easy modification of electrode positions due to the length of time required to calculate the Lagrange multipliers. Furthermore, the published version was limited to 2D, but the method could, in principle, be extended to 3D.

Purpose of This Work

The purpose of this work was to develop and test a simple algorithm in 2D that follows the specifications outlined above. Its main difference compared to preceding work was that it was designed to reconstruct images with data acquired from any electrode positions and any combination of electrodes.

Design

The algorithm was based on an analytical solution to Poisson's equation, from which sensitivity coefficients were calculated using Geselowitz's sensitivity theorem.[10] The inverse problem was solved by weighting the measured voltages by the appropriate sensitivity coefficients. The image quality and sensitivity were tested in a 2D circular tank with and without a plaster of Paris ring intended to simulate the skull.

DESIGN OF ALGORITHM

Background

Poisson's equation can be expressed, in matrix form, as $\mathbf{V} = \mathbf{S}\sigma$. In EIT, we wish to invert this relationship to calculate the conductivity distribution σ given the sensitivity matrix $\mathbf{S}$ and the surface voltages $\mathbf{V}$. This is nonlinear; however, if images of conductivity *change* are reconstructed from *changes* in the measured boundary voltages, then to a first order a linear relationship can be assumed between $\mathbf{V}$ and σ. This has the advantage of only requiring $\mathbf{S}$ to be calculated once and makes the solution less sensitive to electrode placement and electrode-skin impedance.

In this algorithm, the sensitivity matrix is calculated analytically and used to weight the boundary voltages in a single step to produce a linear image of resistivity change.

Solution to Poisson's Equation

The forward problem was solved analytically using the solution to Poisson's equation for current injected from two electrodes on the boundary of a homogeneous circular region, given by equation 1, where r_1 and r_2 are the distances from the two current injection electrodes:

$$V = \ln\left(\frac{r_1}{r_2}\right). \tag{1}$$

This allows the current density (which is proportional to the gradient of voltage) to be calculated for any point inside the region, if the positions of the current injection electrodes are known.

Calculation of Sensitivity Coefficients

The sensitivity coefficients were calculated using Geselowitz's theorem,[10] which states the following: for a four-point impedance measurement with current delivered on electrode pair m and measured on pair n, the sensitivity coefficient $S_{m,n,x,y}$ for a pixel at (x, y) is proportional to the product of the electric field due to the electrode pair m and that due to the pair n (equation 2). This allows the sensitivity matrix to be calculated for any combination of four electrodes anywhere on the head:

$$S_{m,n,x,y} = \nabla V_m \cdot \nabla V_n. \tag{2}$$

Taking the dot product of the electric fields due to electrode pairs m and n is equivalent to assuming that current is injected simultaneously on m and n. This means that equipotential lines exist that connect the two positive electrodes and the two negative electrodes. The gradient of voltage along an equipotential line is zero and, along these lines, the sensitivity coefficient is zero. Between the null lines, **S** is positive; outside them, it is negative. This means that an impedance increase would be expected to produce a voltage increase, decrease, or no change depending on its position. Images reconstructed from a sensitivity matrix calculated in this way have discontinuities and can show positive and negative impedance changes in the image when only a positive impedance change was present in the data. These problems can be avoided by taking the absolute value of the current density before multiplying the components from the two pairs of electrodes. This is equivalent to injecting current on each pair of electrodes separately and then taking the product of the resultant fields (equation 3):

$$S_{m, n, x, y} = |\nabla V_m||\nabla V_n|. \tag{3}$$

The Inverse Problem

The sensitivity matrix **S** relates the normalized measured impedance changes δZ to the actual normalized impedance changes within the body $\delta\sigma$. The forward problem, then, is given by $\delta Z = -S\delta\sigma$ or, equivalently,[11] $\delta V = S\delta\rho$. This follows because, for constant current, $\delta V = \delta Z$ and conductivity is inversely proportional to resistivity; hence $\delta\sigma = -\delta\rho$.

To solve the inverse problem, the matrix **S** must be inverted. However, it is difficult to invert directly, being ill-posed and ill-conditioned. Pseudoinversions are often used,[12–14] but this is time-consuming and unexpected artifacts may be introduced by approximations in the inversion. The application here requires an algorithm that is flexible with regard to electrode position and combination. Instead of inverting **S**, which would have to be repeated for each new electrode combination, **S** is used directly to weight the measured voltages.[15,16] This is equivalent to assuming that a given measured impedance change might be due to a small impedance change where the sensitivity is high, or a high impedance change further from the injection electrodes. By not inverting the matrix, it is simple and quick to try new electrode combinations and even incorporate electrode positions measured directly off each individual's head. Once the positions of the electrodes are decided upon, it may be appropriate to include matrix inversion; however, in the medium term, flexibility is more important than rigor.

The forward problem is solved to generate a matrix of sensitivity coefficients. The value of each pixel is then taken to be the sum of all boundary voltages, weighted by the appropriate sensitivity coefficients. This still leaves the total sensitivity of pixels at the edge of the image being far greater than that for central pixels and each pixel is normalized to the total sensitivity for that pixel. The algorithm can be expressed as equation 4, where $P_{x,y}$ is the pixel value at (x, y), V_k is the voltage measured from the k-th electrode pair, and $S_{x,y,k}$ is the appropriate sensitivity coefficient:

$$P_{x, y} = \frac{\sum_k S_{x, y, k} V_k}{\sum_k S_{x, y, k}}. \tag{4}$$

TESTING THE ALGORITHM

The algorithm was evaluated using a circular tank, 20 cm in diameter and 2 cm deep, with a Perspex rod, 2 cm in diameter, as a test object. A skull was simulated by a ring of plaster of Paris (Vel-Mix stone, Kerr Limited, United Kingdom) of thickness 5 mm and inner diameter 19 cm. The tank was filled with saturated calcium sulfate solution to prevent the plaster of Paris ring from dissolving. The resistivities of the bathing solution and plaster of Paris were approximately 4 Ωm and 110 Ωm, respectively, giving an impedance difference between the simulated "skull" and "brain" of 27:1, similar to that in the human head.[9]

Measurements were made using an EIT system based on a Hewlett-Packard 4284A impedance analyzer.[18] The current was set at the maximum that the instrument could deliver, which in practice was 1–3 mA. The frequency was 10 kHz. Measurements were taken with 16 electrodes using both polar and adjacent protocols so that the two could be compared.

The Perspex rod was moved in steps of 10 mm from the center of the tank to 80% of the diameter. The images were reconstructed using three methods—the sensitivity method with both polar and adjacent current drive and the Sheffield Mark 1 technique.[17] Two images were taken at the start and end of the experiment without the Perspex rod and were used for linear correction of the series of images to compensate for drift due to temperature changes, evaporation, or electrode effects.

Three image parameters were examined in detail:

- Spatial accuracy is the accuracy to which an impedance change can be localized. Even though the resolution of EIT images is poor, the accuracy with which the peak change in the image represents the position of the perturbation is generally good.

- The resolution of an image is defined as the full width at half-maximum (FWHM) of a point spread function. Experimentally, a point spread function is approximated to an image of an object with a diameter much smaller than the expected resolution. A profile was taken across the image at the point of maximum change from which the full width at half-maximum was found.

- The uniformity across an image was examined by plotting the maximum impedance change against the insulator's position in the tank. In an ideal image, the response should be uniform across the image, but this does not occur in EIT images due to the very high current density (and therefore sensitivity) close to the electrodes.

RESULTS

Images were obtained with the perturbation in eight positions along the radius of the tank, both with and without the simulated skull. Three images obtained with the simulated skull in place are shown in FIGURE 1. These images were obtained with no explicit compensation for the skull.

Spatial Accuracy

Without the skull in place, the sensitivity method using polar current drive and the Sheffield Mark 1 adjacent drive technique[17] behave similarly—over most of the radius of the tank, the position of a feature in the image is accurate to within about 5%. The sensitivity method with adjacent drive data consistently underestimates the distance from the center by around 25%.

With the simulated skull, all three algorithms underestimate the radial displacement of the insulator—the sensitivity method with polar current drive by 25%, the Sheffield method by 50%, and the sensitivity method using adjacent drive by up to 70%. FIGURE 2 shows the spatial accuracy when imaging through the simulated skull. The dotted line shows the ideal case where the measured position is the same as the actual position of the insulator.

Resolution

The resolution with the Sheffield Mark 1 algorithm was 15–20% of the image diameter. With the sensitivity method, it was considerably worse: 50% using adjacent protocol and 60–70% with polar protocol. In all three cases, the skull had no noticeable effect on the resolution of the image.

Uniformity

An object at the edge of the tank generates a greater impedance change in the image than one in the center. All three algorithms tested had similar uniformity characteristics, but the uniformity was generally *better* with the simulated skull in place than without. With no skull, the intensity at the center was 50–60% of that at the edge; with the skull, it was 60–70% of the intensity at the edge.

DISCUSSION

Effect of the Simulated Skull on the Image

The effect of the simulated skull is to compress features toward the center of the image. The use of polar current injection reduces this error to 25% of the image radius. In addition, the intensity of the impedance change in an image taken with the simulated skull using polar current injection was of the order of a third of that without the skull. Similar values for the spatial distortion and sensitivity reduction due to the skull have been noted previously.[8,19]

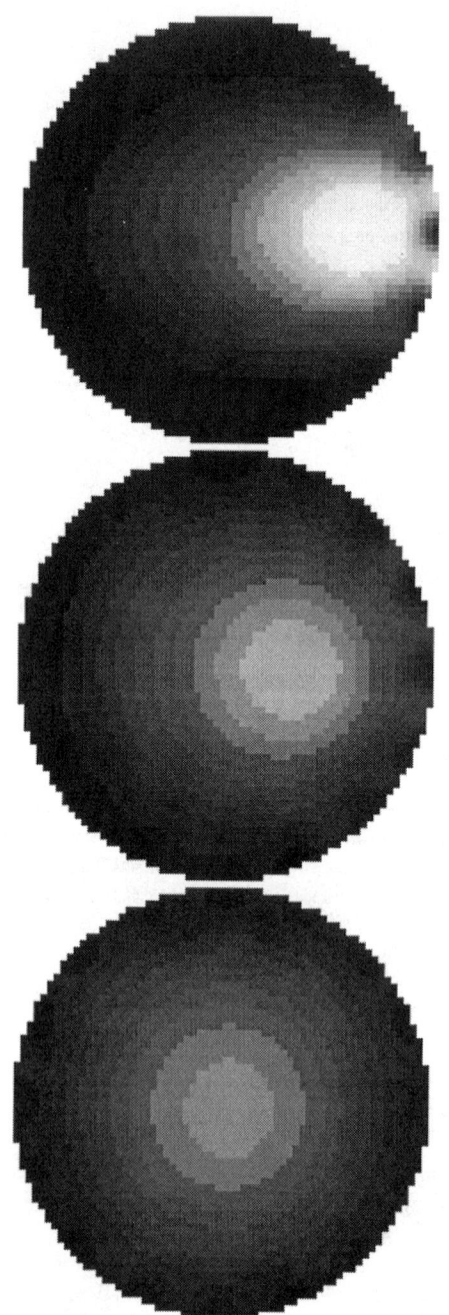

FIGURE 1. Images of an insulator in a calcium sulfate solution–filled tank with a simulated skull in place taken using polar current drive. In the left-hand image, the insulator is in the center, and it moves to the back of the tank (bottom of the image) in the subsequent images.

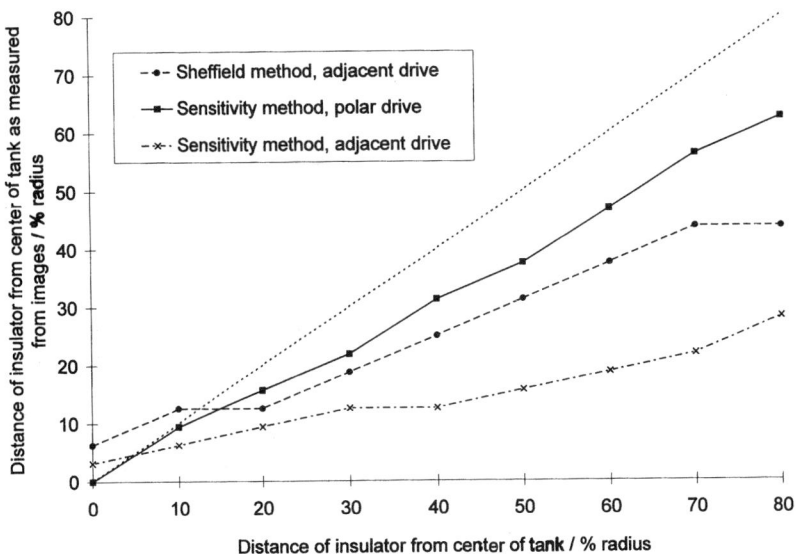

FIGURE 2. Measured position of object in a tank with simulated skull, plotted against position in image.

Skull Compensation

The purpose of this work was to produce an algorithm that can be used to examine whether an impedance change is present or not and to identify from which part of the brain the signal comes. These aims were met without the need for explicit skull compensation.

A possible technique for skull compensation that could be implemented in the future is derived from inverse EEG source modeling, where the head is modeled as concentric spheres (corresponding to the brain, the skull, the scalp, and sometimes the cerebrospinal fluid). The thickness of the shell corresponding to the skull is then increased and its resistivity decreased so that the model becomes homogeneous (FIGURE 3). In EIT, the boundary voltages would then be back-projected into a homogeneous object and the skull is simply not shown. Using this method, it has been demonstrated[20] that localization errors in the EEG can be reduced to those caused by the variability in head anatomy from person to person.

Performance of Algorithm

The performance of the algorithm on *in vitro* data without a simulated skull compares favorably with the Sheffield Mark 1 algorithm,[17] except that the resolution is degraded from 20% of the image diameter to around 60%. The improved resolution of the Sheffield technique is partly due to the resolution-enhancing filter inherent in that method. At this stage, however, poor resolution may not be a problem—it can be improved by Wiener filtering the image after reconstruction.[16] With the simulated skull in place, features in the

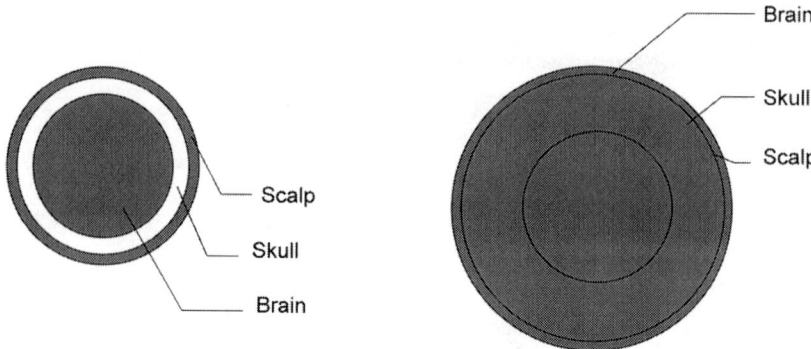

FIGURE 3. Skull compensation technique: To compensate for the skull, the thicknesses of the brain and scalp are kept constant, while that of the skull is increased; thus, the head appears to be a homogeneous medium.

image are compressed toward the center, but using polar current injection reduces the error to 25% of the radius of the image. This work can be extended to 3D by simply taking the appropriate solution to Poisson's equation, and details of the real inhomogeneous head can be included by calculating the sensitivity coefficients from a finite element model of the real head.

The specifications listed in the introduction appear to have been fully met. No potentially misleading artifacts (such as the ring artifacts that result from a resolution-enhancing filter) have been noted and the technique is fully flexible with respect to electrode position.

Drawbacks of This Method

Problems with the technique described here originate largely with the need to be able to incorporate any electrode positions. If the electrode positions were fixed, the sensitivity matrix could be inverted and stored and attempts could be made to implement a nonlinear, iterative solution.

The head is modeled as a homogeneous circle. This has been shown to be a reasonable assumption in a circular tank, which is inhomogeneous, but isotropic and radially symmetric. It is not clear what the effect of the real human head will be, with its complex, anisotropic, nonspherical, 3D geometry.

CONCLUSIONS

A 2D reconstruction algorithm has been written that is optimized for imaging through the skull. The image quality is adequate and any electrode positions and combinations can be used.

No explicit skull compensation appears to be necessary. If the algorithm is used to image through the skull, an impedance perturbation will be placed 25% closer to the center than it actually is and will be around one-third the amplitude that it would have been if it were in a homogeneous medium.

The algorithm will be extended to 3D and tested using a hemispherical saline-filled tank and data acquired from a finite element model of a real head. Trials of imaging visual evoked responses in humans are under way.

REFERENCES

1. HOLDER, D.S., A. RAO & Y. HANQUAN. 1996. Imaging of physiologically evoked responses by electrical impedance tomography with cortical electrodes in the anaesthetised rabbit. Physiol. Meas. **17**(A): 179–186.
2. RAO, A., A. GIBSON & D.S. HOLDER. 1997. EIT images of electrically induced epileptic activity in anaesthetised rabbits. Med. Biol. Eng. Comput. **35**(1): 327.
3. TARASSENKO, L., M. K. PIDCOCK, D.F. MURPHY & P. ROLFE. 1985. The development of impedance imaging techniques for use in the newborn at risk of intra-ventricular hemorrhage. *In* Proc. IEEE Int. Conf. on Electric and Magnetic Fields in Medicine and Biology, p. 83–87.
4. MCARDLE, F.J., B.H. BROWN & A. ANGEL. 1993. Imaging cardiosynchronous impedance changes in the adult head. *In* Clinical and Physiological Uses of Electrical Impedance Tomography, p. 177–183. UCL Press. London.
5. BOONE, K.G. & D.S. HOLDER. 1995. Design considerations and performance of a prototype system for imaging neuronal depolarisation in the brain using "direct current" electrical resistance tomography. Physiol. Meas. **16**(A): 87–98.
6. BOONE, K.G. 1995. The possible use of applied potential tomography for imaging action potential in the brain. Ph.D. thesis, University College London.
7. MORUCCI, J-P., M. GRANIÉ, M. LEI & P.M. MARSILI. 1995. 3D reconstruction in electrical impedance tomography using a direct sensitivity matrix approach. Physiol. Meas. **16**(A): 123–128.
8. MCARDLE, F.J., B.H. BROWN & A. ANGEL. 1989. Imaging resistivity changes of the adult brain during the cardiac cycle. *In* IEEE EMBS 11th Annual International Conference Proceedings, p. 480–481.
9. BAYFORD, R.H., Y. HANQUAN, K.G. BOONE & D.S. HOLDER. 1995. Experimental validation of a novel reconstruction algorithm for electrical impedance tomography based on backprojection of Lagrange multipliers. Physiol. Meas. **16**(A): 237–247.
10. GESELOWITZ, D.B. 1971. An application of electrocardiographic lead theory to impedance plethysmography. IEEE Trans. Biomed. Eng. **BME-18**: 38–41.
11. KOTRE, C. J. 1993. Studies of image reconstruction methods for electrical impedance tomography. Ph.D. thesis, University of Newcastle-upon-Tyne, United Kingdom.
12. MURAI, T. & Y. KAGAWA. 1985. Electrical impedance computed tomography based on a finite element model. IEEE Trans. Biomed. Eng. **BME-32**(3): 177–184.
13. EYÜBOGLU, B. M. 1996. An interleaved drive electrical impedance tomography image reconstruction algorithm. Physiol. Meas. **17**(A): 59–71.
14. KLEINERMANN, F., N. J. AVIS, S. K. JUDAH & D. C. BARBER. 1996. Three-dimensional image reconstruction for electrical impedance tomography. Physiol. Meas. **17**(A): 77–83.
15. GADD, R., P. RECORD & P. ROLFE. 1992. A sensitivity region reconstruction algorithm using adjacent drive current injection strategy. Clin. Phys. Physiol. Meas. **13**(A): 101–105.
16. KOTRE, C. J. 1994. EIT image reconstruction using sensitivity weighted filtered backprojection. Physiol. Meas. **15**(A): 125–136.
17. BARBER, D. C. & A. D. SEAGAR. 1987. Fast reconstruction of resistance images. Clin. Phys. Physiol. Meas. **8**(A): 47–54.
18. BAYFORD, R. H., K. G. BOONE, Y. HANQUAN & D. S. HOLDER. 1996. Improvement of the positional accuracy of EIT images of the head using a Lagrange multiplier reconstruction algorithm with diametric excitation. Physiol. Meas. **17**(A): 91–98.

19. McArdle, F. J., B. H. Brown, R. G. Pearse & D. C. Barber. 1988. The effect of the skull of low-birthweight neonates on applied potential tomography of centralised resistivity change. Clin. Phys. Physiol. Meas. **9**(A): 55–60.
20. Ary, J. P., S. A. Klein & D. H. Fender. 1981. Location of sources of evoked scalp potentials: corrections for skull and scalp thicknesses. IEEE Trans. Biomed. Eng. **BME-28**(6): 447–452.

Monitoring Regional Lung Ventilation by Functional Electrical Impedance Tomography during Assisted Ventilation[a]

INÉZ FRERICHS,[b] GÜNTER HAHN,[b] HOLGER SCHIFFMANN,[c] CORD BERGER,[b] AND GERHARD HELLIGE[b]

[b]*Department of Anesthesiological Research, Center of Anesthesiology, Emergency and Intensive Care Medicine*
[c]*Department of Pediatrics, University of Göttingen, 37075 Göttingen, Germany*

ABSTRACT: A new approach in discriminating the regional air volume changes in the lungs associated with either spontaneous or mechanical ventilation during assisted ventilation is presented. Impedance data are obtained by conventional electrical impedance tomography (EIT). The data are filtered in the range of either the spontaneous or the ventilator rate and processed by the functional EIT (f-EIT) evaluation technique, whereby the variation of the respective EIT data with time is determined and imaged. EIT measurements performed in an infant during synchronized intermittent mandatory ventilation were evaluated with this method and indicated that the specific local lung volume swings related to spontaneous and mechanical inhalations can be separated and imaged as tomograms. This noninvasive approach may become useful in optimizing the ventilatory pattern during advanced forms of artificial ventilation and may help the clinician in the therapy management of individual patients.

INTRODUCTION

Mechanical (i.e., artificial) ventilation is an established tool to secure adequate gas exchange in patients with respiratory insufficiency. In contrast with the conventional controlled mechanical ventilation, delivering a fixed tidal volume at a preselected respiratory rate, modern ventilators enable several ventilation modes that can be better matched with the individual requirements of the patients. Conventional controlled ventilation does not permit spontaneous breathing, which, if present, has to be suppressed by deep sedation and muscle paralysis. Some of the new ventilation patterns allow spontaneous breathing activity and the ventilator only assists the patients in their otherwise insufficient respiratory effort. Such ventilation patterns are extremely important in intensive care medicine as they positively influence the outcome of the patients, reduce the complications, and shorten the weaning period.

Typical forms of assisted ventilation are intermittent mandatory ventilation (IMV) and synchronized intermittent mandatory ventilation (SIMV).[1] During IMV the ventilator-generated inflations occur at regular preset intervals independent of the spontaneous breathing activity, whereas during SIMV the mechanical inflations are triggered by the patient and synchronized with spontaneous ventilation. In both modes, the ventilator settings have to be carefully titrated so as to obtain a proper combination of spontaneous ventilation and

---

[a]This work was supported by the Deutsche Forschungsgemeinschaft, SFB 330, Göttingen, and by the German Aerospace Center, Bonn, Germany.

ventilator assistance that would maintain sufficient alveolar ventilation. The basic characteristics of controlled and assisted ventilation represented by the continuous positive-pressure ventilation (CPPV) and SIMV, respectively, are shown in FIGURE 1.

In clinical settings, arterial blood gas analysis and chest radiographs provide the basic feedback information on the efficacy of assisted ventilation. At present, it is not possible to obtain information on the regional ventilation magnitude and to separate the lung volume changes caused by mechanical and spontaneous inhalations, respectively. Such data would be valuable for a clinician and helpful in optimization of the ventilator performance. We present a new approach to discriminate artificial and spontaneous ventilation on the regional level using the classical electrical impedance tomography (EIT) device[2] with the functional EIT (f-EIT) evaluation technique, which was developed by our research group.[3]

In contrast with the simple EIT, which primarily concentrates on imaging the anatomical information, the f-EIT evaluation focuses on imaging the functional state of organs. In case of thoracic measurements, f-EIT generates images of regional lung ventilation. This method has been shown to identify (1) regional ventilation deficits in artificially induced local airway obstruction in pigs,[3] (2) redistribution of lung ventilation and development of lung edema during experimental lung injury,[4] (3) gravity-dependent variations in regional lung ventilation occurring during postural changes in spontaneously breathing healthy subjects,[5,6] (4) perioperative changes in the distribution of lung ventilation in pulmonary healthy patients,[7] and (5) inhomogeneities of lung ventilation due to lung pathology in intensive care patients.[8] This paper presents the first application of f-EIT in a pediatric patient and the ability of this technique to separate spontaneous and mechanical ventilation during assisted ventilation.

METHODS

General Description of EIT Measurements

EIT measurements were performed with the Sheffield APT System Mk I (IBEES, Sheffield, United Kingdom). This device generates cross-sectional images of regional thoracic impedance changes on the basis of repeated rotating injections of small electrical currents (5 mA_{p-p}, 50 kHz) through a ring of electrodes connected to the circumference of the thorax and subsequent measurements of the resulting potential differences on the same electrodes.[2] The distribution of electrical impedance within the thorax is reconstructed from the obtained surface voltage data using the back-projection algorithm.[9] It determines relative impedance data; that is, the instantaneous distribution of regional thoracic impedance is always referred to the "reference" average thoracic impedance distribution determined during several respiratory cycles and normalized by this reference. In the current settings, each completed EIT measurement consisted of a sequence of relative impedance change values obtained for the thoracic cross section in a 32×32 pixel matrix at a sampling rate of 10 Hz during 100 s. The collected EIT data were then processed by the f-EIT technique.

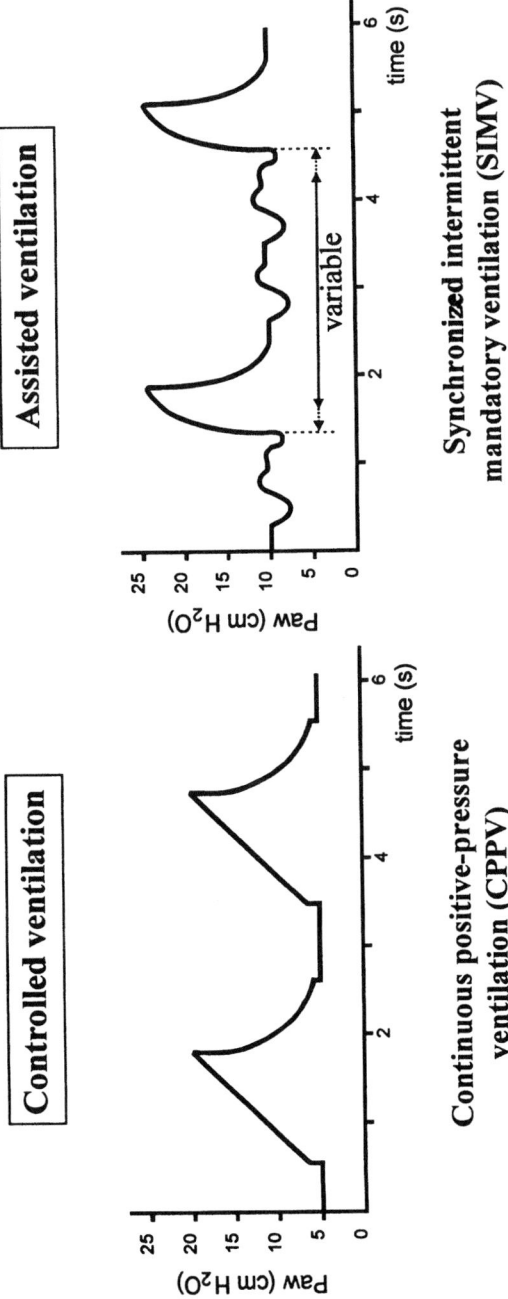

FIGURE 1. The major differences between conventional controlled ventilation (left panel) and assisted ventilation (right panel). The schematic tracings of the airway pressure (Paw) show the typical ventilatory patterns during continuous positive-pressure ventilation (CPPV) and synchronized intermittent mandatory ventilation (SIMV). During CPPV, the ventilator generates the inflations of the lung (see the linear increases in Paw in the left-hand scheme), which are followed by passive expirations (see the decreases in Paw after each peak inflation). No spontaneous breaths occur. In the course of SIMV, the patient is allowed to breathe spontaneously (see the small deflections in the right-hand Paw tracing). The decreases and subsequent increases in Paw correspond with spontaneous inspirations and expirations. The ventilator-generated breaths (see the large deflections) are triggered by the patient (see the initial minute decrease in Paw preceding the mechanical inflation). The time interval between mechanical breaths is slightly variable due to its dependence on the inspiratory effort of the patient. In case of insufficient or absent spontaneous breathing, the ventilator takes over the whole ventilatory activity and the ventilation mode is identical with CPPV. In both forms of ventilation, the end-expiratory airway pressure may be individually adjusted; for example, it is kept positive throughout the whole respiratory cycle (Paw does not fall below 5 cm H_2O and 10 cm H_2O in the left-hand and right-hand tracings, respectively).

Functional EIT (f-EIT)

The f-EIT technique[3] is based on the fact that transthoracic impedance is dependent on the volume of air in the lungs, which typically changes during inspiration and expiration. These variations of regional air content in the course of the respiratory cycle cause variations of regional impedance. The f-EIT technique calculates the variation (~standard deviation) of regional thoracic impedance from a sequence of collected EIT data. The resultant f-EIT image represents this variation of the relative impedance change in each pixel. Light areas in the f-EIT images show high impedance variation due to regional filling and emptying of the lungs with air, whereas dark areas represent low impedance variation in those thoracic areas where no changes in air volume take place. The impedance variation data, originally computed in a 32 × 32 pixel matrix, are interpolated by a factor of four to achieve a better visual effect. A typical f-EIT image and selected tracings of the relative impedance change in three single pixels obtained during spontaneous breathing are shown in FIGURE 2. The spatial orientation of f-EIT images in the transverse plane (i.e., posterior at the top and the left side of the body on the right of the images) is also indicated in this figure.

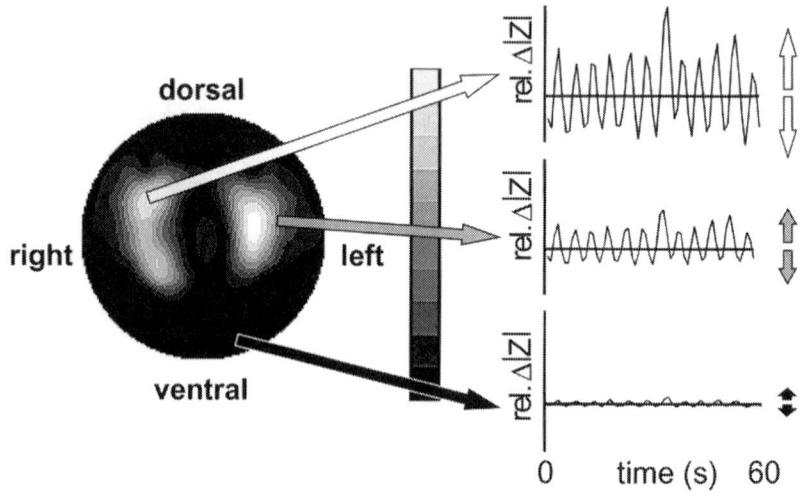

FIGURE 2. General characteristics and orientation of a functional EIT (f-EIT) image of the human thorax. The f-EIT image provides a cross-sectional representation of local lung volume changes occurring in the studied transverse layer of the thorax during the measuring interval. Each pixel of the image shows the local variation of the determined relative impedance change values with time. The relative impedance change values obtained from the lung regions vary largely in the course of the measurement due to the local fluctuations of the air volume (see the upper 60-s course of relative impedance change). Small variation of relative impedance change values is found in those parts of the image where no changes in air volume take place (see the lower course of relative impedance change). The pixels with large impedance variation are depicted in light tone and represent the well-ventilated pulmonary tissue of the right and left lung. Low impedance variation is shown in dark tone.

To discriminate the particular air volume changes caused by either mechanical or spontaneous inhalations during assisted ventilation, a new feature was included in the f-EIT evaluation. Besides the established instantaneous presentation of the local relative impedance changes in the time domain, the new f-EIT software shows the data also in the frequency domain. The artificial and spontaneous breathing rates are not identical. The exact rates can be easily separated and f-EIT images can be subsequently generated from the filtered data in the respective frequency ranges. Consequently, each EIT measurement obtained during assisted ventilation results in two separate f-EIT images, showing the regional lung volume changes elicited by either the mechanical or spontaneous component of assisted ventilation.

Application in a Patient

The efficacy of the new f-EIT imaging approach was checked by EIT measurements in a 13-week-old baby (body weight: 2850 g) in the pediatric intensive care unit (ICU). The measurements in the ICU were performed with the approval of the university ethics committee. The studied baby (birth weight: 2520 g; gestational age: 36 weeks) suffered from a severe cyanotic congenital heart disease (tetralogy of Fallot), stenosis of the left pulmonary artery, and hereditary dysmorphism. The infant was operated on (a palliative procedure with an aorta-pulmonary artery shunt and a patch in the left pulmonary artery).

Sixteen conventional X-ray transparent self-adhesive ECG electrodes (Blue Sensor BR-50-K, Medicotest A/S, Ølstykke, Denmark) were applied on the thoracic circumference approximately in the level of the fifth intercostal space. EIT measurements were performed 27 days after the surgery and lasted 5 days. The baby was always studied in the supine position. Initial EIT measurements were performed during spontaneous breathing. Ten hours later, the baby had to be intubated and thereafter was artificially ventilated with the SIMV mode (Babylog 8000, Drägerwerk, Lübeck, Germany). On the fourth day, extubation followed and the final EIT measurements were again accomplished during spontaneous breathing. During the 5-day period, the array of 16 electrodes was removed twice and new electrodes were attached on the thorax. Chest X-ray films and blood gas analyses were repeatedly obtained during these days.

RESULTS

Altogether, 98 EIT measurements were performed in the baby and evaluated with the f-EIT technique. FIGURE 3 presents the filtered f-EIT images and the time courses of relative impedance change averaged over the image cross section from 8 selected measurements. These measurements represent the most characteristic periods in the clinical course. In the initial measurements 1 and 2, the baby breathed spontaneously. Pulmonary gas exchange was insufficient, and pronounced lung congestion with fluid accumulation affecting predominantly the right lung was found in the chest X-ray (FIGURE 4). A progressive decrease in capillary saturation (S_{O_2}) and partial pressure of oxygen (P_{O_2}), as well as an increase in partial pressure of carbon dioxide (P_{CO_2}), were revealed by blood gas analyses (FIGURE 5). The f-EIT images 1 and 2 indicated predominant ventilation in the left lung corresponding with the chest radiograph. The rapid fluctuations in the respective tracings of the mean rel-

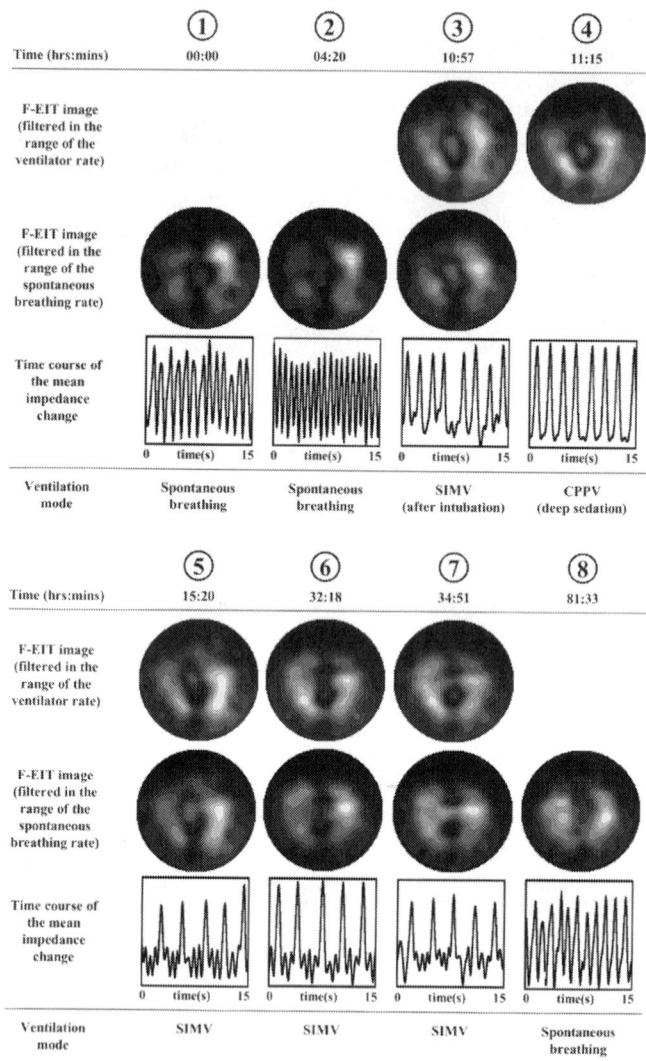

FIGURE 3. Functional EIT (f-EIT) images of a 13-week-old baby. Images 1, 2, and 8 were obtained during spontaneous breathing, while the remaining ones were obtained during artificial ventilation with synchronized intermittent mandatory ventilation (SIMV) or continuous positive-pressure ventilation (CPPV). The images in the lower row show the regional lung volume changes elicited by spontaneous breathing (1, 2, 8) or by the spontaneous breaths in the course of the SIMV ventilation (3, 5–7). The upper images (3–7) show the lung volume swings associated with the ventilator-generated inflations. The corresponding time courses of relative impedance change averaged over the whole thoracic cross section reflect the overall instantaneous lung volume fluctuations. Autoscaled images and time courses showing the first 15 s of the measurement are presented. In the upper and lower parts of the figure, the time of the measurement and the used ventilation mode are indicated, respectively. All measurements were performed in the pediatric intensive care unit.

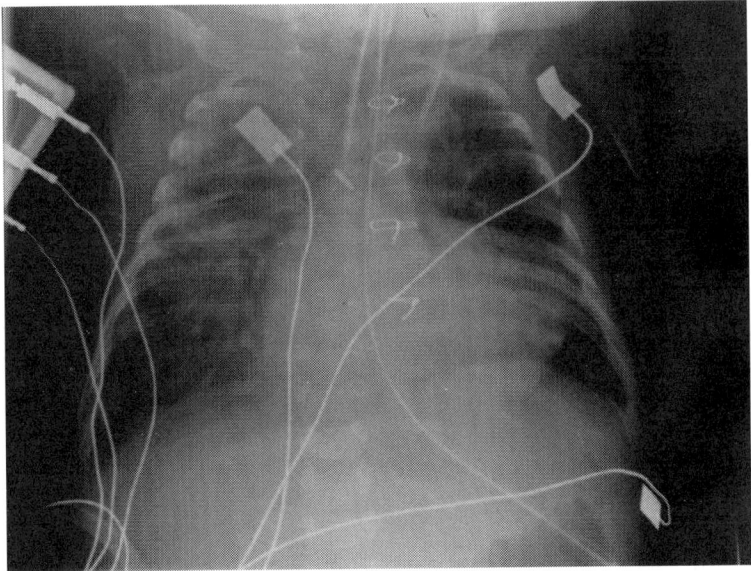

FIGURE 4. Chest X-ray film showing massive lung congestion affecting mainly the right lung in a spontaneously breathing baby. The radiographic examination was performed 27 days after an open-chest surgery and directly preceded EIT measurement 1 (compare with FIGURE 3).

ative impedance change were associated with spontaneous breathing at a rate of about 52 breaths·min^{-1} and, for tachypnea, 76 breaths·min^{-1}.

Due to progressive respiratory insufficiency, the infant had to be intubated and artificially ventilated. The two filtered f-EIT images in the third measurement show separately the regional variations of the impedance change caused by mechanical and spontaneous ventilation, respectively. Both mechanical and spontaneous breaths led to higher volume changes in the left lung. Large and small deflections associated with large mechanical and small spontaneous inhalations were determined in the tracing of the mean relative impedance change. Following deep sedation, the spontaneous breathing activity was suppressed (fourth measurement). Adequate lung ventilation was secured by the controlled mode of ventilation with CPPV, and only mechanical inflations at a rate of approximately 30 breaths·min^{-1} were discernible in the tracing of the mean relative impedance change.

The subsequent measurements 5, 6, and 7 showed the characteristic regional lung air volume changes related to artificial and spontaneous ventilation and the typical pattern of the SIMV ventilation. The spontaneous breathing rate was in the range of 55 to 70 breaths·min^{-1}, and the ventilator rate was about 20 breaths·min^{-1}. The f-EIT images in the sixth and seventh measurements indicated the more pronounced ventilation of the nondependent (i.e., ventral) lung regions during mechanical ventilation and of the dependent (i.e., dorsal) ones during spontaneous breathing. The distribution of air between the left and right lung became symmetrical. The parameters of the blood gas analysis were improved (FIGURE 5).

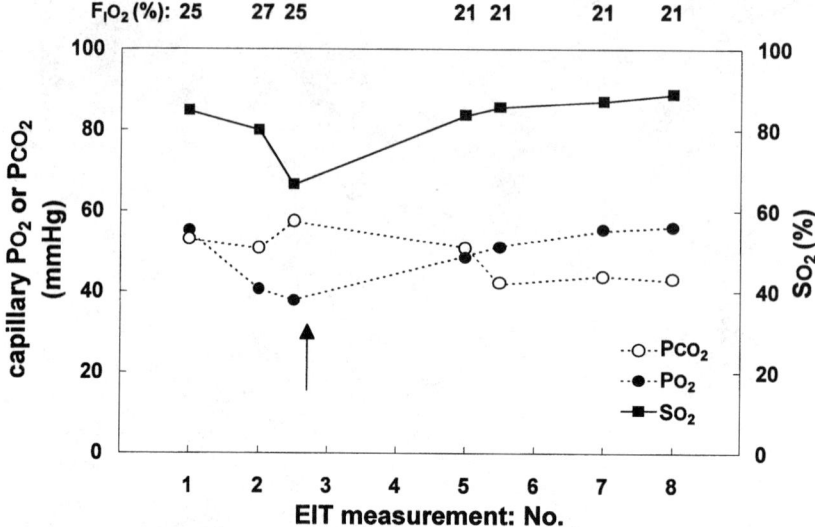

FIGURE 5. Capillary saturation (S_{O_2}) and partial pressures of oxygen (P_{O_2}) and carbon dioxide (P_{CO_2}) in relation to the EIT measurements presented in FIGURE 3. The fraction of oxygen (F_IO_2) in the inspired air at the time of the respective blood gas analysis is shown in the upper part of the figure. The arrow indicates intubation and the onset of artificial ventilation. The final values of P_{O_2}, P_{CO_2} and S_{O_2} differ from those that can be found under physiological conditions in healthy infants of the same age as the studied baby, but are normal in a baby with an aorta-pulmonary artery shunt.

Measurement 8 revealed homogeneous lung ventilation with a balanced distribution of air into the left and right lung after extubation, corresponding with the X-ray film shown in FIGURE 6. The infant breathed spontaneously at a rate of about 48 breaths·min^{-1}.

DISCUSSION

Measurement of bioelectrical impedance is currently being used in several medical applications. In infants, impedance techniques have been applied to determine total body water (e.g., references 10 and 11), cardiac output (e.g., references 12 and 13), gastric emptying or gastroesophageal reflux,[14,15] as well as breath amplitude and respiratory rate (e.g., references 16–18). EIT, which in contrast with the previously mentioned applications offers the new possibility to determine the distribution of impedance within studied parts of the body, has only seldom been applied in children. In harmony with the postulated most probable future clinical use of EIT in respiratory applications,[19–21] the EIT measurements in infants were almost exclusively performed on the thorax. Thoracic EIT images of the neonatal thorax were obtained using electrical current injection of either single[22] or multiple frequencies.[23,24] The quality of the obtained images was rather low due to the difficulties associated with EIT measurements in the intensive care field and the specific features of neonatal impedance measurements.

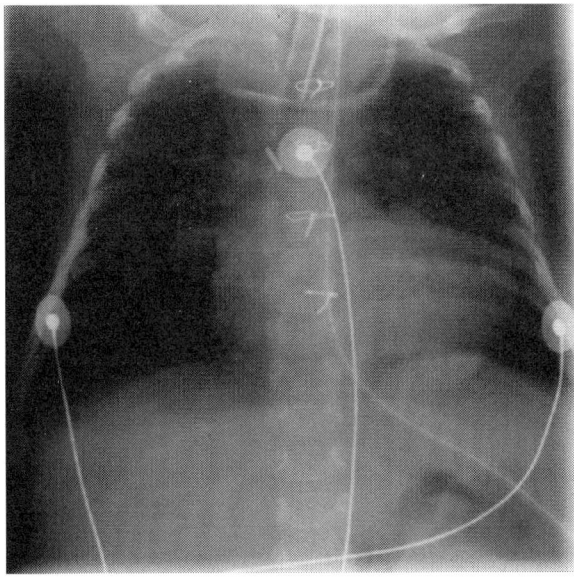

FIGURE 6. Chest radiograph showing clear lung fields of a spontaneously breathing baby performed 32 days after an open-chest surgery. This X-ray film was obtained immediately after EIT measurement 8 (see FIGURE 3).

Although the current EIT measurements were performed in a similar environment, the novel evaluation with the f-EIT technique markedly improved the images. This is apparent in comparison with the low-quality thoracic EIT image[22] obtained under comparable measuring conditions using current injection at a fixed frequency. The simple evaluation of the EIT data using only two instantaneous points from the measurement, expected to correspond with inspiration and expiration,[22] made the generated image strongly dependent on irregularities in the breathing pattern, cardiac events, movement artifacts, or noise. This is not the case when the f-EIT technique is used. All collected impedance data enter the evaluation and the regional variation of impedance in the thoracic cross section with time is imaged. The large gain in image quality achieved by this procedure is related to the reduction of the negative effects due to physiological and environmental noise. Besides, the physiologically relevant information, which is present in the time sequence of cross-sectional distributions of impedance data obtained in the course of the measurement, but hardly accessible by the conventional simple evaluation approach, is condensed into one f-EIT image and visualized as a cross-sectional representation of regional lung ventilation.

As shown by the current results achieved in an infant during artificial ventilation, the clinical relevance of the functional evaluation of EIT data can be further increased by application of filtering procedures. Frequency filtering has been already proposed in EIT data processing (e.g., references 3, 25, and 26) to separate impedance changes related to the cardiac, gastric, or ventilatory activity. However, the application of the method in separating the regional lung volume changes due to spontaneous and mechanical inhalations is unique.

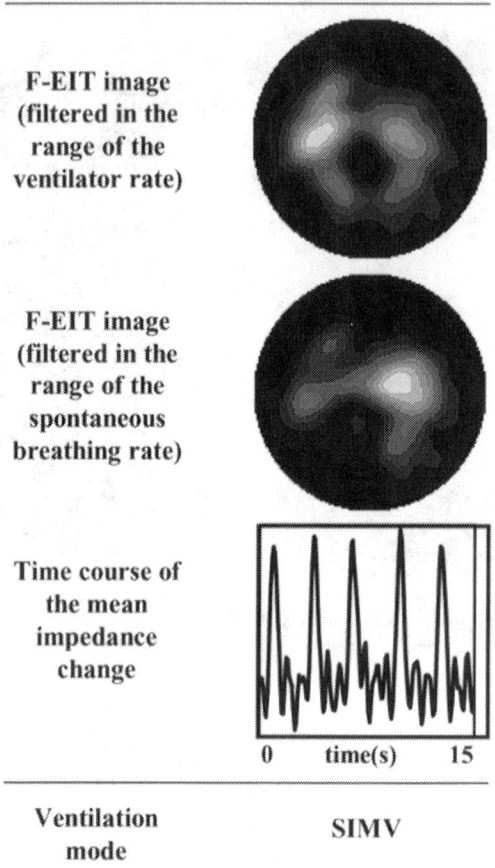

FIGURE 7. Functional EIT (f-EIT) images of an artificially ventilated baby obtained during a single EIT measurement at 1 week before the 5-day series of EIT measurements presented in the text and in FIGURE 3. The baby was ventilated with synchronized intermittent mandatory ventilation (SIMV). The upper f-EIT image shows mechanical ventilation and the lower one shows spontaneous ventilation. The images are autoscaled. The tracing of relative impedance change averaged over the whole thoracic cross section reflects the overall lung volume changes during the first 15 s of the measurement.

Mechanical inflations exhibit a different distribution of air in the lungs compared with spontaneous breathing.[27,28] Radiographic and scintigraphic examinations provided the evidence that the ventilation of the nondependent lung regions dominates during mechanical ventilation, whereas during spontaneous breathing the dependent regions receive the larger portion of the inspired air. This regionally different distribution of air in the lungs during artificial and spontaneous ventilation was also found in our previous measurements in adult patients using the f-EIT technique without filtering procedures.[7] In contrast with the previous studies performed in either awake or anesthetized subjects during the individual forms of ventilation, the current results show the regional differences in lung ventilation during one mixed ventilation mode that is a combination of spontaneous and artificial ventilation. The higher ventilation of the nondependent lung regions during mechanical breaths and of the dependent ones during spontaneous breathing was shown by the filtered f-EIT images during SIMV (see measurements 5, 6, and 7 in FIGURE 3).

The generation of separate f-EIT images representing the regional lung ventilation elicited by either spontaneous or mechanical breaths during assisted ventilation may be of importance in many cases of pathological processes that modify the distribution of ventilation. This is illustrated by the f-EIT images of spontaneous and mechanical ventilation in FIGURE 7. These images were generated from a single measurement performed during SIMV at one week before the complete series of 98 measurements was initiated in the same baby. It is obvious that the regional lung volume changes associated with the spontaneous or mechanical breaths exhibit an opposite distribution between the right and left lung. This is information that is not accessible by any other diagnostic tool. The overall measurement of ventilatory parameters (e.g., tidal volume) may mask such a nonhomogeneous distribution of air in the lungs. The risk of overinflation in some parts of the lungs and reduced ventilation in others may not be revealed and barotrauma may develop. The specific information on the regional ventilation magnitude related to the spontaneous or mechanical ventilation may help the clinician in an early adjustment and optimization of the ventilatory parameters.

At present, no technique exists that would be able to isolate and image the spontaneous and artificial ventilation in the thoracic cross section during assisted ventilation. In the clinical environment, the overall efficacy of ventilation is checked by blood gas analysis and the lung morphology is examined by radiography. A noninvasive bedside method providing information on regional ventilation without radiation load would be desirable in monitoring lung ventilation in small infants. As the gas exchange may vary during assisted ventilation, for example, by variation of the spontaneous breathing activity, by modified proportion between the spontaneous and mechanical inflations, by altered lung mechanics, or by intentional changes of ventilator parameters, rapid feedback information provided by f-EIT would be of benefit.

It remains to be clarified if f-EIT has the potential to become a routine tool for monitoring local lung ventilation. Several features of the EIT measurements, for example, noninvasiveness, inexpensiveness, easy repeatability of the measurements, and no need for the transport of the patient, favor the future use of the method in the clinical field. However, these positive aspects still do not compensate for the negative ones, such as the experimental design of the EIT hardware and software, the unpractical application of single skin electrodes, or the measuring problems associated with the noisy environment. The method is not yet ready for clinical use and its future will largely depend on the development of the EIT hardware and software as well as on the results of indispensable clinical trials.

REFERENCES

1. BANNER, M.J., S. LAMPOTANG, P.B. BLANCH & R.R. KIRBY. 1992. Mechanical ventilation. *In* Critical Care, p. 1391–1417. Lippincott. Philadelphia.
2. BROWN, B.H. & A.D. SEAGAR. 1987. The Sheffield data collection system. Clin. Phys. Physiol. Meas. **8**(suppl. A): 91–97.

3. HAHN, G., I. ŠIPINKOVÁ, F. BAISCH & G. HELLIGE. 1995. Changes in thoracic impedance distribution under different ventilatory conditions. Physiol. Meas. **16:** A161–A173.
4. FRERICHS, I., G. HAHN, T. SCHRÖDER & G. HELLIGE. 1998. Electrical impedance tomography in monitoring experimental lung injury. Intensive Care Med. **24:** 829–836.
5. FRERICHS, I., G. HAHN & G. HELLIGE. 1996. Gravity-dependent phenomena in lung ventilation determined by functional EIT. Physiol. Meas. **17:** A149–A157.
6. HAHN, G., I. FRERICHS, M. KLEYER & G. HELLIGE. 1996. Local mechanics of lung tissue determined by functional EIT. Physiol. Meas. **17:** A159–A166.
7. FRERICHS, I., G. HAHN, W. GOLISCH, M. KURPITZ, H. BURCHARDI & G. HELLIGE. 1998. Monitoring perioperative changes in distribution of pulmonary ventilation detected by functional electrical impedance tomography. Acta Anaesthesiol. Scand. **42:** 721–726.
8. FRERICHS, I., W. GOLISCH, G. HAHN, M. KURPITZ, H. BURCHARDI & G. HELLIGE. 1998. Heterogeneous distribution of pulmonary ventilation in intensive care patients detected by functional electrical impedance tomography. J. Intensive Care Med. **13:** 168–173.
9. BARBER, D.C. 1990. Quantification in impedance imaging. Clin. Phys. Physiol. Meas. **11**(suppl. A): 45–56.
10. TANG, W., D. RIDOUT & N. MODI. 1997. Assessment of total body water using bioelectrical impedance analysis in neonates receiving intensive care. Arch. Dis. Child. **77:** F123–F126.
11. DAVIES, P.S., S.E. JAGGER & J.J. REILLY. 1990. A relationship between bioelectrical impedance and total body water in young adults. Ann. Hum. Biol. **17:** 445–448.
12. BRADEN, D.S., L. LEATHERBURY, F.A. TREIBER & W.B. STRONG. 1990. Noninvasive assessment of cardiac output in children using impedance cardiography. Am. Heart J. **120:** 1166–1172.
13. O'CONNELL, A.J., J. TIBBALS & M. COULTHARD. 1991. Improving agreement between thoracic bioimpedance and dye dilution cardiac output estimation in children. Anaesth. Intensive Care **19:** 434–440.
14. LANGE, A., P. FUNCH-JENSEN, P. THOMMESEN & P.O. SCHIOTZ. 1997. Gastric emptying patterns of a liquid meal in newborn infants measured by epigastric impedance. Neurogastroenterol. Motil. **9:** 55–62.
15. SKOPNIK, H., J. SILNY, O. HEIBER, J. SCHULZ, G. RAU & G. HEIMANN. 1996. Gastroesophageal reflux in infants: evaluation of a new intraluminal impedance technique. J. Pediatr. Gastroenterol. Nutr. **23:** 591–598.
16. RAILTON, R., J. FISHER, I. MITCHELL & R.P.C. BARCLAY. 1983. Long-term respiration monitoring in infants—a comparison of impedance and pressure capsule monitors. Clin. Phys. Physiol. Meas. **4:** 91–94.
17. ADAMS, J.A., I.A. ZABALETA, D. STROH & M.A. SACKNER. 1993. Measurement of breath amplitudes: comparison of three noninvasive respiratory monitors to integrated pneumotachograph. Pediatr. Pulmonol. **16:** 254–258.
18. BAIRD, T.M. & M.R. NEUMANN. 1991. Effect of infant position on breath amplitude measured by transthoracic impedance and strain gauges. Pediatr. Pulmonol. **10:** 52–56.
19. HOLDER, D.S. & B.H. BROWN. 1993. Biomedical applications of EIT: a critical review. *In* Clinical and Physiological Applications of Electrical Impedance Tomography, p. 6–40. UCL Press. London.
20. MORUCCI, J.P. & B. RIGAUD. 1996. Bioelectrical impedance techniques in medicine. Part III: Impedance imaging. Third section: Medical applications. Crit. Rev. Biomed. Eng. **24:** 655–677.
21. KOTRE, C.J. 1997. Electrical impedance tomography. Br. J. Radiol. **70:** S200–S205.
22. TAKTAK, A., A. SPENCER, P. RECORD, R. GADD & P. ROLFE. 1996. Feasibility of neonatal lung imaging using electrical impedance tomography. Early Hum. Dev. **44:** 131–138.
23. HAMPSHIRE, A.R., R.H. SMALLWOOD, B.H. BROWN & R.H. PRIMHAK. 1995. Multifrequency and parametric EIT images of neonatal lungs. Physiol. Meas. **16:** A175–A189.
24. MARVEN, S.S., A.R. HAMPSHIRE, R.H. SMALLWOOD, B.H. BROWN & R.H. PRIMHAK. 1996. Reproducibility of electrical impedance tomographic spectroscopy (EITS) parametric images of neonatal lungs. Physiol. Meas. **17:** A205–A212.
25. LEATHARD, A.D., B.H. BROWN, J. CAMPBELL, F. ZHANG, A.H. MORICE & D. TAYLER. 1994. A comparison of ventilatory and cardiac related changes in EIT images of normal human lungs and of lungs with pulmonary emboli. Physiol. Meas. **15:** A137–A146.

26. Zadehkoochak, M., B.H. Blott, T.K. Hames & R.F. George. 1992. Pulmonary perfusion and ventricular ejection imaging by frequency domain filtering of EIT images. Physiol. Meas. **13:** A191–A196.
27. Rehder, K., A.D. Sessler & J.R. Rodarte. 1977. Regional intrapulmonary gas distribution in awake and anaesthetized-paralyzed man. J. Appl. Physiol. **42:** 391–402.
28. Froese, A.B. & A.C. Bryan. 1974. Effects of anesthesia and paralysis on diaphragmatic mechanics in man. Anesthesiology **41:** 242–255.

Gastric Emptying in Patients with Type I Diabetes Mellitus

NACHUM VAISMAN,[a] NOAMI WEINTROB,[b] ALEXANDER BLUMENTAL,[a] ZEEV YOSEFSBERG,[b] AND PNINA VARDI[b]

[a]*Department of Pediatrics, Kaplan Hospital, Rehovot 76100, Israel, and Hadassah Medical School, Hebrew University, Jerusalem, Israel*

[b]*Division of Endocrinology and Diabetes, Schnieder Children Hospital, Petach-Tikva, Israel, and The Sakler Medical School, Tel Aviv, Israel*

ABSTRACT: Diabetic autonomic neuropathy is a known complication of long-standing diabetes. The present study was designed to study the prevalence of asymptomatic prolonged gastric emptying (GE) in young patients with IDDM and its correlations with disease duration and autonomic nerve function. The study population included 40 poorly controlled patients, mean age 17.6 ± 4.6 years, with a disease duration of 1–17.5 years, and 20 age- and sex-matched controls. Autonomic nerve functions were assessed by standard cardiovascular reflexes, and gastrointestinal (GI) symptoms were assessed by a detailed questionnaire. GE was assessed by electrical impedance tomography (EIT), at 2 hours after a standard semisolid meal. Mean half-time gastric emptying was significantly prolonged in diabetic patients, 54.80 ± 26.63 versus 40.37 ± 8.62 min ($p < 0.05$), with a higher prevalence in the first 3 years and after 10 years of disease duration. No differences were found between diabetics and controls regarding cardiovascular tests. No correlations were found between age, GI scores, cardiovascular tests, and GE. Patients with IDDM may suffer from prolonged GE. This is not always accompanied by autonomic impairments. As impaired gastric emptying may involve poor glycemic control and early satiety, patients with difficulties in metabolic control or poor caloric intake should be studied for the possibility of delayed gastric emptying.

INTRODUCTION

Diabetic neuropathy is a known, often asymptomatic, complication of long-standing diabetes. It affects approximately 40% of the patients, usually correlates with peripheral neuropathy, and has a low prevalence in the first five years of the disease.[1] Diabetic neuropathy may be manifested in several organs, including cardiovascular, gastrointestinal, genitourinary, ocular, and sudomotor systems.[2,3] The symptoms are difficult to evaluate and to quantitate as most of them are nonspecific. Diabetic neuropathy may involve different parts of the nervous system. Several objective measurements of autonomic function have been developed using end-organ response to activation of neural reflexes. The most prevalent are cardiovascular tests, which are believed to also reflect damage elsewhere in the autonomic nervous system.[4–6] These tests study both parasympathetic and sympathetic damage.

Gastrointestinal symptoms are common among diabetic patients and include complaints such as postprandial nausea, epigastric pains, bloating, vomiting, and early satiety.[7–10] Gastric emptying may be one of the main causes of the above symptoms, causing unpredictable blood sugar fluctuations and frequent hypoglycemic episodes, as well as unexplained weight loss.[11,12] Some of the patients are asymptomatic, possibly due to afferent sensory denervation. Delayed gastric emptying results from defects in intrinsic (myenteric) or extrinsic (parasympathetic and sympathetic) neural innervation, as well as from myogenic reasons and hormonal disarrangement.

Most of the studies regarding GI complaints in diabetic patients include symptomatic subjects or descriptions of unusual case reports.[13,14] The present study was designed to study the prevalence of asymptomatic prolonged gastric emptying in young patients with type I diabetes mellitus and its correlation with disease duration, diabetic control, and other parameters of autonomic nerve function.

MATERIALS AND METHODS

Subjects

Forty (22 females) C-peptide-negative patients participated in the present study. The mean age of the patients was 17.59 ± 4.6 years (range, 6–25 years) and disease duration was 1–17.5 years. None of the participants had previous complaints regarding GI symptoms or was previously referred to a gastroenterologist for GI complaints that may have suggested gastroparesis. None of the diabetic subjects had such complaints prior to his or her diagnosis. Twenty age- and sex-matched healthy subjects served as a control group. The study took place in the Nutrition Clinic of Kaplan Hospital, Rehovot, Israel, and in the outpatient Endocrinology and Diabetes Clinic of Schnieder Children Hospital, Petach-Tikva, Israel. Glycosylated hemoglobin (GHb) was essayed by a commercial laboratory kit (SG-6200 Glyc-Affin GHb, ISOLAB Incorporated, Akron, Ohio) with a normal range of 4–8%.[15] The individual GHb was determined by the mean levels of the previous 12 months. Yearly funduscopic examination and 24-hour urine collection for microalbumin were performed on all patients with disease duration longer than 2 years. Prior to each test, blood glucose levels were monitored and, unless in the normal range, subjects were not enrolled in the study. The study was approved by the Human Subject Committee of Kaplan Hospital, Rehovot, Israel.

Assessment of Gastric Emptying

Gastric emptying was assessed by electrical impedance tomography (EIT) (IBEES, University of Sheffield, United Kingdom).[16–18] Each patient was instructed to have his/her regular insulin shot at 07:00 A.M. as well as his/her usual breakfast. At 10:00 A.M., each subject (diabetic or control) had a test meal that included 250 cc of 3% fat milk, 10 g of corn starch, 5 g of sucrose, 1 g of table salt, and 1 slice of bread for patients less than 40 kg, and 375 cc of 3% fat milk, 15 g of corn starch, 5 g of sucrose, 1.5 g of table salt, and 1 slice of bread for subjects above 40 kg. This test represented the midmorning meal of these subjects.

Assessment of Gastrointestinal Symptoms

Each subject was asked to fill out a gastrointestinal questionnaire including complaints regarding postprandial nausea, vomiting, abdominal pains and discomfort, early satiety, heartburn, and bowel habits (six categories). Each topic was rated by five grades of severeness. The minimal possible score was 6 and the maximal was 30. None of the patients or controls ever suffered from GI symptoms in the past.

Assessment of Cardiovascular Reflexes

Autonomic nerve function was assessed by studying standard cardiovascular reflexes as previously suggested.[5] The tests included heart-rate response to Valsalva maneuver, deep breathing, and standing for evaluation of possible parasympathetic damage, and blood-pressure response to standing and sustained handgrip for evaluation of possible sympathetic damage. The results were compared to normal controls.

Statistical Analysis

The different parameters of patients and healthy controls were compared by the Wilcoxon test. Association was measured by the Pearson correlation coefficient.

RESULTS

The mean half-time of gastric emptying was significantly prolonged in diabetic patients as compared to normal controls ($p < 0.05$). The standard deviation was significantly higher in the diabetic group (26.6 vs. 8.6, $p < 0.001$). The distribution of $T_{1/2}$ in patients and controls is illustrated in FIGURE 1. When dividing the patients into five groups according to their disease duration (0–2.5, 2.5–5, 5–7.5, 7.5–10, and more than 10 years), a U-shaped design was observed, but no statistical significant differences were found between groups (FIGURE 2). The score for gastrointestinal complaints was not different between groups and was almost normal in the diabetic group (8.5/30) and normal (6/30) in the healthy controls. No differences were found between diabetic patients and healthy controls in any of the cardiovascular tests regarding both sympathetic and parasympathetic systems. No correlation was found between age, glycosylated hemoglobin, GI score, $T_{1/2}$, or any of the cardiovascular tests.

DISCUSSION

Our results indicate abnormalities in gastric emptying in patients with type I diabetes with no previous gastrointestinal complaints or documented autonomic neuropathy. For 30% of our patients, GE was above normal (>2SD of the mean for the controls). Therefore, these results coincide with previous studies showing prolonged gastric emptying in diabetic patients.[19–22]

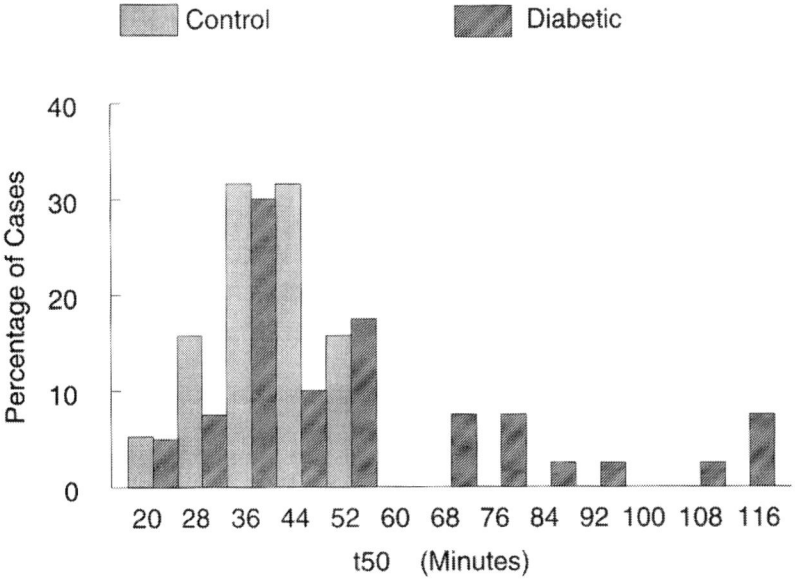

FIGURE 1. Distribution of gastric emptying (minutes) in diabetic patients and controls.

The present study was especially designed to study the effect of disease duration on gastric emptying of fairly young patients (<23 years) with IDDM. When studying gastric emptying as a function of disease duration, a U-shaped occurrence was found (FIGURE 2), with a tendency for higher prevalence of disarrangement in the first 3 years and after 10

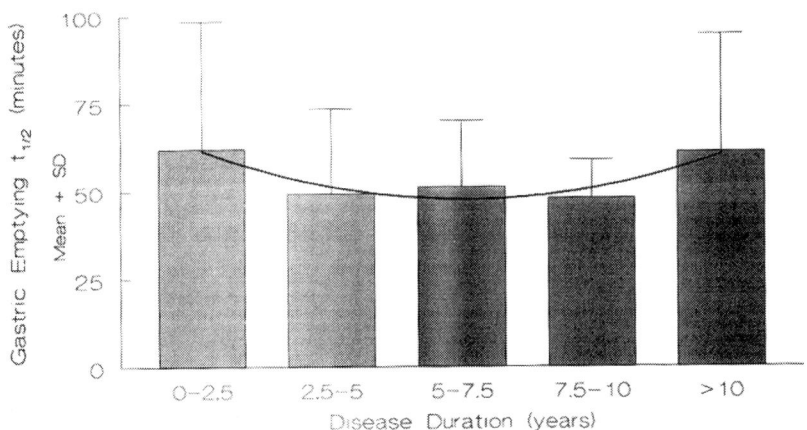

FIGURE 2. Gastric emptying as a function of disease duration in patients with IDDM.

years of disease diagnosis. The large standard deviation in these two periods demonstrates the large variability of our patients. In those two periods, almost half of the patients (4/9) had prolonged gastric emptying (more than the mean ± 2SD of the normal controls) as compared to 4/22 during 2.5–10 years of disease duration. The natural history of diabetic neuropathy is of gradual deterioration. Thus, one would wonder what is the cause for prolonged gastric emptying, especially in the first years after diagnosis.

Recently, it was shown that hyperglycemia slows gastric emptying in normal subjects and in patients with IDDM.[23,24] None of our patients was hyperglycemic during the morning prior to being studied. Yet, postprandial hyperglycemia may have been caused by inadequate insulin administration and we cannot rule out the effect of previous chronic hyperglycemia. On the other hand, we believe that prolonged gastric emptying after 10 years of disease may suggest neuropathic changes caused by the natural history of the disease. The fact that no correlation was found between glycosylated hemoglobin and gastric emptying might be explained by the small number of patients.

Diabetic neuropathy is evident by impaired sensory, motor, and reflex measurements and by impaired autonomic functions. Fraser *et al.*[25] found significant impairment of both peripheral and autonomic nerve function in patients with maturity onset type I and II diabetes mellitus. Peripheral impairments were more prevalent than autonomic impairments, with less prevalence in type I patients. Most of the patients improved with treatment. Our subjects, as a group, were not significantly different from our controls.

Lack of association between gastrointestinal symptoms and autonomic diabetes was also found by other investigators. In general, there is a poor correlation between gastrointestinal symptoms and objective data of gastric emptying in patients with IDDM or NIDDM.[26] Clouse and Lustman[27] found no correlation between the two in a group of adult patients (40.0 ± 15.1 years) with both type I and II diabetes with a mean duration of disease of 12.4 ± 7.6 years. On the other hand, GI complaints correlated with psychiatric illness. One should keep in mind that, in the present study, only the cardiovascular system was studied and no other organs that may be involved in this disorder.

Gastroparesis in diabetic patients in general and in patients with IDDM in particular has been previously documented by many groups,[19–22] yet none of the groups studied the effect of disease duration on gastric emptying in young patients with IDDM and with no previous GI complaints. Our results show that these patients may suffer from prolonged gastric emptying, but unless specifically asked most of the patients will not inform their caretakers about these problems. The prevalence of prolonged gastric emptying increases 10 years after diagnosis, most probably due to diabetic neuropathy as part of the natural history of poorly controlled diabetes. As impaired gastric emptying may involve poor glycemic control and early satiety, patients with difficulties in metabolic control or poor caloric intake should be studied for the possibility of delayed gastric emptying contributing to these symptoms.

REFERENCES

1. THE DCCT RESEARCH GROUP. 1988. Factors in development of diabetic neuropathy. Diabetes **37**: 476–481.
2. ASBURY, A. K. & D. PORTE. 1992. Diabetic neuropathy (consensus panel). Diabetes Care **15**: 62–67.

3. CLARKE, B. F., D. J. EWING & I. W. CAMPBELL. 1979. Diabetic autonomic neuropathy. Diabetologia **17:** 195–212.
4. MACKAY, J. D., M. M. PAGE, J. CAMBRIDGE & P. J. WATKINS. 1980. Diabetic autonomic neuropathy. Diabetologia **18:** 471–478.
5. EWING, D. J. & B. F. CLARKE. 1982. Diagnosis and management of diabetic autonomic neuropathy. BMJ **285:** 916–918.
6. EWING, D. J., C. N. MARTYN, R. J. YOUNG & B. F. CLARKE. 1985. The value of cardiovascular autonomic function tests: 10 years experience in diabetes. Diabetes Care **8:** 491–498.
7. LOO, F. D., D. W. PALMER, K. H. SOERGEL, J. H. KALBFLEISCH & C. M. WOOD. 1984. Gastric emptying in patients with diabetes mellitus. Gastroenterology **86:** 485–494.
8. CABALLERO-PLASENCIA, A. M., M. C. MUROS-NAVARRO, J. L. MARTIN-RUIZ et al. 1994. Gastroparesis of digestible and indigestible solids in patients with insulin-dependent diabetes mellitus or functional dyspepsia. Dig. Dis. Sci. **39:** 1409–1415.
9. CAMPBELL, I. W., R. C. HEADING, P. TOTHILL, T. A. S. BUIST, D. J. EWING & B. F. CLARKE. 1997. Gastric emptying in diabetic autonomic neuropathy. Gut **18:** 462–467.
10. IBER, F. L., S. PARVEEN, M. VANDRUNEN et al. 1993. Realisation of symptoms to impaired stomach, small bowel, and colon motility in long-standing diabetes. Dig. Dis. Sci. **38:** 45–50.
11. CAMPBELL, A. & H. CONWAY. 1960. Gastric retention and hypoglycemia in diabetes. Scott. Med. J. **5:** 167–168.
12. WOOTEN, R. L. & T. W. MERIWETHER. 1961. Diabetic gastric atony: a clinical study. JAMA **176:** 1082–1087.
13. REID, B., C. DILLORENZO, L. TRAVIS, A. F. FLORES, B. B. GRILL & P. E. HYMAN. 1992. Diabetic gastroparesis due to postprandial antral hypomotility in childhood. Pediatrics **90:** 43–46.
14. WEINTROB, N., S. PLAUT, N. SHALEV & C. SHARAN. 1994. Severe neuropathy in a young diabetic. Harefuah **127:** 305–308.
15. ABRAHAM, E. C., R. E. PERRY & M. STALLINGS. 1983. Application of affinity chromatography for separation and quantitation of glycosylated hemoglobins. J. Lab. Clin. Med. **102(2):** 187–197.
16. AVILL, R., Y. F. MANGNALL, N. C. BIRD et al. 1987. Applied potential tomography. Gastroenterology **92:** 1019–1026.
17. NOUR, S., Y. F. MANGNALL, J. A. S. DICKSON, A. G. JOHNSON & R. G. PEARSE. 1995. Applied potential tomography in the measurement of gastric emptying in infants. J. Pediatr. Gastrointest. Nutr. **20:** 65–72.
18. NOUR, S., Y. MANGNALL, J. A. S. DICKSON, R. PEARSE & A. G. JOHNSON. 1993. Measurement of gastric emptying in infants with pyloric stenosis using applied potential tomography. Arch. Dis. Child. **68:** 484–486.
19. BHARUCHA, A. E., M. CAMILLERI, P. A. LOW & A. R. ZINSMEISTER. 1993. Autonomic dysfunction in gastrointestinal motility disorders. Gut **34:** 397–401.
20. URBAIN, J. L. C., M. C. VEKEMANS, R. BOUILLON et al. 1993. Characterization of gastric antral motility disturbances in diabetes using a scintigraphic technique. J. Nucl. Med. **34:** 576–581.
21. HOROWITZ, M., M. EDELBROEK, R. FRASER, A. MADDOX & J. WISHART. 1991. Disordered gastric motor function in diabetes mellitus. Scand. J. Gastroenterol. **26:** 673–684.
22. DRENTH, J. P. H. & L. G. J. B. ENGELS. 1992. Diabetic gastroparesis. Drugs **44:** 537–553.
23. FRASER, R. J., M. HOROWITZ, A. F. MADDOX, P. E. HARDING, B. E. CHATTERTON & J. DENT. 1990. Hyperglycaemia slows gastric emptying in type I (insulin-dependent) diabetes mellitus. Diabetologia **33:** 675–680.
24. SCHWARCZ, E., M. PALMER, J. AMAN, M. HOROWITZ, M. STRIDSBERG & C. BERNE. 1997. Physiological hyperglycemia slows gastric emptying in normal subjects and patients with insulin-dependent diabetes mellitus. Gastroenterology **113:** 60–66.
25. FRASER, D. M., I. W. CAMPBELL, D. J. EWING et al. 1977. Peripheral and autonomic nerve function in newly diagnosed diabetes mellitus. Diabetes **26:** 546–550.
26. HOROWITZ, M., P. E. HARDING, A. F. MADDOX et al. 1989. Gastric and oesophageal emptying in patients with type 2 diabetes mellitus. Diabetologia **32:** 151–159.
27. CLOUSE, R. E. & P. J. LUSTMAN. 1989. Gastrointestinal symptoms in diabetic patients: lack of association with neuropathy. Am. J. Gastroenterol. **84:** 868–871.

Assessment and Calibration of a Low-Frequency System for Electrical Impedance Tomography (EIT), Optimized for Use in Imaging Brain Function in Ambulant Human Subjects

D. S. HOLDER,[a,b] C. A. GONZÁLEZ-CORREA,[c] T. TIDSWELL,[b] A. GIBSON,[b] G. CUSICK,[d] AND R. H. BAYFORD[b,e]

[b]Department of Clinical Neurophysiology, University College London, London W1N 8AA, United Kingdom

[c]Facultad de Medicina, Universidad de Caldas, Manizales, Colombia

[d]Department of Medical Physics, University College London, London W1N 8AA, United Kingdom

[e]Department of Electronic Engineering, Middlesex University, London N11 2NQ, United Kingdom

ABSTRACT: An EIT system has been produced that has been optimized for imaging impedance changes with scalp electrodes during brain activity in ambulant subjects. It can record from 225 Hz to 65 kHz, has a small headbox on a lead 10 m long, and has software programmable electrode selection. In calibration experiments in a small cylindrical tank filled with potassium chloride solution and samples of cucumber, noise was less than 1% with averaging, and acceptable images were produced at frequencies down to 1800 Hz. This suggests that EIT can be performed at low frequencies, which are likely to give larger signals during brain activity. Future work will include trials in humans and improvement of the current source and isolation.

INTRODUCTION

Impedance changes are known to occur in the brain during a variety of physiological and pathophysiological changes, such as stroke,[1] cortical spreading depression,[2] physiologically evoked visual or somatosensory responses,[3] and epilepsy.[4] Impedance changes are due to a combination of the following mechanisms—(1) Cell swelling: At frequencies used in EIT of below a few hundred kHz, most or all of the applied current travels in the extracellular space. During intense brain activity, or because of impaired energy supplies, cells swell when they run out of ATP needed to maintain the cellular volume. Water moves from the extra- to the intracellular compartment, so the extracellular space shrinks. This causes impedance increases of up to 100% or so. (2) Increased blood flow and volume: As the resistivity of blood is approximately one-quarter of that of the brain, increased blood volume during activity lowers the overall resistance. In addition, increased blood flow causes a decrease in resistivity because the higher impedance red cells tend to line up more along the central axis of the cylindrical blood vessels. (See reference 5 for a review.)

[a]D.S. Holder was supported by a Royal Society University Research Fellowship.

Our group at University College London has been interested in developing an EIT system for clinical use—the "UCH EIT system". The intended application is that it could be used to monitor brain function continuously in patients at risk over a period of days. The concept was that the device would comprise a miniaturized headbox, which could be worn in a waistcoat connected by a lead 10 m or so long to a base box attached to a PC.[6,7] Recording would be made from a ring of electrodes placed around the head in the occipitofrontal plane. Particular proposed applications would include monitoring for epilepsy or brain damage in newborn infants, recording physiologically evoked responses in adult humans, and recording in patients undergoing presurgical evaluation prior to resection of parts of the brain as a treatment for severe epilepsy.

Some special considerations are necessary for EIT of brain activity in the human head—(i) Low recording frequency: It has been shown that the impedance change during brain activity due to cell swelling is larger at lower frequencies.[8] This is because impedance changes only if applied current is restricted to the extracellular space. If current enters both the extra- and intracellular compartments, then the movement of water from one to the other will not produce a difference. At frequencies greater than a few kHz, some applied current passes into the intracellular compartment, across the capacitance of lipid cell membranes. As a result, the impedance changes during conditions causing cell swelling are smaller. The UCH EIT system is designed to record at frequencies from 225 Hz to 80 kHz. There is likely to be a trade-off between the increased signal expected from changes in the brain and technical problems because electrode and skin impedances are higher at lower frequencies. The frequency is therefore variable so that the optimum value may be selected in clinical trials. (ii) It is necessary to use current injection through widely separated electrodes[9] in order to inject sufficient current through the resistive skull. The current injection protocol was therefore software-driven so that differing injection protocols could be used.

Most EIT recordings in the literature employ measuring frequencies above 10 kHz on the basis that electrode impedances are larger at lower frequencies.[10] It was therefore uncertain whether our new system would produce acceptable images at low frequencies. This paper is a report of preliminary calibration studies, in saline-filled tanks, in order to determine the accuracy of our system. It is, to our knowledge, the first report of EIT images with applied frequencies in the sub-10-kHz range.

METHODS

The instrumentation employs 16 identical electrodes, of which 4 are used at a time to make a single impedance measurement. Two are used to deliver a test current to the patient, and the other 2 sense the resulting voltage. The system comprises three units: a host PC, used for control, data acquisition, and image reconstruction; a base unit, alongside the PC and connected to it, containing the measurement control and isolation circuitry and the power supplies; and a headbox, connected to the base box via a 10-m-long ribbon cable. The 16 electrodes are connected to the headbox by short, single-core leads (FIGURE 1).

A digitally controlled function generator produced a sinusoidal voltage at the measuring frequency, and a reference signal was used in the demodulator. The amplitude of the sinusoid was passed to an isolated voltage-to-current convertor, based around a current

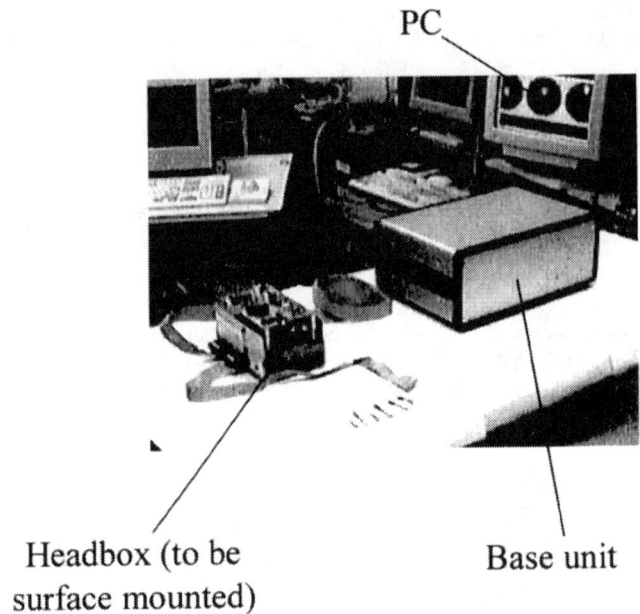

FIGURE 1. The "UCH EIT system" prototype. The headbox is shown with its lid removed. The prototype headbox is designed to be compatible with surface-mounted components. Once tested, it will be enclosed in a small box about the size of a cigarette packet. The headbox is connected to the base unit by a ribbon cable 10 m long.

conveyer integrated circuit. The current source outputs were connected to a selected pair of measuring electrodes via an 8 × 16 cross-point switch. Two further channels of the cross-point were used to connect a second pair of electrodes to the inputs of the sense amplifier. To protect the patient from DC offsets in the current source, multiplexer, or sense amplifier, each electrode was connected to the cross-point switch via a 1-µF nonpolar capacitor. The signal received from the sense electrodes was amplified and then demodulated in a simple synchronous rectifier. The rectifier reference signal was derived from the function generator producing the current drive signal, with an adjustable phase offset.

A Motorola HC11 microcontroller in the base box set the operating frequency, current amplitude, sense amplifier gain, and demodulator phase on the basis of commands from the host PC. The host could also select any 4 electrodes as the current drive and sense pairs, and could set up a sequence of electrode arrangements for automated scanning. The demodulator output was connected to an analog input of an A-D convertor board in the host PC. Conversions were initiated on the active transition of a "data valid" signal generated by the microcontroller.

Data acquisition was controlled by EITWIN 7.0. written in Borland C++ for Windows on a 486 PC. Gain and phase were individually optimized for each electrode combination by selecting the phase at which the greatest nonsaturating output voltage could be obtained with electrodes connected to a tank filled with saline solution. Measurements were made in a Perspex cylindrical tank with an inner diameter of 88 mm, 32 mm deep, and filled with 64 mL of 0.05% or 0.2% potassium chloride solution. The test object was a cylindrical sample of cucumber, cored from the cortex, whose resistivity was determined by direct measurement with a Hewlett-Packard 4284A impedance analyzer (see reference 11 for full experimental details). All measurements were done in room air and at room temperature (27 ± 0.5 °C). A current of 1.5 mA rms was applied at all frequencies for EIT image collection. Each image is the difference between data sets collected with saline alone and with the cucumber present. The fluid level was kept constant.

RESULTS

The resistivity of the cucumber varied with frequency. The contrast ratio, relative to the bathing solution of 0.05% KCl, ranged from 666% at 225 Hz to −29% at 65 kHz (FIGURE 2). Images were acquired with the same test objects (FIGURE 3). The correlation between the cucumber/bathing solution contrast recorded in EIT difference images and that measured directly using the Hewlett-Packard impedance analyzer is shown in FIGURE 4. A monotonic, but nonlinear, relationship may be observed. In all images, the cucumber may be discriminated visually from the background.

Maximum reciprocity errors ranged from 2.0% at 4800 Hz to 44% at 65 kHz. Peak noise in single frames was as high as 10% at 3600 Hz, but was reduced by a factor of about 10 if 36 frames were averaged together (TABLE 1). In general, reciprocity errors at high frequencies were less when the higher conductivity solution was used.

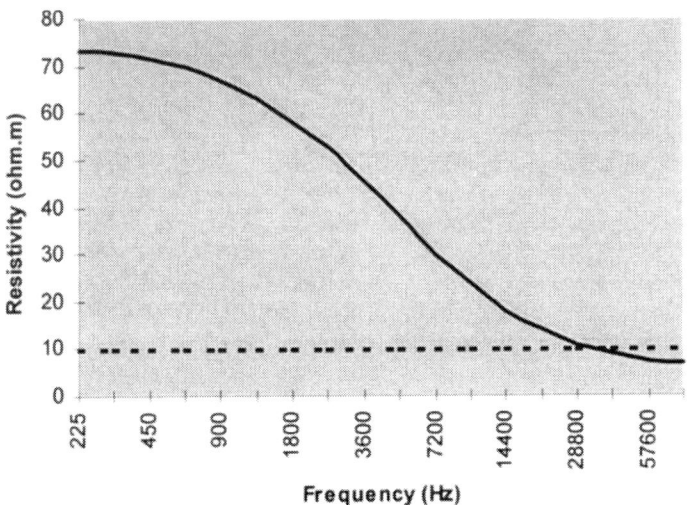

FIGURE 2. Variation of the resistivity of sample cucumbers with frequency (solid line—mean of six samples in three cucumbers), compared to 0.05% KCl solution (dashed line).

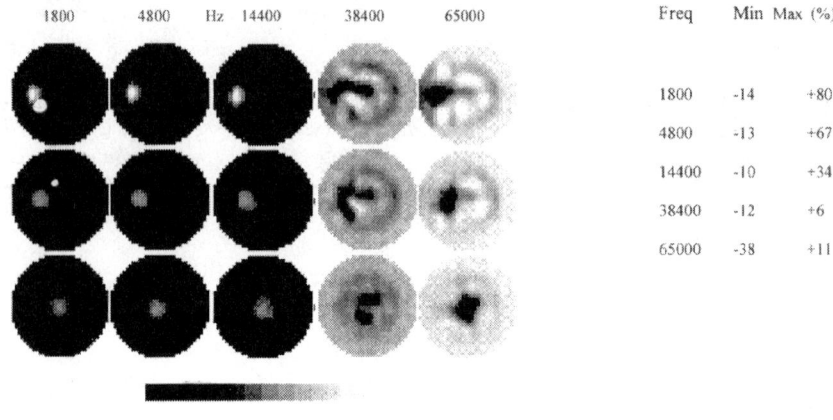

FIGURE 3. EIT images of cucumber in 0.05% KCl solution at different frequencies. The sample was placed at the center (bottom images), midway point (middle images), or edge (top images) of the tank. Impedance changes are normalized for each frequency.

DISCUSSION

The results indicate that it is possible to obtain acceptable images with frequencies as low as 1800 Hz. It therefore appears that the theoretical objection to using lower frequencies, because of increased electrode impedance, is not met with this electronic design, with steel electrodes in a tank. However, these images do not simulate the effect of skin impedance, which will also be greater at lower frequencies. The issue is whether the expected increase in signal due to use of lower frequencies will outweigh the likely instrumentation problems due to the higher skin and electrode impedance.

In a model of the phenomenon of cortical spreading depression (which is closely related to epilepsy), Ranck[8] showed that the impedance change increased from 43% at 50 kHz to 73% at 5 kHz. In contrast, the skin impedance of an area of 1 cm^2 increases from about 300 ohms at 100 kHz to 50 kΩ at 100 Hz.[12] In comparison, the impedance of a silver electrode of 0.5 mm^2 area increased from about 0.5 kΩ at 20 kHz to 4 kΩ at 200 Hz. Success in these experiments does not necessarily indicate that successful images will be possible with skin electrodes, where the series impedance of the skin will probably be considerably larger than that of the metal-saline interface. This series impedance is likely to have deleterious effects on accuracy through mechanisms like the production of common-mode errors.[13] This will be a matter for experimental valuation, and the flexible frequency settings of this device should enable such testing to be easily feasible in human subjects.

The performance of this system in terms of noise is similar to, but not as good as, the Sheffield Mark 1. Image quality in the tank is comparable to that of images acquired with the Sheffield Mark 1 system in a similar tank.[14] This is possibly because the Sheffield system employs transformer coupling, whereas this was not possible in our variable frequency system. The noise in our system can be reduced by averaging, but was roughly three times greater than that of the Mark 1 (using data from a Sheffield Mark 1 system in

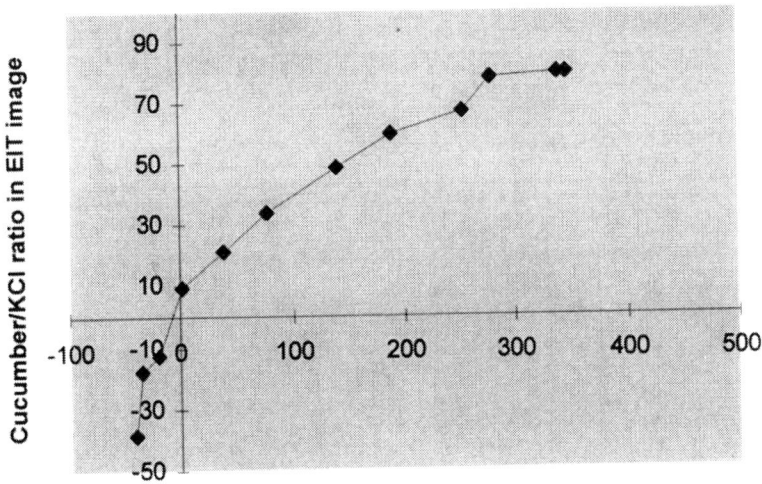

FIGURE 4. Peak impedance change in EIT image (over cucumber) plotted against actual contrast to KCl solution measured directly.

our laboratory in a similar tank). We are currently assessing if performance is significantly improved by simplifying the current source, physically separating the demodulator and amplifier inputs by moving the demodulator to the base box, and isolating the drive and amplifier circuits independently.

The advantage of using a biological test object in a tank is that it is possible to calibrate the accuracy of the system objectively. It is clear that there is not a linear relationship between the true impedance contrast and that seen in the EIT images. The limits of linearity, on theoretical grounds, are for impedance contrasts of about 20%,[14] so it is not surprising that the results presented above were not linear. There are presumably complex reasons for the nonlinearity, besides those expected on theoretical grounds. These will include nonidealities in the electronic components, coupled to instrumentation errors due to interactions with stray capacitance and electrode impedance. However, if these errors are consistent, it may be possible to adjust for them and thus perform multifrequency imaging across a range of frequencies. The advantage of biological test media is that they permit calibration to be performed on test objects with similar impedance properties to those expected in the body.[11]

The novelty of our system, compared to the several excellent existing single and multifrequency systems developed by other groups,[13] is that it can employ low frequencies, has a miniaturized headbox on a long lead, and has software selectable electrode combinations. Differing data collection protocols may therefore be easily performed in a clinical setting. With these improvements, we then plan to use the system for clinical trials of EIT with scalp electrodes for imaging evoked human brain activity in normal subjects and for helping to localize the source of epileptic seizures in patients undergoing preoperative assessment prior to epilepsy surgery.

TABLE 1. Noise and Reciprocity Errors for KCl Solution in the Tank

	0.05% KCl			0.2% KCl		
		Peak Noise			Peak Noise	
Frequency (Hz)	WRE (%)[a]	$n = 1$[b]	$n = 36$	WRE (%)	$n = 1$	$n = 10$
225	4.5	10.8	1.0	4.3	21.2	1.1
300	4.5	6.4	0.9	4.9	4.9	3.2
450	6.0	1.8	1.6	4.6	8.3	1.8
600	2.2	5.2	0.9	3.6	12.7	2.0
900	3.1	8.0	0.9	3.5	5.9	1.7
1200	2.4	12.8	1.5	2.9	8.6	2.3
1800	3.1	6.8	0.6	3.2	4.9	2.1
2400	2.3	6.8	0.6	2.7	5.2	1.8
3600	2.5	10.4	1.0	3.0	9.2	3.1
4800	2.0	4.7	1.0	3.4	5.7	1.5
7200	2.2	5.8	1.0	2.7	8.3	2.4
9600	3.6	4.2	0.5	2.0	4.6	2.5
14,400	4.7	3.6	0.5	3.3	9.1	3.1
19,200	8.7	5.0	0.6	3.1	7.3	1.8
28,800	14.9	6.8	1.5	4.6	8.3	2.3
38,400	18.5	3.8	1.0	4.7	9.2	1.7
57,600	31.6	4.1	1.6	7.2	8.8	3.7
65,000	43.9	7.5	2.0	9.6	7.3	2.2

[a] WRE = worst reciprocity error.

[b] n is the number of frames averaged.

REFERENCES

1. HOLDER, D.S. 1992. Electrical impedance tomography with cortical or scalp electrodes during global cerebral ischaemia in the anaesthetised rat. Clin. Phys. Physiol. Meas. **13:** 87–98.
2. BOONE, K., A.M. LEWIS & D.S. HOLDER. 1994. Imaging of cortical spreading depression by EIT: implications for localisation of epileptic foci. Physiol. Meas. **15:** A189–A198.
3. HOLDER, D.S., A. RAO & Y. HANQUAN. 1996. Imaging physiologically evoked responses by electrical impedance tomography with cortical electrodes in the anaesthetised rabbit. Physiol. Meas. **17:** A179–A186.
4. RAO, A., A. GIBSON & D.S. HOLDER. 1997. EIT images of electrically induced epileptic activity in anaesthetised rabbits. Med. Biol. Eng. Comput. **35**(suppl.): 327.
5. HOLDER, D.S. 1993. Opportunities for EIT imaging in the nervous system. In Clinical and Physiological Applications of Electrical Impedance Tomography, p. 166–175. UCL Press. London.
6. HOLDER, D.S., K. BOONE & G. CUSICK. 1994. Specification for an electrical impedance tomogram for imaging epilepsy in ambulatory human subjects. Innov. Technol. Biol. Med. **15**(SI 1): 33–39.
7. CUSICK, G., D.S. HOLDER, A. BIRKETT & K. BOONE. 1994. A system for impedance imaging of epilepsy in ambulatory human subjects. Innov. Technol. Biol. Med. **15**(SI 1): 40–46.
8. RANCK, J.B. 1964. Specific impedance of cerebral cortex during spreading depression, and an analysis of neuronal, neuroglial, and interstitial contribution. Exp. Neurol. **9:** 1–16.

9. BAYFORD, R.H., K.G. BOONE, Y. HANQUAN & D.S. HOLDER. 1996. Improvement of the positional accuracy of electrical impedance tomography (EIT) images of the head using a Lagrange multiplier reconstruction algorithm with diametric excitation. Physiol. Meas. **17**: A49–A57.
10. RAGHEB, T. & L.A. GEDDES. 1990. Electrical properties of metallic electrodes. Med. Biol. Eng. Comput. **28**: 182–186.
11. HOLDER, D.S., Y. HANQUAN & A. RAO. 1996. Some practical biological phantoms for calibrating multifrequency electrical impedance tomography. Physiol. Meas. **17**: A167–A177.
12. ROSELL, J., J. COLOMINAS, P. RIU, R. PALLAS-ARENY & J.G. WEBSTER. 1988. Skin impedance from 1 Hz to 1 MHz. IEEE Trans. Biomed. Eng. **35**: 649–651.
13. BOONE, K.G. & D.S. HOLDER. 1996. Current approaches to analogue instrumentation design in electrical impedance tomography. Physiol. Meas. **17**: 229–247.
14. HOLDER, D.S. & A. KHAN. 1994. Use of polyacrylamide gels in a saline filled tank to determine the linearity of the Sheffield Mark 1 electrical impedance tomography (EIT) system in measuring impedance disturbances. Physiol. Meas. **15**: A45–A50.

Impedance Mammograph 3D Phantom Studies

JERZY WTOREK, JAROSLAW STELTER, AND ANTONI NOWAKOWSKI

Department of Medical and Ecological Electronics, Technical University of Gdansk, 80-952 Gdansk, Poland

> ABSTRACT: The results obtained using the Technical University of Gdansk Electroimpedance Mammograph (TUGEM) of a 3D phantom study are presented. The TUGEM system is briefly described. The hardware contains the measurement head and DSP-based identification modules controlled by a PC computer. A specially developed reconstruction algorithm, Regulated Correction Frequency Algebraic Reconstruction Technique (RCFART), is used to obtain 3D images. To visualize results, the Advance Visualization System (AVS) is used. It allows a powerful image processing on a fast workstation or on a high-performance computer. Results of three types of 3D conductivity perturbations used in the study (aluminum, Plexiglas, and cucumber) are shown. The relative volumes of perturbations less than 2% of the measurement chamber are easily evidenced.

INTRODUCTION

The presented studies are performed to answer the following question—is there any chance to use electrical impedance tomography (EIT) in tissue recognition, for example, in mammography?

EIT attempts to image the electrical admittivity (or often just resistivity or conductivity) distribution of a body by injecting currents and measuring voltages (potential differences) on its boundary. Since different tissues are characterized by different admittivities, it should be possible to distinguish them in 3D images.

Conventional EIT systems employ the scheme of applying currents and measuring voltages. In general, to set up an electrical field across the examined object, one can choose either to drive a certain amount of current or to establish an electrical potential distribution on the tested object boundary using the attached electrodes. Applied potential tomography (APT)[1] and adaptive current tomography (ACT)[2] are systems belonging to the first group. The APT system sequentially applies electrical current using pairs of adjacent electrodes; voltages between adjacent noncurrent-carrying electrodes are measured. The ACT system simultaneously applies currents to all electrodes of a system, while voltages are measured on each electrode.

To avoid the problems of limited output characteristics of a current source, accurate measurement of currents being delivered to each electrode together with the resultant voltage should be done. It is possible to drive electrodes using voltage sources and to control the driving amplitudes to achieve the desired currents. As for patient safety, the maximum current delivered to each electrode should be limited.

A further improvement can be achieved using compound current-voltage electrodes. These electrodes enable both methods to be implemented in one system. It is possible to apply voltage to the boundary of a tested object and to measure the current distribution, or to apply current and to measure the voltage distribution. In addition, this allows inclusion of electrode contact impedance in the reconstruction process by previous estimation of its value. In the case where the compound electrodes are used, the number of independent measurements is increased to $N(N-1)/2$ as compared to $N(N-3)/2$ for normal electrodes.

Spatial resolution of EIT is limited by the number of independent measurements and by the signal-to-noise ratio. Additional reduction in spatial resolution arises from the nonlinearity of the problem. The physical dependence between the inner complex conductivity and surface voltages is governed by Maxwell's equations. This relationship is nonlinear; therefore, it is impossible to obtain a closed-form expression of the conductivity. Taking into account the examined subjects' electrical properties and the frequency of currents or voltages used in EIT, the resulting equation for the electric potential is the continuity or Laplace equation. In effect, the system spatial resolution may only be found in an experimental way.

The presented paper deals with 3D reconstruction. Very little work has been done up to now on the 3D aspects of EIT.[3-5] This is partly due to the increased computation and hardware complexity over 2D EIT. Electroimpedance 3D reconstruction algorithms and measurement systems involve a great deal of problems to be solved. The correctness of the chosen solutions of these problems can be validated by phantom studies. Two types of phantoms are possible: the first one relies on a network of appropriately connected resistors and capacitors; the second one use tanks filled with electrolyte. The first type of phantom was studied by Griffiths.[6] The phantom was designed for testing and comparing multifrequency EIT data collection systems. The phantom simulated a cylinder of homogeneous conductor with 16 drive and 16 receive electrodes interleaved. Combinations of resistors and capacitors were used to simulate the complex impedance, Z^*, of a typical tissue in the frequency range of 8–2048 kHz, obeying the Cole equation.

In spite of being relatively precise, the resistor-capacitor networks have the drawback of excluding electrode impedances from a measurement process. Measurements of test objects in a tank have the advantage that the clinical environment is simulated more closely as noise generated by the hardware as well as electrode impedances and other imperfections of the measurement channels are included in the reconstruction process.

A relatively difficult task is to create materials of demanded electric properties. Some proposals of solving this problem have been given by the Holder group.[7] They proposed the use of polyacrylamide gel, in which changes of resistivity are produced only by altering the gel concentration; the saline concentration of the test object remained the same as the bathing solution. The impedance change was caused by the obstruction of current flow by the nonconducting polymer that constituted the gel matrix. The advantages were as follows: (i) the impedance increases produced were stable with respect to time; (ii) the interface between the bathing solution and the object was composed of the same medium, saline. Continuing the work, they have studied three groups of phantoms:[8] (1) Inorganic materials, including barium titanate, polystyrene microspheres, and fumed silica, all in aqueous suspension—these had phase angles below 1° and thus were unsuitable. (2) Cucumber in KCl solution—cucumber cortex had a phase angle of 40° at the center frequency of 50 kHz; contrast between the cucumber and bathing solution could be selected by varying the KCl concentration. (3) Polyurethane sponge immersed in packed red cells—the phase angle of packed cells was about 25° at 1 MHz; sponge resistivities and permittivities when immersed in packed cells are 5–20% higher than for the bathing solution itself, for densities of 2–6.2% w/v.

Following this proposal in our experiment, a cucumber without skin (biological tissue), aluminum (conductor), and Plexiglas (insulator) objects were used as perturbations from the uniform conductivity of the electrolyte.

METHODS

Hardware

The study has been performed using the measuring system TUGEM.[9] The TUGEM includes a sensing head, DSP-based signal identification modules, and a PC computer (FIGURE 1). The sensing head contains a measurement chamber and a versatile current and voltage commutator. The measurement chamber is a hemisphere of 16-cm diameter with 64 compound electrodes placed in fixed positions (FIGURE 2). A fixed geometry of the measurement chamber is chosen to minimize any problems introduced by uncertainty of the object geometry. For phantom experiments, the chamber can be filled with saline solution and other materials can be immersed in so as to obtain conductivity perturbations. Additionally, it is expected that the layer of saline solution between the examined object and the surfaces of electrodes will stabilize the electrode impedances in *in vivo* measurements. The TUGEM injects electric currents and measures voltages, or applies voltage and measures currents, on the boundary of the object. The measured voltages or currents are affected by boundary contact impedances, which appear at an interface layer between an electrode and its contacting material. An effective way to avoid the contact impedance problem is the 4-electrode technique. Two electrodes are used to inject current, while 2

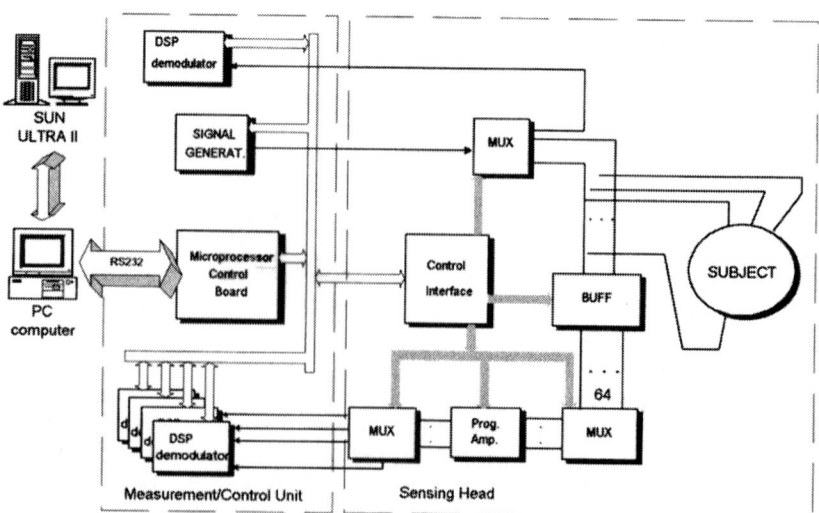

FIGURE 1. Block diagram of the Technical University of Gdansk Electroimpedance Mammograph. See text for details.

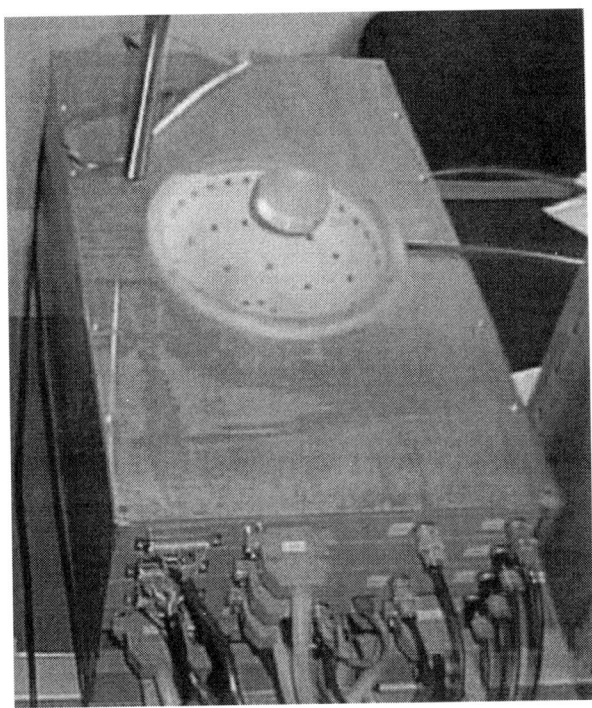

FIGURE 2. View of the sensing head containing the hemispherical measurement chamber. Four rows of compound electrodes are visible.

others are used to measure voltage. There are two possible applications of the 4-electrode method to impedance tomography: the first one is based on an interleaved-drive system and the second relies on using a compound electrode. In TUGEM, annular compound electrodes are used. Current or voltage is applied through the outer electrode, and voltage or current is measured by the inner one, respectively.

The measured values are transferred through the commutator to a measuring cassette. The cassette contains five measuring channels equipped with fast 12-bit A/D transducers and DSP processors. One measurement channel is devoted to measure applied voltage or current, while the other four are used to measure the resulting voltages or currents. Signals can be measured directly or by using the heterodyne technique. Therefore, an additional, synchronized, and spaced in frequency (by 10 kHz) heterodyne generator is used. Amplitudes of measured signals are optimized due to programmable amplifiers placed in front of the A/D convertors. Amplitude and phase shifts of the applied and resultant signals are calculated using specially developed algorithms.[10] The speed of signal identification is 1000 vectors per second and per channel. However, because of switching phenomena, the system speed is reduced and does not exceed a total of 1500 measurements/s.

All measurement processes—including the data transfer from the measuring channels to the PC computer, autocalibration, electrode impedance checking, and system configuration—are controlled by a 16-bit microprocessor controller equipped in a parallel interface for fast communication with a PC computer. Such system construction allows application of different algorithms of data collection and signal identification. The data are preprocessed in the PC computer before sending them to a UNIX graphic station or to a high-performance computer, where the reconstruction is performed.

Software

Software used in the TUGEM can be divided into three main groups: (i) software implemented on the DSP and on the microcontroller board, (ii) software implemented on the PC computer, and (iii) software implemented on the workstation. The main tasks of the microcontroller software are as follows:

- initializing all measurement circuits;
- dynamically changing all programmable parameters, including frequency and amplitude of the input current signal, gain of amplifiers, and selection of injection and measurement electrodes;
- starting of the DSP56001-based detectors;
- collecting data;
- formatting data and sending them to the PC;
- performing autocalibration and testing operations.

In the DSP board, many different types of identification algorithms can be implemented, but typically Nonuniform Sampling Fourier Series Analysis (NSFSA)[10] is used. This algorithm allows one to collect a specified number of samples, to calculate the real and imaginary parts of measured signals, and to send the results of calculations back to the microcontroller board.

Software implemented on the PC computer is written in C++ for Windows. This software is devoted to the following tasks:

- system configuration and calibration;
- data acquisition and preprocessing;
- configuration of experiment and measurement strategy;
- monitoring the progress in the measurement process;
- data transfer via the network.

Reconstruction is done using the Advance Visualization System (AVS). The main reason to use the AVS is its powerful capability of image processing. The software used has a modular structure. The reconstruction modules have been developed in our department. The forward problem for the hemisphere is solved by means of the finite element method.

The developed algorithm of reconstruction is called the Regulated Correction Frequency Algebraic Reconstruction Technique (RCFART).[11] This algorithm is a perturbation one and the formula for the conductivity change calculation is given by the relationship

$$\sigma_e^{(h+1,i)} = \sigma_e^{(hi)} + k\sigma_e^{(hi)} \frac{\sum_{j=1}^{L/H} \sum_{k=1}^{K} c_k^{(li)} s_{p(k,l)e}^{(i)}}{\sum_{j=1}^{L/H} \sum_{k=1}^{K} |s_{p(k,l)e}^{(i)}|}, \tag{1}$$

where $\sigma_e^{(1,i+1)} = \sigma_e^{(H+1,i)}$.

For the prescribed iteration i, in the succeeding corrections h ($h = 1, \ldots, H$), the σ_e terms (conductivities of elements) are modified for the subset of L/H uniformly distributed excitations l. The corrections are proportional to the current value of the conductivity $\sigma_e^{(hi)}$, the normalized covariance $c_k^{(li)}$ of the relative changes of the k-th measured currents to calculated ones for the l-th excitation, and the sensitivity coefficient $s_{p(k,l)e}^{(i)}$ for the element e. The frequency of corrections H should be equal to L/N, where N is a natural number.

A modification of the overrelaxation coefficient is introduced to speed up the reconstruction process. The overrelaxation constant k is dependent on the finite element distance from the surface of electrodes:

$$k(d) = 1 + (k_{max} - 1)\frac{d}{R}, \tag{2}$$

where d is the distance from the center of the element to the electrodes' surface and R is the radius of the hemisphere. An introduction of the dependence of the coefficient k on the element's placement increases the sensitivity for the contrast and the resolution in the center of the examined object, preserving relatively small errors for the superficial elements.

Admittivity Perturbations

In all reported examinations, the measurement chamber was filled with 0.9% NaCl or 0.2% KCl solutions. Three different materials—Plexiglas, aluminum, and cucumber—were used as conductivity perturbations. All perturbations were of cylindrical shape and of volume 2.3%, 0.5%, and 2% of the measurement hemisphere, respectively.

Absolute reference values of the admittivities of all cucumber samples and liquid solutions were measured using a Solartron SI1260 equipped with a measurement cell.[12] The direct impedance measurements were performed in a frequency range from 1 kHz up to 1 MHz. To obtain the mean values of the cucumber tissue parameters, at least three different measurements in the reference cell of three different volumes were performed. Experimental data were corrected by the three-point calibration technique.[13] Reference measurements to correct the results were made for solutions of known conductivities. Conductivities of inorganic perturbations were taken from the literature.[14]

Four different cucumber samples had the maximum phase angles of 35° at a frequency above 100 kHz, while the conductivity varied from 0.878 ± 0.10 mS/cm at 10 kHz to 1.958 ± 0.12 mS/cm at 100 kHz and 4.83 mS/cm at 1 MHz. The variability in the measured parameters between different samples did not exceed 20%. The cucumber samples during EIT measurement were immersed in KCl solution only for a few minutes; thus, the changes of their electrical properties were negligible. The electrical properties of the cucumbers were measured just before and after immersing in KCl solution.

The 0.2% KCl solution was of negligible permittivity and of conductivity equal to 4.43 mS/cm. This gave a cucumber/KCl conductivity ratio of about 66%. The variability in cucumber conductivity was lower than ±2%.

RESULTS

In all cases related here of phantom EIT reconstruction, the measurements were performed at 10 kHz and the RCFART algorithm was used. To obtain reasonable recognition of a sample, only four iterations of the reconstruction algorithm are satisfactory. As the sensitivity of reconstruction may vary with the position of a perturbation, several cases are shown in the following figures. In all cases, the real position of a sample (a), the result of the reconstruction (b), and the discrimination of that object using filtration (c) are indicated.

Even if the conductivity contrast between cucumber and the KCl solution is relatively small, the reconstructions are successful for all presented cucumber placements (FIGURES 3–5). In all cases, the volume of the cucumber sample is the same, equal to 2% of the measurement chamber volume. As absolute values of the conductivities after reconstruction may differ from those received from reference cell measurements, the decision should be made as to what values may be assumed as the sample border recognition. To calculate a perturbation volume in a reconstructed image, we assumed that the sample border is at the value of 50% of the extreme conductivity perturbation. The obtained volumes of the perturbations are dependent on their positions. The average perturbation conductivity is 2 mS/cm with standard deviation (STD) = 20.6%, while the relative perturbation volume is 2.4% for the first placement of the cucumber (FIGURE 3). The background conductivity is 4.4 mS/cm with STD = 14.7%. For the second case (FIGURE 4), the sample is located 5 cm distant from the border of the measurement chamber. The average perturbation conductivity is 3.1 mS/cm with STD = 7.9%, while the perturbation volume is 4.45%. The background average conductivity is 4.5 mS/cm with STD = 13.9%. The average perturbation conductivity is 3.24 mS/cm with STD = 7.35% and the perturbation volume is 6.51% for the cucumber located in the center of the measurement chamber (FIGURE 5); the background average conductivity is 4.45 mS/cm with STD = 9.9%.

Experiments with other objects are performed for the measurement chamber filled with 0.9% NaCl solution. The images obtained for two inorganic cylinders (Plexiglas and aluminum) are presented in FIGURES 6 and 7. In these cases, the conductivity contrast is very high, but it is deformed by interface phenomena. These deformations are not estimated. Both perturbations are visible; however, contrasts depend on mutual placement of the perturbations. In the case of a relatively far distance between the aluminum and Plexiglas cylinders, the obtained contrasts for Plexiglas and aluminum are 41% and 50%, respectively (FIGURE 6). These values are significantly reduced for a shorter distance between perturbations (FIGURE 7). In addition, the shapes of images are changed.

The last example of reconstruction shows the image obtained for the aluminum cylinder kept in two fingers (FIGURE 8). The measurement chamber is filled with 0.9% NaCl solution. The average conductivity of the fingers is lower than that of the solution, while the aluminum conductivity is much higher. A threshold filtration was applied to the obtained image. Fingers are visible as a low conductivity region (FIGURE 8b), while the aluminum cylinder is seen as a high conductivity region (FIGURE 8c).

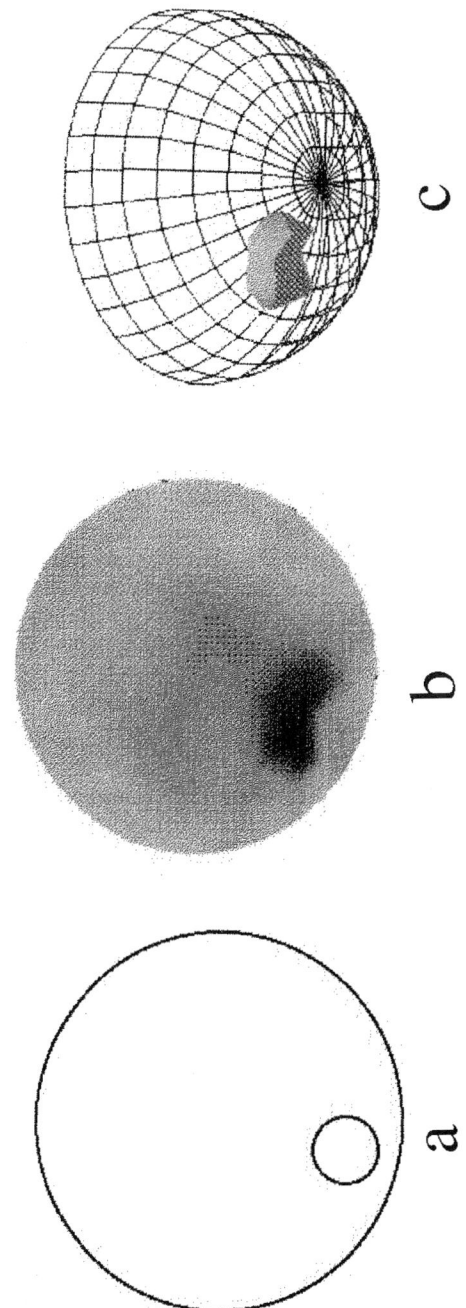

FIGURE 3. Cucumber cylinder with 2% volume of the measurement chamber: (a) position in the chamber; (b) 2D slice of the reconstruction image; (c) 3D view of the region with an average conductivity of 2.04 mS/cm (50% of the minimal value in the reconstructed image).

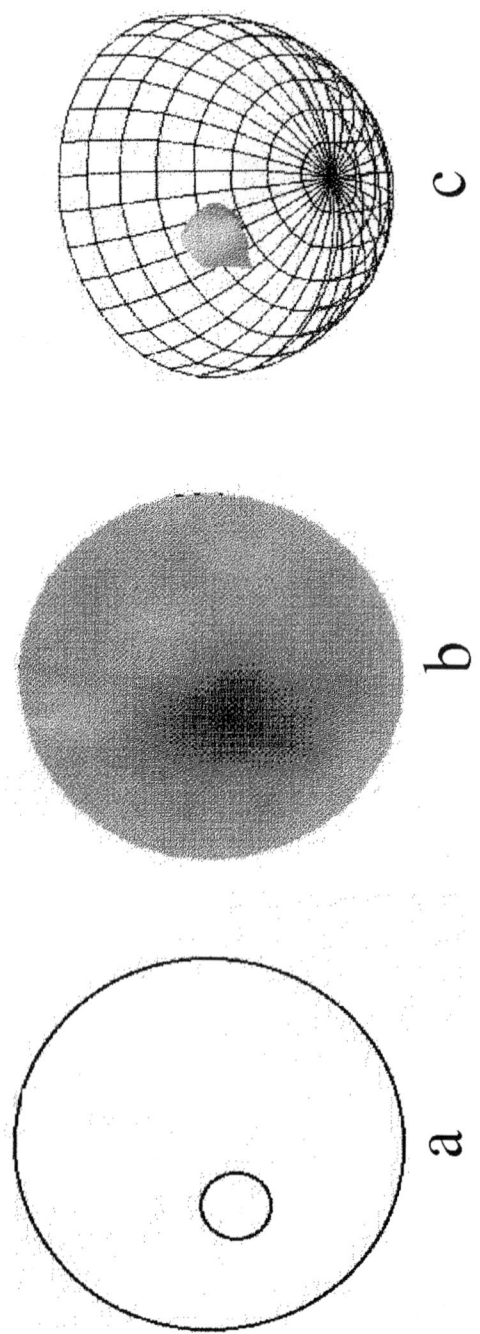

FIGURE 4. Cucumber cylinder with 2% volume of the measurement chamber: (a) position in the chamber; (b) 2D slice of the reconstruction image; (c) 3D view of the region with an average conductivity of 3.08 mS/cm (50% of the minimal value in the reconstructed image).

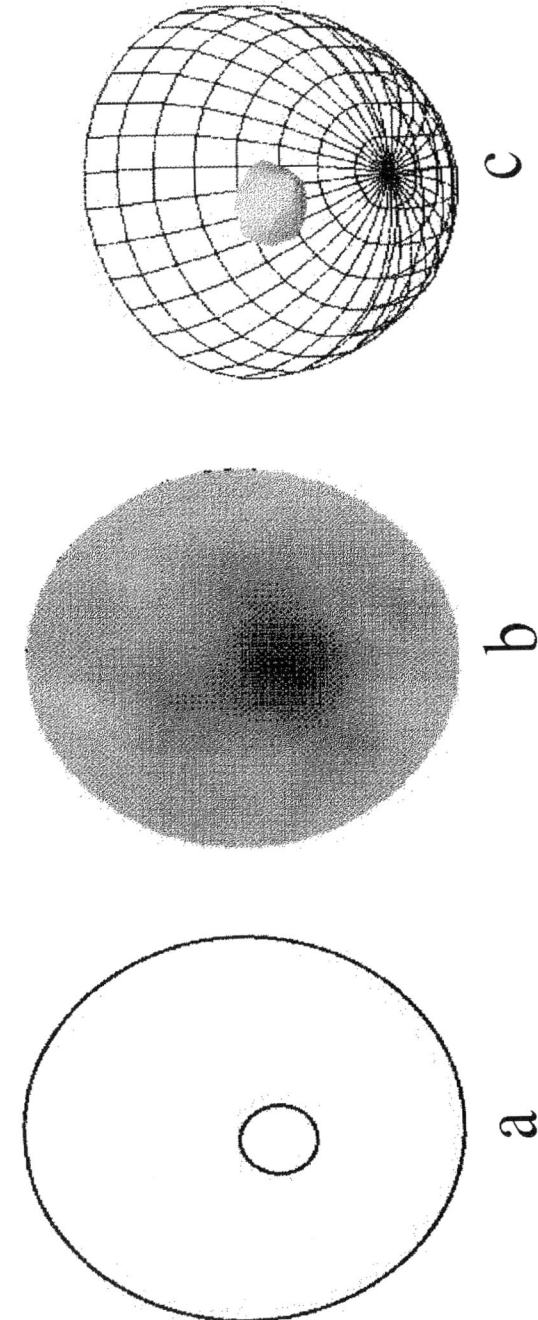

FIGURE 5. Cucumber cylinder with 2% volume of the measurement chamber: (a) position in the chamber; (b) 2D slice of the reconstruction image; (c) 3D view of the region with an average conductivity of 3.24 mS/cm (50% of the minimal value in the reconstructed image).

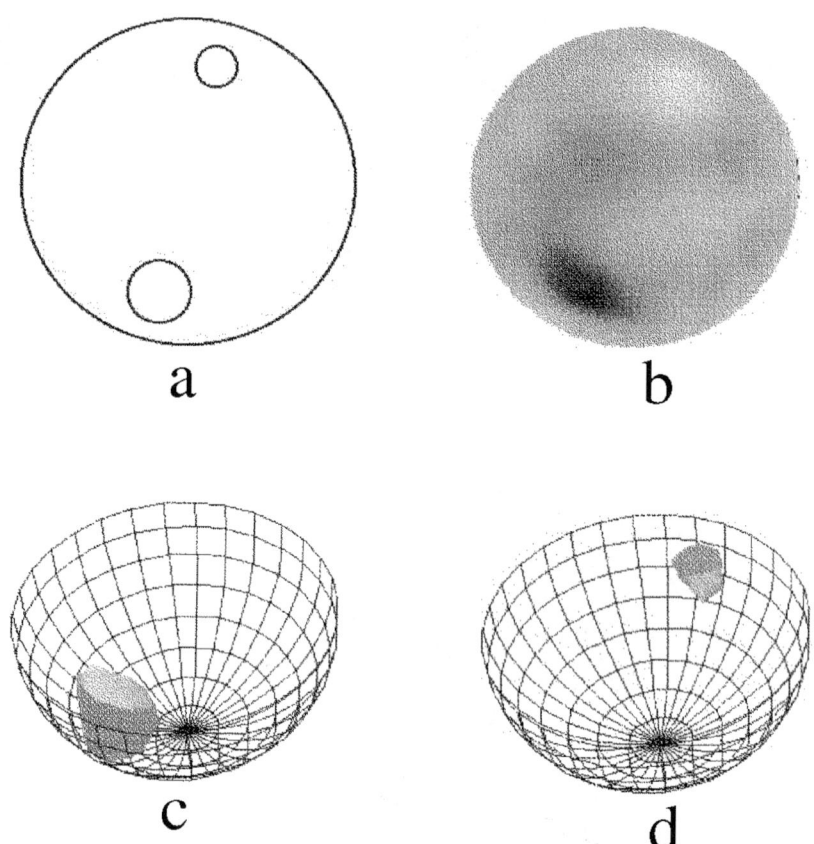

FIGURE 6. Plexiglas cylinder (bigger) and aluminum (smaller) immersed in 0.9% NaCl solution on opposite sites of the measurement chamber: (a) position in the chamber; (b) 2D slice of the reconstruction image; (c) 3D view of the region with low conductivity; (d) 3D view of the region with high conductivity.

DISCUSSION AND CONCLUSIONS

A real 3D EIT measurement system with a 3D reconstruction algorithm is presented. The 3D reconstruction process is relatively complicated and demands high-performance computing resources, including proper memory space and a high-speed processor unit, especially for an increased number of electrodes. The AVS software is applied to reconstruct the object, to process the obtained images, and finally to visualize them. The average time of the RCFART reconstruction on Sun Ultra 1 (170 MHz) of a 3D image, using 64 compound electrodes, is 5 minutes. All results are presented in the form of color images. Those presented in this paper are converted from color to a gray scale; therefore, small changes in the pictures are introduced.

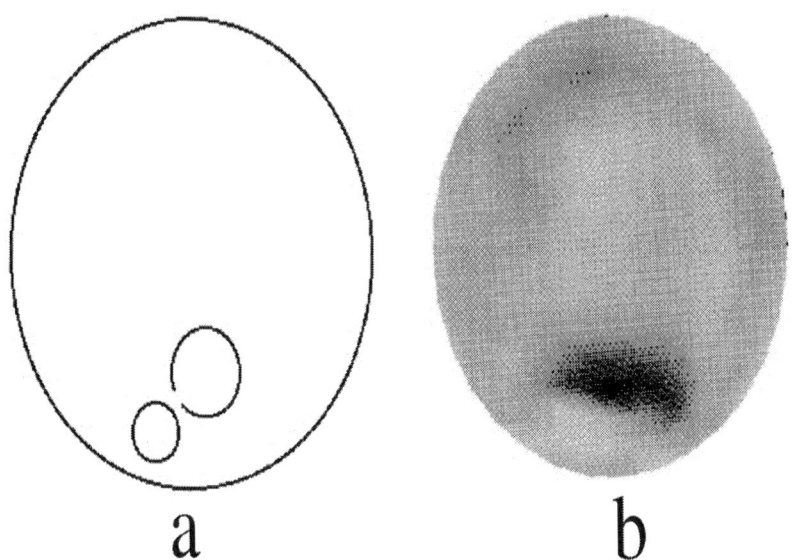

FIGURE 7. Plexiglas cylinder (bigger) and aluminum (smaller) immersed in 0.9% NaCl solution and very close to each other: (a) position in the chamber; (b) 2D slice of the reconstruction image.

Three algebraic reconstruction methods can be used in our system: Algebraic Reconstruction Technique (ART), Simultaneous Iteration Reconstruction Technique (SIRT), and RCFART. The RCFART algorithm differs from ART and SIRT in three points: (i) the number of corrections made during one iteration of the reconstruction process is chosen arbitrarily (one correction per iteration is equivalent to the ART; if the correction number per iteration is equal to the number of electrodes, the method is identical with the SIRT); (ii) instead of the Jacobian matrix, the sensitivity theorem is used; (iii) the value of the overrelaxation coefficient depends on the distance of the corrected element from the boundary of the measurement chamber (the greater this distance, the greater the value of the coefficient used). The reconstruction algorithms differ in memory consumption and computation complexity, which affect the time of reconstruction.

Although the TUGEM hardware is very versatile, it enables satisfactory reconstructions of samples of relative volumes comparable to 0.5%. Further improvement is expected by using averaging methods in the data.

Three types of conductivity perturbations have been used in the study. Different presentations of the results show that objects of relative volume of 2% and not having high contrast can be recognizable. The accuracy of the contrast reconstruction depends on the relative placement of different perturbations. This is a serious drawback of the method. Additionally, which is obvious, the reconstructions are strongly influenced by the relative perturbation location.

The results obtained in our study, when compared with those published by other groups, show an improvement in the reconstruction of relatively small objects characterized by a relatively low contrast. Now, we are involved in the preparation of multifre-

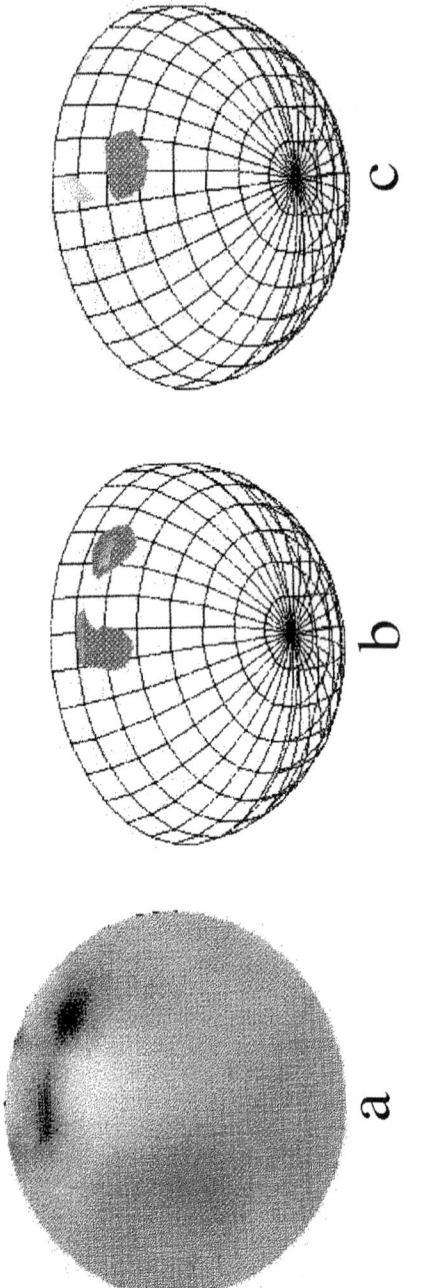

FIGURE 8. Aluminum cylinder kept in two fingers by a human (a). The measurement chamber was filled with 0.9% NaCl solution; thus, fingers are less conductive (dark) than the background and aluminum (light) of course is more conductive. Two further images show the image of the fingers (b) and the aluminum cylinder (c).

quency reconstruction algorithms that should enable us to reconstruct, we hope, even smaller objects.

Almost all the published data have used test objects made of highly different resistivity from the background, such as polythene or metal ones. On the other hand, most of the current algorithms work on the basis of a linear relation between the changes of voltage at the periphery and the impedance inside the object. As the Laplace law is inherently nonlinear, this is only approximately correct for a small impedance change. It cannot be correct for highly resistive or conductive perturbations. A solution to this problem has been attempted by using agar or other gels made up with saline of different concentration to that in the bathing solution. However, such test objects are not adequate for long-lasting studies. The alternative solution is that proposed by Holder.[7] This problem will be studied by our group in future work.

REFERENCES

1. BROWN, B.H., D.C. BARBER & A.D. SEAGAR. 1985. Applied potential tomography: possible clinical applications. Clin. Phys. Physiol. Meas. **6:** 109–121.
2. COOK, R.D., G.J. SAULINER, D.G. GISSER, J.C. GOBLE, J.C. NEWELL & D. ISAACSON. 1994. ACT3: a high-speed, high precision electrical impedance tomograph. IEEE Trans. Biomed. Eng. **41**(8): 713–722.
3. KLEINERMANN, F., N.J. AVIS, S.K. JUDATH & D.C. BARBER. 1996. Three-dimensional image reconstruction for electrical impedance tomography. Physiol. Meas. **17:** A77–A83.
4. GUARDO, R., C. BOULAY, B. MURRAY & M. BERTRAND. 1991. An experimental study in electrical impedance tomography using backprojection reconstruction. IEEE Trans. Biomed. Eng. **38**(7): 617–627.
5. GLIDEWELL, M.E. & K.T. NG. 1997. Anatomically constrained electrical impedance tomography for three-dimensional anisotropic bodies. IEEE Trans. Med. Imaging **16**(5): 572–580.
6. GRIFFITHS, H. 1995. A Cole phantom for EIT. Physiol. Meas. **16:** A29–A38.
7. HOLDER, D.S. & A. KHAN. 1994. Use of polyacrylamide gels in a saline-filled tank to determine the linearity of the Sheffield Mark 1 electrical impedance tomography (EIT) system in measuring impedance disturbances. Physiol. Meas. **15:** A45–A50.
8. HOLDER, D.S., Y. HANQUAN & A. RAO. 1996. Some practical biological phantoms for calibrating multifrequency electrical impedance tomography. Physiol. Meas. **17:** A167–A177.
9. NOWAKOWSKI, A., J. WTOREK & J. STELTER. 1995. A Technical University of Gdansk Electroimpedance Mammograph. *In* Proceedings of the IX International Conference on Electrical Bioimpedance, Heidelberg, Germany, p. 434–437.
10. STELTER, J. & A. NOWAKOWSKI. 1996. Digital demodulator procedure for impedance mammography. *In* Proceedings (CD-ROM) of 18th Annu. Int. Conf. IEEE Eng. Med. Biol. Soc.
11. KOCIKOWSKI, M. & A. NOWAKOWSKI. 1998. RCFART—3D reconstruction algorithm for EIT. *In* Proceedings of the X International Conference on Electrical Bioimpedance, Barcelona, Spain, p. 425–428.
12. STELTER, J., J. WTOREK, A. NOWAKOWSKI, A. KOPACZ & T. JASTRZEBSKI. 1998. Complex permittivity of breast tumor tissue. *In* Proceedings of the X International Conference on Electrical Bioimpedance, Barcelona, Spain, p. 59–62.
13. BAO, J., C.C. DAVIS & R.E. SCHMUKLER. 1993. Impedance spectroscopy of human erythrocytes: system calibration and non-linear modelling. IEEE Trans. Biomed. Eng. **40**(4): 364–378.
14. PASZKOWSKI, B. 1970. Handbook of Electronics. Scientific and technical editions (in Polish).

Can We Optimize Electrode Placement for Impedance Pneumography?

N. KHAMBETE, P. METHERALL, B. BROWN, R. SMALLWOOD, AND R. HOSE

Department of Medical Physics and Clinical Engineering, University of Sheffield, Royal Hallamshire Hospital, Sheffield S10 2JF, United Kingdom

ABSTRACT: In this paper, we discuss issues involved in defining an optimum placement of four electrodes for impedance pneumography. We observed a general trend where the change in impedance (ΔZ) decreased while the sensitivity ($\Delta Z/Z$) increased with distance between the drive and receive electrode pairs. However, the theoretical study indicated that $\Delta Z/Z$ should decrease with distance. The scatter of points in the plots indicated that sensitivity was influenced by factors other than distance. The correlation coefficient between the theoretical and measured $\Delta Z/Z$ was low, but significant. This suggested that the best electrode configuration can be derived from the theoretical data. High $\Delta Z/Z$ was obtained when the drive and receive electrode pairs were placed close to the lungs and in different horizontal planes.

INTRODUCTION

Impedance pneumography is a technique of monitoring respiration by measuring changes in the electrical impedance of the thoracic cavity. The impedance of the thoracic cavity increases with an increase in lung air volume during inspiration and decreases during expiration. This measurement is achieved by injecting a high-frequency, low-amplitude alternating current into the body using a pair of surface electrodes and measuring the resultant changes in voltage by the same or a different pair of electrodes placed at an appropriate location. There exists a good correlation between the volume of inspired air and the impedance of the thoracic cavity.[1]

The impedance of the thoracic cavity has two components. The base impedance (Z) depends upon the impedance of all the tissues within the cavity, while the time-varying component of impedance (ΔZ) depends upon changes occurring due to breathing. The impedance also changes due to the cardiac activity, but these changes are small compared to those caused by breathing. The sensitivity of an electrode configuration to pulmonary changes can be expressed as the ratio $\Delta Z/Z$. This sensitivity is a function of electrode placement for a given subject.[2,3]

In this paper, we have reported results of our work aimed at finding an optimum electrode placement for impedance pneumography. We studied the relationship between ΔZ and $\Delta Z/Z$, and the distance between the drive and receive electrode pairs. Impedance data were recorded from normal human subjects by placing 32 drive and 32 receive electrode pairs around the thoracic cavity. We also studied this relationship theoretically using the sensitivity method of Geselowitz.[4]

METHODS

Experimental Studies

Impedance changes from the thoracic cavity were recorded during spontaneous tidal breathing from eight normal human subjects with a mean age of 27.9 years (range, 22–56) using the Sheffield Mark 3b data collection system.[5] The system consisted of 32 drive and 32 receive electrode pairs separated in 4 horizontal planes, with each plane having 16 equally spaced electrodes forming 8 drive and 8 receive interleaved pairs. This arrangement produced 1024 electrode configurations. The anatomical locations of the planes are shown in FIGURE 1. The current (2 mA peak-to-peak) was injected between one pair of drive electrodes, and the voltage from all the 32 receive electrode pairs was recorded. This was repeated for all the 32 drive pairs, resulting in a set of 1024 measurements. The system was designed to inject current at 8 frequencies in the range of 9.6 kHz to 1.22 MHz in binary steps. We chose measurements at a single frequency (76.8 kHz) for our analysis. The frame rate achieved by the system was 16.7 Hz. Volunteers were asked to relax in an upright sitting position and to perform normal tidal breathing. The data were collected for a duration of approximately 1 minute from each subject.

The data obtained from each electrode configuration were first low-pass filtered (Butterworth filter of order 10, cutoff frequency of 0.8 Hz) to reduce noise and the impedance changes occurring due to the cardiac activity. The mean impedance change with time for breathing was obtained by taking the mean of all the 1024 measurements. This waveform was processed using a peak detection algorithm to determine the frames corresponding to

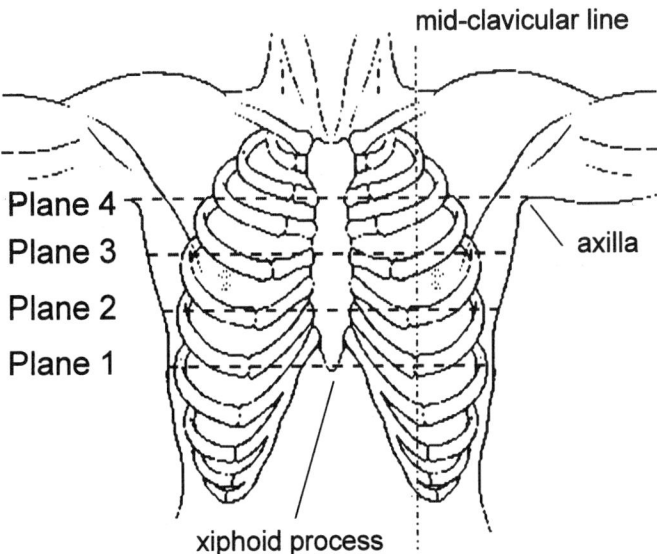

FIGURE 1. Electrode placement in 4 planes. Sixteen electrodes were placed around the thorax in each plane.

instants of maximum inspiration and expiration. The change in impedance (ΔZ) for each of the 1024 measurements was calculated by subtracting the mean value of impedance for the expiration frames from the mean value of impedance for the inspiration frames. The base impedance (Z) was calculated as the mean impedance for the entire time duration. The sensitivity was given by the ratio $\Delta Z/Z$.

The distance between the midpoint of each drive and receive pair was calculated geometrically. The thoracic cavity was assumed to have an elliptical cross section with a ratio of major to minor axis of 1.7.[6] The vertical separation between the electrode planes was assumed to be equal to half the minor axis.

Theoretical Studies

The purpose of our theoretical studies was to determine the same relationships using the sensitivity method of Geselowitz.[4] A simplified model was developed for the thoracic cavity, assuming it to be a homogeneous cylindrical volume conductor consisting of two regions to represent the two lungs as shown in FIGURE 2. It was necessary to generate a sensitivity matrix that could relate impedance changes occurring within these two regions to the voltages recorded by the 32 receive electrodes when a unit current was injected between each of the 32 drive pairs. The finite element modeling (FEM) technique was used for this purpose.

The cylindrical model was meshed into 37,632 "brick" elements, each having 8 nodes, using Ansys software (Ansys Inc., version 5.3.). The node voltages were obtained by solving the finite element model for the 32 drive and 32 receive pairs. The elemental voltage

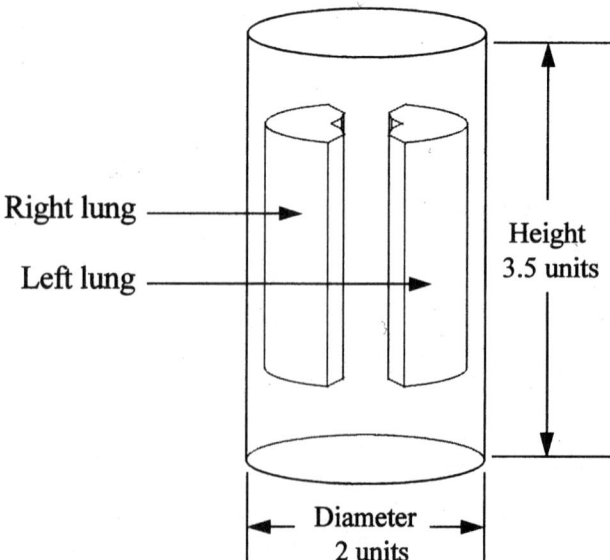

FIGURE 2. Cylindrical volume conductor model for the thoracic cavity showing location of the lungs.

gradient for the *j*-th element for a particular drive or receive electrode pair was calculated from the node voltages using equation 1:

$$\nabla\Phi = \nabla\mathbf{N}\cdot\mathbf{V}_{jn} \quad (1)$$

where

$\nabla\Phi$ = voltage gradient for the *j*-th element,
$\mathbf{N}$ = shape function of the brick element with 8 nodes,[7]
$\mathbf{V}_{jn}$ = node voltages for $n = 8$ nodes of the *j*-th element.

The sensitivity coefficient corresponding to the *j*-th element and *i*-th drive-receive configuration was given by the scalar product of the elemental voltage gradients $\nabla\Phi_i$ (drive pair) and $\nabla\Psi_i$ (receive pair) as shown in equation 2:[8]

$$S_{ij} = -\int_{j\text{-th element}} \nabla\Phi_i \cdot \nabla\Psi_i dv. \quad (2)$$

The integration is over the volume of the *j*-th element.

The base impedance (**Z**) for the 1024 configurations was evaluated by premultiplying the resistivity vector (**c**) by the sensitivity matrix (**S**) as in equation 3:

$$\mathbf{Z} = \mathbf{S}\cdot\mathbf{c}. \quad (3)$$

The resistivity value of all the elements in **c** was set to 1 for evaluating **Z**. The breathing-related impedance changes were simulated by specifying a 10% change from the uniform resistivity value of the elements belonging to the two lung regions. It was assumed that this perturbation of 10% did not affect the isopotential surfaces, and the linearized sensitivity matrix **S** could be used to generate a new set of 1024 boundary voltage measurements ($\mathbf{Z}_{10\%}$) using equation 3. Finally, the $\Delta\mathbf{Z}$ and $\Delta\mathbf{Z}/\mathbf{Z}$ were given by

$$\Delta\mathbf{Z} = \mathbf{Z} - \mathbf{Z}_{10\%} \quad (4)$$

$$\Delta\mathbf{Z}/\mathbf{Z} = (\mathbf{Z} - \mathbf{Z}_{10\%})/\mathbf{Z}. \quad (5)$$

The distance between the drive and receive electrode pair was also calculated geometrically from the electrode coordinates extracted from the FEM model. Thus, this calculation was based on the circular cross section and not on the elliptical cross section, as in the case of experimental data.

RESULTS

Measured Data

FIGURES 3a and 3b plot ΔZ and $\Delta Z/Z$ versus distance for the measured data, respectively. The solid line indicates the regression line of y-axis values on x-axis values. The dashed line indicates the 95% confidence interval and the dash-dot line indicates the 95% prediction interval. The ΔZ and $\Delta Z/Z$ values are the mean of the eight subjects and the distance is expressed as the fraction of the minor axis of the ellipse used to calculate the distance. The plot of ΔZ versus distance, shown in FIGURE 3a, indicates a decreasing trend with distance (slope = -0.157, $p < 0.005$). FIGURE 3b shows the plot of $\Delta Z/Z$ versus dis-

538 ANNALS NEW YORK ACADEMY OF SCIENCES

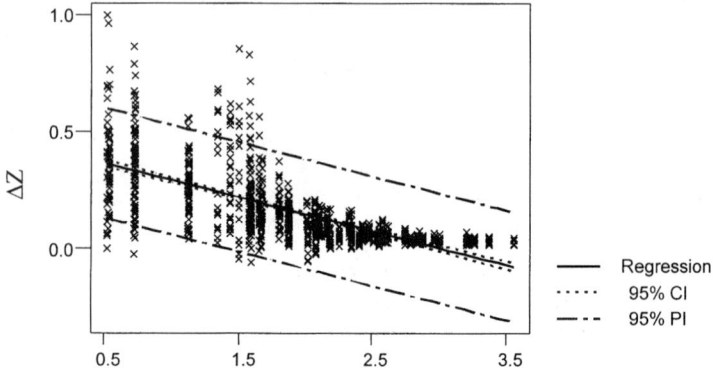

FIGURE 3a. Plot of ΔZ versus distance for measured data.

tance and has an increasing trend (slope = 0.053, $p < 0.005$). The data sets were normalized to their respective maximum values to make them comparable to the theoretical data.

Theoretical Data

FIGURES 4a and 4b show similar plots for the theoretical data. The distance in this case is expressed as the fraction of the cylinder radius. The relationship of ΔZ versus distance shown in FIGURE 4a has a decreasing trend (slope = –0.146, $p < 0.005$) similar to that

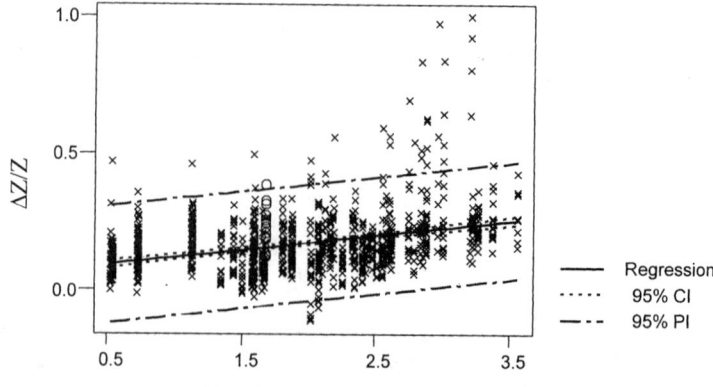

FIGURE 3b. Plot of ΔZ/Z versus distance for measured data. The 16 electrode configurations that gave the highest theoretical sensitivity are marked by open circles in the vicinity of distance 1.5.

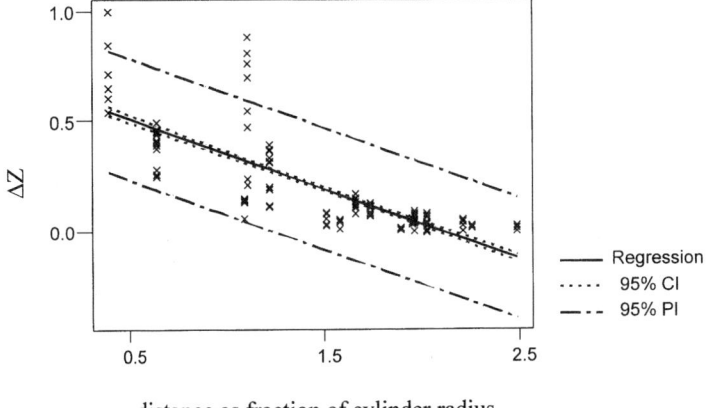

FIGURE 4a. Plot of ΔZ versus distance for theoretical data.

observed in the case of measured data. The plot of $\Delta Z/Z$ versus distance is shown in FIGURE 4b and has a decreasing trend (slope = -0.186, $p < 0.005$). This result is opposite to that obtained for the measured data. The scale limits of this plot are adjusted to make it comparable with the plot shown in FIGURE 3b. As a result, certain $\Delta Z/Z$ values for some electrode combinations corresponding to distance values in the vicinity of 2 units are not seen on the plot. These values were very high and negative and were due to very small magnitude and negative values of Z for the particular electrode combinations.

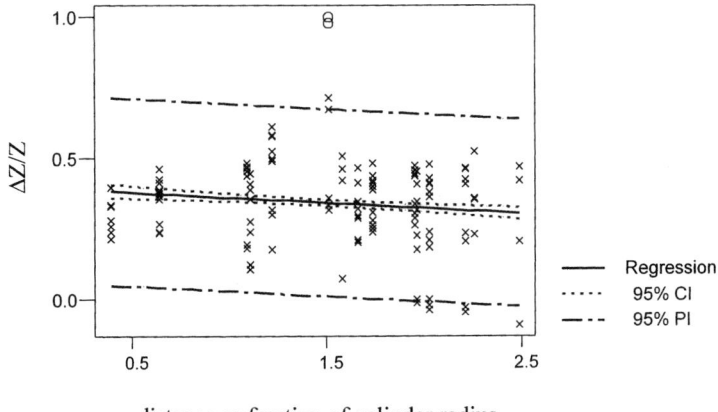

FIGURE 4b. Plot of $\Delta Z/Z$ versus distance for theoretical data. The 16 electrode configurations that gave the highest sensitivity are marked by open circles. Each point has 8 overlapping points.

DISCUSSION

The relationship between ΔZ and $\Delta Z/Z$ and the distance between the drive and receive electrode pair is statistically significant, but there is a large scatter of points in the plots. This indicates that the sensitivity is influenced by factors other than distance.

The purpose of our study was to determine the electrode configurations with high sensitivity. The correlation coefficient between the measured and theoretical values of $\Delta Z/Z$ was obtained in order to find out whether the two results were comparable. The value of the correlation coefficient was low ($r = 0.34$), but significant ($p < 0.005$). We believe that the low value of the correlation coefficient was because a cylindrical cross section was assumed for the FEM model, whereas the thoracic cavity is more elliptical in shape. This also might be the reason for the opposite sign of gradients of the best-fit line describing the relationship between $\Delta Z/Z$ and distance for measured and theoretical data. The significance of the correlation coefficient suggested that it would be possible to find out the electrode combination having high sensitivity by examining the theoretical data. The theoretical data would also be independent of the variations in the shape of the thoracic cavity of different subjects. We observed that there were 16 different electrode configurations that gave high sensitivity. These points are marked in FIGURE 4b by an open circle. Each of the two points has 8 overlapping points. The corresponding points for the measured data are marked also by an open circle and are seen in the vicinity of a distance value of 1.5 in FIGURE 3b. These points also have sensitivity higher than the mean sensitivity. However, these are not the points having the highest sensitivity. The points having the highest sensitivity correspond to electrode configurations separated by larger distances. At these distances, the value of Z is very small in magnitude and is prone to measurement errors due to a poor signal-to-noise ratio.[8] Hence, these highest sensitivity values are not reliable.

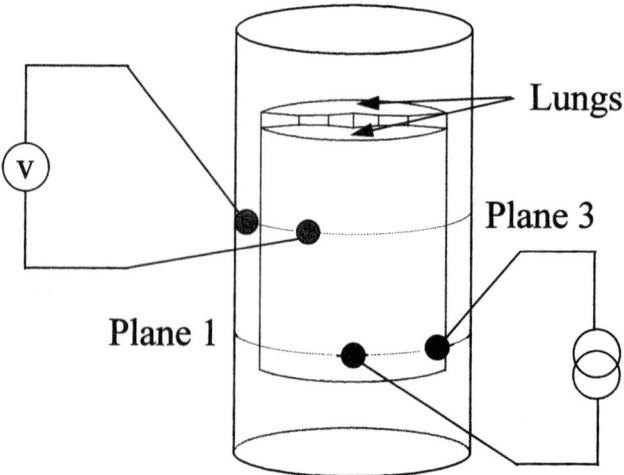

FIGURE 5. Placement of the drive and receive electrode pairs having high sensitivity.

The electrode placement for one of the 16 configurations having the highest theoretical sensitivity is shown in FIGURE 5. The drive and receive electrode pairs for this configuration were located close to one of the lungs. They were placed in two different horizontal planes separated by a vertical distance equal to the radius of the cylinder and displaced by an angle of 67.5°. The high sensitivity for this configuration is because the region of sensitivity in three dimensions for the particular placement of the electrodes has maximum overlap with the region occupied by the lung that is close to the electrodes. The remaining high sensitivity combinations also had a similar placement with respect to the lung proximity. This was due to the symmetry in the model.

CONCLUSIONS

In this paper, we have described our experimental and theoretical studies aimed at defining an optimum placement of 4 electrodes for impedance pneumography. The sensitivity of an electrode configuration depends not only on the distance between the drive and receive electrode pair, but also on the anatomical location of the lungs with respect to placement of the electrode. The maximum sensitivity was obtained when the drive and receive electrode pairs were placed over the same lung, but in different horizontal planes. High sensitivity was obtained in this case because the sensitivity region in three dimensions had maximum overlap with the lung close to the electrodes. Movement artifacts also contribute to the noise and their contribution will also depend on the placement of the electrodes. We are now planning to study the relationship between movement artifacts and electrode placements. These studies will help us to identify the best electrode placement for impedance pneumography.

ACKNOWLEDGMENTS

N. Khambete would like to thank the Association of Commonwealth Universities, United Kingdom, for the financial support provided in the form of a Commonwealth Scholarship. We also wish to thank Action Research and the EPSRC for providing the funds required in the development of the data collection system used in this study. We thank the volunteers who participated in the study.

REFERENCES

1. BAKER, L. E., L. A. GEDDES & H. E. HOFF. 1965. Quantitative evaluation of impedance spirometry in man. Am. J. Med. Electron. **April–June:** 73–77.
2. KHALAFALLA, A. S., S. P. STACKHOUSE & O. H. SCHMITT. 1970. Thoracic impedance gradient with respect to breathing. IEEE Trans. Biomed. Eng. **17:** 191–198.
3. SHEN, L., V. X. AFONSO, J. G. WEBSTER & W. J. TOMPKINS. 1992. The electrode system in impedance-based ventilation measurement. IEEE Trans. Biomed. Eng. **39:** 1130–1141.
4. GESELOWITZ, D. B. 1971. An application of electrocardiographic lead theory to impedance plethysmography. IEEE Trans. Biomed. Eng. **18:** 38–41.
5. METHERALL, P., D. C. BARBER, R. H. SMALLWOOD & B. H. BROWN. 1996. Three-dimensional electrical impedance tomography. Nature **380:** 509–512.
6. KIBER, A. 1991. Determination of object boundary shape for electrical impedance tomography. Ph.D. thesis, University of Sheffield, United Kingdom.

7. BRUCE, I. & A. SOHRAB. 1980. Techniques of Finite Elements. Ellis Horwood. Chichester, United Kingdom.
8. METHERALL, P. 1998. Three-dimensional electrical impedance tomography of the human thorax. Ph.D. thesis, University of Sheffield, United Kingdom.

Index of Contributors

Abboud, S., 360–369
Akond, M. H. R., 408–420
Akter, T., 408–420

Baker, A. T., 353–359
Barber, D. C., 353–359
Bardhan, K. D., 313–321
Barrett, J., 239–244
Bayford, R. H., 482–492, 512–519
Berger, C., 493–505
Bini, M., 454–465
Blumental, A., 506–511
Bragós, R., 51–58, 299–305, 306–312
Brown, B. H., 313–321, 534–542

Cairó, J., 299–305
Carreño, A., 51–58
Casas, O., 51–58, 306–312
Cathignol, D., 396–407
Chauveau, N., 42–50
Cherepenin, V. A., 346–352
Chilcott, T. C., 269–286
Cinca, J., 51–58
Cornish, B. H., 89–93, 370–373
Coster, H. G. L., 269–286
Cusick, G., 512–519

Davey, C., 239–244
de Munck, J. C., 440–453
de Valk–de Roo, G. W., 99–104
Dumler, A., 191–196

Elia, M., 370–373
Emtestam, L., 214–220
Evangelisti, A., 94–98

Faes, Th. J. C., 99–104, 121–127, 128–134, 388–395, 440–453
Fitzgerald, A., 381–387
Francavilla, A., 105–111
Frerichs, I., 493–505
From, A., 143–148
Fujii, M., 77–88, 245–261

Fuller, N., 370–373

Gámez, X., 299–305
Gebhard, M. M., 59–64
Gersing, E., 13–20, 65–71
Gheorghiu, E., 65–71, 262–268
Gheorghiu, M., 65–71
Gibson, A., 482–492, 512–519
Gimsa, J., 287–298
Gòdia, F., 299–305
González-Correa, C. A., 313–321, 512–519
Goovaerts, H. G., 99–104, 121–127, 128–134, 388–395
Gough, W., 335–345
Griffiths, H., 335–345, 381–387
Guglielmi, F. W., 105–111

Haggie, S. J., 313–321
Hagströmer, L., 214–220
Hahn, G., 493–505
Hamzaoui, L., 42–50
Hasegawa, K., 77–88
Heene, D. L, 167–173
Heethaar, R. M., 99–104, 121–127, 128–134, 149–154, 388–395, 440–453
Hellige, G., 493–505
Hermans, A. J., 440–453
Holder, D. S., 381–387, 482–492, 512–519
Hoopes, P. J., 21–29
Hose, R., 534–542
Hutten, H., 322–334
Hyttinen, J. A., 135–142

Ireland, R. H., 353–359

Jacobs, A., 89–93
Jossinet, J., 30–41, 396–407

Kaczmarek, J., 174–181
Kaipio, J. P., 430–439, 472–481
Kalia, N., 313–321

Kanai, H., 77–88, 245–261
Kanai, N., 77–88
Karjalainen, P. A., 430–439
Kauppinen, P. K., 135–142
Kerkkamp, H. J. J., 149–154
Khambete, N., 534–542
Kim, D. W., 112–120
Kim, S. C., 112–120
Kink, A., 155–166
Kirlum, H-J., 59–64
Kööbi, T., 135–142
Korjenevsky, A. V., 346–352
Kovachev, D., 322–334

Lackermeier, A. H., 197–213
Lapaz, C., 374–380
László, P., 421–429
Lavandier, B., 396–407
Lietdke, R. J., 94–99
Lionheart, W. R. B., 466–471
Lukaski, H. C., 72–76

Maggia, G., 94–98
Malmivuo, J., 135–142
Manetta, S., 454–465
Mastronuzzi, T., 105–111
McAdams, E. T., 197–213
Meijer, J. H., 128–134
Metherall, P., 534–542
Min, M., 155–166
Morucci, J. P., 42–50
Moss, G. P., 197–213

Nakajima, K., 245–261
Nakamura, K., 77–88
Nawarycz, T., 174–181
Netelenbosch, J. C., 99–104
Nicander, I., 221–226
Ninaus, W., 322–334
Nowakowski, A., 520–533
Nyrén, M., 214–220

Ollmar, S., 221–226
Olmi, R., 454–465
Osterman, K. S., 21–29
Ostrowska-Nawarycz, L., 174–181

Panarese, A., 105–111
Panella, C., 105–111
Parve, T., 155–166
Patterson, R. P., 143–148
Paulsen, K. D., 21–29
Petrova, G. I., 322–334
Pfleger, S., 167–173
Pietrini, L., 105–111
Pliquett, F., 227–238
Pliquett, U., 227–238
Popov, N., 191–196
Priori, S., 454–465
Puswald, B., 322–334

Raaijmakers, E., 121–127, 128–134, 388–395
Rabbani, K. S., 408–420
Radai, M. M., 360–369
Rigaud, B., 42–50
Riu, P. J., xi, 51–58, 299–305, 374–380
Rochaix, P., 42–50
Rodriguez-Sinovas, A., 51–58
Rogowski, J., 182–190
Rosell, J., 51–58, 306–312
Rosenfeld, M., 360–369

Sakamoto, K., 77–88, 245–261
Sarker, M., 408–420
Sato, Y., 77–88
Savolainen, T., 472–481
Schäfer, M., 59–64
Scharfetter, H., 322–334
Scherhag, A. W., 167–173
Schiffmann, H., 493–505
Schlegel, C., 59–64
Schmitt, M., 30–41
Scholten, R. J. P. M., 121–127
Schwan, H. P., 1–12
Shutov, V., 191–196
Siebert, J., 182–190
Slater, D. N., 313–321
Smallwood, R. H., 313–321, 534–542
Somersalo, E., 430–439
Stastny, J., 167–173
Stelter, J., 520–533
Stephenson, T. J., 313–321
Stewart, W. R., 335–345

INDEX OF CONTRIBUTORS

Stoddard, C. J., 313–321
Sunaga, R., 77–88

Talluri, J., 94–98
Talluri, T., 94–98
ten Bolscher, M., 99–104
Thomas, B. J., 89–93, 370–373
Tidswell, T., 512–519
Todd, R., 239–244
Tozer, J. C., 353–359
Tresànchez, M., 51–58
Tsuchida, T., 77–88

Ueno, A., 77–88

Vaisman, N., 506–511
van der Vijgh, W. J. F., 99–104
Vardi, P., 506–511
Vauhkonen, M., 430–439, 472–481
Vauhkonen, P. J., 472–481
Voelker, W., 167–173
Voigt, J. J., 42–50
Vozáry, E., 421–429

Ward, L. C., 89–93, 370–373
Warren, M., 51–58
Weintrob, N., 506–511
Witsoe, D. A., 143–148
Woolfson, A. D., 197–213
Wtorek, J., 182–190, 520–533

Yelamos, D., 306–312
Yosefsberg, Z., 506–511

Zsivánovits, G., 421–429
Zubarev, M., 191–196